A Manual of Orthopaedic Terminology

Seventh edition

A Manual of Orthopaedic Terminology

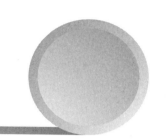

Fred R.T. Nelson, MD, FAAOS

Director Research and Education
Director Osteoarthritis Center
Orthopaedics
Hentry Ford Hospital
Detroit, Michigan

Carolyn Taliaferro Blauvelt

Formerly Writer-Editor, Medical-Dental Publications
National Naval Medical Center
Bethesda, Maryland

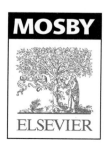

MOSBY

ELSEVIER

1600 John F. Kennedy Blvd
Ste 1800
Philadelphia, PA 19103–2899

A MANUAL OF ORTHOPAEDIC TERMINOLOGY   ISBN: 978-0-323-04503-2

Notice

Knowledge and best practice in this field are constantly changing. As new research and experience broaden our knowledge, changes in practice, treatment and drug therapy may become necessary or appropriate. Readers are advised to check the most current information provided (i) on procedures featured or (ii) by the manufacturer of each product to be administered, to verify the recommended dose or formula, the method and duration of administration, and contraindications. It is the responsibility of the practitioner, relying on their own experience and knowledge of the patient, to make diagnoses, to determine dosages and the best treatment for each individual patient, and to take all appropriate safety precautions. To the fullest extent of the law, neither the Publisher nor the Editors assumes any liability for any injury and/or damage to persons or property arising out or related to any use of the material contained in this book.

Library of Congress Cataloging-in-Publication Data

Nelson, Fred R. T., 1941–
A manual of orthopaedic terminology / Fred R.T. Nelson, Carolyn Taliaferro Blauvelt. – 7th ed.
    p. ; cm.
    Authors' names reversed on previous edition.
    Includes bibliographical references and index.
    ISBN 978-0-323-04503-2
    1. Orthopedics–Terminology–Handbooks, manuals, etc. I. Blauvelt, Carolyn Taliaferro, 1933–
II. Title.
    [DNLM: 1. Orthopedics–Terminology–English. WE 15 N426m 2007]
RD723.B53 2007
616. 7001'4–dc22
                                                                           2007015861

Publishing Director: Kim Murphy
Developmental Editor: Faith Brody
Project Manager: Bryan Hayward
Design Direction: Lou Forgione

Printed in the United States of America.

Last digit is the print number: 9 8 7 6 5 4 3 2 1

Working together to grow
libraries in developing countries

www.elsevier.com | www.bookaid.org | www.sabre.org

ELSEVIER   BOOK AID International   Sabre Foundation

Foreword

Over the last several years the concepts and ideas attributed to and labeled collectively as "Evidence-Based Medicine (EBM)" have become a part of daily clinical lives, and all health care providers, including orthopaedists, increasingly hear about evidence-based guidelines, evidence-based care paths, and evidence-based questions and solutions. The controversy has shifted from whether to implement the new concepts to how to do so sensibly and efficiently. The concepts of hierarchy of evidence, meta-analyses, confidence intervals, study design, and critical appraisal are so widespread that surgeons wishing to apply these terms need to understand both the language and nomenclature of EBM.

The term *evidence-based medicine* first appeared in autumn 1990 in a document for applicants to the Internal Medicine residency program at McMaster University that described EBM as "an attitude of enlightened skepticism" toward the application of diagnostic, therapeutic, and prognostic technologies. As outlined in the text *Clinical Epidemiology*[1] and first described in the literature in the *ACP Journal Club* in 1991,[2] the EBM approach to practicing medicine relies on an awareness of the evidence upon which a clinician's practice is based and the strength of inference permitted by that evidence. The most sophisticated practice of EBM requires, in turn, a clear delineation of relevant clinical questions, a thorough search of the literature relating to the questions, a critical appraisal of available evidence and its applicability to the clinical situation, and a balanced application of the conclusions to the clinical problem. The balanced application of the evidence (i.e., the clinical decision making) is the central point of practicing EBM and involves, according to EBM principles, integration of our clinical expertise and judgement with patients' and societal values, and with the best available research evidence.

Resources associated with EBM should allow clinicians to function more rationally. The ability to follow the path from research to application should also provide more control over what we do and more satisfaction from our daily practice. Although learning to locate, assess, and use new evidence in the original literature can improve physicians' daily practices, limited access to that information and limited time allocated to continuing education may cause their up-to-date clinical knowledge to deteriorate with time. Nelson and Blauvelt realize the need for understandable and efficient resources to assist readers in their daily lives. The 7th edition of the *Manual of Orthopaedic Terminology* provides a comprehensive and quick guide to EBM terminology for the busy clinician, researcher, student, or allied health care professional. This critical resource guides readers through the principles of clinical and experimental research methods.

The practice of EBM means integrating individual clinical expertise with the best available external clinical evidence from systematic research. To provide clinicians with easy access to the best available evidence, several specialized sources include summaries of individual studies, systematic reviews, and evidence-based clinical guidelines. Although readers need to realize the full scope of resources available, Nelson and Blauvelt's *Manual* provides a simple, easy-to-apply compendium of the terms needed to maneuver the EBM resources and the orthopaedic literature at large.

Mohit Bhandari, MD, MSc, FRCSC
Canada Research Chair
McMaster University
Hamilton, Ontario
Canada

Preface

Nearly 30 years ago the authors envisioned a "dictionary" that would serve as a search instrument as well as a hand guide to the myriad of terms unique to orthopaedic surgery and medicine. We had no way of knowing that scientific discovery and technological change would lead to a new edition every 4 years. At the time of publication of the sixth edition, we assumed that work would shortly be underway for the year 2002. However, the call from the publisher never came as it had in the past. In part this was due to merger changes in the publishing industry as it moved to the electronic age of publishing.

During the past 4 years, there has been a continued and consistent demand for this manual. This was brought about by newcomers to orthopaedics, such as medical coders, supportive medical staff, and adjusters, all of whom require better clarification of terms. The authors continued to be greeted with enthusiasm when persons they came into contact with were made aware of this manual. Continued book sales made the authors and executives revisit the matter. In the authors' proposal to the company, it was stated that there was truly a broader audience for a seventh edition, and planned changes were submitted.

With much discretion, an attempt was made to distinguish between recent technology and historical devices or procedures that were no longer in use. We needed to incorporate new materials being used in surgery and prosthetics. Many newer procedures have been developed and are rapidly replacing the procedures that appeared in the sixth edition. We recognized that "jargon" is not recognized officially by certifying organizations, but that it continues to be used in legal reports. There are numerous lawyers and adjusters who concentrate on musculoskeletal matters. The format of this dictionary makes it the only lexicon that can provide a clear definition of terms that are placed close to terminology that is likely to be in the same report or record. The authors also recognized the importance of the manual to sales representatives of pharmaceutical and surgical devices. Their numbers have grown, and many of these "reps" do not have a strong musculoskeletal background and would find this dictionary to be a combined word source and reference. Most importantly, this manual has a track record of being used by orthopaedic technicians and operating room personnel. Revision was the only path to make it useful to this community.

The prediction of therapeutic advances made in the preface of the sixth edition has come to pass. The human genome project, breakthroughs in our understanding of cellular mechanisms and mechanics, and changes in therapies have occurred at a rate that surpassed our imagination. Hence, we have updated the material as follows:

- **Fractures.** We stayed with the same format of fracture classification in order to highlight the intent of the system. Other trauma classifications were added to capture some of the data collection methods being used in large health systems. A traumatologist reviewed the fractures sections, and sprains and strains were reviewed by a sports medicine orthopaedist. The purpose was to capture as much of the terminology as possible. There are several new proposed classification systems that were not included awaiting more general acceptance.

- **Musculoskeletal diseases.** A number of newly named disease processes were included. Of greater importance is the improved understanding of the role of gene products in producing specific disorders. Hence many terms were redefined to reflect this knowledge. The physical appearance caused by a genetic disorder can be considered from the standpoint of the predominant tissue or organ affected, the metabolic gene product affected, or part of the cell affected. A new table has been included to act as a quick guide based on the type of gene product affected. It could not be comprehensive because of space, but it captures 95% of the prevalence of inherited diseases. For the most part, the definitions of disorders were left in the same sections as the previous edition.
- **Imaging.** Several new technologies were inserted. Many changes in radiology technology involve improvements in cost, speed, and resolution where terminology would not be affected. However, there were many new lines, signs, angles, and methods added.
- **Test Signs and Maneuvers.** A sports medicine physician revised this section. It should be recognized that many of these physical exam methods only point the examiner in a certain direction and are not the only means of achieving a diagnosis.
- **Cast, Splints, and Dressings.** The use of preformed removable products is increasingly important in fracture management. For the most part, commercial names have been avoided except in cases where the name is synonymous with the design of the device.
- **Prosthetic and Orthotics.** Extensive revisions were based on third editions of atlases published by the American Academy of Orthopaedic Surgeons. However, information about older devices was maintained since many are still in use.
- **Anatomy and Orthopaedic Surgery.** We continued to struggle with surgical terms that are applicable to general orthopaedics as well as to the subspecialty areas. Where appropriate, terms

isolated to the regions of subspecialization were placed in those chapters. This applied particularly to internal prostheses. However, terms general to all prostheses remain in this chapter. This revision required input from trauma, major joint reconstruction, and sports medicine surgeons. In this chapter, as well as the subspecialty chapters, many brand name terms were eliminated and new ones not listed. The authors felt that each institution has a chosen few devices and that individuals in transcription would be aware of proper spelling. This avoided an excess of pages devoted to "shopping lists." Knee, hip, shoulder, and elbow surgery continue to be listed in this chapter. There are obvious overlaps with subspecialty areas. Where possible, terms are only defined in one part of the book.

- **Spine.** A number of new appliances and surgical procedures are listed. These terms expand the subspecialty terminology introduced in the sixth edition.
- **The Hand and Wrist.** This chapter has expanded extensively to reflect the changes in practice and thinking in hand and upper limb surgery that have occurred over the past 20 years.
- **The Foot and Ankle.** A careful review led to redefining a few terms and the addition of many others. The reviewer is associated with a department that has a podiatric staff, making him aware of the differences and overlap in terminology.
- **Physical Medicine and Rehabilitation: Physical Therapy and Occupational Therapy.** The education and training of these practitioners continues to broaden and many are achieving doctorate level degrees. The result is that their clinical language is becoming broader and would be found in other parts of this book. The terminology in this chapter had some new material as required.
- **Musculoskeletal Research.** This chapter is completely rewritten by a veterinarian clinician scientist with an appreciation of the need for a format that is both clear and instructive. As a teacher of orthopaedic residents, the material included more extensive terminology in the grant application process as well statistics and research design.
- **Appendices.** The appendices continue to have supportive information on: A. Orthopaedic

Abbreviations, B. Anatomic Positions and Directions, C. Etymology—The Origin of Orthopaedic Terms, and D. ICD Eponymic Codes.

As in previous editions, we have invited many qualified contributors to review a chapter or chapters in order to be current and accurate. It is recognized that there are many colloquial terms that may not be defined and others that have been missed. The authors continue to welcome all suggestions and comments. The word "manual" means "to teach," and that is the goal of this seventh edition.

Fred R. T. Nelson
Carolyn Taliaferro Blauvelt

Acknowledgments

For contributions to the last six editions, we wish to acknowledge Alan D. Aaron, MD, The American Occupational Therapy Association, Rockville, MD; The American Physical Therapy Association, Alexandria, VA; Norman Berger, CP; Mark A. Berman, CO; CE Brooks, MD, FRCS(C); Wilton H. Bunch, MD, PhD; John F. Burkart, MD; Robert W. Chambers, MD; David Collon, MD; Joseph Craig, MB, ChB; Helen F. Delaney, OT; J.M. Dennis, DPM; Charles M. Dilla, PT, PA; Terry Elan, Prosthetist; Charles H. Epps, Jr., MD; David Fessell, MD; Jean Flint, Orthotist; Gary E. Friedlaender, MD; David P. Fyhrie, PhD; John J. Gartland, MD; Joshua Gerbert, DPM, MS; Stephen B. Gunther, MD; Stephen F. Gunther, MD, FAAOS; Carole Hays, MA, OTR, FAOTA; Donald L. Hiltz, PT; Donald P. Jenkins, PhD; Emily Jeter, OTR/L; James H. Kimura, PhD; Steve Kramer, CPO; David M. Lichtman, MD, FACS; Frederick G. Lippert, III, MD; Donna M. Mathisen, GPT; W. Patrick Monaghan, PhD; Francesca C. Music, MS, MT; Thomas Neviaser, MD; Jeffrey M. Ogorzalek, MD; Nyana Parikh, BS, Eric L. Radin, MD; Lee H. Riley, III, MD; Leo M. Rozmaryn, MD, FAAOS; James M. Salander, MD, FACS; Barton K. Slemmons, MD, FAAOS; Jeff Virgo, OTC, OPA-C, RSA; Samuel Wiesel, MD; David Q. Wilson, MD, FAAOS; Kent Wu, MD; William D. Wurzel, MHA, MD; and Kae S. Yingling, MD.

We wish to remember the late Charles V. Heck, MD, the former executive director of the American Academy of Orthopaedic Surgeons, who, through his support and encouragement, helped to launch this manual as a supplemental reference for the field of orthopaedics.

The success of the first six editions proved the need for a reference of this kind for this specialty. It is with pleasure that we present this seventh edition with many, many thanks not only to our contributors, but also to the editorial staff and those "behind the scenes" at Elsevier and Mosby, Inc., whose continued guidance, support, and publication skills have contributed much to the book's success.

Fred R. T. Nelson
Carolyn Taliaferro Blauvelt

Contributors

No one can write a book on all areas of orthopaedics and keep it current without the help of many competent people. This manual is no exception. We have chosen contributors whose background and experience make them well qualified to assist in updating material for each edition and who work directly or indirectly in this specialty. These people have generously given their time, in view of other professional commitments, to improve the correctness and accuracy of information, provide an update, and give constructive criticism. We can share in the success of this manual with them, and we wish to express our appreciation and thanks to our past contributors, and the following persons and organizations who participated in the revisions of the sixth edition.

Classifications of Fractures, Dislocations, and Sports-Related Injuries

Paul J. Dougherty, MD
Chief, Orthopaedic Trauma Division
Orthopaedic Surgery Residency Program Director
Department of Orthopaedic Surgery
Henry Ford Hospital
Detroit, Michigan

Musculoskeletal Diseases and Related Terms

Audrey Austin, MD
Assistant Professor of Pediatrics
Children's National Medical Center
Washington, DC

Patricia A. Kolowich, MD
Division Head, Center for Athletic Medicine
Department of Orthopaedics
Henry Ford Hospital
Detroit, Michigan

James M. Salander, MD, FACS
Associate Professor of Surgery
Uniformed Services University of the Health Sciences
Bethesda, Maryland

Susan A. Scherl, MD
Associate Professor
Department of Orthopaedics
The University of Nebraska
Omaha, Nebraska

Imaging Techniques

Joseph Craig, MB, ChB
Staff Radiologist, Department of Radiology
Henry Ford Hospital
Detroit, Michigan

Marnix T. van Holsbeeck, MD
Professor, Department of Radiology
Wayne State Medical School
Director, ER and Musculoskeletal Radiology
Department of Radiology
Henry Ford Health System
Detroit, Michigan

Orthopaedic Tests, Signs, and Maneuvers
Patricia A. Kolowich, MD
Division Head, Center for Athletic Medicine
Department of Orthopaedics
Henry Ford Hospital
Detroit, Michigan

Laboratory Evaluations
Timothy C. Sorrells, MD
Assistant Professor of Pathology
Department of Pathology
Uniformed Services University of the Health Sciences
Captain, Medical Corps U.S. Navy
Head Laboratory Department
National Naval Medical Center
Bethesda, Maryland

Corey Jenkins, MS, MT(ASCP)SBB
Department Head
Armed Services Blood Bank Center
National Naval Medical Center
Bethesda, Maryland

Casts, Splints, Traction, and Dressings
Colleen Ann Collins, COT
Orthopedic Technician
Orthopedics Henry Ford Medical Center,
Fairlane
Dearborn, Michigan

Anatomy and Orthopaedic Surgery
Craig D. Silverton, DO
Associate Professor, Department of Orthopaedics
Rush Medical University
Chicago, Illinois

Chief of Adult Reconstructive Surgery
Department of Orthopaedics
Henry Ford Hospital
Detroit, Michigan

Senior Staff Surgeon
Wilford Hall Medical Center (USAF)
San Antonio, Texas

The Spine
Rahul Vaidya, MD, CM, FRCSc

Chief of Orthopaedic Surgery
Department of Surgery Detroit Receiving Hospital
Detroit, Michigan

The Hand and Wrist
Leo M. Rozmaryn, MD
Assistant Adjunct Professor of Surgery
Department of Orthopaedics
Uniformed Services University Health Science Center
Bethesda, Maryland
Chief Department of Orthopaedics
Shady Grove Adventist Hospital
Rockville, Maryland

The Foot and Ankle
David A. Katcherian, MD
Foot and Ankle Division Head,
Orthopaedic Surgery
Henry Ford Hospital Detroit, Michigan

Physical Medicine and Rehabilitation: Physical Therapy and Occupational Therapy
Amanda Lane Calhoon, MSOT, OTR/L
Occupational Therapist
Hand and Upper Extremity Rehabilitation
Shady Grove Center for Sports Medicine and
    Rehabilitation
Rockville, Maryland

Introduction: The Research Enterprise
Clifford M. Les, DVM, PhD, MRCVS
Associate Professor, Anatomy and Cell Biology
School of Medicine, Wayne State University
Senior Staff Scientist; Head of the Anatomy Section
Bone and Joint Center
Henry Ford Hospital Detroit, Michigan
Affiliate Faculty Clinical Science, College of Veterinary
    Medicine and Biomedical Sciences
Colorado State University Ft. Collins, Colorado

ICD Codes For Eponymic Musculoskeletal Disease Terms
M. Suzanne DeMan, CPC, CPC-H, CCP
Coding Audit Specialist
Department of Orthopaedic Trauma
Detroit Receiving Hospital
Detroit, Michigan

Introduction to the Orthopaedic Specialty

Or''tho-pae'dic. Orthopaedic means correction or prevention of bony deformities (formerly, especially in children). The word comes from the Greek *orthos*, meaning straight, upright, right, or true—hence, also correct or regular—and from the Greek *pais*, meaning child.

The scope of orthopaedic surgery includes the treatment, management, and rehabilitation of patients with musculoskeletal conditions affecting bones, muscles, joints, tendons, ligaments, cartilage, blood vessels, nerves, and related tissues through surgical, nonsurgical, and other medical measures. The nature of these conditions may involve congenital abnormalities, metabolic disease processes, metastatic (tumor) pathology, or traumatic injuries (fractures), to name a few conditions requiring the expertise of the orthopaedic specialty. When surgery is indicated, postoperative rehabilitation is equally important in the continued care and treatment of musculoskeletal conditions.

The orthopaedic surgeon is a specialist on the musculoskeletal system as applied to adult and childrens' orthopaedics and the management of trauma. In addition, he or she possesses a working knowledge of neurology, cardiopulmonary physiology, and bioengineering in the care of the orthopaedic patient. This expertise has expanded to include computed tomography, magnetic resonance imaging, electrical and magnetic bone stimulation, microsurgery, and knowledge of the advances in internal and external fixation devices. Orthopaedic medicine is continually changing, and the orthopaedic surgeon is challenged with the responsibility of keeping informed of new techniques through continuing education in the field.

The orthopaedic surgeon develops many skills in the practice of this specialty. Nonoperative measures include the artful application of casts for immobilization and management of fractures or scoliosis, to the treatment of diseases and disabilities through conservative management. In the operating room, the orthopaedist is skilled in the repair and reconstruction of major skeletal defects, which include replacing diseased joints with plastic implants, inserting metallic rods and other devices for stability, or performing fusions, revisions, or amputations. Of a more delicate nature, he or she performs surgery that applies arthroscopic and microvascular techniques that encompass skin grafts, finger transplantations, nerve repairs, and similar difficult procedures.

From a team approach, the orthopaedic specialty depends on many other disciplines in the treatment of patients. The immediate team members are the professional nurses who provide and participate in the primary care of patients and who are assisted by the services of the orthopaedic technicians, both in the clinic and hospital setting. The second group of team members includes the allied health professionals, the physical therapist, and occupational therapist. These professionals are directly involved in, and may be consulted for, the development of a treatment plan in a patient's rehabilitation and are often headed by a physiatrist, who is a physician that specialized in rehabilitation medicine and interventions. The next group of team members to provide assistance include the prosthetists (artificial limbs) and orthotists (braces), who measure, fit, design, and fabricate devices for the orthopaedic patient. Indirectly, the manufacturer of orthopaedic appliances plays an important role, as does the researcher who tests the biocompatibility of materials used in the musculoskeletal system.

All of these specialties are an important and integral part of the orthopaedic team, and provide a combination of skills that benefits thousands of patients with musculoskeletal problems. Other disciplines that interface with orthopaedics include bioengineering, electrobiology, transplantation, diagnostic imaging, oncology, biochemistry, and similar areas.

Orthopaedic medicine has become so diverse that there is specialization within the specialty. In addition to general orthopaedics, a physician may specialize in diseases and surgery of the spine, soft tissues, the hand, the foot, major joints, trauma, sports medicine, or the ever-changing area of orthopaedic research.

Many physicians are exposed to orthopaedic surgery during their training years, but only a select group actually pursue this difficult and diverse field to the point of certification.

The qualifications for certification by the American Board of Orthopaedic Surgery (ABOS) are 5 or 6 years of post graduate education after medical school. After graduation from an ACGME-approved 5-year program, a candidate sits for Part 1, which is a written examination. After 22 months of practice in the same location, he or she may sit for part 2, which is a practice-based examination reviewing cases and outcomes. The physician must complete all requirements to become "board certified" and a Diplomate of the Board. After completion of the certification requirements, an orthopaedic surgeon becomes eligible for Fellowship in the American Academy of Orthopaedic Surgeons (AAOS), the national organization of the specialty. The admission to fellowship in the Academy requires board certification and recommendations from the community. This is typically 18 months following board certification. The Academy fellowship at present represents about 81% of the practicing orthopaedic surgeons in the United States.

The national organization of the specialty, AAOS, developed the accepted definition of orthopaedics in 1952:

Orthopaedic Surgery is the medical specialty that includes the investigation, preservation, restoration, and development of the form and function of the extremities, spine, and associated structures by medical, surgical, and physical methods.

ORTHOPAEDIC ORGANIZATIONS OF NORTH AMERICA

American Academy for Cerebral Palsy and Developmental Medicine
American Association for Hand Surgery
American Association of Hip and Knee Surgeons
American Board of Orthopaedic Surgery, Inc.
American Orthopaedic Association
American Orthopaedic Foot and Ankle Society
American Orthopaedic Society for Sports Medicine
American Shoulder and Elbow Surgeons
American Society of Orthopaedic Physician's Assistants
American Society of Plastic Surgeons
American Society for Reconstructive Microsurgery
American Society for Surgery of the Hand
American Spinal Injury Association
Arthroscopy Association of North America
Association of Bone and Joint Surgeons
Association of Children's Prosthetic-Orthotic Clinics
Bones Society, Inc.
Cervical Spine Research Society
Clinical Orthopaedic Society
Clinical Orthopaedics and Related Research (journal)
Council of Musculoskeletal Specialty Societies
Eastern Orthopaedic Association
Federation of Spine Associations
Hip Society
International Society of Arthroscopy, Knee Surgery and Orthopaedic Sports Medicine
Irish American Orthopaedic Society
J. Robert Gladden Society
Knee Society
Limb Lengthening and Reconstruction Society
Mid-America Orthopaedic Association

Mid-Central States Orthopaedic Society, Inc.
Musculoskeletal Tumor Society
North American Spine Society
Orthopaedic Rehabilitation Association
Orthopaedic Research and Education
  Foundation
Orthopaedic Research Society
Orthopaedic Trauma Association

Pediatric Orthopaedic Society of North America
Ruth Jackson Orthopaedic Society
Scoliosis Research Society
SICOT (main office)
SICOT (U.S. Chapter)
Society of Military Orthopaedic Surgeons
Southern Orthopaedic Association
Western Orthopaedic Association

Contents

Classifications of Fractures, Dislocations, and Sports-Related Injuries

1

The musculoskeletal reaction to trauma can result in a variety of bone, muscle, and ligamentous disruptions; sometimes fracture and ligamentous injuries occur concurrently. The general types of musculoskeletal trauma are fractures, dislocations, subluxations, sprains, strains, and diastases.

This chapter defines fractures and dislocations by sections. The first part contains general terms that are easily understood by the nonspecialist, followed by classic, descriptive, and eponymic terms by anatomic location. The second section is a brief outline of the AO (Arbeitsge-meinschaft für Osteosynthesefragen) system and Orthopaedic Trauma Association Registry System of fracture classification. The third section defines the many eponymic classification systems by grades, types, and mechanisms. The last section covers the types of dislocations, subluxations, strains and sprains, and sports-related injuries. Many new terms were added to this edition, as were the inclusion of the Trauma Scoring System for soft tissue injuries, to include the Limb Salvage Index and the Mangled Extremity Severity Score (MESS).

Most patients with musculoskeletal injuries present to an emergency room in an acute stage and are treated by the emergency room physician until it is determined that an orthopaedic specialist may be required. Good communication is essential when relating the assessment of acute injuries. A brief and accurate description is vital to the evaluation and immediate treatment of the injured, and familiarity with the classification systems that follow will help in understanding the importance of accurate communication. For example, an "open, midshaft, femur, comminuted fracture" gives a brief description but accurately relates a lot. To achieve this degree of accuracy, learning the classifications is an important tool to the end user.

A uniformed descriptive system also allows accurate coding of specific diagnostic entities. The bony detail is described by the following:

1. Open versus closed
2. Portion of bone involved
3. General appearance
4. Alignment of fragments and position and alignment

Interestingly, fractures have specific terminology that varies from time of occurrence to healing. Fractures may be named for an anatomic location, a person, or a place. They are further defined in terms of how they occurred or reason for the break. As fractures begin to heal, the degree and nature of healing are described.

Contributing factors, such as tumors, infections, and repeated stress, are included in the descriptive terminology. This is important for diagnostic coding. The management of fractures is also clarified. *Closed* management (closed reduction) means that treatment is in the form of a manipulation, cast, or splint/traction application or some combination of the three. *Open* management (open reduction) requires a surgical incision to approximate the fracture fragments into normal position. Often, some form of internal fixation (**osteosynthesis**) is performed with open management of fractures. A **fracture of necessity** is one that requires surgical fixation for reduction.

Many advances have been made in the management of fractures such as immobilization from casting to bracing, or a combination of both. The term **cast brace** has been applied to a form of treatment in which the brace design is incorporated into temporary standard cast materials. This method allows for limited motion in the brace during the early healing stage with "controlled" fracture movement. Its use has shown greater callus weld around the fracture site, improved ligamentous healing, and earlier recovery of joint mobility and muscle control.

Another method of fracture management employs magnetic and electrical bone stimulators, some with *surface electrodes* externally applied to a fracture site. For certain types of fractures, this method has diminished the need for braces.

An option of traumatic fracture management is the use of external fixation devices and frames, also known as "fixateurs" or fixators. External fixation is a diverse system for managing loss of skeletal stability with various components placed in bone. Treatment methods and external skeletal fixation devices are discussed in Chapters 6, 7, and 8.

Terminology of Fractures and Dislocations

diastasis: may be one of two types: (1) disjointing of two bones that are parallel to one another, for example, radius and ulna, tibia and fibula complex or (2) rupture of any "solid" joint, as in a diastasis of the symphysis pubis. Such an injury tends to occur in association with other fractures and is then called "fracture-diastasis."

dislocation (L., *luxatio*): complete displacement of bone from its normal position at the joint surface, disrupting the articulation of two or three bones at that junction and altering the alignment. This displacement affects the joint capsule and surrounding tissues (muscles, ligaments). Dislocation (**luxation**) may be traumatic (direct blow or injury), congenital

(developmental defect), or pathologic (as in muscle imbalance, ligamentous tearing, rheumatoid arthritis, or infection).

fracture (L., *fractura*): structural break in the continuity of a bone, epiphyseal plate, or cartilaginous joint surface, usually traumatic with disruption of osseous tissue.

fracture-dislocation: fracture of a bone that is also dislocated from its normal position in a joint.

sprain-ligament rupture (L., *luxatio imperfecta*): stretching or tearing of ligaments (fibrous bands that bind bones together at a joint), varying in degrees from being partially torn (stretched) to being completely torn (ruptured), with the continuity of the ligament remaining intact. After a sprain, the fibrous capsule that encloses the joint may become inflamed, swollen, discolored, and extremely painful. Involuntary muscle spasm, and sometimes a fracture, may occur. Rest, elevation, and a restrictive bandage, splint, or cast are methods of treating these injuries until properly healed. When a ligament or tendon has been torn completely, dislocation may also occur. Surgical repair may be required in some cases.

strain: stretching or tearing of a muscle or its tendon (fibrous cord that attaches the muscle to the bone it moves) that may result in bleeding into the damaged muscle area, which causes pain, swelling, stiffness, muscle spasm, and, subsequently, a bruise. A strain can be serious because muscle damage (scar tissue) may cause muscle shortening. With rest, strains will subside in 2 to 3 days, but symptoms may persist for months.

subluxation: incomplete or partial dislocation in that one bone forming a joint is displaced only partially from its normal position; also, a chronic tendency of a bone to become partially dislocated, in contrast to an outright dislocation, for example, shoulder, patella, and hip.

Classifications of Fractures

Open Versus Closed (Fig. 1-1)
closed f.: does not produce an open wound of the skin but does result in loss of continuity of bone subcutaneously; formerly called simple f.

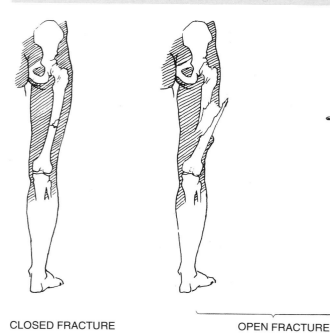
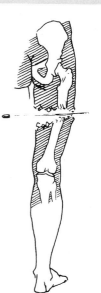

FIG 1-1 Closed versus open fracture. (From Schneider FR: *Handbook for the orthopaedic assistant,* ed 2, St Louis, 1976, The CV Mosby Co.)

CLOSED FRACTURE

OPEN FRACTURE

From within

From without

open f.: one of the fragments has broken through the skin, and there is loss of continuity of bone internally; formerly called compound f.

Portion of Bone Involved

The portion of bone involved or the point of reference of a fracture may be referred to as the distal third, the middle third, and the proximal third. Middle third fractures are commonly known as midshaft fractures. For specific anatomic locations, the following terms are commonly used.

apophyseal f.: avulsion of or fracture through an apophysis (bony prominence) where there is strong tendinous attachment.

articular f.: involves a joint surface; also called joint f. and intra-articular f.

cleavage f.: shelling off of cartilage with avulsion of a small fragment of bone such as the capitellum.

condylar f.: involves any round end of a hinge joint; see sections on femoral and distal humeral fractures.

cortical f.: involves cortex of bone.

diacondylar f.: transcondylar fracture (line across the condyles).

direct f.: results at specific point of injury and is due to the injury itself.

extracapsular f.: occurs near, but outside, the capsule of a joint, especially the hip (**extra-articular**).

intracapsular f.: occurs within the capsule of a joint (**intra-articular**).

nonphyseal f.: any childhood fracture that does not involve a growth plate.

periarticular f.: occurs near but not involving a joint.

transchondral f.: fracture through cartilage, which may not be apparent unless there is a bone fracture line into the joint; not to be confused with transcondylar f.

transcondylar f.: occurs transversely between the condyles of the elbow. This term is also used in fractures of the femur and bones with condyles; also called **diacondylar f.**

tuft f.: involves the distal phalanx (tuft) of any digit.

General Appearance (Fig. 1-2)

avulsion f.: tearing away of a part; a fragmentation of bone where the pull of a strong ligamentous or tendinous attachment tends to forcibly pull the fragment away from the rest of the bone. The fragment is usually at the articular surface.

bursting f.: multiple fragments, usually at the end of a bone; classically, f. of the first cervical vertebra or the body of the vertebra where there is typically displacement of bone into the spinal canal.

butterfly f.: a bone *fragment* shaped like a butterfly and part of a comminuted; usually involves high-energy force delivered to the bone.

chip f.: a small fragment, usually at the articular margin of a joint.

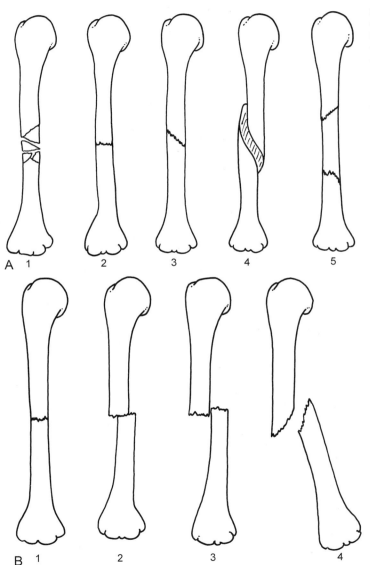

FIG 1-2 A, Midshaft fractures of the humerus. *1,* Comminuted. *2,* Transverse, undisplaced. *3,* Oblique, undisplaced. *4,* Spiral. *5,* Segmental. **B,** Apposition and alignment of midshaft fractures of the humerus, anteroposterior (AP) view. *1,* Perfect end-to-end apposition, perfect alignment. *2,* 50% end-to-end apposition, perfect alignment. *3,* Side-to-side (bayonet) apposition, slight shortening, perfect alignment. *4,* No apposition, approximately 30-degree angulation. (From Mercier LR: *Practical Orthopaedics,* ed 5, St Louis: Mosby, 2000.)

comminuted f.: more than two fragments; lines of fracture may be transverse, oblique, spiral, or T or Y shaped; also called splintered f.

complete f.: the bone is completely broken through both cortices.

compression f.: crumbling or smashing of cancellous bone by forces acting parallel to the long axis of bone; applied particularly to vertebral body fractures.

depressed f.: typically an intra-articular depression of fragments, but may also be applied to depressed skull fractures.

double f.: segmental f. of a bone in two places.

epiphyseal f.: involves the portion of the bone that is distal to the physis, which is the growth plate.

fissure f.: crack in one cortex (surface) only of a long bone.

greenstick f.: in children, incomplete, angulated fracture with a partial break; also called **incomplete f., interperiosteal f., hickory-stick f.,** and **willow f.**

hairline f.: nondisplaced fracture line (crack) in the cortex of bone.

impacted f.: fragments are compressed by force of original injury, driving one fragment of bone into adjacent bone.

incomplete f.: cortices of bone are buckled or cracked, but continuity is not destroyed; the cortex is broken on one side and only bent on the other. Microscopically, the fracture is present on bent side, and resorption and callus will occur on this side as well; types are **greenstick f., torus f.**

infraction f.: small radiolucent line seen in pathologic fractures, most commonly resulting from metabolic problems.

insufficiency f.: a fracture that occurs due to bone that is made insufficient due to osteoporosis or a metabolic process.

linear f.: lengthwise fracture of bone straight line fracture; implies that there is no displacement.

multiple f.: two or more separate lines of fracture in the same bone.

oblique f.: slanted fracture of the shaft on long axis of bone.

occult f.: hidden fracture (undetectable on a radiograph), generally occurring in areas of the ribs, tibia, metatarsals, and navicula.

physeal f: one that involves the cartilaginous growth plate of a bone; also referred to as **epiphyseal slip f., Salter f.,** and **Salter-Harris f.** (Fig. 1-3).

plastic bowing f.: curved deformity of a tubular bone without gross fracture (**bowing f., greenstick f.**).

secondary f.: pathologic f. of bone weakened by disease.

segmental f.: several large fractures in the same bone shaft where the two principal fragments are not adjacent.

spiral f.: fracture line is spiral shaped, usually on shaft of long bones where the mechanism of injury is usually torsion.

stellate f.: numerous fissures radiate from central point of injury.

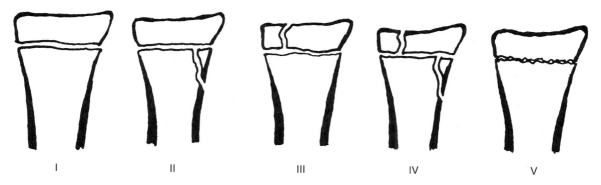

I   II   III   IV   V

FIG 1-3 Epiphyseal fracture types classified by the Salter method.

subperiosteal f.: bone but not its periosteal tube is broken; uncommon, usually the result of a direct blow.

torus f.: usually noticed in children; a stable, often incomplete f. in which one distal cortical surface appears to be wrinkled by compression forces, and the opposite cortex may or may not be infracted by tension forces.

transverse f.: line of fracture across the shaft at right angles to the long axis of a bone.

unstable f.: fracture that most often requires operative intervention due to the likelihood of recurrent deformity despite manipulation.

Position and Alignment of Fragments (Fig. 1-4)

The position of a fragment refers to any displacement of one bone fragment in reference to the next. Displacement, should it exist, can be in any plane. Alignment refers to rotatory and/or angular deviation of the distal fragment in relation to the proximal fragment. For example:

bayonet position: the fragments touch and overlap, but there is good alignment. Internal and external rotation can also be stated in degrees.

bow: the two fragments form an angle where the apex is sometimes described as an anterior or posterior bow.

The descriptive radiographic interpretations of fractures are defined as follows. The *angulation* of the fracture is designated by the direction of the apex of the fracture points. *Fragments* themselves are designated as proximal and distal displacement, which is the amount of offset of the proximal to distal fragment as seen in an anterior to posterior or medial to lateral direction.

When broken ends of the principal fragments are touching, they are said to be in *apposition*. Accuracy or degree of apposition is defined in percentages, such as 50%, indicating at least one radiographic view shows 50% contact and other views may appear to be more.

The *site* may be diaphyseal, metaphyseal, or epiphyseal portions of a specific bone or may be intraarticular. *Extent* may be described as complete, incomplete, cracked, hairline, buckled, or greenstick. The *configuration* may be transverse, oblique, or spiral

and is referred to as comminuted when more than two fragments are present. The *fracture fragments* may be undisplaced or displaced.

Thus, a fracture is described radiographically by its site, bone name, extent, configuration, relationship of fragments to each other and to the external environment (open or closed), and the presence or absence of complications.

Classic and Descriptive Names (By Anatomic Location)

Shoulder Fractures (Proximal Humerus and Scapula)

anatomic neck f.: occurs in the area of tendinous attachments, the true neck of humeral metaphysis.

Bankart f.: detachment of a small piece of bone from the anteroinferior rim of the glenoid; seen with anterior shoulder dislocation, usually called a Bankart fragment. The cartilage rim may detach without a fracture and this is called a **Bankart lesion.**

coracoid f.: fracture of coracoid process of scapula.

greater tuberosity f.: fracture of bone prominence and attachment of supraspinatus.

lesser tuberosity f.: fracture of bone prominence for attachment of subscapularis.

Hill-Sachs (Hermodsson) f.: moderate compression f. or indentation f. of the humeral head usually seen after an anterior dislocation of the shoulder.

surgical neck f.: occurs in area below the anatomic neck of the humerus.

Arm and Elbow Fractures (Distal Humerus)

Boxer's elbow: chip f. at the tip of the olecranon caused by a fast extension of the elbow in a missed jab (punch).

condylar f.: occurs at the medial or lateral articular process of the humerus at the elbow.

epicondylar f.: occurs through one of the two epicondyles, medial or lateral.

Holstein-Lewis f.: involves the humerus at the junction of the middle and distal thirds; associated with radial nerve paralysis because of nerve proximity to posterior septum and bone.

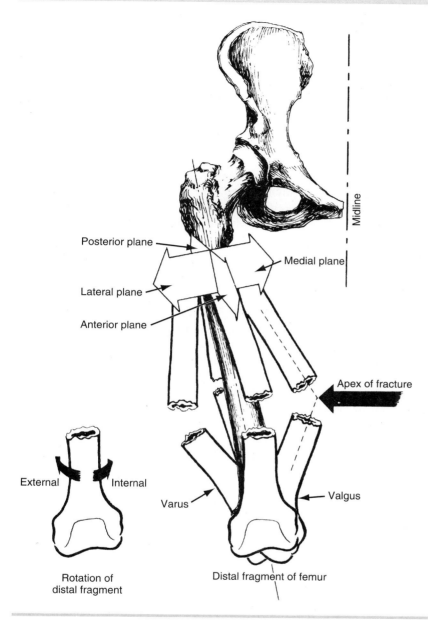

FIG 1-4 Description of fracture deformity. (From Schneider FR: *Handbook for the Orthopaedic Assistant*, ed 2, St Louis, 1976, The CV Mosby Co.)

Kocher f.: semilunar chip f. of capitellum with displacement into joint.

Laugier f.: involves the trochlea of the humerus.

Malgaigne f.: extension mechanism supracondylar f. of humerus; name also applied to a vertically dissociated fracture dislocation of the pelvis and a proximal fibular fracture.

Posada f.: anteriorly angulated fracture of distal humerus associated with posterior dislocation of radius and ulna.

sideswipe f.: comminuted fracture of distal humerus and sometimes radius and ulna caused by direct blow against elbow.

supracondylar f.: occurs through the distal metaphysis of the humerus or femur.

T f.: intercondylar fracture shaped like a T.

Y f.: intercondylar fracture shaped like a Y.

Forearm and Wrist Fractures

Barton f.: an intra-articular fracture of the dorsal rim of the distal radius, usually resulting in subluxation of the radial carpal joint with the fracture site fragment.

chauffeur's f.: oblique fracture of the radial styloid caused by a twisting or snapping-type injury; also called **backfire f., Hutchinson f.,** and **lorry driver's f.**

chisel f.: incomplete, usually involving medial head of radius, with fracture line extending distally about ½ inch.

Colles f.: named prior to x-ray technology, implies a fracture of the distal radius, either articular or nonarticular, with dorsal angulation of the distal fragment producing a silver fork deformity; generally associated with a fracture of the ulnar styloid. (Term becoming archaic.)

corner f.: a small bucket-handle-appearing fracture in the distal metaphyseal corner in a young child, often associated with child abuse.

de Quervain f.: combination of a wrist scaphoid fracture with volar dislocation of scaphoid fragment and lunate.

dye-punch f.: an intra-articular fracture of the ulnar (volar) portion of the distal radius, usually caused by direct impaction of the lunate onto the lunate fossa of the distal radius.

Essex-Lopresti f.: a comminuted radial head fracture with an injury to the distal radioulnar joint due to disruption of the interosseous membrane, which can cause a proximal migration of the radius if the radial head is excised secondarily.

Galeazzi f.: typically a displaced fracture of the distal third or quarter of the radius with disruption of the distal radioulnar joint; called **fracture of necessity** because surgical fixation is required for reduction; also called a **reverse Monteggia f., Dupuytren f.,** or **Piedmont f.**

Kocher f.: fracture of capitellum of distal humerus with possible displacement of fragment into joint.

Laugier f.: isolated fracture of the trochlea of the humerus at the elbow.

lead pipe f: typically in the forearm, a combination of greenstick fracture and torus fracture in the immature skeleton. Such fractures do not penetrate the entire shaft of the bone and have the appearance of a slightly bent lead pipe.

Lenteneur's f.: a distal radial fracture of the palmar rim, similar to Smith's type II fracture.

Monteggia f.: isolated fracture of proximal third of ulna, with posterior or anterior dislocation of radial head allowing angulation and overriding of ulnar fragments.

Moore f.: like a Colles f.; specifically, fracture of distal radius with dorsal displacement of ulnar styloid and impingement under annular ligament.

Mouchet f.: involves humeral capitellum.

nightstick f.: undisplaced fracture of the ulnar shaft caused by a direct blow.

Piedmont f.: oblique f. usually at the proximal portion of distal third of the radius; obliquity runs from proximal ulnar to distal radial aspect, allowing distal fragments to be pulled into the ulna by the pronator quadratus muscle; fracture of necessity requiring operative management.

radial head f.: involves the most proximal part of the radius, a dish-shaped portion of bone called the radial head.

radial styloid f.: involves distal radial tip of radius.

reverse Barton f.: dorsal displacement of carpus on radius, with associated fracture of dorsal articular surface of radius. The mechanism and appearance of this fracture are similar to those of a Colles f.

Skillern f.: open f. of distal radius associated with greenstick f. of distal ulna.

Smith f. (reverse Colles f.): fracture of the distal radius in which the distal fragment is displaced volarly. This fracture was defined before the advent of radiography, and, classically, there are three types:

1. Nonarticular
2. Intra-articular **(volar Barton f.)**
3. Oblique nonarticular fracture near the joint line

Hand Fractures

Bennett f.: fracture of the base of the thumb metacarpal, usually leaving a volar ulnar fragment attached to a retaining ligament with radial subluxation of the metacarpal.

Crush f.: term used for comminuted impaction of any bone, but for the finger is a distal phalanx fracture resulting from a crush injury.

mallet f.: avulsion f. of the extensor tendon from the dorsal base of the distal phalanx of any digit that includes insertion of extensor apparatus, thus allowing distal segment to "drop" into flexion; also called **baseball finger, drop finger, mallet finger deformity.**

Rolando f.: an intra-articular comminuted fracture of the base of the thumb metacarpal resulting in a Y- or T-shaped fracture at the base of the metacarpal.

unciform f.: fracture of the "hook of the hamate," usually caused by direct trauma that may or may not be associated with ulnar neuropathy.

Wilson f.: involves the proximal volar portion of the middle phalanx because of strong attachment of volar plate.

Spine Fractures

Chance f.: involves vertebra, with horizontal splitting of spinous process and neural arch with disruption through vertebral body; an unstable fracture.

clay shoveler's f.: involves spinous process(es) C-6, C-7, T-1, T-2, or T-3.

hangman's f.: posterior element (pedicles) fracture with anterior subluxation of the cervical neck of C-2 on C-3.

Jefferson f.: bursting f. of the ring of the first cervical vertebra (atlas).

posterior element f.: broad term used to describe any fracture of the spinous process, lamina, facets, pars interarticularis, or pedicle.

seatbelt f.: thoracic or lumbar spine fracture due to tensile stress that occurs on spine with forward motion of thorax with abdominal or thoracic restraint resulting in bony and/or ligament disruption. If only the bone is involved called a Chance f.

sentinel f.: a cervical spine fracture characterized by fractures through the lamina on either side of the spinous process. A sentinel of potential instability.

slice f.: an unstable lumbar spine fracture caused by a flexion rotation injury that results in a fracture in the upper body of the lower vertebra and a dislocation of the articular process of the upper vertebra.

spondyloptosis: dislocation of one vertebra from another without any bone fracture.

teardrop f.: exists in two forms: (1) an isolated anteroinferior fracture of the cervical spine (unstable) or (2) a three-part, two-plane fracture of an anteroinferior corner of the vertebral body (the teardrop), a sagittal vertebral body, and the posterior neural arch.

vertebra plana f.: wafer-thin compression f. of a vertebral body resulting from an intrinsic pathologic condition of the bone.

wedge f.: anterior compression f. of any vertebra; most common in the dorsal thoracic spine.

Pelvis, Hip, and Proximal Femur Fractures

basal neck f.: involves base of femoral neck at junction of trochanteric region.

bucket-handle f.: vertical shear fracture of anterior pubis and opposite ilium.

central f.: acetabular fracture, centrally displaced through inner wall of pelvis.

dashboard f.: posterior lip of acetabulum chips when femoral head is driven against it; often caused by a sudden jolt when knee hits dashboard.

dome f.: acetabular fracture involving weight-bearing surface of the acetabulum. This term can also be applied to a fracture of the superior surface of the talus.

Duverney f.: involves ilium just below the anterosuperior spine.

extracapsular f.: occurs outside of joint capsule of humerus or femur.

femoral neck f.: transcervical fracture through midportion of femoral neck.

hip f.: implies a fracture of the femoral neck or intertrochanteric area.

intracapsular f.: commonly used for high femoral neck fractures, but is also used for any fracture within a joint capsule.

intertrochanteric f.: the principal plane of the fracture disrupts the intertrochanteric line.

Malgaigne f.: occurs through wing of the ilium or sacrum with associated fractures through the ipsilateral pubic rami, allowing upward displacement of hemipelvis; often associated with internal injuries.

open book f.: pelvis fracture with symphysis separation and disruption of the sacral pelvic ligaments to give appearance of opening a book.

pertrochanteric f.: involves proximal femur where the fracture line passes through both the lesser and greater trochanters.

ring f.: involves at least two parts of pelvic circumference.

shaft f.: occurs between subtrochanteric and supracondylar area.

sprinter's f.: involves anterosuperior or anteroinferior spine of ilium, with a fragment of bone being pulled forcibly by sudden muscular pull.

straddle f.: double f. or dislocation of the pubis usually caused by a straddling mechanism, for example, falling onto a rail with the point of contact between the legs.

subcapital f.: femoral fracture at head-neck junction.

subtrochanteric f.: transverse f. of femur just below lesser trochanter.

Waddell triad: femoral fracture associated with head and thorax injuries.

Walther f.: transverse ischioacetabular f. where the fracture line passes from ischial spine to acetabular cavity to ischiopubic junction.

Distal Femur, Knee, Tibia, and Fibula Fractures

bumper f.: involves the tibia or femur and is caused by a direct blow in area of the tibial tuberosity; commonly caused by a car bumper accident; may be bilateral.

cartwheel f.: fracture of the distal femoral epiphysis in a child, so named by mechanism of a leg caught in the spokes of a cartwheel.

clipping injury f.: fracture through growth plate of distal femur or proximal tibia due to strike from the lateral side of the knee when the foot is planted.

Hoffa f.: coronal fracture of medial femoral condyle.

patellar f.: involves kneecap.

pillion f.: T-shaped fracture of distal femur with displacement of the condyles posteriorly to femoral shaft, caused by severe blow to knee; so named for pillion back seat position of a motorcycle rider who sustains this injury. Not to be confused with pilon fracture, which is due to a vertical impaction.

Segond f.: small avulsion f. of superolateral tibia caused by tension on the lateral capsule or ligament; usually associated with other severe ligamentous injuries leading to anterolateral knee instability (**lateral capsule sign**).

sleeve f.: involves a small chip of bone from the superior or inferior portion of the patella associated with loss of integrity of quadriceps extensor mechanism.

Stieda f.: avulsion f. of origin of medial collateral ligament on medial femoral condyle.

supracondylar f.: involves the distal shaft of bone above condyles of femur or humerus.

tibial plateau f.: involves proximal tibial articular surface.

toddler f.: nondisplaced fracture of the tibia seen in toddlers beginning to walk.

wagon wheel f.: involves distal femoral epiphysis in children; also called **cartwheel f.**

Y and T f.: combined supracondylar and intercondylar f. of the distal femur.

Ankle and Foot Fractures

ankle mortise diastasis: separation of tibia and fibula at ankle; often associated with a fracture or dislocation.

aviator's astragalus: denotes a talar neck fracture caused by sudden impaction of foot into ankle; may be associated with other fractures about the foot and ankle.

bimalleolar ankle f.: in which both the medial malleolus and distal fibula are fractured (**Pott**).

bimalleolar equivalent: a fracture of the medial or lateral malleolus with ligamentous damage on the opposite side of ankle.

boot-top f.: involves transverse, distal third of tibia, occurring at boot top of old style ski boot; also called **skier's injury.**

Bosworth f.: fracture-dislocation of the ankle, with oblique fracture of the distal fibula and displacement of the proximal fibular fragment out of fibular groove to a place posterior and medial to the posterolateral ridge of the tibia.

bunkbed f.: intra-articular f. of the base of the first metatarsal in children.

Cedell f.: fracture of the posterior process of the talus.

Chaput f.: involves the anterior tubercle of distal tibia because of strong attachment of anterior tibiofibular ligament.

Conrad-Bugg trapping: incarceration of soft tissue, usually the posterior tibial tendon, between fragments of an ankle fracture. This produces an injury that usually is reduced by open methods.

Cotton f.: partial forward dislocation of the tibia to produce a fracture of the posterior inferior margin of the tibia, sometimes called the **posterior malleolus.** This is most commonly associated with a fibular fracture.

Descot f.: involves the posterior lip of tibia.

dome f.: involves the superior articular surface of talus or the weight-bearing portion of the acetabulum.

Dupuytren f.: spiral f. of the distal end of fibula; associated with ankle diastasis.

Gosselin f.: V-shaped fracture of the distal tibia into the tibiotalar joint.

Henderson f.: trimalleolar fracture of the ankle.

Jones f.: fracture of the base of the fifth metatarsal such that the fracture line extends from lateral to medial cortex 1½ inches distal to the apophyseal tip. This term has been misapplied to fractures in the proximal apophyseal portion.

Kohler f.: involves the navicular and is associated with avascular necrosis; seen in children.

Lisfranc f.: usually a fracture-dislocation, with displacement of the proximal metatarsals.

Maisonneuve f.: spiral f. of proximal end of fibula, near the neck, associated with a tear of the anterior tibiofibular ligament and the potential for ankle diastasis.

march f.: stress f. of metatarsal caused by excessive marching; also called **fatigue f.**

midnight f.: open, oblique fracture of proximal phalanx of little toe caused by stubbing the toe on a solid object.

Montercaux f.: fracture of fibular neck with associated diastasis of ankle mortise.

paratrooper f.: involves posterior articular margin of tibia and/or lateral malleolus.

Pott f.: spiral oblique f. of distal fibula with associated rupture of the deltoid ligament; avulsion of the medial malleolus and lateral displacement of foot on tibia.

plafond f.: any fracture that involves the surface of the tibia that comes in contact with the dome of the talus.

Shepherd f.: involves posterior talus with sheared off piece of bone and, in some instances, a separate piece of bone (os trigonum).

Tillaux Kleiger f.: involves distal lateral tibia, vertically extending into the joint; sometimes associated with diastasis and other fractures about the ankle.

tongue f.: involves the posterosuperior portion of calcaneus.

trimalleolar f.: fracture of medial, lateral, and posterior malleolus.

triplane f.: involves the ankle in three planes: coronally through the posterior tibial metaphysis, transversely through the growth plate, and sagittally through the distal tibial epiphysis.

Volkmann f.: involves a triangular portion of the posterior lateral tibia into the joint, leaving a triangular bone fragment sometimes called **Volkmann's triangle.**

Wagstaffe f. (Le Fort f.): separation of a distal anterior fragment of the fibula, that is, the portion of attachment of the anterior tibiofibular ligament.

Contributing Factors

Aside from a single obvious traumatic event, there are other factors contributing to fractures.

dyscrasic f.: results from weakening of bone by a disease process.

endocrine f.: occurs in bone weakened by an endocrine disorder.

fatigue f.: spontaneous fracture in healthy bone resulting from fatigue or stress produced by excessive physical activity in a short period of time; seen in fibulas/tibias of young long-distance runners, the hips and heels of young military recruits, and in the metatarsals; also called **stress f., march f.**

hoop stress f.: involves the medial or anteromedial femoral neck and occurs during broaching of the femoral canal for a prosthesis or during the actual impaction of the prosthesis.

inflammatory f.: occurs in association with inflammation secondary to an infection, such as syphilis.

insufficiency f.: stress f. that occurs in bone because of its diminished volume (i.e., osteopenia).

neoplastic f.: a form of pathologic f. Presence of a tumor in bone, whether originating in the bone or metastatic from elsewhere, causes sufficient weakening to allow it to fracture spontaneously or with less trauma than it would normally take to break a healthy bone.

neuropathic f.: fracture due to overuse trauma to bone that occurs because of lack of pain perception.

pathologic f.: occurs with or without trauma where bone has been weakened by a local or systemic process. The most common causes are a tumor (benign or malignant), local infection, or bone cyst. This term is less widely applied to congenital disorders such as osteogenesis imperfecta, osteopetrosis, and neurofibromatosis. The term is applied more to congenital or acquired disorders such as osteomalacia, rickets, Paget disease, scurvy, and osteoporosis.

pseudofracture: radiographic finding of a line through bone that is due to abnormal mineralization that occurs in osteomalacia.

spontaneous f.: fracture that occurs without abnormal force. Usually due to a pathologic condition of the bone or the cumulative overuse of a bone where the response to repeated stress is sufficient for a fracture to occur.

stress f.: crack in bone from overexertion placed on bone structure of limb or metatarsals and from pull of muscle on bone. Not noticeable on initial radiograph but is on later radiographs when callus formation has taken place at the site. A bone scan or magnetic resonance imaging (MRI) will show the fracture; also called **march f., fatigue f.** More recently, the term **stress reaction to bone** has been used because fracture lines often do not appear and because the term more accurately describes the condition.

tension f.: bone fails at right angle to the direction of a tension force resulting in a transverse fracture.

Degree and Nature of Healing

The quality of bone healing is stated in terms of the solidarity of adhesiveness of the bone fragments. As most fractures heal, a surrounding "sleeve" of bone, or **callus,** is formed. This new bone formation is composed of cartilage, bone, blood vessels, and fibrous tissue and is often referred to in discussing bone healing.

If the bone is completely healed, the term **healed** is used. Anything less is considered a *state of healing,* unless there is *a failure of progression of healing with expectation of no further healing.* This is then considered a **nonunion.**

The absence of complete union is called **ununited,** but this term by some users implies an expectation of failure to unite. In **delayed union** the speed of callus formation (fracture healing) is slower than anticipated, but this does not imply expectancy of either total healing or nonunion. A **pseudoarthrosis** is the formation of a joint-like structure at the old fracture site and is a type of nonunion. It consists of fibrocartilaginous tissue and a synovial fluid sac. If a bone unites but in abnormal position and/or alignment, the term **malunion** is used. If two bones parallel to one another unite by osseous tissue, such as the tibia/fibula or ulna/radius complex, the result is a **crossunion,** or **synostosis.**

For example, in a simple fracture of the midshaft of the radius and ulna, assume that the radius adheres to the ulna at the distal fracture site and that the radius does not heal because of angulated healing of the ulna. Such a situation can be described as a **malunited fracture** of the **midshaft** of the ulna with a nonunion of the radius and crossunion of the distal radius and ulna. When the diagnoses are listed, they might be given as (1) malunion, fracture, closed, midshaft, ulna, right, or (2) nonunion, fracture, closed, midshaft, radius, right, associated with crossunion.

Secondary union is a term that has multiple meanings. It implies delayed healing either by the eventual adhesion of granulating surfaces of bone fragments or surgical intervention late in the course of fracture healing to promote union.

Nutritional support is important in bone healing to augment medical and surgical care. Bones need mineral and protein to heal, another consideration in treatment.

International Classification System and Trauma Registry System

AO/ASIF (Long Bone Fractures)

A scheme of fracture classification for research purposes and a more uniform description in the literature. The scheme has not been validated or used by all investigators.

- The system defines bones by number (**1**, humerus; **2**, radius and ulna; **3**, femur; **4**, tibia and fibula; **5**, spine, jaw, clavicle, and scapula; **6**, pelvis and sacrum; **7**, hand; **8**, foot).
- Nature of fracture by letter (**A**, simple involving at least 90% of the cortex or extra-articular; **B**, wedge with some contact between fragments or partial articular; **C**, complete with no contact between fragments or complete articular).
- Degree of comminution by number (**A**—1, spiral; 2, oblique; 3, transverse less than 30 degrees. **B**—1, spiral wedge; 2, bending wedge; 3, fragmented wedge. **C**—1, spiral; 2, segmental; 3, irregular).

The subgroups .1, .2, and .3 further define the complexity of each of the above groupings.

Limitation: agreement among raters.*

AO/ASIF (Soft Tissue Classification)
For uniform description in the literature.

Integumentary Injury (I)
Closed (C)
IC1: no skin lesion.
IC2: contusions but no skin laceration.
IC3: circumscribed degloving.
IC4: extensive closed degloving.
IC5: necrosis from contusion.
Open (O)
IO1: skin breakage from inside out.
IO2: skin breakage from outside in < 5 cm, contusion at edges.
IO3: skin breakage > 5 cm, increased contusion, devitalized edge.
IO4: considerable full thickness contusion, abrasion, extensive open degloving, skin loss.

Muscle/Tendon Injury (MT)
MT1: no muscle injury.
MT2: circumscribed muscle injury, one compartment only.
MT3: circumscribed muscle injury, two compartments.

---

*Müller ME et al, 1991.

MT4: muscle defect, tendon laceration, extensive muscle contusion.
MT5: compartment syndrome, crush syndrome with wide injury zone.

Neurovascular Injury (NV)
NV1: no neurovascular injury.
NV2: isolated nerve injury.
NV3: isolated vascular injury.
NV4: extensive segmental vascular injury.
NV5: combined neurovascular injury, subtotal and total amputation.*

Classification Systems by Grades, Types, and Mechanisms

The trend toward standard classification of fractures and dislocations is certainly a step forward, but such a system is designed for computer storage and is sometimes difficult to apply when viewing a fracture for the first time. It should not be forgotten that most of these specific classification systems were developed to address a specific set of circumstances. Attempting to apply them to other areas frequently leads to misinterpretation and erroneous conclusions. The authors, therefore, feel that these systems should be interpreted as meant by the original author(s). The reference is indicated at the end of the definition (see Bibliography for full reference citations).

Allman (Clavicle Fractures)
To define location of most common sites of occurrence and of nonunion.

Group I: fractures of middle third.
Group II: fractures distal to coracoclavicular ligament, nonunion frequent.
Group III: fractures of proximal end, nonunion and displacement rare.

Limitations: does not incorporate other factors such as degree of trauma.

Reference: Allman FL.

---

*Müller ME et al, 1991.

Anderson and d'Alonzo (Odontoid Fractures of the Second Cervical Vertebra)

Based on location of fracture; to define fracture pattern likely to require surgery for healing.

Type I: avulsion fracture of tip of odontoid.
Type II: fracture at junction of odontoid to body of vertebra.
Type III: fracture line extends downward into cancellous bone of body of vertebra.

Reference: Anderson LD and d'Alonzo RT.

Ashurst (Ankle Sprain/Fractures)

Based on direction or mechanism of force.

External Rotation Injuries (Supination)

first degree: transsyndesmotic fracture of the fibula.
alternate first degree: rupture of the anterior tibiofibular ligament with or without spiral fracture of the proximal fibula.
second degree: rupture of the deltoid ligament.
alternate second degree: avulsion of the medial malleolus.
third degree: fracture of the entire lower end of the tibia and fibula with external rotation.

Abduction Injuries (Pronation)

first degree: transverse fracture of the medial malleolus at or below its base.
second degree: rupture of the deltoid ligament or fracture of the medial malleolus followed by a fracture of the distal fibula.
third degree: fracture of both lower tibia and medial malleolus lateral displacement.

Adduction Injuries (Supination)

first degree: avulsion of the fibular malleolus at or below its base.
second degree: avulsion of the fibular malleolus at or below its base with medial malleolus below plafond, a shear vertically into tibial shaft.
third degree: supramalleolar fracture in both the tibia and fibula with medial displacement.

Fracture by Compression in Long Axis of Leg

first degree: isolated marginal fracture of the distal weight-bearing plate of the tibia.
second degree: comminution of the tibial plafond.
third degree: T or Y fractures (V fracture of Gosselin).

Limitations: fracture patterns overlap.

Reference: Ashurst APC.

Badelon (Lateral Condylar Fractures of the Humerus in Children)

Roentgenographic basis for stability versus displacement, which requires surgical reduction.

Type I: nondisplaced fracture that can be seen only on one view.
Type II: visible fracture line with minimal displacement.
Type III: displacement of more than 2 mm on all views.
Type IV: severe displacement with complete separation of fracture edges.

Reference: Badelon O et al.

Bado (Fractured Ulna with Dislocation of the Radial Head [Monteggia])

Based on mechanism of injury; to help define management.

Type 1: fracture of any portion of the ulna diaphysis with anterior angulation and anterior dislocation of the radial head.
Type 2: fracture of the ulnar diaphysis with posterior angulation and posterior or posterolateral dislocation of the radial head.
Type 3: fracture of the ulnar metaphysis with lateral or anterolateral dislocation of the radial head.
Type 4: proximal fracture of both bones at the same level with anterior dislocation of the radial head.

Limitations: some controversy as to relationship to treatment; types I and II have equivalents that involve dislocation radial head only (type 1) and fractured radial head.

Reference: Bado JL.

Brendt and Harty (Modified); (Fractures or Development of Osteochondritis Dissecans of the Dome of the Talus)

To define stages of "posttraumatic" necrosis of bone.

Stage I: normal x-ray but positive bone scan or change seen on magnetic resonance imaging (repeated minitrauma).
Stage II: incomplete separation of subchondral fragment (single injury event).
  Stage IIA: cyst formation (repeated minitrauma).
Stage III: complete separation of fragment, which is in anatomic position (single injury event).
Stage IV: separation of fragment (single injury event).

Reference: Anderson IF.

Boyd and Griffin (Extracapsular Fractures of Proximal Femur from Neck to 5 cm Distal to Lesser Trochanter)

To define surgical approach and prognosis for fractures near and around the femoral neck.

Type 1: intertrochanteric f., simple to reduce and maintain.
Type 2: intertrochanteric f. with comminution and additional coronal seen from lateral.
Type 3: subtrochanteric f. with at least one fracture line passing just distal to or through lesser trochanter.
Type 4: fractures of the trochanteric region and proximal shaft and fracture in two planes requiring two-plane fixation.

Limitations: crosses over from subtrochanteric fracture type to intertrochanteric and neck fractures.

Reference: Boyd HB and Griffin LL.

Bryan and Morrey

To define shape and direction of elbow capitellar fractures.

Type 1: shear fracture in plane of capitellum involving none or little of the trochlea.
Type 2: a variable amount of the cartilage of the capitellum with minimal attached subchondral bone.
Type 3: comminuted or compression fracture of the capitellum.

Canale-Kelly (Talar Fractures)

Based on location of fracture and association with displacement and effect on blood supply; to define prognosis for long-term outcome with particular reference to avascular necrosis.

Type I: minimal displacement, only one source of blood supply might be disrupted.
Type II: subtalar subluxation or dislocation, two or three sources of blood supply might be affected.
Type III: body of talus dislocated from the ankle and the subtalar joint.
Type IV: fracture of talar neck associated with dislocation of the body from the ankle, or subtalar joint and additional subluxation or dislocation of the head of the talus from the talonavicular joint.

Reference: Canale ST and Kelly FB.

Cervical Spine Injury Score System

Four columns: anterior, right pillar, left pillar, and posterior.
    For each column, an analogue scale using fracture displacement and ligament disruption is given:

Fracture nondisplaced with mild ligamentous 1–3 mm (analogue scale 0–1)
Fracture displaced 1–3 mm, mild ligamentous 1–3 mm (analogue scale 1–2)
Fracture displaced 1–3 mm, moderate ligamentous 3–5 mm (analogue scale 2–3)
Fracture displaced 3–5 mm (analogue scale 3–4)
Fracture displaced > 5 mm, severe ligamentous > 5 mm (analogue scale 4–5)

Chadwick and Bentley (Distal Tibia Fractures Affecting Epiphysis in Children)

Based on x-ray analysis; reflects the mechanism of type IV Salter fractures of the distal tibia and fibula and helps predict retardation of growth.

Group I: epiphysis not fractured.
  Group 1a: abduction injury with fracture of the distal fibular shaft and lateral displacement.
  Group 1b: supination/hyperplantar flexion injury with posterior metaphyseal fragment of the tibia and posterior displacement.

Group 1c: supination/external rotation injury with large anteromedial metaphyseal component, tibia, and posterior displacement.

Group 1d: adduction injury (rare), posteromedial metaphyseal fragment of the tibia with fracture of the distal fibular shaft and medial displacement.

Group II: vertical fracture through epiphysis with shift of lateral fragment.

Group III: adduction injury, Salter type I or II fibular slip with type IV medial malleolar fracture.

Reference: Chadwick CJ and Bentley G.

Colonna (Delbet) (Hip Fractures in Children)
Attributes classification to Delbet; no purpose given.

Type I: transepiphyseal separations with or without dislocation of femoral head.

Type II: transcervical fractures, displaced and nondisplaced.

Type III: cervicotrochanteric fractures, displaced and nondisplaced.

Type IV: intertrochanteric fractures.

Reference: Colonna PC.

Colton (Olecranon Fractures)
To define treatment.

Avulsion group: transverse fracture line separates a small fragment of olecranon with or without displacement.

Oblique group: primary failure being an oblique line from the trochlear notch to the distal outer ulnar shaft, degree of comminution staged a to d.

   Stage a: single fracture line, displaced and nondisplaced.

   Stage b: nondisplaced single central large V-shaped fragment.

   Stage c: displaced single central large V-shaped fragment.

   Stage d: highly comminuted central pieces of bone with displacement.

Fracture dislocation (Monteggia group): fracture line at or slightly proximal to coronoid, which may result in anterior fracture/dislocation of the elbow.

Unclassified group: high energy, highly comminuted fractures not matching the above descriptions.

Reference: Colton CL.

Dias-Tachdjian (Ankle Fractures in Children)
Uses Lauge-Hansen guidelines, foot position, and direction of force in correlation with the Salter-Harris classification to plan surgical and other treatment approaches.

Supination-inversion: inversion force applied to supinated foot.

   Grade I: Salter-Harris type I or II of distal fibular epiphysis.

   Grade II: grade I with Salter-Harris type III or IV of tibial epiphysis.

Supination-plantar flexion: plantar flexion force on supinated foot.

   Grade I: Salter-Harris type I or II of distal tibia, usually with posterior displacement.

Supination-external rotation: external rotation ankle force on fully supinated foot.

   Grade I: Salter-Harris type II of distal tibia with long spiral fracture of distal tibia.

   Grade II: grade I with spiral fracture of fibula.

Pronation-eversion-external rotation: a combination of eversion and external rotation force on pronated foot.

   Grade I: posterolateral displacement of Salter-Harris type II tibial fracture with short oblique fibular fracture above physis.

Limitations: fractures not covered under this system include Salter-Harris type III distal tibia and triplane fracture (as described by author).

Reference: Dias LS and Tachdjian MO.

Essex-Lopresti (Os Calcis Fractures)
Based on direction of injury force (A-C superior to inferior, and D-F anterosuperior to posteroinferior); helps define method of closed and open management.

Type A: nondisplaced fracture inferior to lateral process of talus and through lateral cortex.

Type B: type A with shearing of sustentaculum tali along with one-third to one-half of the posterior facet.

Type C: type B with depression of joint and superior posterior displacement of distal portion.

Type D: affects lateral half or two-thirds of subtalar joint and fracture of the lateral cortex without displacement.

Type E: type D with superior displacement of anterior portion of calcaneus.

Type F: type E with displacement of posterior facet of calcaneus and further superior migration of anterior portion.

Reference: Essex-Lopresti P.

Evans-Wales (Intertrochanteric Fractures of Femur)

Grouped by stable or unstable and expected response to treatment.

Type I: fracture line extends upward and outward from lesser trochanter:
Undisplaced stable.
Displaced reduced with stable medial apposition.
Displaced unreduced with no medial apposition.
Comminuted unstable with no medial apposition.

Type II: reversed obliquity with line from lesser trochanter to inferior lateral cortex.

Limitations: directed at open versus closed management, which is no longer used.

Reference: Evans EM and Wales SS.

Ferkel-Cheng (Arthroscopic Classification of Osteochondral Lesions of the Talus)

To define stages of appearance and attachment of lesion to subchondral bone.

Stage A: smooth, intact, but soft or ballottable.
Stage B: rough surface.
Stage C: fibrillations or fissures.
Stage D: flap present or bone exposed.
Stage E: loose, nondisplaced fragment.
Stage F: displaced fragment.

Reference: Ferkel RD et al, 1995.

Ferkel-Sgaglione (CT Classification of Osteochondral Lesions of the Talus)

To define stages of attachment of subchondral bone.

Stage I: cystic lesion within dome of talus.
Stage IIA: cystic lesion with communication to talar dome surface.
Stage IIB: open articular surface lesion with overlying nondisplaced fragment.
Stage III: nondisplaced lesion with lucency.
Stage IV: displaced fragment.

Reference: Ferkel RD et al, 1990.

Fielding-Magliato (Subtrochanteric Fractures of Femur)

Based on distance from lesser trochanter for selection of method of surgical fixation.

Type 1: at level of lesser trochanter.
Type 2: between 2.5 and 5 cm below lesser trochanter.
Type 3: 5–7.5 cm below lesser trochanter.

Limitations: oblique and comminuted fractures involve more than one level, newer appliances cover a wider spectrum of conditions.

Reference: Fielding JW and Magliato HJ.

Frykman (Distal Radial and Ulnar Fractures)

Based on radial joint involvement with and without ulnar styloid fractures to define method of fixation.

Type I: radial extra-articular without ulnar styloid fracture.
Type II: radial extra-articular with ulnar styloid fracture.
Type III: radiocarpal joint only without ulnar styloid fracture.
Type IV: radiocarpal joint only with ulnar styloid fracture.
Type V: distal radioulnar joint only without ulnar styloid fracture.
Type VI: distal radioulnar joint only with ulnar styloid fracture.

Type VII: both radiocarpal and distal radioulnar joint without ulnar styloid fracture.

Type VIII: both radiocarpal and distal radioulnar joint with ulnar styloid fracture.

Reference: Frykman G.

Garden (Subcapital Fractures of Femoral Neck)

Based on anteroposterior (AP) and lateral radiographic guidelines for reduction and likelihood of avascular necrosis.

Stage 1: incomplete, impacted, head tilted in posterolateral direction.

Stage 2: complete but undisplaced.

Stage 3: complete, displaced, but fragments remain in contact.

Stage 4: fracture fragments completely displaced, no contact between fragments.

Reference: Garden RS.

Gartland (Supracondylar Fractures of the Humerus in Children)

Based on displacement; to define surgical treatment.

Type I: undisplaced.

Type II: displaced and difficult to hold with cast immobilization.

Type III: posteromedial or posterolateral displacement with difficult reduction that is hard to maintain due to periosteal stripping.

Reference: Gartland JJ.

Gustilo (open fractures)

Based on intraoperative assessment of size of wound and soft tissue involvement; to determine fixation types and limb salvage.

Type I: clean wound < 1 cm minimal contamination.

Type II: laceration > 1 cm without extensive soft tissue damage, flaps, or avulsions.

Type IIIA: despite extensive soft tissue damage or high energy trauma soft tissue coverage of the bone is adequate. Also includes segmental or highly comminuted fractures regardless of size of wound.

Type IIIB: extensive soft tissue laceration with periosteal stripping, exposed bone, usually massively contaminated, typically requiring soft tissue coverage.

Type IIIC: arterial injury, requires repair regardless of size of wound.

Limitations: types II and III have interobserver variation.

Reference: Gustilo RB et al, 1990.

Hawkins (Talar Neck Fractures)

Based on location of fracture and association with displacement and effect on blood supply; prognosis for long-term outcome with particular reference to avascular necrosis.

Type I: minimal displacement, only one source of blood supply might be disrupted.

Type II: subtalar subluxation or dislocation, two or three sources of blood supply might be affected.

Type III: body of talus dislocated from the ankle and the subtalar joint.

Reference: Hawkins LG.

Herbert and Fisher (Wrist Scaphoid Fractures)

To differentiate between fractures that are likely to unite in 6 to 8 weeks and those that would not; to define need for surgery.

Type A1: nondisplaced tubercle hairline fracture.

Type A2: nondisplaced hairline wrist fracture.

Type B1: oblique fracture of distal third.

Type B2: displaced middle wrist fracture.

Type B3: proximal pole fracture.

Type B4: fracture dislocation of carpus.

Type B5: comminuted fractures.

Type C: delayed union.

Type D1: fibrous union.

Type D2: sclerotic nonunion (pseudoarthrosis).

Limitations: type B5 and C have been deleted; D2 changed to pseudoarthrosis; D3 sclerotic pseudoarthrosis; D4 avascular necrosis.

Reference: Herbert TJ and Fisher WE. (Modified *J Bone Joint Surg* 1996; 78-B:519–528).

Hohl-Moore (Tibial Plateau Fractures)
Based on pattern; designed for surgical planning.

Type 1: minimally displaced.
Type 2: local compression.
Type 3: split compression.
Type 4: total condyle.
Type 5: both condyles.

Limitations: does not take into account ligament injury.

Reference: Hohl M and Moore TM.

Ideberg (Glenoid Fractures of the Scapula)
To define mechanism and to compare surgical and nonsurgical treatment.

Type I: avulsion of the anterior margin.
Type II: transverse fracture through glenoid fossa with inferior triangular fragment displaced with the humeral head.
Type III: oblique fracture through the glenoid exiting on the midsuperior border of the scapula; often associated with acromioclavicular fracture or dislocation.
Type IV: horizontal, exiting through medial border of the blade.
Type V: type IV with a separation of the inferior half of the glenoid.

Reference: Ideberg R.

Jensen (Intertrochanteric Femur Fractures)
Modified Evans system to determine possibility of stable reduction and secondary fracture displacement.

Type I: single fracture line, nondisplaced, stable on fixation.
Type II: single fracture line, displaced, stable on fixation.
Type III: comminuted, not involving the lesser trochanter; risk of loss of reduction.
Type IV: unstable, lesser trochanteric fragment, portion of greater trochanter attached to neck; greater risk of loss of reduction.

Type V: unstable lesser and greater trochanteric fragments; greatest risk of loss of reduction.

Reference: Jensen JS.

Johansson (Femoral Fractures Following Total Hip Replacement)
To define fracture pattern that is likely to require surgery for healing.

Type I: fracture proximal to tip of the prosthesis.
Type II: fracture extends from proximal shaft to point distal to tip of prosthesis.
Type III: fracture lines entirely below distal tip of prosthesis.

Reference: Johansson JE et al.

Key and Conwell (Pelvic Fractures)
Based on stability and location; to define need for stabilization.

I: fractures without break in pelvic ring.
  A: avulsion fractures.
    1: anterosuperior spine.
    2: anteroinferior spine.
    3: ischial tuberosity.
II: single break in pelvic ring.
  A: fracture of two ipsilateral rami.
  B: fracture near or subluxation of symphysis pubis.
  C: fracture near or subluxation of the sacroiliac joint.
III: double break in pelvic ring.
  A: double vertical fractures or dislocation of pubis (straddle).
  B: double vertical fractures or dislocation (Malgaigne).
  C: severe multiple fractures.
IV: fractures of the acetabulum.
  A: small fragment with dislocated hip.
  B: linear fracture associated with nondisplaced pelvic fracture.
  C: linear fracture associated with hip joint instability.
  D: fracture secondary to central dislocation of the acetabulum.

Reference: Key JA and Conwell HE.

Kilfoyle (Medial Condylar Fractures of the Humerus in Children)

To define need for closed (first two types) versus open treatment (type III).

Type I: greenstick impacted fracture on medial condylar apophyseal region, stable.

Type II: fracture through the medial condyle into the joint with little or no displacement.

Type III: intra-articular fracture of medial epicondyle with displacement and rotation.

Reference: Kilfoyle RM.

Kyle (Femoral Trochanteric Fractures)

Based on stability and displacement; to define nail-type management.

Type I: stable, undisplaced intertrochanteric fractures.

Type II: stable, displaced varus deformity with fracture of the lesser trochanter.

Type III: unstable, displaced fracture of greater trochanter with posteromedial comminution and varus deformity.

Type IV: type III with subtrochanteric component.

Limitations: designed to compare sliding versus rigid nail; other devices now available.

Reference: Kyle RF et al.

Lauge-Hansen (Ankle Fractures)

Patterns that describe the position of the foot and the forces across the ankle that produced the fracture; to identify surgical and other treatment approaches.

supination-eversion: external or lateral rotation.
supination-adduction.
pronation-abduction.
pronation-adduction.

Limitations: interobserver disagreement; eversion a misnomer—it should be "external rotation" or "lateral rotation"; mechanism not consistent in producing specific injury.

Reference: Lauge-Hansen N.

Letournel and Judet (Acetabular Fractures)

(Fig. 1-5)

Based on division into five basic groups (fractures of the posterior wall, posterior column, anterior wall, anterior column, and transverse fractures) to define best surgical approach for reduction.

Elementary

A: posterior wall
B: posterior column
C: anterior wall
D: anterior column
E: transverse

Associated

F: posterior column and posterior wall
G: transverse and posterior wall
H: T-shaped
I: anterior and posterior hemitransverse
J: complete, both columns

Reference: Judet R et al.

Letts-Vincent-Gouw ("Floating Knee" Fracture in Children Involving Both Femur and Tibia)

For descriptive purposes.

Type A: both bones diaphyseal closed.

Type B: one bone metaphyseal and other diaphyseal closed.

Type C: epiphyseal and diaphyseal closed.

Type D: one open fracture.

Type E: two open fractures with major soft tissue injury.

Reference: Letts M et al.

Levine-Edwards (Axis Fracture)

Treatment based on location, displacement, and mechanism of injury.

Type I: through neural arch, no angulation, displacement to 3 mm.

Type II: through neural arch, angulation, and translation.

Type IIa: through neural arch, slight, or no translation but very severe angulation.

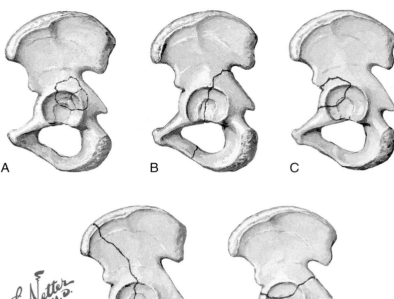

FIG 1-5 Acetabular fractures. **A,** Fracture of posterior wall. Repair with plate and lag screw. **B,** Fracture of posterior column. Repair with plate and lag screws. **C,** Wedge fracture of anterior wall. Repair with lag screws. **D,** Fracture of anterior column. Repair with plate and long screws. **E,** Transverse fracture. Repair with plate and lag screws.

A   B   C

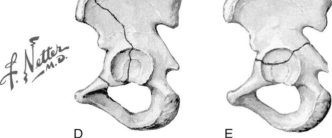

D   E

(Continued)

Type III: severe angulation and displacement with concomitant unilateral or bilateral facet dislocation at second and third cervical vertebrae.

Reference: Levine AM and Edwards CC.

Mallory (Femoral Shaft Fractures Occurring During Total Hip Replacement Surgery)

Based on location, prognosis, and degree of internal and external fixation required for healing.

Type I: fracture includes areas of lesser trochanter and calcar.
Type II: fracture extends beyond lesser trochanter to a point up to 4 cm proximal to the prosthetic tip.
Type III: fracture line extends below a point 4 cm above prosthetic tip.

Reference: Mallory TH et al.

Mason (Radial Head Fractures)

Prognosis based on displacement and comminution.

Type I: undisplaced marginal fracture.
Type II: displaced segmental.
Type III: comminuted.
Type IV: comminuted with posterior elbow dislocation.

Reference: Mason ML.

Mast-Spiegel-Pappas (Distal Tibial Fractures Affecting Tibial Plafond, Pilon)

Based on mechanism of deforming load to help define a clear prognosis.

Type I: essentially malleolar fracture with large posterior plafond fragment.
Type II: spiral extension mechanism includes a spiral shaft fracture with no comminution plafond.

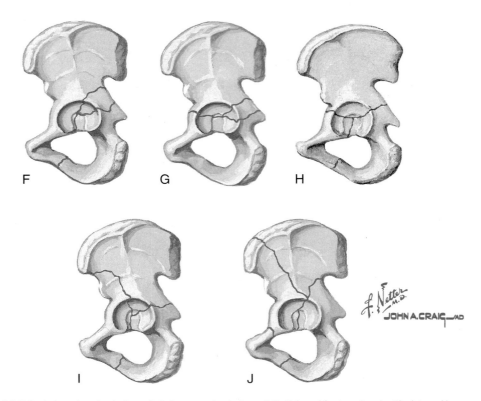

FIG 1-5 Cont'd. F, Posterior column/posterior wall. **G,** Transverse/posterior wall. **H,** T-shaped fracture. Repair with plate and lag screws. **I,** Anterior column/posterior hemi transverse. **J,** Both columns. (Reprinted from *Netter Anatomy Illustration Collection* © Elsevier Inc.)

Type III: central compression with impaction of talus into distal tibia, graded A to C per Rüedi and Allgöwer:

Type IIIA: cleavage fracture of articular surface without displacement.

Type IIIB: significant fracture and dislocation of articular surface without comminution.

Type IIIC: type IIIB with significant comminution and impaction.

Limitations: the word pilon implies impaction into a surface, which is more a posterior or rotatory displacement in types I and II.

Reference: Mast JW et al.

Mayo (Olecranon Fractures)

Surgical and closed management based on location, comminution, and stability.

Type I: undisplaced.

IA: noncomminuted.

IB: comminuted.

Type II: displaced, stable.

IIA: noncomminuted.

IIB: comminuted.

Type III: unstable.

IA: noncomminuted.

IB: comminuted.

Reference: Cabenela ME and Morrey BF.

Meyers-McKeever (Intercondylar Eminence Fractures of the Tibia in Children)

For surgical planning.

Type I: nondisplaced avulsion.

Type II: anterior one-third to one-half lifted with posterior rim intact.

Type III: completely displaced.

Reference: Meyers MH and McKeever FM.

Milch (Medial and Lateral Condylar Fractures of the Humerus in Children)
To define closed versus open treatment.

Type 1: fracture line from trochlear groove to lateral superior or trochlear sulcus to medial superior; more stable on reduction (compression fracture mechanism).

Type 2: fracture line from trochlear sulcus to lateral superior or trochlear groove to medial superior; more unstable (compression fracture-dislocation mechanism).

Reference: Milch H.

Monteggia (Fracture of Ulna with Dislocation of Radial Head)
Type I: Volar bow of ulnar fracture with radial head dislocation superior.

Type II: dorsal bow ulnar fracture with inferior radial head dislocation.

Type III: lateral bow ulnar fracture with lateral radial head dislocation.

Type IV: midshaft radius and ulnar fractures with radial head dislocation.

Neer (Humeral Head Fractures)
Based on location and number of fragments; to define method of treatment. Note: a part is not a part unless it is separated by 1 cm or more or there is 40-degree angulation.

Anatomic neck: two part (neck and shaft only).

Surgical neck: below tuberosity; considered two part even if comminuted.

Greater tuberosity: may be two part, three part with anatomic neck, or four part with anatomic neck and lesser tuberosity.

Lesser tuberosity: may be two part, three part with anatomic neck, or four part with anatomic neck and greater tuberosity.

Fracture-dislocation, anterior: two part with greater tuberosity, three part with anatomic neck and greater tuberosity, four part with lesser tuberosity.

Fracture-dislocation, posterior: two part with lesser tuberosity, three part with anatomic neck, four part with greater tuberosity.

Limitations: interobserver disagreement on x-ray interpretation.

Reference: Neer CSI.

Neer-Horowitz (Proximal Humeral Physeal Fractures in Children)
Based on location.

Grade I: < 5 mm displacement.

Grade II: displaced up to one-third the width of the shaft.

Grade III: displaced from one- to two-thirds the width of the shaft.

Grade IV: displaced more than two-thirds the width of the shaft.

Reference: Neer CSI and Horowitz BS.

Ogden (Fractures with Injury to All Bone and Cartilage Components that May Affect Growth)
To better define effects on growth, including nonphyseal growth areas.

Type 1: entirely through physis.
  1A: undulates through provisional calcification of hypertrophic zone; no effect on growth.
  1B: more into degenerative cartilage zone and primary spongiosa; no effect on growth.
  1C: affects a portion of germinal layer of physis leading to bridging bar.
Type 2: through provisional calcification and hypertrophic zone with piece of metaphysis.
  2A: attached metaphyseal fragment.
  2B: comminuted metaphyseal fragment.
  2C: shorter metaphyseal fragment that traverses most of metaphysis.
  2D: similar to type 1C; affects germinal layer of physis with growth effect.
Type 3: fracture extends from articular surface through epiphysis up to, but not across, physis.
  3A: transverse fracture line entirely through physis.

3B: transverse fracture line through spongiosa, leaving small portion of metaphysis with epiphysis.

3C: local compression of physis.

3D: nonarticular epiphysis such as ischial tuberosity.

Type 4: fracture extends from articular surface, through epiphysis and past physis to metaphysis.

    4A: basic transepiphyseal physeal fracture.

    4B: 4A with line across portion of physis, similar to type 3.

    4C: involves nonarticular cartilaginous region such as proximal femur.

Type 5: affects germinal layer without bony fracture.

Type 6: involves zone of Ranvier (ring of cells at margin of physis from local contusion).

Type 7: completely intraepiphyseal.

    7A: involves both articular cartilage and bone of secondary ossification center.

    7B: injury to cartilage growth surface on articular surface of epiphysis.

Type 8: injury to metaphyseal growth and remodeling mechanism.

Type 9: selective injury to diaphyseal growth mechanism, appositional.

Limitations: complexity.

Reference: Ogden JA.

Ogden (Tibial Tuberosity Fractures in Children)

Need for surgical reduction and fixation.

Type 1: injury to most distal part of tuberosity.

    1A: mild displacement, relatively stable, possible propagation into main ossification center.

    1B: separation of fragment from metaphysis with or without separation from rest of the secondary ossification center.

Type 2: separation of entire ossification center of tuberosity with possible propagation into main ossification center of proximal end of tibia; fracture of tuberosity segment at juncture of main ossification centers of tibia and tuberosity.

    2A: without communication of ossification center.

2B: with communication of ossification center.

Type 3: more severe separation of fragments; propagation of fracture through main proximal tibial epiphysis into joint; disruption of articular surface under anterior attachments of medial or lateral meniscus or both.

    3A: single displaced fragment.

    3B: comminuted displaced fragments.

Reference: Ogden JA et al.

Olecranon Fractures (No Eponym)

Type I: involves only proximal third of articular surface or no articular surface.

Type II: involves middle third of articular surface.

Type III: may occur in conjunction with anterior displacement of the radius.

Reference: Crenshaw AH.

Pauwels (Femoral Neck Fractures)

Based on angle of fracture to define stability of fracture in management.

Type I: angle of fracture line is 30 degrees from the horizontal.

Type II: angle of fracture line is 50 degrees from the horizontal.

Type III: angle of fracture line is 70 degrees from the horizontal.

Reference: Pauwels F.

Pipkin (Hip Dislocations with Femoral Head Fracture)

Based on location of fracture head and neck when associated with a posterior hip dislocation (type V Epstein Thompson); to determine prognosis for long-term outcome.

Type I: posterior dislocation of the hip with fracture of the femoral head caudad to fovea centralis.

Type II: posterior dislocation of the hip with fracture of the femoral head cephalad to fovea centralis.

Type III: type I or II with femoral neck fracture.

Type IV: type I, II, or III with associated acetabular fracture.

Reference: Pipkin G.

Poland (Childhood Fractures Involving Epiphysis)

Entirely descriptive, written at time of development of radiographs.

Type I: separation across physis only.
Type II: separation across physis with fragment metaphysis.
Type III: separation of portion of epiphysis across physis.
Type IV: separation of both portions of epiphysis from physis.

Reference: Poland J.

Quénu and Küss Modified (Fractures-Dislocations of Tarsometatarsal Articulation)

To determine the magnitude of soft tissue injury, displacement plane, prognosis, and treatment.

Type A: total incongruity; all five metatarsals displaced in same direction.
Type B: partial incongruity:
  medial dislocation.
  lateral dislocation.
Type C: divergent usually between first and second ray:
  total—all five rays involved.
  partial—some lateral rays intact.

Reference: Hardcastle PH et al.

Riseborough and Radin (Distal Humeral Intercondylar T Fractures)

Based on roentgenographic analysis to compare closed versus open treatment.

Type 1: undisplaced fracture between capitellum and trochlea.
Type 2: nondisplaced T or Y fracture, with fracture exiting from groove proximally between condyle and then dividing transversely or obliquely across the shaft separating the condyles from each other and the shaft; no appreciable separation or rotation on AP roentgenogram.
Type 3: significant separation with rotational displacement of condyles.
Type 4: severe comminution of articular surface and wide condylar separation.

Reference: Riseborough EJ and Radin EL.

Rockwood (Acromioclavicular Separations)

To determine degree of injury or need for surgical intervention.

Type I: neither acromioclavicular nor coracoclavicular ligament torn.
Type II: acromioclavicular ligament torn but coracoclavicular ligament intact.
Type III: both acromioclavicular and coracoclavicular ligament torn.
Type IV: both ligaments torn and clavicle displaced posteriorly through trapezius.
Type V: both ligaments torn and wide superior separation of the clavicle.
Type VI: both ligaments torn and distal clavicle caught inferior to coracoid and posterior to conjoined tendon.

Reference: Rockwood CA.

Rowe and Lowell (Central Fracture Dislocations of Acetabulum)

To define surgical planning and risk of complications.

Type I: undisplaced (single line or stellate).
Type II: inner wall fractures.
  Type IIA: femoral head reduced under acetabular dome initially.
  Type IIB: femoral head out, reduced under acetabular dome initially.
Type III: superior dome fractures.
  Type IIIA: acetabulum generally congruent with femoral head.
  Type IIIB: acetabulum incongruent with femoral head.
Type IV: bursting fracture (all elements of acetabulum involved).

Type IVA: fractures with congruity between femoral head and acetabular dome.
Type IVB: fractures with incongruity between femoral head and acetabular dome.

Reference: Rowe CR and Lowell JD.

Rüedi and Allgöwer (Distal Tibial Pilon Fractures)
Degree of comminution and displacement of articular fragments; to define nature of management of pilon fractures of the distal tibia.

Type A: cleavage fracture of the articular surface without major dislocation of the fragments.
Type B: significant fracture and dislocation of the articular surface without comminution.
Type C: severe comminution and impaction of tibial articular surface.

Reference: Rüedi T and Allgöwer M.

Russell-Taylor (High Proximal Femoral Fractures)
To predict effectiveness of closed nailing techniques.

Group I: does not involve piriformis fossa.
 Group Ia: comminution and fracture line extends from below lesser trochanter to femoral isthmus.
 Group Ib: fracture line and comminution involving area from lesser trochanter to femoral isthmus.
Group II: involvement of piriformis fossa.
 Group IIa: fracture extends from lesser trochanter to isthmus with involvement of piriformis fossa (seen on lateral roentgenogram).
 Group IIb: fracture extends into the piriformis fossa (seen on lateral roentgenogram) with significant medial comminution and loss of lesser trochanteric continuity.

Reference: Russell TA.

Salter-Harris (Fractures Involving the Physis in Children)
To predict growth disturbance and need for exact reduction.

Type I: fracture line across physis only.

Type II: fracture line across physis with portion through metaphysis.
Type III: fracture through physis and portion of epiphysis.
Type IV: fracture line through epiphysis, crosses physis, and out metaphysis.
Type V: crush injury to physis.

Reference: Salter RB and Harris WR.

Samilson-Preito (Degenerative Change Associated with Shoulder Dislocation)
Relating degenerative change to timing of treatment.

mild: inferior exostosis of humeral head or glenoid < 3 mm in size on AP radiograph.
moderate: inferior exostosis of humeral head or glenoid between 3 and 7 mm in size with slight joint irregularity.
severe: > 8 mm osteophyte with joint narrowing and sclerosis.

Reference: Samilson RL and Preito V.

Schatzker (Tibial Plateau and Proximal Tibial Fracture Patterns)
Based on pathoanatomic factors, etiologic factors, and therapeutic features; to determine treatment of fracture of the tibial plateau and proximal tibia.

Type I: pure cleavage.
Type II: cleavage combined with depression.
Type III: pure central depression.
Type IV: fracture of medial condyle.
Type V: bicondylar fractures.
Type VI: plateau fracture with dissociation of tibial metaphysis and diaphysis.

Limitations: type V could be divided into axial, laterally tilted, and medially tilted.

Reference: Schatzker J et al.

Seinsheimer (Femoral Intertrochanteric and Subtrochanteric Fractures)
Based on number of fragments and the location and configuration of fracture lines; to select method of surgical fixation.

Type I: nondisplaced or < 1 mm displacement.
Type II: two-part fractures.
   Type IIA: transverse.
   Type IIB: spiral with lesser trochanter attached to proximal fragment.
   Type IIC: spiral with lesser trochanter attached to distal fragment.
Type III: three-part fractures.
   Type IIIA: spiral with lesser trochanter a part of the proximal fragment.
   Type IIIB: spiral with lesser trochanter a butterfly fragment.
Type IV: comminuted with four or more fragments.
Type V: subtrochanteric-intertrochanteric configuration.

Limitations: lesser trochanteric continuity and involvement of piriformis fossa a major factor of stability.

Reference: Seinsheimer FI.

Stewart and Milford (Hip Dislocation with Associated Acetabular and Femoral Head Fracture)

For prognosis.

Grade I: simple dislocation without acetabular fracture.
Grade II: dislocation with one or more large acetabular fractures but stable after reduction.
Grade III: explosive or blast fracture with disintegration of acetabular rim, unstable after reduction.
Grade IV: dislocation with fracture of head or neck of femur.

Reference: Stewart MJ and Milford LW.

Stress Injury to Bone (Stress "Fractures")

To grade relative state or level of effect on bone.

Grade O: positive bone scan in an asymptomatic subject with negative radiographs. Seen only in research surveys.
Grade I: local symptoms associated with a positive bone scan and negative radiographs.
Grade II: local symptoms with a positive bone scan and minimal findings on radiographs.
Grade III: local symptoms with a positive bone scan and clear evidence of bone absorption on radiographs.

Grade IV: local symptoms with a positive bone scan and actual bone fracture.

Thompson and Epstein (Hip Dislocation with Acetabular Fracture)

Based on size and stability of associated fractures to determine outcome of treatment.

Type I: with or without minor fracture.
Type II: with a large single posterior acetabular rim fracture.
Type III: with comminution of the posterior rim with or without a major fragment.
Type IV: with fracture of the acetabular floor.
Type V: with fracture of the femoral head.

Limitations: does not take into account size and place of femoral head fragment (see Pipkin classification).

Reference: Thompson VP and Epstein HC.

Tile (Pelvic Fractures)

Numbers used by the AO group based on mechanism and letters based on vertical and rotational stability (A, stable; B, rotationally unstable and vertically stable; C, rotationally and vertically unstable); to determine if surgical or closed treatment is indicated.

Type A1: does not involve pelvic ring such as avulsion fracture and fractured ilium.
Type A2: stable pelvic ring such as low energy fall in elderly; minimal displacement.
Type B1: "open book" or anterior compression injury.
Type B2: lateral compression force with ipsilateral fracture.
Type B3: lateral compression force with contralateral fractures.
Type C1: unilateral fracture with both anterior and posterior complex.
Type C2: bilateral injuries.
Type C3: vertical shear fracture with fractured acetabulum.

Reference: Tile M.

Torode and Zieg (Pelvic Fractures in Children)

Type I: avulsion of the bony elements of the pelvis.

Type II: iliac wing fractures.

Type III: simple ring fracture including pubic rami or disruption of pubic symphysis.

Type IV: unstable ring fracture including straddle (bilateral pubic rami) fractures, pubic rami or symphysis with posterior elements or sacroiliac joint disruption, anterior fracture with acetabular fracture.

Reference: Torode I and Zieg S.

Tronzo (Intertrochanteric Fractures)

Based on reduction potential.

Type I: incomplete trochanteric fracture reduced anatomically with traction.

Type II: uncomminuted fracture of both trochanters, with or without displacement, reduced with traction; anatomic reduction usually achieved.

Type III: comminuted fracture with large lesser trochanteric fragment, posterior wall exploded, fracture line makes beak of inferior femoral neck unstable.

Type IV: comminuted and unstable disengaged trochanteric fractures with explosion of posterior wall and medial displacement of femoral neck spike.

Type V: trochanteric fracture with reverse obliquity (downward from a medial to lateral direction).

Reference: Tronzo RG.

Tscherne (Classification for Tibial Fractures with Associated Soft Tissue Injury and Extent of Contamination)

To define risk of surgical management.

Grade CO: simple fracture configuration with little or no soft tissue injury.

Grade CI: superficial abrasion, mild to moderately severe fracture configuration.

Grade CII: deep contaminated abrasion with local damage to skin or muscle, moderately severe to severe fracture configuration.

Grade CIII: extensive contusion or crushing of the skin or destruction of the muscle, severe fracture.

Limitations: definition of severity is lacking, no vascular annotation.

Reference: Oestern HH and Tscherne H.

Watson-Jones (Tibial Tuberosity Fractures in Children)

To determine need for surgical reduction and fixation.

Type I: small fragment displaced superiorly.

Type II: larger fragment hinged upwards involving secondary center of ossification.

Type III: displaced fracture passes posteriorly and proximally across epiphyseal plate.

Limitations: does not account for potential entry of type II into knee joint.

Reference: Watson-Jones.

Weber (Danis-Weber) (Ankle Fractures)

Based on the appearance of the fibular fracture; to define direction of causative and thus reducing forces.

Type A: caused by internal rotation and adduction, produces a transverse fracture of the lateral malleolus below the plafond.

Type B: caused by external rotation resulting in an oblique fracture of the lateral malleolus.

Type C-1: abduction injury with oblique fracture of fibula proximal to disrupted tibiofibular ligament (medial malleolus or deltoid ligament may be affected).

Type C-2: abduction-external rotation injury with more proximal fracture of fibula and more extensive disruption of interosseous membrane (medial malleolus or deltoid ligament may be affected).

Reference: Weber BG.

Winquist-Hansen (Femoral Shaft Fractures)

Based on comminution and stability; to determine if static locking nail is necessary.

Grade O: transverse.

Grade I: comminuted with small piece not affecting stability.

Grade II: comminuted with $\geq 50\%$ abutting major cortex sufficient to prevent rotation and shortening with good proximal and distal nail purchase.

Grade III: < 50% major cortex contact allowing rotation or shortening; requires proximal and distal cross-fixation.

Grade IV: no fixed contact between major proximal and distal fragment; requires proximal and distal crossfixation.

Reference: Winquist RA and Hansen ST.

Young-Burgess (Pelvic Fractures) (Fig. 1-6)
Radiologic assessment based on probable mechanism to recognize pattern at high risk for hemorrhage or related injury in acute setting.

LC: transverse fracture of pubic rami, ipsilateral, or posterolateral to posterior injury.
  I: sacral compression on side of impact.
  II: crescent (iliac wing) fracture on side of impact.
  III: LC-I or LC-II injury on side of impact: contralateral open-book (APC) injury.
APC (anterior-posterior compression): symphyseal diastasis and/or longitudinal rami fractures.
  I: slight widening of pubic symphysis and/or anterior sacroiliac (SI) joint; stretched but intact SI, sacrotuberous, and sacrospinous ligaments; intact posterior SI ligaments.
  II: widened anterior SI joint; disrupted anterior SI, sacrotuberous, and sacrospinous ligaments; intact SI posterior ligaments.
  III: complete SI joint disruption with lateral displacement; disrupted anterior SI, sacrotuberous, sacrospinous ligaments; disrupted posterior SI ligaments.
VS (vertical shear): symphyseal diastasis or vertical displacement anteriorly and posteriorly, usually through the SI joint, occasionally through the iliac wing and/or sacrum.
CM (combination): combination of other injury patterns, LC/VS being the most common.

Reference: Young JW et al.

Zickle (Subtrochanteric Fracture)
To define a method of fixation.

Type IA: short oblique fracture from above the lesser trochanter to the lower lateral shaft.
Type IB: long oblique fracture from above the lesser trochanter to the lower lateral shaft; comminution may be present.

Type IC: transverse fracture just below lesser trochanter to a point near the isthmus.

Reference: Zickle RE.

Dislocations

This section is divided into two parts: The first is a general list of terms applied to all joints, and the second is a list by specific anatomic location. Posttraumatic arthritis, recurrent dislocation, limitation of joint motion, joint mice, instability, and/or avascular necrosis may accompany various dislocation types. Hand and wrist dislocations are very complicated and, therefore, are discussed separately in Chapter 10.

General Dislocations
closed d.: one in which the skin is not broken; formerly called **simple d.**
complete d.: one that completely separates the joint surfaces.
complicated d.: associated with surrounding tissue injuries.
consecutive d.: the luxated bone has changed its position since its first displacement.
developmental dysplasia: exists in infancy with or without dislocation of the hips; formerly called **congenital d.**
frank d.: a complete dislocation in any area.
habitual d.: one that repeatedly recurs; usually congenital.
incomplete d.: subluxation with only slight displacement.
old d.: inflammatory changes have occurred.
open d.: one in which the skin is broken; formerly called **compound d.**
partial d.: incomplete dislocation.
pathologic d.: results from paralysis or disease in the joint or surrounding area.
primitive d.: bones remain as originally displaced.
recent d.: there is no complicating inflammation.
recurrent d.: repetitive dislocation with or without adequate trauma.
traumatic d.: caused by serious injury.
voluntary d.: dislocation that is caused by will of the person and can be reduced as well by the will of the person.

CLASSIFICATION OF PELVIC FRACTURES (YOUNG AND BURGESS)

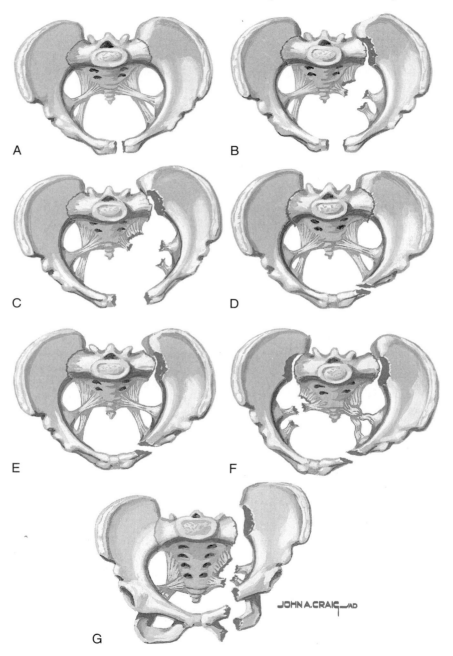

FIG 1-6 Pelvic fractures. **A,** Anteroposterior compression type I (APC-I). **B,** Anteroposterior compression type II (APC-II). **C,** Anteroposterior compression type III (APC-III). **D,** Lateral compression type I (LC-I). **E,** Lateral compression type II (LC-II). **F,** Lateral compression type III (LC-III). **G,** Vertical shear. (Reprinted from *Netter Anatomy Illustration Collection* © Elsevier Inc.)

Specific Dislocations (By Anatomy)
Cervical Dislocation
Bell-Dally d.: nontraumatic dislocation of the first cervical vertebra (atlas)

Shoulder Dislocations
A/C joint separation: acromioclavicular joint disruption and separation.

anterior shoulder d.: involves the glenohumeral joint with the humeral head displaced anteriorly and inferiorly; may be associated with one of the following:

Bankhart lesion: seen surgically as detachment of the glenoid labrum and sometimes a bone fragment from the glenoid. **Perthes-Bankhart lesion.**

Hill-Sachs lesion: seen radiographically as an indentation of the posteromedial humeral head, which occurred at the time of the dislocation; also called **hatchet head deformity.**

locked scapula: rare scapulothoracic dissociation with entrapment of scapula into chest wall or with anterior displacement; usually associated with severe neurovascular injury.

luxatio erecta: dislocation of shoulder so that the arm stands straight up over the head with humerus locked in 110 to 160 degrees abduction.

multidirectional instability: shoulder that is unstable in multiple planes, commonly anterior inferior and posterior inferior.

posterior shoulder d.: involves the glenohumeral joint with the humeral head displaced posteriorly.

reverse Bankhart lesion: seen surgically as a detachment of the rim of the posterior labrum from the glenoid rim.

reverse Hill-Sachs lesion: defect of anteromedial humeral head; may be seen on radiographs or at surgery.

sternoclavicular joint separation: disruption of the sternoclavicular joint.

subcoracoid d.: glenohumeral dislocation with the humeral head displaced medially.

subglenoid d.: glenohumeral dislocation with the humeral head displaced inferiorly.

Elbow Dislocations
direct injury d.: posterior displacement of the olecranon.

divergent d.: ulna and radius are dislocated separately.

milkmaid's d.: dislocation of radial head superiorly and anteriorly; also called **superior radial head d., milkmaid's elbow.**

Monteggia f.-d.: fracture of the ulna with a radial head dislocation.

Spine Dislocations
spondylolisthesis: not a true dislocation, because it rarely occurs as a result of trauma or muscle imbalance, but is a forward displacement of one vertebral body over another; usually occurs as a result of a defect in the pars interarticularis.

spondylolysis: acute (traumatic) dissociation of pars interarticularis or posterior elements (lamina) with or without spondylolisthesis.

unilateral facet subluxation: dislocation of one of the two facets at any level; most common in the cervical region.

Hip Dislocations
anterior d.: involves the femoral head anteriorly.

central d.: one in which the femur jams into the acetabulum; also called **bursting d.**

developmental dysplasia of the hip (DDH): formerly called **congenital dysplasia of the hip (CDH), congenital d., luxatio coxae congenita.**

luxatio perinealis: dislocation of femoral head into the perineum.

Monteggia d.: involves femoral head to near the anterosuperior spine of the ilium; hip joint dislocation.

Otto pelvis: gradual central displacement of the femur by unknown causes.

posterior d.: femoral head slips posteriorly; more common than anterior d. **(dashboard d.)**

posterior f.-d.: chip f. of the acetabulum with a posterior d. of the femoral head.

Patella (Dislocation vs. Subluxation)
One of the most common dislocations is a patellar dislocation, erroneously called a dislocated knee. The dislocated patella simply goes out of the femoral groove. A subluxation is a tendency for the patella to move partially out of the groove. The most common direction is lateral, but may be medial.

Knee Dislocations

horseback rider's knee: dislocation of fibular head; injury associated with rider hitting leg against a post.

knee d.: slippage of the femur off the tibia; commonly called a **true knee d.** to distinguish it from a dislocated patella.

parachute jumper's d.: anterior dislocation of proximal fibula.

Ankle and Foot Dislocations

Chopart d.: navicula and cuboid dislocate across talus and calcaneus (Chopart joint).

fracture-dislocation of ankle: any combination of tibial and fibular fractures resulting in a displaced talus.

Lisfranc d.: tarsometatarsal dislocation; not to be confused with a **frank dislocation,** which denotes a complete dislocation in any area.

medial swivel d.: navicula is displaced medially on a fracture of the midtalus, but the calcaneocuboid joint stays intact and the subtalar joint is not dislocated. The calcaneus rotates on the intact interosseous talocalcaneal ligament.

metatarsophalangeal joint d.: occurs at the base of the toe.

Nélaton d.: dislocation of the ankle in which the talus is forced between the end of the tibia and fibula.

Smith d.: upward and backward dislocation of the metatarsals and medial cuneiform bone.

subastragalar d.: separation of the calcaneus and navicular bone from the talus.

tarsal d.: usually an ankle dislocation associated with a fracture of the neck of the talus; commonly an open injury. This term may also denote other tarsal bone dislocations, such as of the cuneiform and cuboid.

Subluxations

Subluxations are categorized by anatomic location as there are no eponymic terms.

facet s.: malalignment of opposing facet, allowing one cervical body to rotate around another.

patellar s.: most commonly in a lateral direction.

radioulnar s.: involves the distal ulnar radial joint.

sacroiliac s.: involves the sacroiliac joint; usually associated with a pelvic fracture and other dissociations of the pelvic ring.

shoulder s.: involves the glenohumeral joint (as opposed to the acromioclavicular joint).

wrist s.: involves the proximal carpal bones on the radius and ulna.

Strains and Sprains

The term **strain** applies to an injury of muscle or its tendon. The term **sprain** applies to ligamentous injury. However, the term *strain* is often interchanged with the word *sprain*. In part, this is because both injuries can occur at the same time, such as a low back strain. It is clear at the time of injury that there is an acute tear or stretching of a back muscle, but there can also be a concurrent injury to the ligaments or disk tissue. If the symptoms continue, the sprain component becomes more apparent because the muscle normally recovers very rapidly.

Strains are often associated with injury to muscle caused by strenuous exercise without preconditioning and are usually referred to the back region. **Sprains** and ruptures of ligaments occur in the knee, ankle joints, and, sometimes, shoulder. At the ankle, a sudden twisting motion with full weight on the side of the foot can cause a sprain. A fracture may occur as well. There are many terms for muscle, tendon, and ligament injuries as follows.

Shoulder Sprain

acromioclavicular s.: stretching of the ligaments of the acromioclavicular joint and/or the coracoclavicular ligaments. The grades are from I to VI. When there is separation (grades II to VI), it is termed a **shoulder separation**. Often the term **shoulder sprain** implies this specific condition, as opposed to an effect on the glenohumeral joint.

Type I: no disruption of acromioclavicular joint.

Type II: less than joint height separation of acromioclavicular joint.

Type III: joint height separation of acromioclavicular joint.

Type IV: posteriorly displaced incarceration of clavicle into trapezial muscle.

Type V: very wide superior separation of clavicle from acromion.

Type VI: inferior incarceration of clavicle under acromion.

Knee Sprains

anterior cruciate s.: commonly associated with a medial collateral ligament tear, dislocated patella, or torn meniscus; may occur as an isolated injury; allows the femur to slide backward on the tibia (tibia slides forward on the femur).

lateral collateral s.: isolated injury that may be associated with rupture of the biceps femoris tendon, anterior and/or posterior cruciate ligament, and iliotibial tract; allows the joint to open laterally, and with some associated injuries allows the lateral femur to slide backward on the tibia (tibia slides forward on the femur). Also, the peroneal nerve, fabellar-fibular ligament, popliteus, and popliteal-fibular ligament may be at risk in a posterolateral complex injury.

medial collateral s.: occurs as a result of a clipping injury; may be associated with a cruciate ligament tear, patellar dislocation, or torn medial meniscus; allows the joint to open medially, and with some associated injuries allows the medial femur to slide backward on the tibia (tibia slides forward on the femur).

posterior cruciate s.: allows the tibia to slide backward on the femur; often seen alone; allows the femur to slide forward on the tibia (tibia slides backward on the femur).

posterior oblique ligament s.: part of the medial collateral ligament s. or rupture complex; allows the medial femur to slide backward on the tibia (medial tibia slides forward on the femur).

Ankle Sprains

deltoid s.: commonly occurs with a fibular fracture; rarely an isolated rupture.

fibular collateral s.: general term for sprain or rupture of one or more of three ligaments on the lateral side of the ankle.

anterior talofibular s.: most common sprain or rupture of the ankle ligaments.

calcaneofibular s.: sprain or rupture of middle of three lateral ankle ligaments, usually associated with other injuries.

tibiofibular s.: without rupture, there is no spreading of the tibia and fibula; with rupture, a diastasis occurs; syndesmotic sprain, high ankle sprain.

Sports-Related Injuries

Injuries from vocational and avocational sports activities have greatly increased over the years. In the United States, more than 2 million sports-related injuries occur annually. So much time and effort have been devoted to the more immediate identification and treatment of these athletic injuries that the development of the subspecialty of sports medicine became an integral part of orthopaedics.

Sports medicine has had a dramatic effect on the activities themselves. Exercise as a science has opened new dimensions in health care. Improved sports equipment and design have been developed through the combined efforts of engineers and medical support personnel, and "rule changes" are often made in consideration of the safety of the players.

Many sports injuries are a result of muscle and tendon overuse rather than a specific sprain or strain. Some of these conditions are so common in certain sports that they are named after the sport, for example, baseball finger.

This terminology applies to the nonathletic population, as well, who experience similar conditions. This may be the result of an increase in activity from a previously sedentary, nonactive lifestyle, or other factors such as degenerative joint disease. The classic example is that of tennis elbow. Many people with this problem cannot attribute it to a change in activity, such as painting or tennis, but have a condition of the cervical spine that causes the muscle of the forearm to tighten, resulting in overuse of the tendon.

The following terms are related mostly to athletic injuries of the soft tissues. Fracture-related sports injuries are listed in the preceding section.

ALPSA lesion: anterior labrum of the glenoid tears during anterior shoulder dislocation and strips the glenoid periosteum, leaving labrum attached to periosteum. This gives the shoulder the arthroscopic appearance of an intact labrum (ALPSA: *a*nterior *l*abrum *p*osterior *s*uperior to *a*nterior).

archer's shoulder: recurrent posterior dislocation or subluxation of the shoulder.

backpack palsy: similar to Erb palsy, a brachial plexus compression caused by a heavy pack with shoulder straps, resulting in palsy of the fifth and sixth cervical nerve muscle distribution.

BAGHL: *b*ony *a*vulsion of *g*leno*h*umeral *l*igament.

baseball elbow: condition of baseball pitchers in which overstress on the medial side of the elbow causes medial collateral ligament bone spurs, myositis, ulnar nerve injuries, or posterior compartment loose bodies. Also referred to as **javelin thrower's elbow, throwers elbow, posteromedial impingement.**

baseball finger: acute rupture of the terminal end of the distal extensor tendon. This may be either intra-tendinous or bony and is a result of a direct axial blow to the digit. The injury causes an inability to extend the distal interphalangeal joint (extensor lag). There is usually full passive movement of the digit; also called **mallet finger.**

basketball foot: subtalar dislocation of the foot.

bicycle spoke injury: bruising, swelling, and some-time necrosis seen in ankle 24–48 hours after foot and ankle get caught in spoke of a bicycle tire.

BIL lesion: *b*iceps *i*nterval *l*esion seen in rotator cuff at biceps tendon and subscapularis muscle. Pain and swelling occur over intertubercular groove.

black-dot heel: small dark spot on the heel fat pad caused by blood under the skin on the lateral side where there is repeated trauma to heel in athletic activity or shear stress in running; also called **black heel syndrome.**

bowler's thumb: irritation of the flexor tendon of the thumb with increased nerve sensation on the lateral side caused by the repeated grasping of a large bowling ball.

boxer's f.: fracture of the fifth metacarpal head with volar angulation. This is usually seen due to punching a wall or hard object.

breaststroker's knee: irritation of the medial capsule of the knee, tibial collateral ligament, or patellar cartilage caused by repeated thrusts of the limbs by a breaststroke swimmer.

charley horse: cramping, stiffness of quadriceps muscles due to muscle overuse, contusion, or direct blow to the thigh as in a sports injury.

coach's finger: proximal interphalangeal joint dislocation in finger.

coracoid impingement syndrome: specific impingement of the rotator cuff and lesser tuberosity by the coracoid process.

cross-over syndrome: extensor tendon inflammation at the wrist seen in kayak and canoe sports enthusiasts.

flexor origin syndrome: tendonitis originating at the flexor wad of five at the medial elbow; Also called **medial epicondylitis, reverse tennis elbow, golfer's elbow.**

football ankle: area of ill-localized pain in midmetatarsophalangeal part of foot above malleoli. X-ray changes show exostosis or loose bodies.

football finger: avulsion of the deep flexor tendon of the distal phalanx of the ring finger; often occurs when trying to tackle an opponent by hooking the finger over the pants belt line; **ruger jersey finger.**

gamekeeper's thumb: a traumatic rupture of the ulnar collateral ligament of the metacarpophalangeal (MCP) joint of the thumb; usually a hyperabduction injury; skier's thumb.

gobies: rock-induced skin abrasions that are observed on the fingers and dorsal surfaces of hands in rock climbers; also known as **bouldering** and **face climbing.**

golfer's elbow: inflammation at the origin of the wrist and finger flexor muscles of the inner elbow; also called **thrower's elbow, medial epicondylitis,** and **reverse tennis elbow.**

HAGL: *h*umeral *a*vulsion of *g*lenohumeral *l*igament.

handlebar palsy: palsy of the muscles of the hand innervated by the ulnar nerve, caused by pressure against bicycle handlebar.

heel spur: ossification in area of inflammation of the proximal attachment of the plantar fascia; usually involves the median tubercle of the plantar surface of the calcaneus; often seen in runners and commonly the result of excessive joint pronation. Anything that causes stress on the plantar fascia (weakened feet, structural deformity, or excessive pronation of the subtalar joint) will encourage the development of a heel spur.

hip pointer: very painful irritation of the insertion of abdominal muscles along the superior iliac crest. Pain localized here can also represent the pull of a thigh muscle in that region.

hockey player's hip: painful bone bruise of the greater trochanter caused by landing on the ice.

horseback rider's knee: a posterior dislocation of the proximal fibula on the tibia.

iliotibial band syndrome: condition seen in distance runners and other endurance athletes; pain on the lateral side of the knee just anterior to the lateral collateral ligaments due to swelling in a bursa or thickening of the distal expansion of the iliotibial band.

impingement syndrome: alludes to symptomatic compression on the rotator cuff by overhanging acromioclavicular structures, the anterolateral acromion, and acromioclavicular ligament; graded according to the **Neer staging system.**

> **Stage I:** inflammation and edema of the rotator cuff.
>
> **Stage II:** degenerative fibrosis.
>
> **Stage III:** partial or full thickness tear.

Jersey finger (rugger jersey finger): an injury to the ring finger seen commonly in football and rugby players. This is a closed rupture of the flexor digitorum profundus (FDP). There are three types:

1. FDP retracted to the palm with total loss of blood supply.
2. FDP retracts to the PIP joint with partial loss of blood supply.
3. FDP retracts to the A4 pulley with a large bone fragment; blood supply is usually intact.

jogger's heel: irritation of the fibrous and fatty tissue covering the heel due to striking the ground surface when jogging.

jogger's toe: dark nail that develops in some distance runners, due to impaction of the nail into the shoe with long distance running and blood under nail.

jumper's knee: infrapatellar tendonitis or quadriceps tendonitis, often seen in athletes who jump as part of that sport, for example, basketball, skiing, and volleyball.

linebacker's arm (tackler's arm): a myositis ossificans reaction in the lateral brachial muscle; usually seen in the midarm of tacklers.

Lisfranc injury: low velocity injury of tarsometatarsal joints (Lisfranc joint) due to forced plantar flexion in rotation with or without abduction, as seen in runners and basketball players. The injury was first described as one sustained during a fall from a horse while the foot is caught in the stirrup. The injuries may be severe enough to include fractures or dislocations as opposed to a lesser sprain.

little leaguer's elbow: in children, a traction injury of the elbow on the medial epicondyle caused by prolonged pitching or throwing. Serious in that it may lead to fragmentation of the bone and disturbance of growth.

little leaguer's shoulder: traction injury to the shoulder in the growth plate of the proximal humerus that may lead to a painful shoulder and eventual deformity if throwing is continued.

muscle cramps: a sudden cramp in the hamstring and calf muscles usually during athletic activities. Occurs often in athletes because of overuse of an undertrained muscle or inadequate salt or water intake during hot weather. This term is used diversely to specify a hamstring and calf muscle spasm or a contusion to the quadriceps.

PASTA: *p*artial *a*rticular *s*ide *t*endon *a*vulsion.

RHAGL: *r*everse *h*umeral *a*vulsion of *g*lenohumeral *l*igament injury.

ring man shoulder: bony resorption or sclerosis at the insertion of the pectoralis major muscle of upper arm; seen in gymnasts who use rings.

rotator cuff injury: inflammation or rupture of one or more of the tendons that lie deep in the shoulder and bridge the glenohumeral joint. This type of injury is inhibiting in pitchers and tennis players, in particular, and can be caused by excessive use (repetitive microtrauma), direct blow, or stretch injury.

runner's bump: prominence of the posterior heel at the point of insertion of the Achilles tendon; associated with distance running.

runner's knee: tight and tense condition of quadriceps muscle of thigh that directs pain to anterior knee.

sailboarder's injury: stirrup-type injury that occurs when surfer falls from board with foot caught in strap, causing a forced equinus position with disruption of dorsal stabilizers at Lisfranc joint; also found in horseback riders.

shin splints: pain in the anterior lower limbs (shins) that follows repeated stress such as running or walking long distances without conditioning; describes a painful condition rather than a specific anatomic lesion. The most common causes are posterior tibial tendonitis, stress fracture of tibia, muscle strain, periostitis, periosteal avulsion, fascial hernia, stress fracture, and anterior tibial compartment syndrome with the inability of blood to reach the muscle (ischemia) because of compartmental swelling during increased activity; also known as **medial tibial stress syndrome.**

shoulder apprehension: apprehension of the patient during shoulder abduction and external rotation due to glenohumeral subluxation (usually in patients with a previous shoulder dislocation).

shoulder pointer: a tearing of the anterior deltoid muscle leading to a distinct point of discomfort at the origin (immediate vicinity of the acromioclavicular joint) of the deltoid muscle.

SLAP lesion: *s*uperior *l*abrum from *a*nterior to *p*osterior tear that occurs along a line from biceps tendon attachment to superior labrum; condition causes shoulder pain with throwing motion.

spear tackler's spine: cervical spine injury in contact sports (e.g., football) where an individual spear tackles opponent head-on (with top of helmet); findings may include cervical cord or brachial plexus neuropraxia or preexisting posttraumatic abnormalities; condition may lead to posttraumatic arthritis.

surfer's knots: lower limb and foot nodular swelling with possible bony changes due to trauma and pressure from using a surfboard.

swimmer's shoulder: overuse of rotator cuff muscle usually due to training errors in swimming training.

tennis elbow: inflammation of the wrist and finger extensor muscles near their origin at the elbow; also called **lateral epicondylitis.**

tennis leg: tear of the medial head of the gastrocnemius or plantaris muscle; often seen in tennis players.

tennis toe (marathoner's toe): subungual hematoma causing a black toenail; usually painless and requires no treatment.

turf-toe: an acute injury of the first metatarsal phalangeal joint as a result of hyperextension leading to separation of the medial and lateral sesamoid occurs. This is classically described in football players on artificial turf, but it can occur in any sport where sudden push-off on the foot and great toe occur.

weight-lifter's shoulder: osteolysis of the lateral aspect of the clavicle as seen in weight lifters.

whiplash: a stretch injury to the neck that includes the muscles, ligaments, and disks of the cervical spine; caused by an acceleration (forward movement) or deceleration (backward movement) of the head as in a vehicular accident. A direct head injury may also cause a whiplash because of the resultant forces on the neck. Damage may involve minor neck ligament sprain, rupture, or subluxation (partial dislocation). This term denotes a complex of symptoms including pain and stiffness and is sometimes biomechanically inaccurate because there are many mechanisms that can produce these symptoms.

Trauma Scoring Systems and Associated Soft Tissue Injuries

Injury Scales and Scores
Limb Salvage Index
To assess the likely success of attempts at limb salvage in severe injury.

Artery

0 Contusion, intimal tear, partial laceration or avulsion (pseudoaneurysm) with no distal thrombus and palpable pedal pulses; complete occlusion of one of three shank vessels or profunda.

1 Occlusion of two or more shank vessels, complete laceration, avulsion or thrombus of femoral or popliteal vessels without palpable pulses.

2 Complete occlusion of femoral, popliteal, or three of shank vessels with no distal runoff available.

Nerve

0 Contusion or stretch injury; minimal clean laceration of femoral, peroneal, or tibial nerve.

1 Partial transection transaction Partial transaction or avulsion of sciatic nerve; complete or partial transaction of femoral, peroneal, or tibial nerve.

2 Complete transaction or avulsion of sciatic nerve; complete transaction or avulsion of both peroneal and tibial nerves.

Bone

0 Closed fracture one or two sites; open fracture without comminution or with minimal displacement; closed dislocation without fracture; open joint without foreign body; fibula fracture.

1 Closed fracture at three or more sites on same extremity; open fracture with communication or moderate to large displacement; segmental fracture; fracture dislocation; open joint with foreign body; bone loss < 3 cm.

2 Bone loss > 3 cm; type III-B or II-C fracture (open fracture with periosteal stripping, gross contamination, extensive soft tissue injury-loss).

Skin

0 Clean laceration; single or multiple, small avulsion injuries, all with primary repair; first degree burn.

1 Delayed tissue closure due to contamination; large avulsion requiring split thickness skin graft or flap closure. Second and third degree burns.

Muscle

0 Laceration or avulsion involving a single compartment or single tendon.

1 Laceration or avulsion involving two or more compartments; complete laceration or avulsion of two or more tendons.

2 Crush injury.

Deep vein

0 Contusion, partial laceration or avulsion; complete laceration or avulsion if alternate route of venous return is intact, superficial vein injury.

1 Complete laceration, avulsion, or thrombosis with no alternate route or venous return.

Warm ischemia time

0 < 6 hours
1 6–9 hours
2 9–12 hours
3 12–15 hours
4 > 15 hours

Mangled Extremity Severity Score (MESS) (Degree of Injury to Soft and Hard Tissue of a Limb)

To assess the prognostic effects of injury, ischemia, shock, and age.

Skeletal/Soft Tissue

Group 1: low energy stab wounds, low caliber gun shot, simple fractures—1 point.

Group 2: medium energy, open, or multiple level fractures, moderate crush injury—2 points.

Group 3: high energy, close range shotgun blast, or high velocity gunshot wound—3 points.

Group 4: massive crush injury, industrial accident—4 points.

Shock Group

Group 1: normotensive; blood pressure stable at scene and during surgery—0 points.

Group 2: transient hypotension; unstable blood pressure at scene but stable when given intravenous drugs—1 point.

Group 3: prolonged hypotension; systolic blood pressure < 90 mm Hg with recovery in operating room (OR) only.

Ischemia Group

Group 1: none; no signs of ischemia, pulses intact—0 points.

Group 2: mild; diminished pulses without ischemia—1 point.

Group 3: moderate; no pulse by Doppler, sluggish capillary refill and other activity, paresthesias—2 points.

Group 4: advanced; no pulse, cool, no capillary refill—3 points.

Age

Group 1: < 30 years—0 points.

Group 2: > 30 to < 50 years—1 point.

Group 3: > 50 years—2 points.

Reference: Helfet DL et al.

Predictive Salvage Index

System predictive of amputation based on arterial, bone, muscle, and skin injury.

Level of arterial injury	
Suprapopliteal	1
Popliteal	2
Infrapopliteal	3
Degree of bone injury	
Mild	1
Moderate	2
Severe	3

Degree of muscle injury

    Mild   1

    Moderate   2

    Severe   3

Interval from injury to arrival in the operating room

    < 6 hours   0

    6–12 hours 2

    > 12 hours 4

$$A + B + C + D = \text{predictive salvage index}$$

NISSSA Score

System predictive of amputation based on *n*erve, *i*schemia, *s*oft tissue, *s*keletal injury, as well as *s*hock and *a*ge.

Nerve injury

    Sensate   0

    Dorsal   1

    Plantar partial   2

    Plantar complete 3

Ischemia

    None   0

    Mild   1

    Moderate   2

    Severe   3

Soft tissue/contamination

    Low   0

Medium   1

High   2

Severe   3

Skeletal

    Low energy   0

    Medium energy 1

    High energy   2

    Severe energy   3

Shock

    Normotensive   0

    Transient hypotension 1

    Persistent hypotension 2

Age

    < 30 years   0

    30–50 years   1

    > 50 years   2

Associated Soft Tissue Injuries

degloving: term applied to stripping or loss of skin and subcutaneous tissue from site of injury to point distal to the injury site.

Morel-Lavallee lesion: seen usually with severe pelvic fractures where there is a closed soft tissue degloving injury, where the skin and soft tissue around the area of the pelvis is separated from the underlying fascia.

Musculoskeletal Diseases and Related Terms

2

This chapter addresses the nontraumatic musculoskeletal disorders. The standard way of trying to categorize disorders based on a specific anatomic part or specific organ or tissue that is affected has always been a challenge. As we continue to learn more precise ways that specific genetic changes can affect a variety of musculoskeletal tissues, we recognize that a wide spectrum of changes may have quite divergent genetic origins. The basic categories of disease remain reasonably intact and have been kept consistent from the sixth to the seventh edition. However, there are very similar disorders that have varied genetic sources. The terminology has been changed to reflect those findings. A table has been created to demonstrate genetic effects based on whether the controlling element of the gene is on DNA, receptors, intracellular signaling, matrix protein products, or posttranslational changes.

The musculoskeletal reaction to bone and soft tissue lesions can be due to many factors: bones fracture or dislocate; joints become arthritic; bursae around joints become inflamed; muscles, ligaments, and tendons become strained, stretched, weakened, or torn; muscles may spasm or atrophy; cartilage may degenerate; disks become compressed; and vascular and metabolic changes may occur that affect both bone and soft tissue. All of these areas of the musculoskeletal system can be affected temporarily or permanently.

The terms *disease* and *syndrome* are sometimes used interchangeably but to be precise they have different meanings.

A **disease** is a specific result of a pathologic condition that presents as a group of symptoms associated with physical and/or psychologic changes. A disease may be classified acute or chronic, congenital or acquired, focal or systemic, malignant or benign, and contagious or noninfectious. Diseases may also be characterized as hereditary, inflammatory, metabolic, degenerative, or idiopathic.

A **syndrome** is a group of symptoms that occur together and are associated with any morbid condition that constitutes the scenario for a specific disease.

Many diseases of the musculoskeletal system overlap into other specialties, such as neurology, neurosurgery, and vascular surgery, and the patient's symptoms often present as an orthopaedic problem. Therefore terminology of other specialties is included as it relates to orthopaedics.

Both soft tissue and skeletal disorders can be associated with **referred pain,** which means that the pain is felt at a site other than its origin. Pain is a perception, and as with all perceptions, illusions are possible. For example, pain can originate at the lumbar region but be felt at some point in the lower limb. Referred pain can also occur with direct pressure on a spinal nerve root in the back (a form of sciatica). In most cases of a back disorder with pain perceived to be in the lower limb, actual pressure is not on a spinal nerve root. Pain in the distribution of the muscles supplied by a specific spinal nerve is called **sclerotomal** pain. Pain in the sensory distribution of a spinal nerve is called **dermatomal** pain. The distinction is important in that a dermatomic distribution of pain tends to be more distinctive of actual nerve root irritation.

The goal in the treatment of musculoskeletal diseases and conditions is to help the patient become functional and productive as quickly as possible through a conservative approach, surgery, or other measures. The musculoskeletal diseases are defined here by tissue type and anatomic location.

Bone Diseases

Osteo-, the Greek root for bone, can be used in various combinations that include more than one root, for example, osteochondral (bone and cartilage), or in terms in which *osteo-* is preceded by other terms, for example, *polyostotic fibrous dysplasia*. The "os" terms relate to small bones **(ossicles),** especially those in the foot, and are named in Chapter 11.

Bone disease types are grouped together for purposes of identifying similar or related processes by anatomic or eponymic terms. However, eponyms that are used more often than the common (Greek or Latin) terms are listed separately. The bone diseases are divided as follows: *osteo-* root diseases, infectious bone diseases, tumors of bone, miscellaneous Latin and English terms, and eponymic bone diseases.

Osteo- Root Diseases

hyperosteoidosis: excess osteoid tissue due to defective mineralization (osteomalacia) and to normal but delayed mineralization; **hyperparathyroidism, hyperthyroidism, Paget d.**

ostealgia: pain within bone. (archaic)

osteitis: inflammation of bone with enlargement, tenderness, dull aching; many varieties.

osteitis condensans (piriform sclerosis ilium): increased density of the ilium near the sacroiliac joint of unknown etiology; may be associated with back pain.

osteitis deformans: disease of unknown origin resulting in bowing of long bones and deformation of flat bones; **Paget d.**

osteitis fibrosa cystica: bone disease caused by hyperfunction of parathyroid gland; **osteoplastica.**

osteitis ossificans: an older general term denoting an inflammatory process in bone that results in increased bone density. (archaic)

osteitis pubis: increased bone density seen at symphysis pubis; may be associated with pain or increased physical activity.

ostemia: abnormal congestion of blood in bone. (archaic)

ostempyesis: suppuration (pus) within bone. (archaic)

osteoaneurysm: aneurysm in bone.

osteoarthritis: Osteoarthritic diseases (OA) are a result of both mechanical and biological events that destabilize the normal coupling of degradation and synthesis of articular cartilage chondrocytes and extracellular matrix, and subchondral bone. Although they may be initiated by multiple factors, including genetic, developmental, metabolic, and traumatic, OA diseases involve all of the tissues of the diarthrodial joint. Ultimately, OA diseases are manifested by morphologic, biochemical, molecular, and biomechanical changes of both cells and matrix, which lead to a softening, fibrillation, ulceration, loss of articular cartilage, sclerosis, and eburnation of subchondral bone osteophytes and subchondral cysts. When clinically evident, OA diseases are characterized by joint pain, tenderness, limitation of movement, crepitus, occasional effusion, and variable degrees of inflammation without systemic effects.

osteoarthropathy: a condition of increased bone formation at the joints; sometimes used to refer to osteoarthritis. Variations of osteoarthropathy are hypertropic, hypertrophic pulmonary, pulmonary trophic, and secondary hypertrophic.

osteoarthrosis: same as the term **arthrosis;** "a heterogeneous group of conditions that lead to joint symptoms and signs associated with defective integrity of articular cartilage, in addition to related changes to the underlying bone at the joint margins"* (Fig. 2-1).

osteoarticular: pertaining to or affecting bones and joints.

osteocachexia: chronic disease of bone resulting in the wasting of bone. (archaic)

osteochondritis: inflammation of bone. Formerly called **osteochondrosis.** Osteochondritis applies to a number of conditions in which the pathologic findings and cause may vary. In children, the disease affects the ossification centers at the *pressure epiphysis* (joints) or *traction epiphysis* (e.g., the patellar

---

*American College of Rheumatology. *Arth Rheum* 33(11): 1601-1610, 1990.

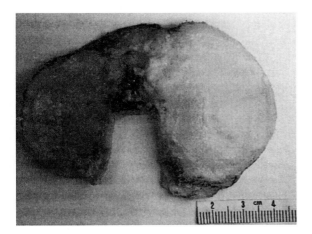

FIG 2-1 Surface of tibia following excision for total knee replacement. Joint surfaces are rough with loss of cartilage and formation of new bone and cartilage at margin (osteophytes). (Courtesy of the Orthopaedic Research Laboratory, Good Samaritan Medical Center, West Palm Beach, FL.)

tendon to the tibia or the Achilles tendon attachment to the heel). In a pressure epiphysis, an area of avascular necrosis or similar process can occur. In the absence of a clear etiologic relationship or consistent pathologic findings, the osteochondritis diseases (as specified by areas affected) can be separated into traction and pressure epiphyses as follows:

Traction Epiphyses

Osgood-Schlatter d.: patellar tendon to tibia.

Scheuermann d.: epiphysitis of vertebral body.

Sever d.: Achilles tendon to calcaneus.

Sindig-Larsen-Johansson d.: patellar tendon to patella.

Pressure Epiphyses

Blount d.: epiphyseal plate of tibia.

Avascular Necrosis Types

Brailsford d.: radial head.

Burns d.: humeral trochlea.

Freiberg d.: second metatarsal head.

Haas d.: head of humerus.

Kienböck d.: lunate.

Köhler d.: midpatella.

Köhler d.: tarsal navicular.

Konig d.: femoral condyle.

Legg-Calvé-Perthes d.: femoral head.

Mauclair d.: metacarpal heads.

Panner d.: capitellum.

Thiemann d.: proximal phalanx.

osteochondrodesmodysplasia: a mucopolysaccharide disorder associated with multiple deformities of bone, joints, and tendons; **Rotter-Erb syndrome.**

osteochondrodystrophy: dwarfing disease mainly affecting spine and hips with little or no mental disturbance; **Morquio syndrome.**

osteochondrofibroma: tumor containing elements of osteoma, chondroma, and fibroma.

osteochondrolysis: osteochondritis dissecans.

osteochondromatosis: Transformation of synovial villi into bone and cartilage masses, causing loose bodies in the joint. This condition occurs in joints affected by trauma or other degenerative diseases. A condition specifically called **synovial osteochondromatosis** and **Henderson-Jones chondromatosis.**

osteochondropathy: condition affecting bone and cartilage; marked by abnormal enchondral ossification.

osteochondrophyte: an archaic term synonymous with osteochondroma.

osteochondrosis: term being replaced by **osteochondritis;** condition in children that affects the epiphyseal and apophyseal regions where increased stress occurs.

osteochondrosis dissecans: formation of a separate center of bone and cartilage on an epiphyseal surface. The osteochondral fragment may remain in place, be absorbed and replaced slowly, or break loose and become a loose body. Multiple etiologies probably exist. This was originally believed to be an inflammatory lesion, but there is no clear evidence for this, hence the change of the term from osteochondritis to osteochondrosis. Another probable etiology is a demarcation of an area of avascular necrosis; **osteochondritis dissecans.**

osteoclasia: breaking down and absorption of bone tissue.

osteocope: syphilitic bone disease with severe pain within bone. (archaic)

osteocystoma: cystic tumor in bone. (archaic)

osteodiastasis: abnormal separation of bones.

osteodynia: pain in bones. (archaic)

osteodystrophy: defective bone formation.

osteofibrochondrosarcoma: malignant tumor containing bone and fibrous and cartilaginous tissue.

osteofibroma: tumor containing both osseous and fibrous elements.

osteofibromatosis: formation of multiple osteofibromas.

osteofibrous dysplasia: lesion that has a histologic appearance similar to fibrous dysplasia, except that the bone is being formed by osteocytes rather than by fibrocyte-like cells; **campanacci lesion; ossifying fibroma of long bones.**

osteogenesis imperfecta: condition in which bones are abnormally brittle and subject to fractures; inherited and usually is a function of abnormal type I collagen. There are a few rare osteogenesis imperfecta disorders that are not associated with type I collagen. Classifications are based on physical appearance and not the type of mutation, **osteitis fragilitans, fragilitas ossium congenita, osteopsathyrosis idiopathica,** and **brittle bones.**

Shapiro Classification System

congenita A: fractures at birth, bones radiographically abnormal.

congenita B: fractures at birth, bones radiographically normal.

tarda A: first fracture before or at walking stage, bones narrow andosteopenic.

tarda B: first fracture before or at walking stage, bones radiographically normal.

Sillence (Modified)

Type IA: mild, dominant inherited, associated with blue sclerae and no skeletal deformity.

Type IB: mild, dominant inherited, associated with blue sclerae, no skeletal deformity, and dentinogenesis imperfecta.

Type II: lethal, recessive inherited, associated with multiple fractures and a short survival. **Bauze:** Lethal OI.

Type III: severe, inherited recessive, associated with progressive deformity, white or blue sclerae, and nonambulatory status. **Bauze:** Severe OI.

Type IVA: moderate, inherited dominant new mutation, associated with some deformity and white sclerae in adults. **Bauze:** Mild OI.

Type IVB: moderate, new mutation, associated with some deformity, white sclerae in adults, and dentinogenesis imperfecta.

These groups were formerly called:

osteogenesis imperfecta congenita: severe form of brittle bone disease and deformity expressing itself in infancy or even at birth; can be fatal.

osteogenesis imperfecta tarda: brittle bone disease expressing itself when child begins to walk; **Lobstein d.** or **syndrome.**

osteohalisteresis: loss or deficiency of mineral elements of bones, producing softening.

osteolipochondroma: cartilage tumor with bone and fatty elements.

osteolipoma: fatty tumor containing osseous elements.

osteolysis: dissolution of bone.

familial expansile osteolysis: an autosomal dominant bone dysplasia with general and focal skeletal changes occurring in the second decade of life. There is usually pain, osteoclastic resorption, bowing, and a tendency toward pathologic fracture. Deafness and early loss of teeth may also occur.

massive osteolysis: rare condition characterized by prevalent monostotic unilateral, localized, concentric osteolysis. **Gorham d., phantom bone d., vanishing bone d., disappearing bone d.,** *hemangiomatosis, lymphangiomatosis,* and *hemo-lymphangiomatosis.*

pubic osteolysis: in adults, a worrisome-appearing lesion that may be mistaken for chondrosarcoma of the pubic bone area. Characterized by progressively destructive radiographic changes, soft tissue mass with calcification, histologic features of metaplastic cartilage, bone formation, and granulation tissue with myxoid and angiomatoid patterns.

osteomalacia: a reduction of physical strength of bone caused by decreased mineralization of osteoid;

may result from a deficiency of vitamin D, calcium, or phosphorous with or without renal disease. Osteomalacia in the child is associated with the growth deformities of rickets.

osteomesopyknosis: autosomal dominant disorder characterized by osteosclerosis similar to that in pyknodysostosis but localized to the axial spine, pelvis, and proximal part of the long bones.

osteomyelitis: inflammation of bone marrow, cortex, tissue, and periosteum; can be caused by any organism, but usually bacteria. (See Infectious Bone Diseases section.)

osteomyelodysplasia: thinning of osseous tissue of bone with increase in size of marrow cavities, accompanied by leukopenia (low white blood cell count) and fever.

osteonecrosis: death of bone tissue, usually of vascular origin.

osteoneuralgia: nerve pain in bone. (archaic)

osteopathia striata: affection of bone giving distinct striped appearance on radiographs; lesions characterized by multiple condensation of cancellous bone tissue, sometimes said to be in association with osteopetrosis; **Voorhoeve d.**

osteopathy: any disease process of bone.

osteopenia: any state in which bone mass is reduced below normal. This would include conditions of osteoporosis and osteomalacia. The World Health Organization (WHO) redefined this to mean that bone density is significantly diminished (<-0.1 standard deviation below normal but greater than -2.5 standard deviation below normal). It is preferred to use the term "low bone mass" in place of the term osteopenia.

osteoperiostitis: inflammation of bone and periosteum.

osteopetrorickets: the association of rickets and osteopetrosis in children characterized by hypophosphatemia, hypocalcemia, widened growth plates, and increased skeletal mass.

osteopetrosis: areas of condensed bone within bone due to a variety of gene disorders, which include an autosomal recessive disorder of macrophage colony-stimulating factor, an autosomal recessive disorder of carbonic anhydrase receptor in a malignant infantile form, an autosomal dominant disorder of the carbonic anhydrase receptor in a less severe form, and an autosomal recessive disorder of beta 3 integrin. **Albers-Schönberg d., osteosclerosis fragilis.**

osteophlebitis: inflammation of the veins in bone.

osteophyte: bony excrescence or osseous outgrowth, usually found around the joint area of bone. Around margins of arthritic joints, osteophytes are formed by new cartilage and bone. Around the spine and at strong ligamentous attachments, a portion of the ligament may turn to bone.

osteoplastica: inflammatory bone changes seen in cystic fibrosis.

osteopoikilosis: presence of multiple sclerotic foci in ends of long bones and scattered stippling in round and flat bones; usually without symptoms but noted on radiographs.

osteoporosis: the current definition by National Osteoporosis Foundation is "a systemic disorder characterized by decreased bone mass, micro-architectural deterioration, and increased susceptibility to fracture in the absence of other recognizable causes." Primary osteoporosis is an age-related disorder characterized by decreased bone mass and increased susceptibility to fractures in the absence of other recognizable causes of bone loss. The secondary cause of osteoporosis is most commonly immobilization, such as casting. The WHO definition is bone density that is -2.5 standard deviations below normal.

osteoradionecrosis: necrosis (death) of bone following irradiation.

osteosclerosis: hardening or abnormal denseness of bone.

osteosis: formation of bone tissue with infiltration of connective tissue within bone.

osteospongioma: spongy tumor of bone. (archaic)

osteosynovitis: inflammation of synovial membranes and neighboring bones.

osteotabes: condition in which bone marrow cells are destroyed and marrow disappears; usually in infants. (archaic)

osteothrombophlebitis: inflammation through intact bone by progressive thrombophlebitis of small venules.

osteothrombosis: blood clots or plugging of veins of bone.

parosteitis: inflammation of tissues around a bone.

parosteosis: ossification of the tissue outside the periosteum.

Infectious Bone Diseases

Osteomyelitis (Fig. 2-2) may be caused by bacteria or fungi. (Viruses have been suggested as a cause, but this has not been proved.)

- Bacteria associated with osteomyelitis
  Staphylococcus aureus
  Streptococcus organisms
  Escherichia coli
  Pseudomonas organisms
  Klebsiella organisms
  Salmonella organisms
  Neisseria gonorrhoeae
  Mycobacterium tuberculosis

- Fungal types (rare)
  Actinomycosis
  Blastomycosis
  Histoplasmosis

Terms Related to Osteomyelitis (Bone Infection)

acute o.: possibly up to 6 weeks, radiographs may be negative for first 2 weeks.

chronic o.: more than 6 weeks; may last for years.

chronic multifocal o.: multiple foci of bone infection in same period, with a fastidious, slow-growing bacterium the most likely causative agent.

chronic sclerosing o. of Garré: minimally symptomatic, long-term osteomyelitis associated with radiographic findings of densely scarred bone but not the usual abscess formation.

cloacae: in osteomyelitis, these are the openings in the infected sequestra of bone.

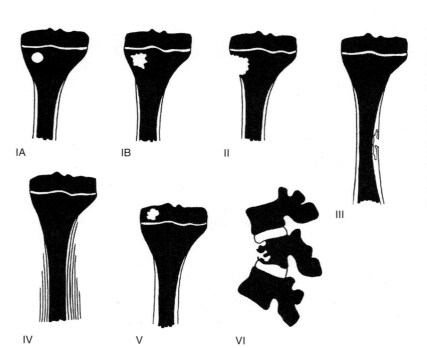

IA IB II

IV V VI

III

FIG 2-2 Different radiographic presentations of subacute osteomyelitis with classification scheme. Growth plate (physis) is below joint surface. Type IA is a punched out lucency suggestive of eosinophilic granuloma. Type IB has a sclerotic margin (not depicted) as seen in a more chronic form called Brodie's abscess. Type II has loss of metaphyseal cortical bone. Type III has loss of diaphyseal cortical bone. Type IV has onion skin layering of subperiosteal bone. Type V has an epiphyseal lesion. Type VI is an osteomyelitic lesion of the vertebral body.). (From Dormans JP, Drummond DS: *J Am Assoc Orthop Surg* 2:340, 1994.)

cystic o.: the radiographic appearance of an aborted osteomyelitis where a fluid-filled cystic cavity remains in the bone.

iatrogenic o.: an infection brought about by surgery or other treatment.

involucrum: bone formation around infected cortical bone.

mastocytosis: rare condition associated with accumulation of histamine-producing cells called "mastocytes" or mast cells. Painless, sclerotic bone lesions can occur.

nonsuppurative o.: term applied to tuberculosis of bone.

primary subacute o.: osteomyelitis that presents as localized, progressive bone pain with periods of remission. There is usually little or no systemic illness and no temperature elevation. Radiographic changes are identifiable on the first visit.

SAPHO: *synovitis-acne-pustulosis-hyperostosis osteo*myelitis syndrome related to the pustulotic arthrosteitis syndrome.

sequestrum: detached piece of dead bone from sound healthy bone during process of necrosis.

sinus: drainage tract extending from an area of infected bone to skin.

suppurative o.: infection of bone with active production of pus; may be acute or chronic.

Tumors of Bone (Fig. 2-3)

A staging system for musculoskeletal tumors has gained wide acceptance and is applied to both bone and soft connective tissue. It has been adopted by the American Joint Committee Task Force on Bone Tumors. The system is based on the relationship of the following factors: grade (G), site (T), and metaphysis (M). Staging is based on the scales in Tables 2-1 and 2-2.

- Histologic grade.
  - G_0: benign.
  - G_1: low-grade malignant.
  - G_2: high-grade malignant.
- Site.
  - T_0: lesion confined within a capsule.
  - T_1: lesion has extracapsular extensions.
  - T_2: lesion extends beyond compartmental barriers.

Benign

Stages 1-3. Histologically benign (G_0); variable clinical course and biologic behavior

Stage 1. Remains static or heals spontaneously with indolent clinical course. Well encapsulated

Stage 2. Active; progressive, symptomatic growth. Remains intracapsular. Limited by natural boundaries but may often deform them

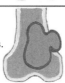

Stage 3. Aggressive; locally aggressive but not limited by capsule or natural boundaries. May penetrate cortex or compartment boundaries. Higher rate of recurrence

Malignant

Stage I. Histologically low grade (G_1); well differentiated; few mitoses; moderate nuclear atypia. Tends to recur locally. Radioisotope uptake moderate

Intraosseous or intracompartmental

Extraosseous or extracompartmental; penetrates cortex or compartment boundaries

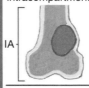 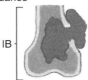

IA   IB

Stage II. Histologically high grade (G_2); poorly differentiated; high cell-to-matrix ratio; many mitoses; much nuclear atypia, necrosis, neovascularity; permeative. Radioisotope uptake intense. Higher incidence of metastases

Intraosseous or intracompartmental

Extraosseous or extracompartmental; penetrates cortex or compartment boundaries

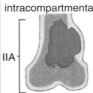 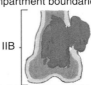

IIA   IIB

Stage III. Metastases; regional or remote (visceral, lymphatic, or osseous)

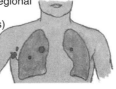

FIG 2-3 Staging of the musculoskeletal tumors. (Reprinted from *Netter Anatomy Illustration Collection*, © Elsevier Inc.)

TABLE 2-1 Stages of Benign Musculoskeletal Lesions

	1	2	3
Grade	G_0	G_0	G_0
Site	T_0	T_0	T_{1-2}
Metastasis	M_0	M_0	M_{1-2}
Clinical course	Latent, static, self-healing	Actively progressing, expands bone or fascia	Aggressive, invasive, breaches bone or fascia
Radiographic grade	I_A	I_B	I_C
Isotope scan	Background uptake	Increased uptake in lesion	Increased uptake beyond lesion
Angiogram	No neovascular reaction	Modest neovascular reaction	Moderate neovascular reaction
CT/MRI*	Crisp, intact margin—well-defined capsule, homogeneous	Intact margin "expansile"—thin capsule, homogeneous	Indistinct broached margin—extracapsular and/or extracompartmental extension, nonhomogeneous

From Enneking WF: A system of staging musculoskeletal neoplasms, Clin Orthop 204:9-24, 1986.
*A magnetic resonance imaging (MRI) study is now used in addition to the computed tomography (CT) study.

TABLE 2-2 Stages of Malignant Musculoskeletal Lesions*

	I_A	I_B	II_A	II_B	III_A	III_B
Grade	G_1	G_1	G_2	G_2	G_{1-2}	G_{1-2}
Site	T_1	T_2	T_1	T_2	T_1	T_2
Metastasis	M_0	M_0	M_0	M_0	M_1	M_1
Clinical course	Symptomatic, indolent growth	Symptomatic, mass, indolent growth	Symptomatic, rapid growth	Symptomatic, rapid growth, fixed mass, pathologic fracture	Systemic symptoms, palpable nodes, pulmonary symptoms	
Isotope scan	Increased uptake	Increased uptake	Increased uptake beyond radiographic limits	Increased uptake beyond radiographic limits	Pulmonary lesions, no increased uptake	
Radiographic grade	II	II	III	III	III	
Angiogram	Modest neovascular reaction, involvement of neuromuscular bundle	Modest neovascular reaction, involvement of neurovascular bundle	Marked neovascular reaction, no involvement of neurovascular bundle	Marked neovascular reaction, involvement of neurovascular bundle	Hypervascular lymph nodes of neurovascular bundle	
CT/MRI*†	Irregular or broached capsule but intracompartmental	Extracompart-mental extension or location	Broached (pseudo) capsule, intracompartmental	Broached (pseudo) capsule, extracompartmental	Pulmonary lesions or enlarged nodes	

From Enneking WF: A system of staging musculoskeletal neoplasms, Clin Orthop 204:9–24, 1986. (Used by permission.)
*A magnetic resonance imaging (MRI) study is now used in addition to the computed tomography (CT) study.
†MRI is now a standard part of the radiologic evaluation.

- Metastasis.
  M$_0$: no metastasis.
  M$_1$: metastasis.

The term *osteogenic sarcoma* formerly defined all the bone sarcomas (e.g., osteosarcoma, chondrosarcoma, and fibrosarcoma). Currently, more specific terms are preferred.

Benign tumors of bone are classified by the type of neoplastic tissue within the lesion. Nine general categories of tumors are described in the classification system of the WHO.

I. Bone-forming tumors
  1. Osteoma
  2. Osteoid osteoma
  3. Osteoblastoma
II. Cartilage-forming tumors
  1. Chondroma
  2. Osteochondroma
  3. Chondroblastoma
  4. Chondromyxoid fibroma
III. Giant cell tumors
IV. Marrow tumors (none)
V. Vascular tumors
  1. Hemangioma
  2. Lymphangioma
  3. Glomus tumor
VI. Other connective tissue tumors
  1. Desmoplastic fibroma
  2. Lipoma
  3. Fibrous histiocytoma
VII. Other tumors
  1. Neurilemmoma
  2. Neurofibroma
VIII. Unclassified tumors (none)
IX. Tumor-like lesions
  1. Solitary bone cyst
  2. Aneurysmal bone cyst
  3. Metaphyseal fibrous defect
  4. Eosinophilic granuloma
  5. Fibrous dysplasia
  6. Osteofibrous dysplasia
  7. Myositis ossificans
  8. Brown tumor of hyperparathyroidism
  9. Intraosseous epidermoid cyst
  10. Giant cell (reparative) granuloma

General Terms

tumor capsule: a layer of compressed normal tissue surrounding a tumor.

tumor pseudo-capsule: a layer of compressed normal tissue and neoplastic tissue surrounding a tumor.

Bone Cell Tumors

osteoblastoma: a benign tumor composed mostly of osteoblasts, occasional giant cells, fibrovascular tissue, and new bone formation. Generally located in the spine or diaphysis of long bones.

osteoid osteoma: a benign tumor characterized by increased osteoblasts and osteoid and fibrovascular tissue. Located in the cortex of long bones. Often surrounded by a thick sclerotic border as seen both radiographically and histologically.

osteoma: benign tumor characterized by dense bone production. Usually located in the skull.

osteosarcoma: a high-grade malignant bone tumor (sarcoma) generally located in the medullary cavity of the distal femur, proximal tibia, and proximal humerus. Characterized by osteoid production by malignant osteoblasts, with variable amounts of cartilage being present.

  parosteal osteosarcoma: a low-grade malignant bone tumor characterized by osteoid formation by malignant osteoblasts. This tumor is located on the outer surface of the periosteum, without involvement of the medullary cavity. Posterior cortex of the distal femur is a common location.

  periosteal osteosarcoma: a moderate-grade malignant bone tumor located beneath the periosteum but outside the cortex characterized by osteoid production by malignant osteoblasts. These osteosarcomas contain a large amount of cartilage.

  secondary osteosarcoma: osteosarcoma that arises in preexisting pathologic bone, such as in Paget's disease or following irradiation treatment.

telangiectatic osteosarcoma: intramedullary high-grade osteosarcoma characterized by abundant vascular changes and mesenchymal tissue in conjunction with sparse malignant osteoid production; **osteotelangiectasia.**

Cartilage Tumors

chondroblastoma (Codman tumor): benign tumor composed of chondroblasts, giant cells, and chondroid material. Calcification often appreciated surrounding the chondroblasts (chicken-wire calcification). This tumor generally is located in the epiphysis.

chondroma: an extraosseous benign tumor that contains mature chondrocytes in a cartilage matrix often surrounded by a rim of reactive bones. Varying degrees of calcification can be appreciated on radiographs and histology.

chondromyxoid fibroma: a benign tumor composed of cartilage and myxomatous and fibrous tissue. Commonly located in the proximal tibia.

chondrosarcoma: a malignant tumor characterized by cartilage production by malignant chondrocytes.

clear cell chondrosarcoma: cartilage tumor that histologically is characterized by clear, vacuolated cells.

dedifferentiated chondrosarcoma: malignant tumor in which a well-differentiated low-grade cartilaginous component, sometimes of long duration, is associated with a poorly differentiated noncartilagenous neoplasm of recent development and higher malignant grade.

enchondroma: an intraosseous benign tumor; similar both radiographically and histologically to a chondroma.

enchondromatosis: proliferation of multiple benign cartilaginous neoplasms within the metaphysis of several bones. It can result in thinning of the overlying cortices and distortion of length in growth. Higher risk of malignant transformation into secondary chondrosarcoma than a single enchondroma. **Ollier d.**

epiphyseal osteochondroma: development of intraosseous chondromas within the epiphysis with occasional extension beyond epiphyseal margins. May occur from infancy to adulthood. Formerly called **osteomatosis, epiphyseal exostosis, intraarticular osteochondroma, epiarticular osteochondroma, dysplasia epiphysealis hemimelica,** and **epiarticular osteochondromatous dysplasia.**

mesenchymal chondrosarcoma: tumor with well-differentiated cartilaginous component associated with highly malignant round cell component of recent development.

multiple osteochondromatosis: multiple osteochondromas located in the metaphysis of long bones and pelvis resulting in growth abnormalities, with an autosomal dominant inheritance pattern.

osteochondroma: a cartilage-capped extraosseous benign tumor with a bony stalk. Generally located in the distal femur, proximal tibia, or proximal humerus.

parosteal chondrosarcoma: malignant cartilage-producing tumor arising from the surface of the bone.

periosteal chondroma: an extraosseous benign cartilage tumor located between the periosteum and bone cortex characterized by cartilage and active chondrocytes.

secondary chondrosarcoma: usually well-differentiated cartilage malignancy occurring in a previously benign cartilage tumor, such as an osteochondroma or enchondroma.

Round Cell Tumors

eosinophilic granuloma (formally histiocytosis X): tumor-like process in bone composed of masses of histiocytes, cholesterol, and eosinophils. Common locations include the pelvis, scapula, and diaphysis of long bones in children; *Hand-Schüller-Christian d., Letterer-Siwe d.*

Ewing's sarcoma: high-grade malignant tumor commonly presenting in children; characterized by monotonous sheets of small round cells.

Hand-Schüller-Christian d.: one of the so-called histiocytosis X group of diseases; a complex of bony tumors caused by either accumulation of cholesterol, metabolic error, or neoplasm; characterized by eosinophilic granuloma, exophthalmos, and diabetes.

Hodgkin tumor: low-grade malignant process involving the lymphatic system, with rare 13% bone involvement characterized by Reed-Sternberg cells.

Langerhans cell histiocytosis: formerly known as histiocytosis X; a nonneoplastic condition characterized by monocyte-macrophage lineage cell infiltration of multiple organs including bone. The cause is unknown, and there are many forms of the disease with uncertain outcome. When a bony lesion occurs, it may involve one or a few **eosinophilic granulomas.** When associated with cranial disorder, diabetes, and exophthalmos, it may be **Hand-Schüller-Christian d.;** in infants with a poor prognosis associated with wasting it is called **Letterer-Siwe d.**

lymphoma: a general term for new tissue growth in the lymphatic system. There are many types.

multiple myeloma: common malignant tumor characterized by multiple plasma cell-containing bone lesions.

myeloblastoma: benign tumor of bone marrow.

plasmacytoma: uncommon malignant tumor characterized by a single focus of plasma cells in a bone. Often progresses to multiple myeloma.

primary lymphoma: distinguishes this rare malignant solitary bone tumor from the more common soft tissue or systemic presentation of lymphoma. Characterized by multiple malignant lymphocytes. A slower growing tumor seen in adults.

Fibrous Tumors

desmoplastic fibroma of bone: an aggressive but benign fibrous tumor characterized by dense bands of collagenous tissue.

fibrosarcoma: a malignant tumor characterized by fibroblastic cells and dilated vessels. More commonly presents as a soft tissue malignancy.

malignant fibrous histiocytoma: malignant tumor consisting of pleomorphic fibrous and histiocytic cell proliferation without osteoid or chondroid production.

nonossifying fibroma: common benign fibrous tumor presenting in childhood; located in the metaphysis of long bones. Characterized by whorl patterns of spindle cells, fibrous tissue, numerous xanthoma cells, and, occasionally, giant cells.

Other Tumors

adamantinoma: a malignant epithelial tumor located in the tibia.

chordoma: a malignant tumor commonly located in the sacrum or cervical spine; arises from residual notochord tissue.

epithelioid sarcoma: tumor composed of a nest of epithelial-like cells but with sarcomatous activity.

giant cell tumor (osteoclastoma): benign but aggressive lesion consisting of osteoclast-like giant cells originating in the metaphysis of long bones. Expansile on radiographs without any reactive bone formation.

liposarcoma: malignant soft tissue tumor composed of lipoblasts.

rhabdomyosarcoma: a malignant tumor composed of muscle cell precursors (rhabdomyoblasts).

synovial cell sarcoma: a malignant tumor composed of tissue that resembles synovium.

synovioma: a benign tumor of the synovial membrane.

Miscellaneous Bone Conditions

acroosteolysis: resorption of bone that involves the distal regions of the limbs but most commonly the phalanges of the fingers.

algodystrophy syndrome: association of pain and dystrophic changes in bone.

aneurysmal bone cyst: single or multiple benign, blood-filled cysts of bone.

apophysitis: inflammation of an apophysis. Depending on the location, specific types may be referred to as:

> **Osgood-Schlatter d.:** tibial apophysis at the insertion of the patellar tendon.
>
> **Sever d.:** apophysitis of the heel bone at the insertion of the Achilles tendon.
>
> **Scheuermann d.:** osteochondrosis of the vertebral epiphysis in juveniles.

aseptic necrosis: osteonecrosis (bone death) caused by vascular insult, usually at the end of a bone. In adults, the most common symptom producing aseptic necrosis occurs in the femoral head (avascular necrosis). In children, aseptic necrosis is called epiphyseal ischemic necrosis or epiphyseal aseptic necrosis. The precise pathologic condition of these diseases is debatable; therefore the term is used here in reference to epiphyseal osteochondritis or by area:

> *Assmann d.:* head of first metatarsal.
>
> *Buchman d.:* medial cuneiform.
>
> *Freiberg d.* second metatarsal head.
>
> *Iselins d.:* base of the fifth metatarsal.
>
> *Kappis d.:* talus.
>
> *Kienböck d.:* lunate bone of wrist.
>
> *Köhler d.:* tarsal navicular; sometimes of the patella.
>
> *Lance d.:* cuboid.
>
> *Legg-Calvé-Perthes d.:* femoral head; *Legg-Perthes d., Perthes d., coxa plana.*
>
> *Panner d.:* capitellum of the humerus.
>
> *Silfverskiöld d.:* calcaneus.

Thiemann d.: proximal phalanges.
Wagner d.: base of the first metatarsal.

Also known as **avascular necrosis** the following are classification systems for aseptic necrosis.

International Classification (for Femoral Head)

Stage 0: bone biopsy results consistent with avascular necrosis; normal findings in all other tests.

Stage I: positive scintiscan and/or magnetic resonance image (MRI); lesions subdivided into medial, central, or lateral depending on location and involvement of femoral head.

I-A: < 15% involvement of femoral head.
I-B: 15%–30% involvement of femoral head.
I-C: > 30% involvement of femoral head.

Stage II: radiographic abnormalities (mottled appearance of femoral head, osteosclerosis, cyst formation, and osteopenia); no signs of collapse of femoral head on radiographs or computerized tomography scan; positive scintiscan and MRI; no changes in acetabulum; lesions subdivided into medial, central, or lateral depending on location of involvement of femoral head.

II-A: < 15% involvement of femoral head.
II-B: 15%–30% involvement of femoral head.
II-C: > 30% involvement of femoral head.

Stage III: crescent sign; lesions subdivided into medial, central, or lateral depending on location of involvement of femoral head.

III-A: < 15% crescent sign or < 2-mm depression of femoral head.
III-B: 15%–30% crescent sign or 2- to 4-mm depression of femoral head.
III-C: > 30% crescent sign or 4-mm depression of femoral head.

Stage IV: Articular surface flattened radiographically and joint space shows narrowing; change in acetabulum with evidence of osteosclerosis, cyst formation, and marginal osteophytes.

Lichtman (for the Lunate in the Wrist)

Stage I: linear line possibly seen across lunate or no radiographic finding.

Stage II: definite density changes in lunate compared with other carpal bones.

Stage III: lunate collapse with proximal migration of capitate.

Stage IV: stage III plus degenerative changes in the carpus.

Ratcliff (for Pediatric Fractures of Femoral Head)

Type I: total head involvement.

Type II: segmental head involvement.

Type III: involvement of the fracture line to the physis.

Steinberg (for the Hip) (Fig. 2-4)

Stage 0: normal radiograph, bone scan, and MRI.

Stage I: normal radiograph; abnormal bone scan and/or MRI.

Stage II: sclerosis and/or cyst formation in femoral head.

A: mild (15% of head)
B: moderate (15%–30%)
C: severe (> 30%)

Stage III: subchondral collapse (crescent sign) without flattening.

A: mild (15% of surface)
B: moderate (15%–30%)
C: severe (> 30%)

Stage IV: flattening of femoral head without joint narrowing or acetabular involvement.

A: mild (15% of surface and < 2-cm depression)
B: moderate (15%–30% of surface and 2- to 4-mm depression)
C: severe (> 30% of surface or > 4-mm depression)

Stage V: flattening of head with joint narrowing and/ or acetabular involvement.

A: mild (15% of surface and < 2-cm depression)
B: moderate (15%–30% of surface and 2- to 4-mm depression)
C: severe (> 30% of surface or > 4-mm depression)

Stage VI: advanced degenerative changes.

---

bone infarct: area of bone where blood supply is interrupted.

bone island: small areas of compact but microscopically normal bone that appear as 0.5- to 1-cm areas on radiographs.

bone spur: ossification of ligamentous or muscular attachment to bone. Generally applied to any bony excrescence seen on radiographs, but specifically refers to a portion of ligament or tendon that has turned to bone at the attachment to bone. The most common areas include the heel, patella, humeral epicondyles, and vertebral body margins.

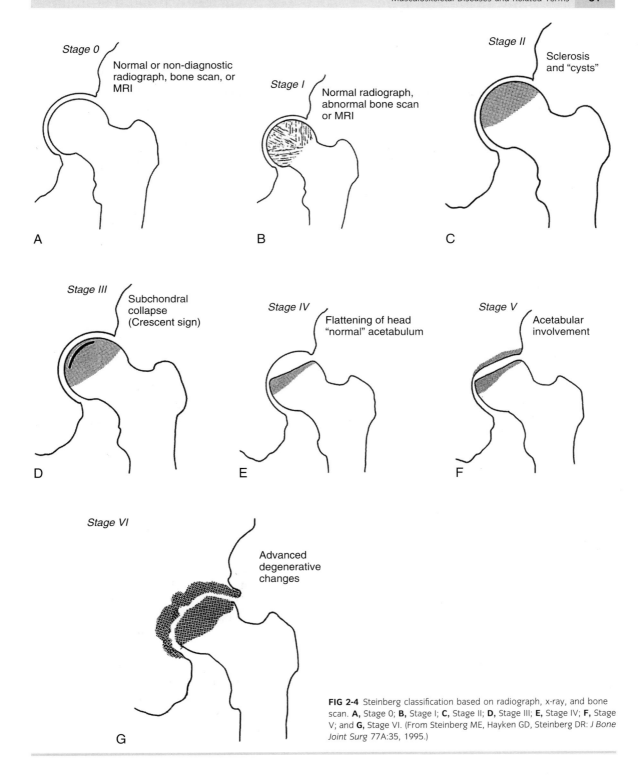

Stage 0
Normal or non-diagnostic radiograph, bone scan, or MRI

A

Stage I
Normal radiograph, abnormal bone scan or MRI

B

Stage II
Sclerosis and "cysts"

C

Stage III
Subchondral collapse (Crescent sign)

D

Stage IV
Flattening of head "normal" acetabulum

E

Stage V
Acetabular involvement

F

Stage VI
Advanced degenerative changes

G

FIG 2-4 Steinberg classification based on radiograph, x-ray, and bone scan. **A,** Stage 0; **B,** Stage I; **C,** Stage II; **D,** Stage III; **E,** Stage IV; **F,** Stage V; and **G,** Stage VI. (From Steinberg ME, Hayken GD, Steinberg DR: *J Bone Joint Surg* 77A:35, 1995.)

brown tumor: brown-appearing lesion in bone secondary to hyperparathyroidism; **osteoclastoma.**

caisson disease: avascular necrosis of bone (and soft tissue) caused by sudden increase and release in air pressure causing infarct; **diver's disease.**

cleidocranial dysostosis: autosomal dominant defect of a core binding protein (cfba-1, RUNX2) resulting in failure to form collarbones and portions of the skull.

condensing osteitis of the clavicle: rare and benign disorder of unknown origin affecting the medial clavicle, characteristically in women of late childbearing age. The level of discomfort varies, and radiographs reveal a slight expansion of the medial one third of the clavicle.

congenital pseudarthrosis: inborn propensity for breakdown of integrity of midshaft of tibia with formation of a false joint. There are six types:

Type I: congenital anterior bowing and defect in tibia. There may be other congenital deformities.

Type II: congenital anterior bowing and hourglass deformity of tibia. Fracture occurs usually before 2 years of age.

Type III: bone cyst forms first, then bowing or fracture.

Type IV: sclerotic bone, then fracture occurs.

Type V: dysplastic fibula. May develop pseudarthrosis of tibia or fibula.

Type VI: intraosseous neurofibroma or schwannoma may develop but usually does not result in pseudarthrosis.

cortical fibrous dysplasia (ossifying fibroma of long bone, intracortical fibrous dysplasia): benign anomaly of bone cortex, usually found in children and characterized by a cystic-appearing lesion on radiographs. Microscopically, this lesion is characterized by a fibrous replacement of cortex with some trabecular bone.

exostosis: excess bone formation, usually near a joint.

hypertrophic e.: sometimes used to describe excess bone formation in osteoarthritis.

multiple hereditary exostosis: autosomal dominant disorder of EXT or EXT2 genes resulting in multiple bony excrescences growing from cortical surfaces and forming tubular extensions roughly transverse to the long axis of bone involved; *Jaffe d.*

fibrodysplasia ossificans progressiva: autosomal dominant disease of BMP 4 and autosomal recessive disorder of BMP 1 receptor type 1A (ACVR1) resulting in connective tissue disease in which soft tissue ossification leads to skeletal malformation and disability; **myositis ossificans progressiva, hyperplasia fascialis ossificans progressiva, myositis fibrosa generalista,** and **fibrositis ossificans progressiva.**

fibrogenesis imperfecta ossium: rare inherited disorder in which bone in adults is replaced with collagen-deficient tissue throughout the skeleton, resulting in multiple fractures.

giant cell reparative granuloma: common benign lesion of jaw characterized by a fibrous background within which there are scattered multinucleated giant cells. A multicentric form is seen in the small bones of the hands and feet.

heterotopic ossification: formation of normal bone at ectopic soft tissue locations. In the acquired form, abnormal bone formation usually follows trauma or surgery and will sometimes occur around joints after a closed head injury. Two rare heritable and developmental forms are fibrodysplasia ossificans and progressive osseous heteroplasia.

A system to classify ectopic ossification is often referred to as the **Brooker** classification:

Class I: islands of bone within the soft tissues about the hip.

Class II: bone spurs from the pelvis or proximal end of the femur, leaving at least 1 cm between opposing bone surfaces.

Class III: bone spurs from the pelvis or proximal end of the femur, reducing the space between opposing bone surfaces to less than 1 cm.

Class IV: apparent bone ankylosis of the hip.

Another system is the **Hamblen** classification:

Grade 0: no ossification.

Grade I: formation of new bone involving less than one third of the area of the hip occupied by the femoral head and capsule.

Grade II: formation of new bone involving between one- and two-thirds of the same area of the hip.

Grade III: formation of new bone involving more than twothirds of that area of the hip.

hypophosphatasia: rare (1 in 100,000) usually autosomal recessive bone disorder due to deficient alkaline phosphatase activity, characterized by defective mineralization of the skeletal and dental structures leading to an appearance of rickets and very low alkaline phosphatase. There are four types based on the severity of alkaline phosphatase abnormality: **perinatal hypophosphatasia** with neonatal death, **infantile hypophosphatasia** presenting in the first year of life with severe skeletal fractures, **childhood hypophosphatasia** with rickets appearance and abnormal teeth, and **adult hypophosphatasia** with osteoporosis and fractures.

infantile cortical hyperostosis: painful hyperostosis with involvement of long bones and the mandible. This usually occurs in infants 5 months of age and younger and is associated with irritability, fever, and soft tissue swelling.

intraosseous lipoma: rare condition of benign fatty tumor that develops in the medullary canal of a long bone.

intraosseous lipomatosis: very rare disorder of progressive systemic development of leg and foot lipomas in medullary canals, producing bone pain and pathologic fractures.

intraosseous pneumatocyst: rare benign small pocket of air that appears usually in iliac bone. No treatment is required.

longitudinal epiphyseal bracket: ossification anomaly in which an abnormal arcuate or C-shaped secondary ossification center brackets a tubular bone in the hand or foot.

malacoplakia: disease that usually involves the gut and has a probable infectious cause. Histiocytes respond with the formation of Michaelis-Gutmann bodies. Bone lesions are rare and can be destructive.

melorheostosis: form of osteosclerosis or hyperostosis (dense bone); linear longitudinal thickenings of the shaft of long bones, very rare, resulting in a candle wax (dripping) appearance of the bone.

milk-alkali disease: excess calcium in tissue resulting from heavy ingestion of milk and certain antacids.

myelofibrosis: replacement of bone marrow by fibrous tissue.

nonossifying fibroma: an anomaly of bone that appears in youngsters as a sharply circumscribed, eccentrically located lesion in the metaphysis of long bones; microscopically, this lesion is characterized by whorl patterns of spindle cells, fibrous tissue, numerous xanthoma cells, and, occasionally, giant cells; **fibroxanthoma, fibrous cortical defect, subcortical defect.**

ochronosis: hereditary error of protein metabolism marked by accumulation of homogentisic acid resulting in degenerative arthritis and a characteristic blackening of cartilage.

ossifying fibroma of the jaw: fibroma of the jaw with histologic appearance of small areas of ossification. This is in distinction to the rare ossifying fibroma of long bones.

pachydysostosis: enlargement of fibular length resulting in bowing of the leg.

periostitis: inflammation of bone covering (periosteum); usually the result of an infection such as syphilis.

progressive diaphyseal dysplasia: neuromuscular dystrophy associated with general wasting; abnormally formed shafts of long bones; *Engelmann d.*

progressive osseous heteroplasia: heritable disease characterized by focal dermal ossification with progression to intramembranous ossification of subcutaneous fat and deeper tissues leading to ankylosis. **Hemimelic progressive osseous heteroplasia** is a very rare condition in which only one side of the body is involved.

pulmonary osteodystrophy: hypertrophic cortical bone changes occurring near joints in the long bones of patients with chronic lung disease.

pyknodysostosis: condition marked by patchy areas of thickening of the cortex of bone.

regional migratory osteoporosis: most often seen in middle-aged men; characterized by arthralgias of lower limb joints, severe intercurrent osteoporosis, with symptoms lasting 6 to 9 months with recovery.

rickets: failure of deposition of bone salts within the organic matrix of cartilage and bone associated with stunting of growth and bone deformities.

skeletal amyloidosis: deposition of amyloid β-microglobulin material in bone that produces bubbly appearing lesions on radiographs. Condition is associated with plasma cell dyscrasias, primary systemic amyloidosis, focal amyloidosis, and those undergoing hemodialysis for chronic renal insufficiency.

slipped capital femoral epiphysis: gradual or sudden movement of the femoral head toward a posterior and medial direction; usually occurs in preteenage children. The condition is also called **slipped capital femoral epiphysis (SCFE)** or **slipped upper femoral epiphysis (SUFE).** In America, the acronym SCFE is so common that the slang word "skiffy" is used for SCFE.

solitary fibromatosis of bone: similar to generalized fibromatosis except bone lesion is isolated to one location. Systemic symptoms do not occur.

solitary osteoma of long bone: a benign periosteal or endosteal tumor composed predominantly of cortical-type bone.

subperiosteal giant-cell reparative granuloma: self-limited condition seen in older adults characterized by subperiosteal bony lesions located in cortical bone of the diaphysis with giant cells and reparative cells with bone formation; **subperiosteal ABC, periostitis ossificans, florid reactive periostitis, pseudomalignant fibroosseous tumors.**

transient osteopenia: decreased bone mass usually following immobilization or injury. Most often bone mass is recovered. May be seen as a spontaneous event in the juvenile hip.

uncommitted metaphyseal lesion: benign but radiologically aggressive-appearing lesion seen in the proximal metaphysis of children, microscopically characterized by whorls of fibrous tissue, new bone, giant cells, and vascular components.

unicameral bone cyst: benign bone anomaly in which a fluid-filled cavity is seen in the metaphysis of a long bone of a child. Microscopically, the cavity is lined with fibrous stroma, curlicues of trabecular bone similar to fibrous dysplasia, and cholesterol clefts.

weaver's bottom: ischial gluteal bursitis often seen in patients with a sedentary occupation.

Eponymic Bone Diseases

Albers-Schönberg d.: osteopetrosis affecting the ends of bone; *chalk bones, thick bones, marble bones.*

Albright syndrome: spontaneous mutation of gene for GS alpha protein for adenylate cyclase (GNAS-1) resulting in hypophosphatemic precocious puberty associated with bone deformities resulting from fibrous dysplasia; **polyostotic fibrous dysplasia, Albright-McCune-Sternberg syndrome,** and **McCune-Albright syndrome.**

Apert d.: autosomal dominant disease due to fibroblast growth factor receptor 2 disorder that results in early fusion of the skull (craniosynostosis) and fusion of the digits, multiple deformities, and mental retardation; **acrocephalosyndactylism.**

Assmann d.: avascular necrosis of the head of the first metatarsal.

Blount d.: lesion of the medial proximal tibial epiphysis causing valgus (lateral bowing) deformity of the tibia; **osteochondrosis deformans tibia, tibia vara** (Fig. 2-5).

Boeck sarcoid: condition usually affecting small bones of hands and feet with granulomatous inflammatory reaction in lymph nodes, spleen, lungs, and liver.

Bouchard nodes: cartilaginous and bony enlargement of the proximal interphalangeal joints of fingers in degenerative joint disease.

Brailsford d.: avascular necrosis of the radial head seen in children.

Brodie abscess: chronic infection of bone resulting in a characteristic coin-sized sclerotic lesion with a lucent center.

Buchman d.: avascular necrosis of the medial cuneiform.

Burns d.: avascular necrosis of the humeral trochlea head seen in children.

Caffey d.: subperiosteal cortical defect; infantile cortical hyperostosis; self-limited process of excess bone formation seen in newborns to 2-year-olds.

Stage I   Stage II   Stage III

Stage IV   Stage V   Stage VI

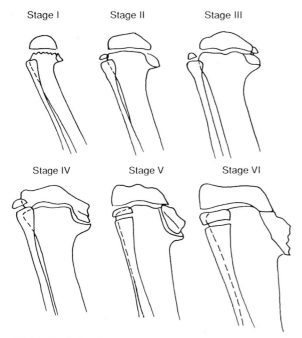

FIG 2-5 Blount disease.

Crouzon d.: autosomal dominant disease due to fibroblast growth factor receptor 2 disorder that results in early fusion of the skull (craniosynostosis) and facial deformities that vary widely in severity.

Engelmann d. (Camurati-Engelmann dysplasia): primarily a disorder of intramembranous ossification that usually affects the cortex of long bones and the skull with less frequent effects on the face; **progressive diaphyseal dysplasia.**

Freiberg d.: aseptic (avascular) necrosis of the second metatarsal head.

Fröhlich adiposogenital dystrophy: slipped capital femoral epiphysis; **Babinski-Fröhlich syndrome.**

Gardner syndrome: multiple osteomas concurrent with intestinal polyps, fibromas, and epidermal cysts.

Gaucher d. (cerebroside reticulocytosis): autosomal dominant bone disorder resulting from lipid storage disease that is due to an absence of glucocerebrosidase. Excessive production of histiocytes with interference of marrow function and destruction of bone occurs. There are three clinical forms: Type

I is associated with an enlarged liver and spleen with longer life and no brain effect, Type II leads to death by age two due to severe liver and brain disorder, and Type III is associated with seizures and sometimes liver and spleen are affected.

Type 1: Adult—chronic, nonneuronopathic form associated with hypersplenism, bone lesions, skin pigmentation, and pingueculae.

Type 2: Infantile—acute neuronopathic form that is manifested in infancy and is associated with severe neuronal abnormalities and early demise.

Type 3: Juvenile—subacute neuronopathic form that has the features of the adult form but with neurologic symptoms that develop in the first decade of life.

Gorham d.: rare condition characterized by monostotic, unilateral, localized, concentric osteolysis.

Haas d.: avascular necrosis of the head of the humerus seen in children.

Hajdu-Cheney syndrome: rare syndrome of resorption of bone of the distal part of the limbs with associated skeletal dysplasias.

Heberden nodes: cartilaginous and bony enlargement of the distal interphalangeal joints in osteoarthritis.

Iselins d.: avascular necrosis of the base of the fifth metatarsal.

Jaffe d.: osteoid osteoma; hereditary multiple exostosis.

Kappis d.: avascular necrosis of the talus.

Kienböck d.: aseptic necrosis affecting lunate or ilium.

Klippel-Feil syndrome: congenital bone abnormalities of neck associated with dental, scapular, and other abnormalities.

Köhler d.: aseptic necrosis of tarsal navicular (scaphoiditis) or patella.

König d.: osteochondrosis dissecans of the knee; a separate formation of bone and cartilage segment at the joint surface.

Lance d.: avascular necrosis of the cuboid.

Lateral Pillar (Herring) Classification of Legg-Calvé-Perthes Disease

A. The lateral pillar of the femoral head is intact.

B. The lateral pillar of the femoral head is less than 50% collapsed B/C. Border: The lateral pillar of the femoral head is thin or poorly ossified or has collapsed exactly 50%.

C. The lateral pillar of the femoral head is greater than 50% collapsed.

Legg-Calvé-Perthes d.: aseptic epiphyseal ischemic necrosis of the capital femoral epiphysis in children; **coxa plana; Perthes d.; Legg-Perthes d.**

Letterer-Siwe d.: histiocyte tumor of bone, usually fatal in infants and small children; *eosinophilic granuloma*.

Marie-Bamberger d.: hypertrophied joints resulting from lung disease.

Mauclair d.: avascular necrosis of the metacarpal heads seen in children.

Milkman syndrome: bone disease in which multiple transparent stripes are seen on radiograph.

nail-patella syndrome: autosomal dominant disorder characterized by hypoplastic patella, deformed fingernails, elbow deformities, and pelvic "horns."

Niemann-Pick d.: fatal fat storage disease affecting bone marrow in infancy, marked by absence of sphingomyelinase.

Ollier d.: enchondromatosis.

Osgood-Schlatter d.: osteochondritis affecting anterior tibial tuberosity.

Paget d.: disease of excess bone removal and replacement with deformity; seen in older people; *osteitis deformans*.

Panner d.: aseptic necrosis; osteochondritis dissecans of capitellum of humerus.

Perthes d.: aseptic necrosis of the hips in children.

Pott d.: osteomyelitis; tuberculosis of the spine.

Ribbing d: rare bone dysplasia associated with painful long bone central sclerosis after skeletal maturity; often resolves spontaneously.

Scheuermann d.: osteochondritis affecting anterior vertebral body apophysis.

shepherd's crook deformity: characteristic deformity of proximal femur seen in fibrous dysplasia. The deformity has the appearance of a shepherd's crook.

Silfverskiöld d.: avascular necrosis of the calcaneus.

Sinding-Larsen-Johansson d.: secondary center of ossification of inferior pole of patella.

Stewart-Morel syndrome: hyperostosis of frontal bone; **Morel syndrome.**

Thiemann d.: avascular necrosis of proximal phalanges.

Tietze syndrome: chronic inflammation of the costochondral junction of a rib or ribs, causing pain; **chondropathia tuberosa.**

Van Neck d.: nonspecific ischiopubic osteochondritis.

Volkmann deformity: congenital dislocation of the ankle due to absent or defective fibula, not to be confused with **Volkmann ischemic contracture.**

von Recklinghausen d.: autosomal dominant disorder of nuclear factor neurofibromin (NF1) resulting in fatty tumors, peripheral nerve tumors, areas of skin pigment changes, and other disorders; **neurofibromatosis.**

Voorhoeve d.: osteopathia striata.

Wagner d.: avascular necrosis of the base of the first metatarsal.

Waldenström d.: osteochondrosis of distal humerus at the radial site of elbow (capitellum).

Muscle Diseases

Myo- (Gr. *mys*) is a combining form denoting relationship to muscle. The *myo-* root diseases are followed by miscellaneous muscle diseases, the muscular dystrophies (listed together for comparison), and other muscle disorders. Eponymic terms are included.

Myo- Root Diseases

myasthenia: lack of muscle strength; **amyosthenia.**

myasthenia gravis: syndrome of attacks of muscle weakness that are episodic and reversible, **Erb-Goldflam d.**

myatrophy: muscle wasting.

myoblastoma: tumor of striated muscle consisting of groups of granular-appearing cells resembling primitive myoblasts.

myobradia: sluggish muscle reaction to electric stimuli.

myocele: herniation and protrusion of muscle through its ruptured muscle sheath.

myocelialgia: pain in abdominal muscles.

myocelitis: inflammation of abdominal muscles.

myocellulitis: myositis with cellulitis.

myocerosis: waxy-appearing degeneration of muscle.

myoclonus: any disorder in which rapid rigidity and relaxation alternate; **myoclonia.**

myocoele: the cavity within a myotome.

myocytoma: benign muscle tumor.

myodegeneration: muscle degeneration.

myodemia: fatty degeneration of muscle. (archaic)

myodiastasis: separation of muscle. May be congenital or traumatic.

myodynia: pain in the muscles; **myalgia, myosalgia.**

myodystonia: disorder of muscle tone.

myoedema: edema, muscle swelling. (archaic)

myofascitis: inflammation of muscle and its fascia, particularly of fascial insertion of muscle into bone.

myofibroma: muscular and fibrous tumor; fibroma containing muscular elements.

myofibrosis: replacement of muscle tissue by fibrous tissue.

myogelosis: area of hardening in a muscle. (archaic)

myoglobinuria: protein myoglobin that appears in urine after vigorous activity; may lead to renal shutdown.

myohypertrophia: muscular hypertrophy.

myoischemia: local deficiency of blood supply in muscle.

myokerosis: waxy degeneration of muscle tissue; **myocerosis.**

myolipoma: fatty tumor of muscle.

myolysis: disintegration of degeneration of muscle tissue.

myoma: tumor made up of muscular elements.

myomalacia: pathogenic softening of muscle. (archaic)

myomatosis: formation of multiple muscle tumors.

myomelanosis: black pigmentation of a portion of muscle.

myoneuralgia: muscular nerve pain.

myoneurasthenia: relaxed state of the muscular system in neurasthenia (lack of strength due to muscle nerve supply loss).

myoneuroma: nerve tumor containing muscle tissue.

myoneurosis: any abnormal nerve condition of the muscles. (archaic)

myopachynsis: hypertrophy of muscle; thickening. (archaic)

myopalmus: muscle twitching. (archaic)

myoparalysis: paralysis of muscle; **myoparesis.**

myopathy: any disease of the muscles.

myophagism: atrophy or wasting away of muscle tissue, with removal of tissue by inflammatory cells. (archaic)

myopsychopathy: any muscular nerve affection associated with mental weakness or disorder.

myorrhexis: muscle rupture.

myosarcoma: malignant muscle tumor.

myosclerosis: hardening of muscle. (archaic)

myoseism: jerky, irregular muscle contractions. (archaic)

myositis: inflammation of a voluntary muscle.

myositis ossificans: ossification of muscle in response to trauma. To distinguish the traumatic form of myositis ossificans from the generalized form, the term **myositis ossificans circumscripta,** proliferative myositis, is sometimes used.

myospasia: clonic contraction of muscle. (archaic)

myospasm: muscle spasm. (archaic)

myospasmia: disease characterized by uncontrolled muscle spasms. (archaic)

myostasis: stretching of muscle. (archaic)

myosteoma: bony tumor in muscle. (archaic)

myosynizesis: adhesions of muscle. (archaic)

myotenositis: inflammation of muscle and its tendon insertion.

myotonia: increased muscular irritability and contractility with decreased power of relaxation; tension and tonic spasm of muscle.

Miscellaneous Muscle Diseases and Conditions

amyoplasia congenita: disorder of fascia and muscle resulting in contracted joints during growth. A specific form of arthrogryposis.

amyotonia congenita: muscle disorder of the newborn, usually fatal; characterized by muscle degeneration with failure of replacement (**congenital hypotonia, Oppenheim d.**); several types including **Werdnig-Hoffmann d.** (central nervous system [CNS] origin), rod d. (microscopic rods forming within muscle cells), and central core d., which is not fatal.

congenital myotonia: disorder found at birth, in which initiation and cessation of voluntary movement are delayed; **Thomsen d.**

delayed-onset muscle soreness (DOMS): muscle weakness, restricted range of motion, and tenderness on palpation that occurs 24 to 48 hours after intense or prolonged muscle activity.

eosinophilia-myalgia syndrome: severe myalgia associated with elevated eosinophile count in blood in the absence of any infection. Has been felt to be associated with high doses of tryptophan.

familial periodic paralysis: disorder of muscle metabolism in which periods of partial to nearly complete paralysis occur; **myotonia intermittens.**

mitochondrial myopathy: slowly progressive muscular weakness associated with abnormal mitochondria, a cell structural component important in oxygen metabolism. The onset of symptoms is usually between birth and 10 years of age, but the disorder may not appear until adulthood.

muscle atrophy: general loss of muscle from various causes; **muscle wasting.**

muscle contracture: condition of fixed high resistance to passive stretch of a muscle resulting from fibrosis of the tissues supporting the muscles or the joints or from disorders of the muscle fibers such as trauma or a congenital disorder.

   ischemic c.: contracture and degeneration of muscle due to interference with circulation from pressure, as by a tight bandage or from injury or cold.

   organic c.: contracture that is permanent and continuous.

   postpoliomyelitic c.: any distortion of a joint following an attack of poliomyelitis.

muscle cramps: uncontrolled contraction of muscle; **charley horse.**

muscle guarding: involuntary contraction of muscle in effort to avoid pain that would be produced by moving the body part.

muscle ischemia: decreased blood supply to a muscle; can be spontaneously reversible; if not, ischemic contracture may develop.

muscle spasm: sudden contraction of muscle, usually in reflexive response to stimulus from external source, for example, back spasm caused by a herniated disk.

muscular dystrophy: group of degenerative disorders of muscle resulting in atrophy and weakness; **Erb d.**

dystrophinopathy: autosomal recessive form of muscular dystrophy due to failure of formation of dystrophin resulting in a severe form; **Duchenne muscular dystrophy,** or a less severe form, **Becker muscular dystrophy.**

pseudohypertrophic: dystrophy of shoulder girdle and sometimes pelvic girdle muscles, beginning with hypertrophy in childhood, followed by atrophy; **Erb paralysis.**

fascioscapulohumeral: marked atrophy of face, shoulder girdle, and arm muscles with autosomal dominant inheritance; **Landouzy-Dejerine disease.**

limb girdle: slow, progressive dystrophy, affecting mostly the back and pelvic muscles. There are a number of types including: **type I:** autosomal dominant; **type IIA:** autosomal recessive with lack of calcium-activated neutral protease-3 (calpain-3); **type IIB,** autosomal recessive; **type IIC and D:** autosomal recessive lack of gamma-sarcoglycan; and **type IIE:** autosomal with lack of beta-sarcoglycan.

distal: dystrophy affecting mostly the distal muscles of the extremities and usually slowly progressive proximally.

ocular: dystrophy usually confined to the levator and other facial muscles; **progressive dystrophic ophthalmoplegia.**

myotonic dystrophy: myotonia followed eventually by atrophy of face and neck muscles, ultimately extending to muscles of trunk and extremities due to autosomal dominant lack of myotonin-protein kinase.

pyomyositis: infection of muscle in which an abscess forms.

rhabdomyolysis: destruction of muscle following excessive activity, crush, or compartment syndrome. Can cause renal failure due to high levels of myoglobulin in blood.

Stewart-Morel syndrome: intermittent progressive muscular rigidity; **stiff man syndrome.**

trigger points: this term has several different meanings. In general, these are specific points of muscle or muscle attachment that are very tender and related to muscle spasm. Pressure on these points may cause pain referred distal to those points.

These point areas may be the result of chronic spinal disorders or caused by overuse of specific muscle groups.

Cartilage Diseases

Chondro- (Gr. *chondros*, gristle or cartilage). Cartilage serves a very important function in the growing process and joint motion. Healthy cartilage is essential for normal growth.

A growth plate called the epiphysis, a cartilage layer near or outside the joint, is essential to most of the longitudinal growth of bone during childhood. Disorders of this structure can lead to dwarfism or deformity. Cartilage is not apparent on radiographs, and many cartilage diseases are not detected until sufficient degeneration to cause joint narrowing takes place. Often a disorder that affects cartilage affects bone as well, such as osteo/chondr/itis (inflammation of bone and cartilage) or osteo/chondr/oma (bone and cartilage tumor).

Because diseased cartilage cells affect the combined function of bones and joints, many cartilage disease terms are found in the sections on bone tumors and joint diseases. The cartilage-related diseases are categorized in this section as follows:

1. *Chondro-* root diseases
2. Miscellaneous cartilage diseases
3. Abnormalities of the epiphyses
4. Mucopolysaccharidoses (proteoglycan abnormalities)

Chondro- Root Diseases
chondralgia: pain in cartilage. This is an old term because there are no nerve pain fibers in cartilage. However, the perception is that pain comes from the cartilage; **chondrodynia.** (archaic)

chondritis: although implies inflammation of cartilage, the term alludes to pain from a cartilage bone interface such as ribs, costochondritis, where inflammation may not be present.

chondrodysplasia: hereditary deforming abnormal cartilage formation; **dyschondroplasia.**

chondrodysplasia punctata: X-linked dominant or recessive disorder.

chondrodystrophia: rare condition of nutritional abnormality of cartilage development; **dwarfism.**

chondroepiphysitis: inflammation of epiphyseal cartilage.

chondrofibroma: fibroma with cartilaginous elements.

chondrolipoangioma: a well-circumscribed tumor in which there is a predominance of mature cartilage, mature blood vessels, and mature fat.

chondrolipoma: fatty tumor containing cartilaginous elements.

chondrolysis: degeneration of cartilage cells, ending in cell death.

chondromalacia: softening of cartilage, as of the patella.

chondromatosis: multiple formation of chondromas.

chondrometaplasia: condition in which cells that would normally form cartilage function abnormally.

chondromyoma: muscle tumor with cartilaginous elements.

chondromyxoma: mucous tumor of bone with cartilaginous elements.

chondromyxosarcoma: sarcoma containing cartilaginous and mucous elements.

chondronecrosis: necrosis (death) of cartilage.

chondroosteodystrophy: nutritional abnormality of bone and cartilage.

chondropathology: diseased state of cartilage.

chondropathy: disease of cartilage.

chondrophyte: excess cartilaginous growth at bone ends, at the margins of a joint.

chondroporosis: normal growth process in childhood; in adults, the formation of empty space in cartilage is a part of a disease process. (archaic)

chondrosarcomatosis: multiple chondrosarcomas; abnormal tumor cartilage.

chondrosteoma: tumor made up of bone and cartilaginous tissue.

Miscellaneous Cartilage Diseases
achondroplasia: autosomal dominant disorder affecting fibroblast growth factor-3; resulting in congenital dwarfism associated with deformed long bones and misshapen epiphyses; **achondroplastic dwarfism, chondrodystrophia fetalis.**

cartilage-hair hypoplasia: autosomal recessive mutation in RMRP, a non-encoding RNA resulting in short stature and abnormal facial appearance; **McKusick-type metaphyseal chondrodysplasia.**

diastrophic dwarfism: autosomal recessive dwarfism with flattening subluxation of various epiphyses due to defect in sulfate transporter; **diastrophic dysplasia.**

Henderson-Jones chondromatosis: synovial formation of multiple loose pieces of cartilage within a joint, often associated with pain and swelling. The condition can spontaneously resolve with absorption of the cartilage bodies.

hypochondrodysplasia: autosomal dominant condition due to mutation of fibroblast growth factor-3, resulting in milder dwarfing than achondroplasia and normal facial appearance.

Jansen d.: autosomal dominant disease of parathyroid hormone-related peptide receptor associated with mental retardation, short limb dwarfism, exophthalmia, hypercalcemia, and long bone bowing; **metaphyseal chondrodysplasia, Jansen type.**

Maffucci syndrome: dyschondroplasia with hemangiomas, some of which have calcified walls as seen on radiographs.

Ollier d.: multiple enchondromatosis, usually unilateral benign cartilage tumors of bone.

precocious osteoarthritis: degenerative arthritis that develops at a very young age, often a genetic defect such as type II collagen.

Schmid d.: autosomal disorder affecting type X collagen and characterized by short stature, bowed lower extremities, coxa vara, flared metaphyses, and a waddling gait; **metaphyseal chondrodysplasia, Schmid type.**

Stickler syndrome: autosomal dominant disorder of type II collagen associated with small lower jaw, nearsightedness, thin limbs, mild scoliosis, and early degenerative arthritis. In another form, type XI collagen is affected and there is no eye disorder.

synchondrosis: fusion of cartilage surfaces in a joint. This may be a disease state or a normal maturation process, depending on the location.

synoviochondromatosis: process in which the joint lining forms small nodules of cartilage, which may break loose and be free in the joint. Synonymous with **synovial osteochondromatosis** or **osteochondromatosis.**

Abnormalities of the Epiphyses (Fig. 2-6)

The epiphyses are the cartilaginous layers at the end of long bones at the joints responsible for growth. Any dysfunction of metabolic origin or injury can cause deformity or dwarfism such as the following.

dysplasia epiphysealis hemimelia: osteochondroma arising from an epiphysis and projecting from the articular surface. This will usually interfere with joint function.

epiphyseal hyperplasia: condition in which the epiphyses form from multiple centers and become enlarged and misshapen.

epiphysiodesis: premature fusion of the epiphysis to diaphysis. This can be due to injury or surgical intent.

epiphysiolysis: separation of an epiphysis from the shaft of the bone.

epiphysiopathy: any disease of the epiphyses.

epiphysitis: inflammation of joint cartilage or epiphyses in contrast to the rest of the bone.

hatchet head shoulder: flattening of humerus seen in multiple epiphyseal dysplasia. Not to be confused with hatchet head deformity seen after an anterior shoulder dislocation.

multiple epiphyseal dysplasia: multiple irregular epiphyseal ossification centers causing enlargement and flaring. **Type I multiple epiphyseal dysplasia** is due to an autosomal dominant disorder affecting oligomeric protein of cartilage (COMP), and **type II-IV multiple epiphyseal dysplasia** is due to an autosomal dominant disorder affecting type IX (A1, A2, and A3) collagen. **Type V** due to autosomal dominant disorder of matrilin 3. There are additional dominant as well as recessive forms; **dysplasia epiphyseal multiplex congenita.**

slipped epiphysis: subluxation or dislocation of the epiphysis from the shaft of the bone. This may not

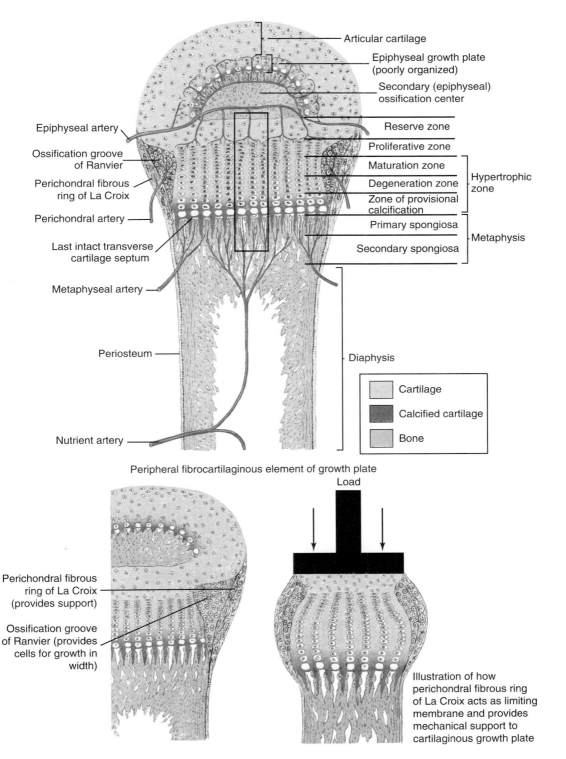

- Articular cartilage
- Epiphyseal growth plate (poorly organized)
- Secondary (epiphyseal) ossification center
- Reserve zone
- Proliferative zone
- Maturation zone — Hypertrophic zone
- Degeneration zone — Hypertrophic zone
- Zone of provisional calcification
- Primary spongiosa — Metaphysis
- Secondary spongiosa — Metaphysis

- Epiphyseal artery
- Ossification groove of Ranvier
- Perichondral fibrous ring of La Croix
- Perichondral artery
- Last intact transverse cartilage septum
- Metaphyseal artery
- Periosteum
- Diaphysis
- Nutrient artery

	Cartilage
	Calcified cartilage
	Bone

Peripheral fibrocartilaginous element of growth plate

Load

Perichondral fibrous ring of La Croix (provides support)

Ossification groove of Ranvier (provides cells for growth in width)

Illustration of how perichondral fibrous ring of La Croix acts as limiting membrane and provides mechanical support to cartilaginous growth plate

FIG 2-6 Disease conditions that affect the epiphysis often also affect the physis, which is the growth plate or epiphyseal plate. (Reprinted from *Netter Anatomy Illustration Collection*, © Elsevier Inc.)

necessarily be a single traumatic event but may occur gradually.

spondyloepiphyseal dysplasia: autosomal dominant and recessive disorders of type II collagen causing a spectrum of changes including inability to ossify normal epiphyseal centers, resulting in dwarfing and/or precocious osteoarthritis, primarily in spine and hips. There are four forms: **spondyloepiphyseal dysplasia congenita** (autosomal dominant); **spondyloepiphyseal dysplasia tarda** (autosomal recessive); dominant X-linked due to a defect in sedlin; and **Kniest dysplasia** (autosomal dominant).

spondyloepiphyseal dysplasia of Maroteaux: disorder of development of vertebrae and hips but without associated biochemical and eye changes seen in Morquio syndrome.

stippled epiphysis: radiologic sign of chondrodystrophia calcificans, a disease associated with multiple calcifications of epiphyseal cartilage. A mild form of the condition may be called **epiphyseal dysplasia.**

Mucopolysaccharidoses (Metabolic Effects)

The mucopolysaccharidoses (MPSs) are a variety of hereditable metabolic disorders of mucopolysaccharides presently called *proteoglycans*. Glycosaminoglycan chains are sugars that contain amino and sulfate components, are attached to a protein core molecule, and are formed by posttranslational pathways in the cell. Specific enzymatic failures are responsible for the accumulation of specific chemicals. *Muco-* originally signified the gelatinous appearance of the pure aggregate of these molecules. Most disorders of mucopolysaccharide metabolism are autosomal recessive. For many types, the eponymic designations are preferred because the metabolic nomenclature is complex.

Hunter s.: similar to Hurler syndrome, but less severely deforming; sex-linked dominant inheritance affecting sulfoiduronate sulfatase; *MPS II*. There are severe and mild forms of the disease.

Hunter-Scheie s.: condition that has mixed clinical appearance of Hunter and Scheie syndrome; *MPS I H/S*.

Hurler s.: autosomal recessive severely deforming condition associated with blindness, mental retardation, and early death; due to a deficiency of alpha-L-iduronidase; *MPS I H*. Formerly called **gargoylism, lipochondrodystrophy.**

Maroteaux-Lamy s.: growth retardation, lumbar kyphosis, sternal protrusion; no mental retardation; *MPS VI*.

McArdle s: autosomal recessive disorder caused by deficiency of muscle phosphorylase B glycogen phosphorylase leading to muscle weakness, cramps, and muscle pain on exercise.

Morquio s.: dwarfing disease affecting mostly the spine and hips; little or no mental retardation. There are two forms that have similar clinical appearance—*MPS IV A* and *MPS IV B*; **chondroosteodystrophy.** Both types are autosomal recessive inherited disorders; A due to defects in galaxtosamine-6-sulphate sulfatase; and B due to a defect in beta-galactosidase.

Sanfilippo s.: four forms of this autosomal recessive disease resulting in accumulation of heparan sulfate exist and all have profound mental retardation, hyperactivity, and relatively mild somatic manifestations—*MPS III A, MPS III B, MPS III C*, and *MPS III D*.

Scheie s.: autosomal recessive disorder due to dysfunction of alpha-1-iduronidase with no mental impairment but noted corneal clouding, aortic disease, and stiff joints; *MPS I S*.

Sly s.: autosomal recessive disorder of glucuronidase, which causes multiple long bone growth abnormalities associated with liver and spleen enlargement; wide spectrum of severity; *MPS VII*.

Diseases of (Specific) Soft Tissue

In addition to bone, muscle, and cartilage, other tissues surround a joint. The root terms for these tissues (*fibro-, lipo-, myxo-, muco-*) denote the relationship to certain disease processes and disorders.

Fibro- Root Diseases

Fibro- (L. *fibra*, fiber) is a combining form indicating fibrous tissue such as tendons and ligaments. Such tissue contains collagen, which is the major supportive protein of bone, tendon, cartilage, and connective tissue. Fibrous-like tissues and structures can arise in a number of places.

elastofibroma: benign tumor-like growth usually seen in the back. It is a painless, slow-growing, firm, subcutaneous mass not attached to skin, and microscopically it appears as a nonencapsulated proliferation of collagen and elastin fibers with few fibroblasts. The most common location is subscapular.

fibroma: benign fibroblastic tumor.

fibromatosis: formation of multiple fibromas. This term is used for a variety of conditions including plantar and palmar fibromatosis, neurofibromatosis, and a more aggressive and locally invasive fibromatosis.

fibrosis: proliferation of fibrous tissue as a result of reaction to a reparative process.

fibrositis: inflammation of fibrous tissue.

fibrous histiocytoma: benign tumor of bone containing fibrous stroma, xanthomatous cells, and a round and spindle cell component. There is a malignant form called *malignant fibrous histiocytoma.*

Garrod fibromatosis (Garrod pads): thickening of the skin almost always confined to the dorsal aspects of the proximal interphalangeal joints of the hand.

juvenile hyaline fibromatosis: disease that develops in early childhood and is characterized by multiple fibromatous lesions of the skin, muscle, bone, and ligaments, possibly leading to joint contractures. It is not necessarily progressive; histologically, it is characterized by multiple spindle cells with an amorphous matrix or collagenous tissue.

malignant fibrous histiocytoma: highly malignant soft tissue tumor of later adult life that is initially seen as a subcutaneous to deep muscle lesion; **malignant fibrous xanthoma, fibroxanthosarcoma, malignant giant cell tumor of soft tissue.**

monostotic fibrous dysplasia: disease of bony remodeling, causing deformity of only one bone.

polyostotic fibrous dysplasia: disease due to a defect in GS alpha protein of adenylate cyclase (GNAS-1) marked by fibrous tissue replacement of bone with resultant deformities and clinical appearance of café-au-lait skin pigmentation and precocious puberty; **Albright syndrome.**

neurofibroma: abnormal proliferation of nerve sheath cells; **Schwann tumor.**

periarticular fibrositis: inflammatory condition of fibrous tissue surrounding a joint.

periosteal fibroma: fibrous tumor of bone-covering tissue.

pseudosarcomatous fibromatosis: disease of extensive subcutaneous fibroma formation; **subcutaneous pseudosarcomatous fibromatosis, proliferative fasciitis.**

Lipo- Root Diseases

Lipo- (Gr. *lipos*, fat) is a combining form denoting relationship to fat and fatty tissue. There are several disease processes based on this root.

lipochondrodystrophy: lipodystrophy as it affects cartilage.

lipodystrophy: defective metabolism of fat that results in the absence of subcutaneous fat, either partial or total. May be congenital or acquired.

lipofibroma: fibrous fatty tumor.

lipoma: fatty tumor; tumor made up of fat cells.

Myxo- Root Diseases

Myxo- (Gr. *myxa*, mucus) is a combining form denoting relationship to mucus. Myxomatous cells contain mucous material that is clear in appearance. These cells are naturally found in the intervertebral disks, but when seen elsewhere they usually represent an abnormality. Myxomatous cells contain the mucopolysaccharide (proteoglycan) material, which could rupture, causing mucous cysts to form. Terms containing *myxo-* indicate the presence of this type of cell.

myxofibroma: tumor containing both fibrous and myxomatous tissue.

myxoma: tumor containing myxoid cells.

myxosarcoma: sarcoma containing myxomatous tissue.

Muco- Root Diseases

The Latin word *mucus,* for the purposes of orthopaedics does not imply secretions but rather the association of tissues that contain certain chemicals called *mucopolysaccharides,* which, when sufficient collection of material occurs, are in the form of a clear jelly and seen in certain cysts. Elsewhere in medicine, the terms *mucus* and *mucous* relate particularly to the gut and respiratory tract.

ganglion cyst: a sac, usually 1 mm to more than 5 cm in size, commonly near a joint; contains a mix of collagen, proteoglycans, and other proteins with water such that the content appears clear and gelatinous. Ganglion cysts may occur anywhere, including within bone (intraosseous ganglion) and just under the periosteum (periosteal ganglion).

mucopolysaccharidosis: any of a variety of heritable disease states resulting from abnormalities in mucopolysaccharide (sugars containing SO_4, COOH, and NH_2) metabolism. These mainly affect cartilage in terms of orthopaedic diseases and cause stunted growth.

mucous cyst: in orthopaedics, a benign cyst under the fingernail.

Ligament, Tendon, Bursa, and Fascia Diseases

Desmo- Root Diseases

Desmo- (Gr. *desmos*, ligament)is a combining form denoting relationship to a band, bond, or ligament. Ligaments are composed of fibrous tissue that binds the joints together. Desmogenous dysfunctions and diseases may be any of the following:

desmectasis: stretching of a ligament. (archaic)

desmitis: inflammation of a ligament. (archaic)

desmocytoma: now called *fibrosarcoma*. (archaic)

desmodynia: pain in a ligament; **desmalgia.** (archaic)

desmoid: collection of fibrous tissue occurring at the insertion of a tendon (cortical desmoid) or arising from soft tissue of an extremity. The latter is a true tumor, recurrent but not malignant; **periosteal desmoid, extraabdominal desmoid.**

desmoma: a fibroma; a benign fibrous tumor.

desmopathy: any pathologic disease of a ligament.

desmoplasia: formation and development of fibrous tissue.

desmoplastic: producing or forming adhesions.

desmorrhexis: rupture of a ligament.

desmosis: disease of connective tissue. (archaic)

extraabdominal desmoid (aggressive fibromatosis): a desmoid tumor that recurs with extensions in fascial planes but with no metastasis.

Eponymic Ligamentous Diseases

Duplay d.: capsulitis of the glenohumeral joint area; **frozen shoulder.**

MGHL cord: pattern where the *m*iddle gleno-*h*umeral *l*igament is cord-like and enlarged.

Pellegrini-Stieda d.: ligamentous calcification of the medial collateral ligament of the knee following trauma.

Tendo-/Teno- Root Diseases

Tendo- and *teno-* (L. *tendo*; Gr. *tenōn*) are combining forms denoting relationship to a tendon. A tendon is a fibrous cord of connective tissue in which the fibers of a muscle end and by which the muscle is attached to bone.

tendonitis: although this term implies an inflammation of tendons or of tendon-muscle attachments, it is now clear that many tendons that have focal swelling and soreness do not have evidence of the increased blood supply seen with inflammation. The biologic effects to the tendon that creates the symptoms in these cases has no apparent effect on the blood supply; **tenontitis, tenonitis, tenositis.**

  bicipital t.: inflammation of a biceps muscle at tendon insertion of shoulder.

  calcific t.: inflammation associated with calcium deposits in the tendon and/or bursa (i.e., subacromial or subdeltoid bursa) producing pain and tenderness and limiting motion of shoulder.

  tendonitis ossificans traumatica: development of ossification in areas of tendons due to trauma.

tenodynia: pain in a tendon; tenontodynia.

tenontagra: gouty affection of tendons. (archaic)

tenontophyma: tumorous growth in tendon. (archaic)

tenontothecitis: inflammation of a tendon sheath. (archaic)

tenoperiostitis: inflammation of muscle-tendon attachment to bone, for example, tennis elbow and golfer's elbow.

tenophyte: growth or concretion in tendon.

tenositis: inflammation of a tendon.

tenostosis: ossification of a tendon.

tenosynovitis: inflammation of a tendon sheath and synovial sac; tendosynovitis.

Other Tendon-Related Diseases

acute calcific tendonitis: rapid onset of pain and occasionally fever associated with swelling and redness. Most commonly confused with infection. Radiographs reveal subtle soft tissue calcification. Seen most commonly in the hands and wrist but may be seen in the shoulder, elbow, hip, or knee. Rarely seen in the small, deep anterior neck muscles. This condition may be called **acute calcific retropharyngeal tendonitis** and is important to orthopaedics because it is a rare but benign cause of severe neck pain.

Albert achillodynia: discomfort felt around terminal segment of heel cord; **achillodynia, achillobursitis.**

de Quervain d.: tenosynovitis of the abductor pollicis longus and extensor pollicis brevis.

enthesopathy: degenerative disorders of ligaments, muscles, and tendon attachments to bone, the central structure in the disease process. **Enthesis** is the site of a tendon, ligament, or muscle attachment to bone. However, the term is more specifically applied to certain degenerative disorders of tendons such as supraspinatus and Achilles tendonitis. Because a neighboring bursa may be involved, it is sometimes called a bursitis.

enthesitis: inflammation resulting from stress on muscle or tendon that is attached to bone. There is a strong tendency toward fibrosis, calcification, and even rupture.

epicondylitis: inflammation of the tendon origins on the medial epicondyle (*golfer's elbow, thrower's elbow*) or the lateral epicondyle (*tennis elbow*).

Bursa-Related Diseases

Bursae (pl.) are closed sacs of fibrous tissue lined with synovial membrane, filled with viscid fluid, and situated in places in tissue where friction would otherwise inhibit function, such as near joints. Most disorders of bursae are part of another disease process.

bursitis: inflammation of a bursa at site of bony prominences between muscles or tendons.

  calcific bursitis: deposition of calcium in a bursa, usually associated with inflammation; can often be seen on a radiograph.

bursolith: calculus or concretion in a bursa.

bursopathy: any pathologic condition of bursae.

Fascia-Related Diseases

Fasciae (L. *fascia*, band) are bands of fibrous tissue that lie deep to the skin and form an investment for muscles and various organs of the body. *Retinacula* (*retinaculum,* sing.) are also thickened bands that bind muscles and tendons of distal portion of limbs into position. There are several processes that are disease related.

Dupuytren contracture: thickening and contracture of the palmar fascia of the hand resulting in flexion deformities of the fingers.

fasciitis: inflammation of fascia. Usually an anatomic structure is named when describing the location of the fasciitis, for example, plantar fasciitis, inflammation of the fascia of the sole of the foot.

nodular fasciitis: fasciitis resulting in the formation of nodules.

Joint Diseases (Arthro-, Synovio-, Capsulo-, Ankylo-)

The joint (*arthro-*) has a smooth inner lining or fluid sac (synovium) and a strong fibrous outer connective tissue enclosure (*capsulo-*). Affections of the joint cartilage, synovium, and capsule may result in transient or permanent functional changes. When motion is severely or completely lost, **ankylosis** (an abnormal fusion of a joint) is the result. The terms in this section relate to loss of joint function or a change in appearance of the joint. Joint function depends on its surrounding tissue. Diseases or dysfunctions affecting the joint spaces are presented here.

Arthro- Root Diseases

Arthro- (Gr. *Arthron,* joint) is a combining form denoting relationship to a joint, the junction where two bones meet and articulate with one another. Articulatio (Latin) is a general term for joint. The *arthro-* root diseases are as follows:

arthralgia: pain in a joint; arthrodynia.

arthrempyesis: infection in a joint; arthroempyesis.

arthritis: pathologic inflammation of a joint; may be crippling; can become a degenerative joint disease. Various types are **osteoarthritis, gouty a., rheumatoid a., septic a., traumatic a., infectious a., allergenic a.,** and **hemophilic a.**

arthrocace: infected cavity of a joint; caries. (archaic)

arthrocele: swollen joint. (archaic)

arthrochalasis: abnormal relaxation or flaccidity of a joint. (archaic)

arthrochondritis: inflammation of the cartilages of a joint. (archaic)

arthrodysplasia: deformity of various joints; hereditary condition. (archaic)

arthrogryposis: due to a variety of sex-linked recessive and autosomal recessive disorders that lead to decreased fetal movement that leads to soft tissue contractures affecting two or more joints.

arthrokatadysis: limitation of motion of the hip resulting from protrusio acetabuli (deep-shelled acetabulum).

arthrokleisis: ankylosis of a joint. (archaic)

arthrolith: deposit of calculus in a joint. (archaic)

arthromeningitis: synovitis; inflammation of the membranous lining of a joint. (archaic)

arthroncus: joint swelling; arthrophyma. (archaic)

arthroneuralgia: nerve pain in a joint. (archaic)

arthronosos: disease of joints. (archaic)

arthropathy: any joint disease.

arthrophyte: abnormal growth in a joint cavity.

arthropyosis: suppuration, or formation of pus, in a joint cavity.

arthrorheumatism: articular rheumatism. (archaic)

arthrosclerosis: hardening or stiffening of a joint. (archaic)

arthrosis: disease or abnormal condition of a joint.

arthrosteitis: inflammation of any bony joint structure. (archaic)

arthrosynovitis: inflammation of the synovial membrane of a joint. (archaic)

arthroxerosis: chronic osteoarthritis. (archaic)

Other Joint Diseases and Conditions

cystic arthrosis: development of large cysts just under the bony surface of a joint. It is not clear whether this is due to cystic degeneration within the bone that leaves the articular cartilage intact or to synovial invasion from the joint. Condition progresses to degenerative arthritis. This condition is probably separate from ganglions that form within the bone and are not associated with arthritic progression.

diffuse idiopathic sclerosing hyperostosis (DISH): excess bone formation at the margins of large joints, particularly the lumbar spine and hips.

flail joint: complete loss of ligamentous stability.

frozen shoulder: severe loss of motion in the shoulder joint resulting from inflammation of the capsule.

hemarthrosis: extravasation of blood into a joint or synovial cavity.

hydrarthrosis: accumulation of watery fluid in the joint cavity.

hypertrophic arthritis: increased bone formation around the joint, as seen on radiographs; *osteoarthritis.*

internal derangement of joint: commonly named "internal knee injuries," particularly when the precise nature of the injury is unknown.

joint mice: loose pieces of cartilage or other organic material in the joint.

pannus: growth of blood vessels onto margin of articular cartilage surface.

pauciarticular: involving a few joints as opposed to many joints.

polyarthritis: inflammation of many joints.

pseudoarthrosis: false joints that result from nonunion of a fracture or from a pathologic bone condition.

pustulotic osteoarthropathy: pain, swelling, and radiographic findings of hypertrophy and sclerotic changes involving the sternum, ribs, and clavicle associated with the skin condition pustulosis palmaris et plantaris. The sacrum, spine, and peripheral joints may also show radiographic changes. The cause is unknown.

rice bodies: small, glistening, soft, loose bodies either in joints or bursae; *loose fibrocartilage tissue.*

suppurative arthritis: bacterial infection causing pain, swelling, tenderness, redness, and effusion; **pyarthrosis.**

synarthrosis: ankylosis and contracture; usually caused by arthritic joint disease.

villous lipomatous proliferation: rare disorder of synovial joint lining in which there is fatty proliferation with the formation of numerous villous formations. The term **lipoma arborescens** was applied to this condition. Because it is not a neoplasm, the villous lipomatous proliferation term is preferred.

Eponymic Joint Diseases

Behçet syndrome: disease of undetermined etiology that may produce joint complaints predominantly in young people in the third decade of life. Marked by oral and genital ulcerations and eye and skin lesions. Often arthritis, thrombophlebitis, gastrointestinal lesions, and central nervous system lesions also occur.

Kawasaki d.: mucocutaneous lymph node syndrome in children characterized by fever, exanthematous skin disease, and sometimes arthritis (30%–40%).

Lyme d.: inflammatory arthritis involving usually a few joints, particularly the knees, caused by an organism that is transmitted by a tick.

Reiter syndrome: arthritis of various joints, usually associated with one or more of the triad of urethral drip, conjunctivitis, and oral mucosal lesions.

Synovio-Related Diseases

Synovial fluid, or synovia, is an alkaline viscid transparent fluid resembling egg white that is found in joint cavities, tendon sheaths, and bursae and is responsible for lubrication and nourishment of these joint structures. Synovial membrane is the inner lining of a joint, which is a two-layer membrane on a bed of fat composed of certain cells that produce synovial fluid; other cells act as phagocytes. Related disease processes are the following:

synovial cyst: accumulation of fluid in any bursa forming a firm cystic structure. The fluid often becomes gelatinous as seen in a ganglion. The contents and structures of these cysts are often indistinguishable from a ganglion. Some can communicate with a joint or tendon sheath.

> **popliteal cyst:** seen behind the knee, this cyst usually involves the gastrocnemius-semimembranosus bursa.
>
> **antefemoral cyst:** located in the suprapatellar area.
>
> **anteromedial cyst:** found in association with the pes anserinus bursa below the anteromedial joint line.
>
> **tibiofibular cyst:** associated with the tibiofibular joint, which in 10% of people communicates with the knee.

synovial osteochondromatosis: formation by the synovium of cartilage bodies, which develop into bone.

synoviochondromatosis: synovial formation of cartilage bodies.

synovitis: inflammation of synovial membrane, which may be associated with swelling.

Miscellaneous Synovial Diseases

pigmented villonodular synovitis: inflammation of synovium with production of pigment, giant cells, and other characteristic cell types.

villous synovitis: inflammation of joint lining, resulting in long fronds of synovium.

Capsulo-Related Diseases

The capsule is the thick fibrous tissue enclosing the cavity of the synovial joint and defines the limits of the joint; more *joint c., synovial c.* There are two related dysfunctions.

adhesive capsulitis: adhesive inflammation between joint capsule and the peripheral articular cartilage of the shoulder, obscuring the subdeltoid bursa. It produces a painful shoulder, stiffness, and may result in limited joint motion; *frozen shoulder, adhesive bursitis.*

capsulitis: inflammation of the capsule.

Ankylo-Root Diseases

The combining form *ankylo-* means bent or deformed. It was originally used to describe untreated deforming loss of joint function. Now such terms apply to joints fused congenitally or those that are aligned normally because of a surgical process. Therefore the implication of *ankylo-* is not necessarily bent or deformed but rather complete fusion or restricted motion of a joint.

ankylodactylia: adhesions of fingers or toes to one another.

ankylosis: consolidation and abnormal immobility of a joint caused by fibrous or bone tissue bridging the joint space.

> *bony a.:* abnormal union of bones at joint site; **true ankylosis.**
>
> *extracapsular a.:* caused by rigidity of structure exterior to joint capsule, usually a surgically implanted piece of bone.
>
> *false a.:* results from other causes not related to the abnormal union of bones comprising the joint.
>
> *fibrous a.:* caused by formation of fibrous bands within the joint.
>
> *intracapsular a.:* caused by undue rigidity of structure within the joint capsule.
>
> *ligamentous a.:* results from rigidity of ligaments.
>
> *spurious a.:* false ankylosis.

Vascular Diseases and Conditions

Blood Vessels

All tissues of the body are supplied with nutrients and oxygen by blood vessels. These vessels are subject to an assortment of disease processes. The larger named arteries are usually impaired by arteriosclerosis or trauma; the larger named veins are usually impaired by trauma or thrombosis; and the smaller, unnamed vessels (on either side of the circulation) can be injured by arteriosclerosis, trauma, or systemic degenerative disorders (e.g., collagen vascular diseases). In addition to these, the heart itself can be afflicted by diseases of the arteries that feed the heart muscle, causing deterioration of the muscle (cardiomyopathy).

Trauma and arteriosclerosis (hardening of the arteries) are the two most frequent arterial conditions that are seen by the orthopaedic surgeon. However, the orthopaedist will often see a host of other vascular disorders or symptoms that influence the treatment of a musculoskeletal problem. Often, patients with these specific disease entities are referred to the peripheral vascular surgeon, and a combined effort is made to restore function. The venous and arterial disorders, collagen vascular disorders, and blood vessel tumors are considered here.

Venous Disorders

deep venous thrombosis (DVT): blood clots in the deep venous circulation usually of the lower extremity, in the calf, thigh, or pelvis. Portions of these clots may break off and lodge in the lungs, causing pulmonary emboli. These clots in the veins eventually destroy the valves of the veins and can cause chronic problems related to venous insufficiency.

phlebitis: inflammation of a vein; may be a result of infection, inflammation, or trauma and is usually associated with thrombus in that vein (thrombophlebitis).

phlebothrombosis: clot in a vein; phlebitis with secondary thrombosis.

postphlebitic syndrome: chronic venous insufficiency of lower limbs resulting from deep venous thrombosis. Develops with loss of function of valves in veins, allowing blood to pool and cause swelling, pain, leg ulceration, and varicose veins. Also the result of scar-thickened deep veins.

pulmonary embolism (PE): acute obstruction to circulation in lungs as a result of a clot that has migrated from the pelvic or leg veins and lodged in the lung. A life-threatening problem requiring anticoagulant, thrombolytic therapy, and sometimes surgery.

thrombophlebitis: inflammation of a vein associated with thrombosis (blood clots) usually in the lower limbs. The clot can also become infected, becoming septic thrombophlebitis.

thrombosis: formation of a clot (thrombus) within a blood vessel that results in occlusion or stenosis of the vessel, which may cause infarction of tissue supplied by that vessel.

varices (*sing.* **-ix**): enlarged and tortuous (twisted) veins or lymphatic vessels, usually of the lower limbs; many types; **varicose veins.**

varicose veins: a degenerative condition of veins whereby the muscle fibers in the walls of the vessel become stretched out and baggy, like the elastic in an old pair of underpants. The valves become incompetent and blood falls back the wrong way creating a reflux and further wall failure. Return flow becomes inefficient, producing pain, tenderness, and swelling.

venous insufficiency (reflux): malfunction of venous valves that allow blood to flow in a retrograde (backward) direction; **postphlebitic syndrome.**

Arterial Disorders

aneurysm: thin-walled, dilated segment of a vessel wall that may be caused by degeneration from arteriosclerosis, congenital abnormality, or trauma. Complications of aneurysms include rupture, thrombosis, or breakoff of a blood clot that has collected in the aneurysm.

arterial insufficiency: inadequate blood flow to an organ or extremity often caused by arteriosclerotic narrowing or occlusion of the blood vessel restricting blood flow. In severe cases, necrosis and gangrene may develop, requiring amputation of a limb.

arterial occlusive disease: hardening of the arteries; **arteriosclerosis.**

arteriosclerosis: name for degenerative process that affects most blood vessels in most people (in varying degrees) and begins in early teens. Its progression is related in part to genetics, diet, smoking, and high blood pressure. It can be exacerbated by injuries such as trauma or surgery; it causes narrowing and irregular surfaces in blood vessels, where fatty plaque forms on vessel walls and occludes the blood supply, which leads to ischemia. It is the most frequent problem in arteries; **atherosclerosis.**

arteriovenous fistula (AVF): abnormal communication between an artery and a vein; **AV fistula.** May be the result of trauma or may be created intentionally for dialysis access. See **malformation, arteriovenous.**

atheroma: localized collection of arteriosclerosis (thickened arterial intima—plaque) that has degenerated.

blue toe syndrome: bluish or black tender and painful discoloration of a toe. It is the result of a localized acute ischemia of the toe caused by distal embolization of platelet aggregates or arteriosclerotic plaque, which then occludes the small end vessels. This represents a proximal emboligenic source, for example, aneurysm or significant arteriosclerotic plaque.

Buerger disease: thromboangiitis obliterans: an inflammation of the arteries (and veins) in extremity causing severe ischemia; occurs usually in young smokers and is a pathologic variant of arteriosclerosis.

cerebrovascular accident (CVA): (outdated term) See stroke.

chilblains: breakdown of skin and swelling of the hands and feet from overexposure to cold moisture; *thermal injuries.*

claudication: inadequate blood flow to large muscle groups of lower limbs resulting from hardening of the arteries, causing pain, numbness, or heaviness in muscle groups brought on by exercise and relieved promptly by rest; may produce similar symptoms in the upper limbs after prolonged use; *intermittent claudication.*

compartment syndrome: compromise of circulation and function of tissue within a closed space caused by increased pressure within that space, with diminished oxygenated blood supply; may be due to overexertion of leg muscles, a tight bandage, or trauma-related injury. The syndrome may self-correct or progress, with eventual muscle necrosis (ischemia), loss of arterial blood supply, nerve palsy, or loss of limb. The most commonly affected compartments are the anterior leg **(anterior compartment syndrome),** volar forearm (leading to Volkmann ischemic contracture), and anterior thigh **(rectus femoris syndrome).**

diabetic foot infection: diabetes alters the hormonal and cellular response to infection both by recognition of the invading bacteria and the attempts to destroy bacteria. Secondly, blood flow can be limited by thickened blood vessels and arteriosclerosis producing relative ischemia. Thirdly, the neurologic response is blunted, creating sensory deficit and decreased shunting of blood to the affected area. Additionally, altered anatomy, such as tightened tendons, bony changes, dry skin, and deformed nails can create a foot susceptible to infection, ulceration, osteomyelitis, and progression to limb loss.

embolus (*pl.* **emboli**): blood clot or piece of atheromatous debris that blocks an artery or vein. Can also be made up of an air bubble, fat, portion of tumor, or piece of prosthetic material. An embolus may cause a heart attack if in the heart, a stroke if in the brain, and acute ischemia if in the lower limbs.

fibromuscular dysplasia (FMD): uncommon degenerative disease of the arteries often affecting the renal arteries of young females. The problem causes narrowing of the vessel with weblike deformities that appear as a string of beads on an arteriogram. Can also cause aneurysm.

fistula: abnormal communication between any two structures that normally do not communicate; can be the result of trauma, arteriosclerosis, or surgical procedure. An arteriovenous fistula may be created and used for hemodialysis. (See AVF.)

frostbite: damage to tissue resulting from exposure to cold; may lower blood supply sufficiently to cause permanent sensory loss, chronic pain, or partial limb loss.

gangrene: sign of substantial ischemia involving death of tissue. May be dry (not infected) or wet (infected).

Hollenhorst plaque: cholesterol emboli in a small retinal eye artery. Usually indicative of carotid arteriosclerosis. May represent a transient ischemic attack (TIA) or warning for a stroke.

infarct: area of ischemic necrosis resulting from acute interruption of blood supply. This term is often applied to areas of the brain or heart.

ischemia: acute or chronic decreased blood flow (perfusion) to organ or limb caused by obstruction of inflow of arterial blood or by vasoconstriction. Acutely, the symptoms include the six *P*s: pain, pallor, pulselessness, paresthesias, paralysis, and poikilothermia (coldness).

kinking: bending of an artery, causing pain; result of trauma or body position.

malformation, arteriovenous (AVM): congenital arteriovenous connection often resulting in disfigurement or malfunction. Often seen as a discolored area on the skin, but may represent a much larger diversion of blood such that it interferes with organ function. Its continuing presence may interfere with the heart because of the large alteration in flow that it creates.

pallor: loss of color of skin representing a markedly decrease in blood flow, either acute or chronic; may be present only with the elevation of the extremity.

peripheral arterial occlusion (PAO): results from buildup of atherosclerosis (fatty tissue) that can cut off blood supply to the limbs and feet.

popliteal cyst: degeneration of the wall of the popliteal artery resulting in a cystic-like structure within the wall of the artery that can partially or completely obstruct the artery. Popliteal arterial cyst is a more complete term to avoid confusion with the more common synovial or ganglion type.

popliteal entrapment: partial or complete obstruction of popliteal artery as a result of abnormal location of adjacent medial head of the gastrocnemius muscle. It may include an artery, vein, and/or nerve.

pseudoaneurysm: an aneurysm that does not include all three layers of the blood vessel wall. True aneurysms contain all three layers. Pseudoaneurysms can be the result of a traumatic partial disruption of a blood vessel wall, or the result of an infection that allows a surgical anastomosis to come apart slowly. An infected prosthetic graft is a typical example.

rest pain: distal foot pain caused by acute or chronic arterial ischemia representing a significant decrease in blood flow, usually from hardening of the arteries. The pain is burning and sharp in nature. Symptoms may be relieved temporarily by a dependent position.

rubor (dependent): dark purplish-red color to foot when foot is hung over the edge of bed. It represents maximally dilated capillary beds that are responding to decreased arterial inflow and their subsequent fill by gravity.

stroke: ischemia of a portion of the brain as a result of an occluded blood vessel from an embolus arising from the heart or great vessels of the neck; often the result of hardening of the arteries, a rupture of the blood vessel in the brain, or a tumor. (Formerly called a cerebrovascular accident [CVA].)

Sudeck atrophy: vascular reflex in a limb, caused by trauma, resulting in a red, stiff, and severely painful limb; referred to as "causalgia" when caused by trauma involving a large area or affecting a large nerve.

subclavian steal syndrome: reversed blood flow down the vertebral or carotid artery neck vessels away from the brain. Produced by arm activity in the face of a blocked subclavian artery. Flow is "stolen" down these vessels to meet the needs of the arm muscles, producing dizziness, syncope, or visual symptoms because of transient decreased blood flow.

transient ischemic attack (TIA): transient neurologic deficit that clears within 24 hours. Usually the result of decreased blood flow to the portion of brain from a blood clot from either the heart or extracranial carotid vessels. Usually from hardening of the arteries—atheromatous plaque breaks off and lodges in the vessels of the brain or eye.

venous thromboembolic d.: a clot in the venous system, usually the legs or lungs, caused by stasis, endothelial injury, or hypercoagulable state.

Volkmann contracture: final state of an unrelieved forearm compartment syndrome; decreased blood supply to forearm muscles resulting in muscle death, contractures of tendons to wrist and hand, and a claw-hand deformity. This usually starts out as a compartment syndrome that develops after an elbow or forearm fracture.

Collagen Vascular Disorders

Collagen vascular diseases are a series of disorders relating to the basic building blocks of the body, that is, collagen. The walls of blood vessels are made up of collagen, a type of protein seen in all connective tissue such as bone, cartilage, and tendon. Certain diseases affect the collagen, particularly in scattered blood vessels.

Through a variety of mechanisms, the immune system of the body begins to attack, thereby causing degeneration in small blood vessels and/or parts of the bony anatomy (joint capsule, synovial fluid of joint and synovium). The systemic inflammatory condition that results can be mildly inconvenient or severely disabling or can result in death. Certain diseases such as rheumatoid arthritis affect this collagen and, as a result, interfere with the function of bones, joints, and blood vessels. The term *inflammatory joint disease* is often used to describe arthritis, but this general term is also applied to gout, pseudogout, and some other systemic causes of arthritis.

Dyscollagenosis and **systemic connectivitis** are older terms specifically related to the collagen vascular disorders that are due to immune processes such as rheumatoid arthritis, systemic lupus erythematosus, Sjögren syndrome, progressive systemic sclerosis, polyarteritis nodosa, polymyositis, dermatomyositis, and eosinophilic fasciitis. This spectrum of disorders represents the effects on the different collagens of the joint lining and vascular walls.

The treatment of these disorders is often complicated and frustrating for both patient and physician. Medication often involves corticosteroids (antiinflammatory drugs) and nonsteroidal antiinflammatory drugs (ibuprofen, aspirin), and often drugs that directly interfere with the immune mechanism of the body (antimetabolites). **Rheumatology** is the specialty devoted to the diagnosis and treatment of these systemic conditions. A rheumatologist is an internal medical specialist. Although rheumatologists often deal with nonsystemic joint diseases, specialty training in this field equips them with the pharmacologic knowledge required to diagnose the broad spectrum of autoimmune and metabolic joint disorders.

Terms associated with these various conditions are discussed here along with a series of other miscellaneous disorders.

acrosclerosis: thickening of the skin and other soft tissues of the distal part of a limb. This is usually a part of a larger disease complex such as scleroderma or CREST syndrome.

ankylosing spondylitis: inflammatory joint disease mainly affecting the spine, hips, and pelvis. Seen most commonly in young men, this can lead to fusion of the spine with deformity, depending on the position of the spine during the fusion process. Seen in the child, the disorder is called Marie-Strümpell disease or rheumatoid spondylitis.

arteritis: inflammation of small arteries.

calcinosis circumscripta: quadrad of calcium deposits in the skin (calcinosis cutis), Raynaud phenomenon, scleroderma, and telangiectasia is seen in this collagen disease that has been considered a variant of scleroderma.

CREST syndrome (limited scleroderma): complex of calcinosis of articular tissue associated with

*R*aynaud phenomenon, *e*sophageal dysmotility, *s*clerodactyly, and *t*elangiectasia. This condition appears to be less aggressive than scleroderma.

dermatomyositis: idiopathic, autoimmune, inflammatory myopathy characterized by proximal limb and neck weakness. Muscles may become painful, weak, and stiff. A rash can appear on the knees, knuckles, and elbows. The pathologic findings are muscle necrosis and regeneration.

ergotism: acute or chronic effects of ergot alkaloids on the blood flow to an organ such as the brain or limbs. Ergot alkaloids are in some plants and medicines that are taken for headaches.

Felty syndrome: a combination of chronic rheumatoid arthritis, enlarged spleen, and a reduced number of granulocytes in the white blood count.

focal scleroderma: disease of unknown etiology characterized by circumscribed areas of fibrosis of the skin, subcutaneous fat, fascia, and muscle into bone. It is usually restricted to a limb and usually occurs in children and young adults; **Addison's keloid.**

intermittent hydrarthrosis: rare disorder characterized by recurrent swelling in joints with no associated problems or deformity.

Jaccoud syndrome: deformity of hands and feet as a result of recurrent episodes of rheumatic fever or lupus synovitis. Often mistaken for rheumatoid arthritis.

lupus erythematosus: disease affecting not only the joints but also heart, heart lining, and circulation in bone. It is life threatening, although a protracted mild course is possible. This disease may be called **systemic lupus erythematosus** to distinguish it from discoid lupus, a more benign process.

Marie-Strümpell d.: begins in childhood, similar to rheumatoid arthritis, usually resulting in ankylosis of the spine and involvement of the liver and spleen; **rheumatoid** or **ankylosing spondylitis.**

Mönckeberg sclerosis: calcification of the middle coat of small and medium-sized muscular arteries; **medial arteriosclerosis.**

palindromic rheumatism: recurrent acute arthritis and periarthritis with symptom-free intervals of days to months. A number of patients with this disorder develop rheumatoid arthritis.

polyarteritis nodosa: disease causing nodules in small arteries with some microscopic clotting, resulting in muscle cramps and eventual loss of muscle tone; can be severe.

progressive systemic sclerosis: spectrum of disorders that are characterized by fibrosis and degenerative changes in the skin. This includes scleroderma and CREST syndrome.

Raynaud d. or phenomenon: small arterioles of upper limbs, particularly of the fingertips, become extremely sensitive to cold, and the vessels undergo segmental spasm, interrupting blood flow to tissue; occasionally progresses to necrosis and dry gangrene in fingertips.

rheumatoid arthritis: generalized inflammatory joint disease. In children, it is called **juvenile rheumatoid arthritis** and **Still disease.** The disease may result in mild, lifelong discomfort, or it may become severely crippling; in some cases, there is associated skin nodularity. Certain laboratory studies confirm the diagnosis (positive rheumatoid factor).

scleroderma: disease causing a waxy thickening of the skin and classically affecting swallowing; tends to be severely progressive.

Sjögren syndrome: a group of conditions including keratoconjunctivitis sicca (dry eyes), arthritis, dry mouth, and enlargement of the parotid glands.

vasoconstriction: narrowing of vessel lumen caused by contraction of muscular vessel walls.

vasodilatation: enlargement of vessel lumen caused by relaxing of muscular vessel wall.

vasospastic: localized intermittent contraction of a blood vessel.

Blood Vessel Tumors

hemangioendothelioma: tumor composed mostly of endothelial cells of the inner walls of capillary vessels.

hemangioma: any benign small-vessel tumor of dilated blood vessels; may be flush with the skin with a violescent, patchy discoloration or elevated like a violescent or red mole. Size may vary from 1 mm to large area of the body.

hemangiopericytoma: spindle cell tumor with a rich vascular network; arises from pericytes.

hemangiosarcoma: malignant blood vessel tumor; **angiosarcoma.**

Associated Vascular Conditions

acrocyanosis: mottling of the skin of the extremity not produced by major vascular occlusions. May be related to an emotional change or temperature.

atrophy: reduction in size of an anatomic structure, often related to disuse or decreased blood supply.

arrhythmia: abnormal rhythm of the heart.

bradycardia: abnormal slowing of heart rate, usually less than 60 beats/minute.

bruit: abnormal sound on mediate auscultation over a blood vessel or the heart that indicates turbulence.

congestive heart failure: condition in which heart is unable to pump out venous blood returning to it, resulting in pooling of venous blood and accumulation of fluid in various parts of the body (lungs, legs, etc.).

cyanosis: bluish-purple discoloration of the skin or nail beds; represents decreased blood flow to that area.

hypercholesterolemia: elevated blood cholesterol level; **hypercholesteremia, hypercholesterinemia.**

hypertension: elevated blood pressure, either temporary or permanent; may be an elevation of the systolic or diastolic blood vessels or pressure.

hypotension: blood pressure below normal.

hypovolemia: loss of normal amount of circulating blood volume; could be the result of hemorrhage from trauma (or from ulcer).

hypoxia: decreased amount of oxygen in any given tissue.

myocardial infarction (MI): acute or chronic blockage of blood vessels to the heart, resulting in localized area of ischemia (heart attack).

necrosis: pathologic definition of death of tissues caused by lack of blood supply to that part.

normotensive: referring to normal blood pressure.

occlusion: closed or shut, such as an occluded artery or vein.

palpitation: sensation either by patient or examiner of irregular heartbeat.

phlegmasia cerulea dolens: an acute, rare condition that includes a nonpitting edema (swelling that cannot be indented with pressure) in the legs associated with a cyanotic mottled appearance and high muscle compartment pressures. This has been associated with the use of vena cava filters.

stasis: decrease or absence of flow in the venous circulation.

stenosis: narrowing of lumen of blood vessel; a stricture.

tachycardia: abnormal increase in heart rate, usually more than 100 beats/minute in an adult.

Neurologic Diseases

Neuro- (Gr. *neuron*, nerve) is a combining form denoting the relationship to a nerve or nerves, or to the nervous system in general. Of all the specialties in medicine, neurology interrelates with orthopaedics more often than any other. The presenting symptoms of certain neurologic disorders may be quite similar to those of some orthopaedic disorders or diseases in that they result in muscular loss, altered function, and possible deformities, particularly in growing individuals.

In orthopaedic diagnoses, the nervous system is considered in two portions, the central and the peripheral. The central portion is composed of the brain and spinal cord and their covering soft tissues. The peripheral portion is composed of all the nerves in the body. Because some diseases affect both the central and peripheral nervous systems simultaneously, discussion of both is presented in an alphabetic listing of nerve disorders, except for some eponymic terms that belong to a specific category. The same term may be defined several times in this chapter to avoid cross-referencing.

General Neurologic Diseases

amyotrophic lateral sclerosis (ALS): disease principally of the spinal cord, seen in adult life; results in loss of motor control and eventual death; **Charcot d., Lou Gehrig d.**

apoplexy: old term used to describe a stroke, a bleeding into or loss of blood supply to the brain. (archaic)

apraxia: inability to perform purposeful movements where there is no sensory or motor impairment; **kinetic a., motor a.**

arachnoiditis: inflammatory disease of the covering, spiderweb-like membrane of the spinal cord and nerves. In the lumbar spine, this condition can lead to fibrosis that will bind the roots of the cauda equina.

ataxia: motor incoordination.

atonia: lack of tone or tension; relaxation, flaccidity.

autonomic dysreflexia: syndrome marked by muscle spasms, low blood pressure, headache, sweating, goose bumps, and other signs of autonomic nervous system instability. Can be associated with spontaneous joint dislocation.

axonotmesis: disruption of nerve plasma without disruption of the axon sheath, resulting in a recovery of nerve function over a period of up to 3 years.

Barre-Lieou syndrome: degenerative or arthritic changes of C3, C4, and intervertebral disks, often involving the fifth and sixth cervical nerves. Affects mainly middle-aged and older patients, many of whom have associated complaints of dizziness, nausea, headaches, transitory deafness, blurred vision, and loss of balance because of presumed involvement of the cervical sympathetic nervous system and the vertebral artery.

causalgia: lesion of a peripheral nerve containing sensory fibers manifested by burning pain, hypersensitivity, and paresthesias in the limb. A painful condition that occurs after trauma, infection, or vascular inflammation of extremity; associated with a fracture or dislocation with soft tissue, nerve, and vascular injury. To distinguish this from similar disorders in which a nerve is not involved, the term causalgia has been used. The terms **reflex sympathetic dystrophy, posttraumatic reflex dystrophy, Sudeck atrophy, mimocausalgia,** and **algodystrophy** are used for those disorders in which there is a similar exaggerated response to an injury such as fracture, sprain, laceration, or other minor insult.

cerebral palsy (CP): very general term applied to central nervous system disorders found at birth or infancy that affect muscle control; can range from being almost undetectable to totally incapacitating and extremely deforming. There is mild to severe loss of motor control, which is called **diplegic CP** if it seems to affect primarily the lower extremities.

spastic CP: most common form; attempts by victim to use affected muscles result in uncontrolled contractions.

ataxic CP: additional elements of incoordination.

athetoid CP: uncontrolled writhing movements.

flaccid CP: very severe form in which muscle contractions cannot be initiated.

cheiroarthropathy: seen in peripheral neuropathy such as diabetic neuropathy, the person is unable to touch the palms together in the prayer position.

chorea: continuing uncontrolled jerking motions caused by brain disease; may occur as a result of rheumatic fever or other diseases; may be inherited, which is called **Huntington chorea; St. Vitus dance.**

dysautonomia: an often familial condition characterized by labile blood pressure, insensitivity to pain, abnormal gastrointestinal motility, ataxia, and spinal deformity.

dural ectasia: often seen with neurofibromatosis, thickening of the dural tissues may occur. This can lead to dissolution of the spinal elements and eventual spinal instability.

entrapment syndrome: symptoms caused by entrapment of a nerve in soft or hard tissue, for example, occipital nerve entrapment syndrome, a chronic muscle irritation of the neck, causing impingement on occipital nerve.

epilepsy: disorder of nervous system characterized by seizures in which there may be clonic and tonic muscular contractions and loss of consciousness.

grand mal e.: epilepsy marked by major convulsions, usually first tonic then clonic, oscillating eyeballs, feeble pulse, stupor, and unconsciousness.

petit mal e.: mild or minor attack (small seizures) of epilepsy without convulsions other than slight twitching of muscles of the face or extremities.

jacksonian e.: recurrent episodes of localized convulsive seizures or spasms limited to a part of the body, without loss of consciousness.

familial dysautonomia: autosomal recessive disorder of autonomic system causing loss of control of multiple organs including bowel, bladder, heart, and lungs.

ganglioneuroma: tumor made up of ganglion cells.

glioma: tumor arising from specialized connective tissue found in brain and spinal cord.

glomus tumor: benign tumor consisting of nerve and small-vessel components. These small lesions often produce severe pain and local vascular effects. They are often found near the tips of digits of the hands and feet.

Gross Motor Function Classification System (GMFCS): For cerebral palsy function based on self-initiated movement with emphasis on function

Level I: Walk indoors and outdoors and climb stairs without limitation. With running and sports, speed and balance are impaired.

Level II: Walk indoors and outdoors and climb stairs holding onto a railing but have limitation with uneven walking, inclines, crowds, and confined spaces.

Level III: Walk indoors or outdoors on a level surface with an assistive mobility devise. May climb stairs holding onto a railing. May propel a wheelchair manually or are transported when traveling for long distances, outdoors, or on uneven terrain.

Level IV: May walk for short distance on a walker or rely more on wheeled mobility at home, school, and community.

Level V: Unable to maintain antigravity head and trunk postures. No independent mobility.

hemiplegia: paralysis of one side of the body.

Klumpke palsy (lower obstetrical palsy): palsy of the lower cervical nerve roots C8 and T1; usually seen following an infant delivery but may be seen in adult life after trauma.

locomotor ataxia: see tabes dorsalis.

lumbar thecoperitoneal shunt syndrome: occurs after a thecoperitoneal shunt for idiopathic communicating hydrocephalus, characterized by severe, rigid, and progressive lumbar lordosis, severe bilateral restriction of straight leg raising, and abnormalities of stance and gait.

meralgia: pain in the thigh, usually caused by irritation of lateral cutaneous nerve of the thigh.

mononeuritis multiplex: impairment of sensation, usually in the foot, where there is increased or decreased sensitivity associated with a vasculitis, usually seen in rheumatoid vasculitis.

motor neuron d.: any disease caused by destruction of the nerve cells involved in voluntary muscle function.

upper motor neuron d.: any brain disorder that affects the normal pathways leading to voluntary muscle function.

lower motor neuron d.: disorder of the cells in the spinal cord, resulting in loss of motor function.

multiple sclerosis: slowly progressive disease of nervous system in which scattered areas of degeneration of the myelin occur; common in the spinal cord; cause unknown.

myopathy hand: characteristic hand dysfunction due to spinal cord injury. A loss of adduction power, extension of the ulnar two or three fingers, and an inability to grip and release rapidly with these fingers distinguishes this hand weakness from other hand dysfunctions due to peripheral nerve disorders.

neural tube defect: group of malformations of the brain and spinal cord that originate at various times during fetal development. The most commonly seen kind is meningomyelocele.

neuralgia: pain along the course of a nerve or nerves.

neuritis: inflammation of any nerve; usually painful.

neurogenic: occurring because of a nervous system disorder.

neurologic d.: any disease of the nervous system.

neurolysis: dissolution of the nerve tissue in disease process.

neuroma: this condition is not an actual tumor but is due to a tumescence in the nerve due to hypertrophy of the cells covering the inside and outside of the nerve.

traumatic n.: neuroma caused by a complete cutting of the nerve or by sufficient injury to cause excess scarring in the nerve.

amputation n.: a traumatic neuroma occurring after an amputation.

neuropathy: any disease of the peripheral nerves (those outside the brain and spinal cord).

neuropraxia: contusion of a nerve resulting in transient disruption of nerve function; less severe than axonotmesis or neurotmesis.

neurotmesis: complete transection of a nerve, resulting in cell death.

paralysis: loss or impairment of voluntary muscle function; palsy.

paralysis agitans: chronic nervous disease in later life marked by muscular tremor or by a peculiar gait; Parkinson disease.

paraplegia: paralysis of lower part of body or lower extremities.

paresis: incomplete loss of voluntary muscle function.

paresthesia: abnormal sensations such as numbness, burning, tickling, and crawling due to central or peripheral nerve lesions such as multiple sclerosis or locomotor ataxia.

pellagra: vitamin B_6 deficiency disease manifested by disorders of skin, alimentary tract, and nervous system.

peripheral neuropathy: diseases at or distal to the nerve root.

poliomyelitis: inflammation of gray matter of spinal cord; may result in loss of voluntary muscle control.

polyneuritis: inflammation of multiple nerves.

quadriplegia: loss of voluntary muscle function in both arms and legs.

radial tunnel syndrome (supinator syndrome): peripheral nerve syndrome due to compression of radial nerve as it passes through region between radial head and the arcade of Frohse.

radiculitis: inflammation of intradural portion of a spinal nerve root before its entrance into the intervertebral foramen, or of the portion between that foramen and the nerve plexus.

radiculoneuritis: inflammation of nerve root and nerve.

Rett syndrome: genetically determined disorder of the extrapyramidal system manifested by scoliosis, hip dislocation, and lower limb contractures. It expresses itself in the second year of life in girls.

syncope: fainting or swooning caused by lack of oxygen or blood flow to the brain.

syringomyelia: disorder of spinal cord, marked by abnormal cavities filled with liquid.

tabes dorsalis: severe progressive disease of the central nervous system, caused by syphilis and characterized by demyelination of the dorsal columns of the spinal cord; **locomotor ataxia, Duchenne d.**

taboparesis: condition in which symptoms of tabes dorsalis and general paresis are associated; **neurosyphilis.**

tic: involuntary and usually quick, repetitious contractions of a muscle or muscle groups; repeated twitching.

tic douloureux: painful affliction (neuralgia) involving the trigeminal nerve.

tremor: involuntary trembling or quivering; shaking.

vertigo: loss of equilibrium.

Eponymic Neurologic Diseases

Bell palsy: loss of function of the facial nerves.

Brown-Séquard syndrome: injury to only one side of the spinal cord, resulting in loss of motion on one side of the body and loss of sensation on the opposite side.

Charcot joint d.: joint destruction caused by loss of normal sensation.

Charcot-Marie-Tooth d.: spontaneous degeneration of the neuromuscular complex, most commonly peroneal nerve, but also ulnar nerve, generally starting in childhood; **Marie-Charcot-Tooth d.**

   type I motor and sensory neuropathy: a slowly progressive peripheral neurologic condition of childhood that can result in recurrent dislocation of the patella, peroneal muscle atrophy, high-arched/turned-in foot, and scoliosis. This is autosomally inherited and due to a failure of normal peripheral myelin protein 22 (type 1A) a failure of myelin protein 0 (type 1B), unknown defect (type 1C), and early growth response gene *EGR2* (type 1D).

   type II motor and sensory neuropathy: a neuronal disorder associated with peroneal muscular atrophy. Type IIA is inherited as an autosomal dominant. Other types being defined include type 2, an autosomal recessive, and two x-linked, one of which is associated with a disorder of connexin-32.

Dejerine d.: spontaneous local hypertrophic interstitial neuropathy of a peripheral nerve, cause unknown.

Dejerine-Sottas syndrome (familial interstitial hypertrophic neuritis): familial neuritis associated with high-arched feet and marked sensory changes in all limbs.

Erb palsy (upper obstetrical palsy): to be distinguished from Erb paralysis (form of muscular dystrophy). Palsy affects muscles supplied by upper cervical nerve roots C5 and C6; usually due to a distraction injury such as a difficult infant delivery but may occur in adult life after trauma.

Friedreich ataxia: autosomally recessive inherited disease due to lack of frataxin in mitochondria resulting in oxidative stress leading to sclerosis of the dorsal and lateral columns of the spinal cord, attended by loss of coordination; usually apparent in early childhood; can be fatal.

Guillain-Barré syndrome: viral disorder involving spinal cord, peripheral nerves, and nerve roots; recovery of lost voluntary muscle function usually occurs, but the disease can be fatal.

Morton neuroma: excessive proliferation of perineural tissue, usually at the third and fourth metatarsal heads.

Naffziger syndrome: scalenus anticus syndrome; pain in brachial plexus distribution, caused by muscle impingement.

Parkinson d.: see **paralysis agitans.**

Parrot pseudoparalysis: decreased movement of the extremity due to syphilitic bone covering inflammation (periostitis) in infants.

Parsonage-Andrew-Turner syndrome: condition of the brachial plexus resulting in sudden onset of pain and muscle weakness in upper limbs that may lead to muscle wasting (atrophy). Pain may occur simultaneously or after several weeks, and last 1 to 4 weeks or persist for 18 months. Cause unknown; **neuralgic amyotrophy.**

Refsum syndrome: hypertrophic neuropathy that begins in childhood and progresses with repeated remissions and reactivation consisting mostly of distal sensory and motor loss.

Roussy-Lévy syndrome (hereditary areflexic dystasia): disease of peripheral nerves that is associated with a tremor and becomes arrested at puberty.

schwannoma: neoplasm of a nerve sheath.

von Recklinghausen disease: multiple neurofibromatosis.

Metabolic Diseases

There are thousands of chemicals in the body. Most of them are being rapidly destroyed and replaced as part of the essential chain of events that supplies energy, growth, and normal tissue replacement. There are conditions in which some of these chemicals may accumulate or be produced in inadequate quantity for normal function. Not all metabolic diseases can be identified at birth.

Gout is a disease in which uric acid accumulates in the soft tissues and joint spaces; it usually does not occur until middle adult life. **Sickle cell anemia** is the result of production of the wrong kind of chemical, causing changes in the shape of red cells and a subsequent decreased oxygen supply; this disorder is usually detected in infancy.

Many such disorders of chemical production and destruction (metabolism) have been defined elsewhere in this text because of certain characteristic tissues or extremity appearances. Some terms will be re-defined here, with greater emphasis placed on the metabolic aspects.

Osteopenia is a term that defines abnormally diminished bone content. It may occur regionally after immobilization or be due to a systemic effect involving the entire skeleton. The term does not define the quality of the bone, but simply states that there is less of it. The WHO definition of osteopenia refers to T scores between −1.0 and −2.5. Normal bone density is present if the T score is greater than −1.

Osteoporosis is a condition in which the mineral and organic content is normal, but there is less bone. The most common generalized osteoporosis is associated with aging (*senile osteoporosis*). Some metabolic conditions such as the postmenopausal state and abnormal gastrointestinal absorption are associated with a generalized osteoporosis. If no specific cause is found, the condition is often referred to as *idiopathic osteoporosis*. In children it is called *juvenile osteoporosis*. The WHO Working Group defines osteoporosis according to measurements of bone mineral density (BMD) using dual-energy x-ray absorptiometry (DEXA). They define osteoporosis as a bone density T score at or below 2.5 standard deviations (T score) below normal peak values for young adults. One or more fragility fractures in conjunction with a T score less than −2.5 is called established or severe osteoporosis. The WHO definition of osteoporosis only takes into consideration measurement of bone density, with no component of bone quality. The NIH Consensus Development Panel on Osteoporosis in 2001 defined osteoporosis as a skeletal disorder characterized by compromised bone strength predisposing a person to an increased risk of fracture. This definition takes into consideration that there are other factors that influence bone quality such as the microarchitecture of bone.

Osteomalacia describes softening of bone, resulting from vitamin D deficiency or kidney disease. Milk allergy, liver disease, excision of the ovaries, kidney disorders, and chronic intestinal problems may interfere with vitamin D metabolism, absorption of calcium, or other processes, resulting in abnormal bone formation and mineralization.

Diseases Associated with Osteomalacia

autosomal dominant hypophosphatemic rickets: autosomal dominant disorder due to a dysfunction in FGF 23 receptor with a range of disorders present in childhood with limb deformity to adult onset bone pain due to osteomalacia secondary to renal phosphate loss.

Fanconi syndrome: severe form of vitamin D–resistant rickets, often fatal, and characterized by the presence of glucose, amino acids, and other chemicals in the urine.

hyperparathyroidism: abnormal increase in the level of parathyroid hormone, resulting in loss of calcium from bones.

hypoparathyroidism: abnormal decrease in the level of parathyroid hormone, either congenital or acquired, resulting in decreased bone formation and lowered serum calcium.

hypophosphatasia: autosomal recessive inherited disease characterized by severe skeletal defects resulting from a failure of calcification of bone.

milk-alkali syndrome: osteoporosis and/or osteomalacia, usually resulting from excessive intake of milk and alkali to treat ulcer disease; changes in therapy have reduced the prevalence of this disorder.

pseudohypoparathyroidism (PHPT): deficient hormone action due to target tissue resistance. Associated with short stature, shortened metacarpals and metatarsals (particularly the fourth), obesity and rounded face, reduced intelligence, subcutaneous calcification and ossifications, and some less common bone abnormalities; *Albright hereditary osteodystrophy.* Specific forms include PHPT as a result of guanine nucleotide deficiency, parathyroid hormone (PTH) receptor abnormality, and circulating antagonists to PTH action type II with normal bone responsiveness (hypohyperparathyroidism).

renal osteodystrophy: descriptive of a specific bone resorptive pattern seen in children and adults who have chronic kidney disease.

rickets: refers to the specific appearance of stunted growth, prominent rib cartilage (rachitic rosary), skull deformity (hot cross bun skull), and bowlegs; these appear during childhood and are characteristic of a variety of disorders that lead to a failure of normal calcification of bone. In the United States, the cause is rarely nutritional, but the disease is still seen because children can be born with kidney problems that produce a bone salt loss.

vitamin D–resistant rickets (VDDR1): rickets due to an autosomal recessively inherited deficiency of the vitamin D enzyme 25-α-hydroxycholicaliferol-1-hydroxylase, resulting in severe rickets **(pseudo deficiency rickets).**

vitamin D–resistant rickets (VDRR2): autosomal recessive disease due to dysfunction of 25-α-hydroxycholicaliferol receptor resulting in rickets marked by normal-appearing kidneys that excrete excessive phosphorus into the urine; resistant to usual vitamin D therapy but responds to very high doses of vitamin D **(pseudo deficiency rickets).**

x-linked hypophosphatemic rickets: sex-linked dominant disorder due to a disorder of intracellular signaling of a phosphate endopeptidase homolog (PHEX) leading to postnatal rickets with growth retardation and dental abnormalities.

Diseases Associated with Osteoporosis

Cushing d.: disease caused by increase in corticosteroids from the adrenal glands or medication; may result in a characteristic vertebral body appearance and generalized osteoporosis.

hyperthyroidism: increased thyroid hormone production and increased general metabolism; may result in osteoporosis.

hypothyroidism: decreased thyroid hormone; may result in less bone production and osteoporosis.

Other Metabolic Genetic Conditions (Table 2-3)

acrocapitofemoral dysplasia: rare autosomal recessive condition cue to abnormality of indian hedgehog (IHH) function, characterized by short stature and short limbs. Radiographs show cone-shaped epiphyses mainly in hands and hips.

Angelman syndrome: Failure of production of UBE3A, is a component of this ubiquitin pathway a protein that helps degrade proteins in the brain. This results in a stiff, jerky gait, absent speech, excessive laughter, and seizures.

beta$_2$-microglobulin amyloidosis: intraosseous and soft tissue deposition of beta$_2$-microglobulin seen in long-term hemodialysis patients.

Coffin-Lowry syndrome: heritable disorder characterized by pronounced mental retardation, peculiar facies, short stature, and a clumsy, broad-based gait. There are multiple skeletal abnormalities.

diabetes: disorder of insulin and sugar metabolism, resulting in high blood glucose levels. Does not necessarily cause bone disorders, but in later life causes vascular compromise to the legs, possibly leading to amputation.

Down syndrome: mongolism; the condition is produced by chromosomal abnormality; *trisomy 21.*

dyssegmental dysplasia: rare lethal form of short-limbed dwarfism with different abnormal shapes of the vertebral bodies.

Ehlers-Danlos syndrome (EDS): spectrum of disorders marked by laxity of joints, velvety skin that is soft and hyperextensible, and vessel fragility. Some of these have known specific collagen defects. Because of an improved understanding of the consequence of the various genetic defects, the classification system has been reorganized to incorporate related conditions and reassign others:

New Classification

Classic type (EDS I & II): (I) autosomal dominant, easy bruising, mitral valve prolapse, premature rupture of the fetal membranes, and/or premature birth, type V collagen disorder. (II) autosomal dominant, similar to type 1, but the effects are milder; type V collagen disorder.

Hypermobility type (EDS III): autosomal dominant, striking joint hypermobility and minimal skin changes, multiple gene; type III collagen being one.

Vascular type (EDS IV): autosomal dominant, vascular/ecchymotic form, prominent venous markings, which are readily visible through the skin. Patients are subject to spontaneous rupture of the bowel, the medium-sized arterial structures, or both; type III collagen disorder.

Kyphoscoliosis type (EDS VI): autosomal recessive, retinal detachments, microcornea, myopia, scoliosis, and neonatal hypotonia due to deficiency of lysine hydrocyclase effect on collagen.

Arthrochalasia type (EDS VIIB): both types VIIA and VIIB, autosomal dominant, multiplex congenita (overflaccidity of the joints without hyperelasticity of the skin), short stature, and micrognathia. Dermatosparaxis (EDS VIIC) is autosomal recessive, multiplex congenita overflaccidity of the joints without hyperelasticity of the skin, short stature, and micrognathia.

Types not included in new scheme include the following: EDS type V a sex-linked recessive form described only in a single family some what similar to type 2 EDS.

EDS type VIII: classic type with periodontitis, autosomal dominant. Multiple skin striae and significant dental problems, including early tooth loss, periodontitis, and alveolar bone loss.

EDS type IX: allelic to Menkes syndrome X-linked recessive. Occipital exostoses, bladder diverticula or rupture, bony dysplasias, and decreased copper and ceruloplasmin. The gene is related to a condition termed *cutis laxa* or occipital horn syndrome, due to failure of the activity of lysyl oxidase, a copper-dependent enzyme involved in cross-link formation in collagen.

EDS type X: Described in one family; autosomal recessive, fibronectin-1 disorder. Patients exhibit poor wound healing, petechiae, and a platelet aggregation defect, which can be corrected by fibronectin supplementation.

gout: disease process in which uric acid crystals are deposited into the joint lining or inflammatory cells within the joint and soft tissue. The most common form is urate (monosodium urate monohydrate). Other forms include pyrophosphate (calcium pyrophosphate dihydrate), apatite (various calcium

TABLE 2-3 Genetic Musculoskeletal Disorders

Musculoskeletal Disorder	Mutation	Site	Inheritance	Notes
Osteogenesis imperfecta	Type I collagen	Protein product in matrix	Most autosomal dominant	COL1A1 or COL1A2
Type IA; IB (teeth affected, more severe	Type I collagen	Protein product in matrix		IA mild to moderate, blue sclera
Type II Lethal	Type I collagen	Protein product in matrix	Autosomal dominant	
Type III	Type I collagen	Protein product in matrix	Autosomal dominant	Early childhood fx, dentogenesis
Type IV	Type I collagen	Protein product in matrix	Autosomal dominant	Later childhood, sclera normal or pale blue
Ehlers-Danlos VIIA and B	Type I collagen	Protein product in matrix	Autosomal dominant	
Ehlers-Danlos VIIC	Type I collagen (synthesis enzyme)	Protein product in matrix	Autosomal dominant	
Ehlers-Danlos VI	Type I collagen (synthesis enzyme)	Protein product in matrix		
Kniest dysplasia	Type II collagen	Protein product in matrix	Autosomal dominant	
Stickler dysplasia	Type II collagen	Protein product in matrix	Autosomal dominant	
Stickler dysplasia without involvement of eyes	Type XI collagen	Protein product in matrix	Autosomal dominant	Minor collagen associated with fibrillar assemblies
Precocious osteoarthritis	Type II collagen	Protein product in matrix	Autosomal dominant	
Spondyloepiphyseal dysplasia, congenita	Type II collagen	Protein product in matrix	Autosomal dominant	
Spondyloepiphyseal dysplasia, tarda	Type II collagen	Protein product in matrix	Autosomal recessive	
Ehlers-Danlos IV	Type III collagen	Protein product in matrix	Autosomal dominant	
Ehlers-Danlos I	Type V	Protein product in matrix		
Ehlers-Danlos 2	Type V	Protein product in matrix		
Multiple epiphyseal dysplasia	Type IXA1,23 COMP, Matrilin 3	Protein product in matrix	Autosomal dominant	
Schmid metaphyseal dysplasia	Type X collagen	Protein product in matrix		
Spondyloepiphyseal dysplasia, x-linked	Sedlin	Protein product in matrix	X-linked dominant	
Marfan's	Fibrillin 1	Protein product in matrix	Autosomal dominant	Not all are fibrillin
Marfan-like	Fibrillin 2	Protein product in matrix	Autosomal dominant	Joints stiff

TABLE 2-3 Genetic Musculoskeletal Disorders—Cont'd

Musculoskeletal Disorder	Mutation	Site	Inheritance	Notes
Pseudoachondroplasia	COMP, Matrilin	Protein product in matrix	Autosomal dominant	
Ehlers-Danlos X	Fibronectin-1	Protein product in matrix	Autosomal dominant	
Hypophosphatasia: neonatal, infantile, childhood, adult	Decreased alkaline phosphatase	Protein product in matrix	Autosomal recessive	
Neurofibromatosis	Neurofibrilin	Protein product in matrix	Autosomal dominant	
Type I Hurler	Alpha-1-iduronidase	Posttranslation in matrix	Autosomal recessive	Enlarged heart
Type II Hunter	Sulfoiduronidase	Posttranslation in matrix	X-linked dominant	
Type III Sanfilippo	Accumulation of heparan sulfate	Posttranslation in matrix	Autosomal recessive	
Type IVA Morquio A	Galactosamine 6 sulphate sulfatase	Posttranslation in matrix	Autosomal recessive	
Type IVB Morquio B	Galactosidase	Posttranslation in matrix	Autosomal recessive	
Type V Scheie (MP 1S)	Alpha-l-iduronidase	Posttranslation in matrix	Autosomal recessive	
Type VII Sly	Beta glucuronidase	Posttranslation in matrix	Autosomal recessive	
McArdle	Glycogen phosphorylase	Posttranslation in matrix	Autosomal recessive	
Ehlers-Danlos VI	Lysine hydrocylase	Posttranslation in matrix	Autosomal recessive	
Gaucher type I, II, and III	Excess glucocerebroside	Posttranslation in matrix	Autosomal recessive	
Diastrophic dysplasia	Sulfate transporter	Posttranslation in matrix	Autosomal recessive	
Pfeiffer	FGF receptor 1	Cell surface receptor	Autosomal dominant	
Apert's syndrome	FGF receptor 2	Cell surface receptor	Autosomal dominant	Type 1 acrocephalosyndactyly
Crouzon syndrome	FGF receptor 2	Cell surface receptor	Autosomal dominant	
Thanatophoric dysplasia	FGF receptor 3	Cell surface receptor	Spontaneous mutation	
Hypochondrodysplasia	FGF receptor 3	Cell surface receptor	Autosomal dominant	
Vitamin D–resistant rickets (VDDR2)	25-α-hydroxycholicaliferol receptor	Cell surface receptor	Autosomal recessive	
Osteopetrosis	Carbonic anhydrase type II; proton pump in humans	Cell surface receptor	Autosomal dominant; autosomal recessive in malignant infantile form	
Jansen metaphyseal chondrodysplasia	PTH/PTHrP receptor	Cell surface receptor	Autosomal dominant	
Osteopetrosis	Beta 3 integrin	Cell surface receptor	Autosomal recessive	
Fibrodysplasia ossificans progressiva	Activin receptor type IA (ACVRI)	Cell surface receptor	Autosomal dominant	
Autosomal dominant hypophosphatemic rickets	FGF23	Cell surface receptor	Autosomal dominant	

(Continued)

TABLE 2-3 Genetic Musculoskeletal Disorders—Cont'd

Musculoskeletal Disorder	Mutation	Site	Inheritance	Notes
McCune-Albright polyostotic fibrous dysplasia	GS alpha protein of adenylate cyclase (GNAS-1)	Intracellular signaling	Mosaic spontaneous	
Duchenne muscular dystrophy	Dystrophin	Intracellular signaling	X-linked recessive	
Autosomal limb girdle dystrophy	Part of dystrophin-glycoprotein complex	Intracellular signaling	Autosomal recessive	
Multiple hereditary exostosis	EXT, EXT2 genes	Intracellular signaling	Autosomal dominant	
Vitamin D–resistant rickets (VDDR1)	25-α-hydroxycholicaliferol-1-hydroxylase	Intracellular signaling	Autosomal recessive	
Neurofibromatosis	NF-1 (neurofibromin)	Nucleus	Autosomal dominant	
Cleidocranial dysostosis	cbfa1 (core binding protein) RUNX2	Nucleus	Autosomal dominant	
McKusick metaphyseal chondrodysplasia	Mutations in RMRP, a nonencoding RNA	Nucleus	Autosomal recessive	
X-linked hypophosphatemic rickets	PHEX, a Zn metallopeptidase	Nucleus	X-linked dominant	
Osteopetrosis	MCSF	Paracrine factor	Autosomal recessive	
Fibrodysplasia ossificans progressiva	BMP-4	Paracrine factor	Autosomal recessive	Muscular dystrophy
Acrocapitofemoral dysplasia	IHH	Paracrine factor	Autosomal recessive	
Friedreich's ataxia	Frataxin	Microsome	Autosomal recessive	
Angelman syndrome	UBE3A		Autosomal recessive	
Prader-Willi	Chromosome 15	Spontaneous	Uniparental disomy	
Trichorhinophalangeal syndrome	Zinc finger protein chromosome 8q		Autosomal dominant	Combined nose, hair, joint effect
Charcot-Marie-Tooth	Connexin 32		Sex linked	In general, different gene product can produce axonal wrapping disorder or demyelination
Type IA	PMP 22 gene		Autosomal dominant	
Type IB	PMP φ gene		Autosomal dominant	
Type II	Gene kinesin (K1F1B)		Autosomal dominant	
Type II recessive	LMNA gene		Autosomal recessive	

crystals), cholesterol, and oxalate (calcium oxalate monohydrate and dihydrate).

gouty arthritis: inflammatory joint changes associated with gout; may be associated with tophi.

gouty node: collection of uric acid crystals near joints.

hemophilia: inherited disorder of coagulation; sex-linked; repeated hemorrhages may result in bone and joint deformity.

infantile hypophosphatasia: autosomal recessive disorder affecting alkaline phosphatase affecting bone formation seen in infants.

Kashin-Beck disease: endemic in eastern Siberia and northern China and Korea; abnormalities in enchondral bone growth leading to osteoarthrosis.

Klinefelter syndrome: failure of full sexual development in males, with development of some female characteristics; results from the fertilized egg receiving both female X chromosomes and the male Y chromosome.

lipid storage disease: inherited disorder resulting in multiple problems; bone disorders are secondary to displacement of the marrow by abnormal cells, resulting in avascular necrosis of the hip or irregular patterns on radiographs; also called **lipid reticuloendotheliosis.**

lipocalcinogranulomatosis: probable metabolic-based disorder with lipid-filled histiocytes and associated tumoral calcinosis.

Marfan syndrome: autosomal dominant disorder of fibrillin-1 resulting in elastic inherited defect in elastic tissue resulting in ligamentous laxity and spider-like fingers, with joint and vessel disorders.

Marfan-like syndrome: autosomal dominant disorder of fibrillin-2 resulting in elastic inherited defect in elastic tissue resulting in ligamentous laxity and spiderlike fingers, with joint and vessel disorders.

Menkes kinky-hair syndrome: X-linked recessive disorder that is fatal in infancy or early childhood; associated with depigmented and kinky hair, hypertrophic gingiva, loose joints, vascular tortuosity, seizures, and severe mental retardation. Similar to types V and IX Ehlers-Danlos syndrome.

metallosis: in orthopaedics, the term is applied to conditions resulting from very tiny microscopic particles that come from internal prosthetic devices.

Milroy d.: swelling of distal parts caused by a congenital disorder in which there is a retention of lymph fluid; *familial lymphedema.*

Pfeiffer syndrome: an autosomal dominant disorder of fibroblast growth factor receptors (FGFR 1 & FGFR 2) resulting in early fusion of the skull (craniosynostosis), dental problems due to crowded teeth, often a high palate, poor vision, and hearing loss in about 50% of children.

prune belly syndrome: undescended testicles, urinary tract obstructions, and hypoplastic abdominal muscles that result in a prune belly appearance and assorted musculoskeletal abnormalities; **Eagle-Barrett syndrome.**

pseudoachondroplasia: autosomal dominant condition due to defect in collagen oligomeric protein (COMP) affecting major joints with deformity and short stature.

pseudogout: more appropriately called **calcium pyrophosphate deposition disease (CPPD).** Usually occurs after age 60. Joint symptoms are consistent with degenerative arthritis development and x-rays reveal deposition of calcium within the cartilage. Can be, but not necessarily is, associated with mineral metabolic disorders such as renal disease or hyperparathyroidism.

Shwachman syndrome: pancreatic exocrine insufficiency associated with cyclical low white blood cell production in children. Orthopaedic conditions include profound short stature.

sickle cell anemia: autosomal recessive inherited disease that affects the shape of red cells (oat-shaped erythrocytes); the result that most concerns orthopaedists is *salmonella bone infection* in infancy and bone infarcts in adults, particularly of the hip.

thalassemia: autosomal recessive inherited disease of red cell structure; may result in skeletal deformity.

thanatophoric dysplasia: autosomal dominant mutations in the fibroblast growth factor receptor 3 gene (*FGFR3*) most common form of skeletal dysplasia that is lethal in the neonatal period due to respiratory insufficiency and compression of the brainstem. TD type 1 (TD1, TD I), is more, has a normally shaped skull and curved long bones. TD type 2 (TD2, TD II) has a cloverleaf-shaped skull and straight femurs.

trichorhinophalangeal syndrome: There are two types: TRPSI and TRPSII.

> **TRPSI Sugio-Kajii syndrome**: characterized by unique facial features, cone-shaped epiphysis, and mild growth retardation.
>
> **TRPSII Langer Giedion syndrome**: similar to **TRPSI** with exostosis and redundant skin.

tumoral calcinosis: probable metabolic disorder in which there is massive accumulation of calcium phosphates, pyrophosphates, or calcium carbonates in the soft tissues, particularly around joints.

Turner syndrome: failure of development of some female characteristics in girls; results from failure of the fertilized egg to receive both female X chromosomes.

Diseases and Conditions by Anatomic Area

The back and neck disease section is found in Chapter 9.

Miscellaneous Shoulder and Elbow Conditions

Buford complex: shoulder joint anatomic variance consisting of a cord-like middle glenohumeral ligament that blends with a loosely attached superior labrum. The third variance is a large sublabral hole.

hooked acromion: hooked appearance of the anterolateral acromion sometimes associated with impingement of the underlying rotator cuff. This is a condition that develops in adult life. The appearance has been categorized into three types seen on radiographs:

> **type I acromion:** normal flat appearance of undersurface of acromion.
>
> **type II acromion:** slight hooked or roughened undersurface of acromion.
>
> **type III acromion:** markedly curved appearance of undersurface of acromion.

impingement syndrome: when used in reference to the shoulder this term denotes symptoms that are related to the bursa or rotator cuff changes that result in pain in the acromial, subacromial, and lateral arm produced by abducted positions where bursal impingement occurs.

painful arc syndrome: pain in the acromioclavicular (A/C) area on active shoulder abduction; a sign of arthritis of the A/C joint.

patella cubiti: compatible with good function a rare developmental variant in which the proximal part of the olecranon appears like a patella separate from the remaining olecranon.

snapping scapula: grinding sensation felt by the patient on specific motions of the scapula. May be a sign of a prominent rib or an osteochondroma of the scapula.

winged scapula: winging of scapula and prominence of interior angle at rest or on active range of motion. May be a sign of muscle paralysis, particularly palsy of the long thoracic nerve.

Hip (Coxa) Diseases

The Latin term *coxa* refers to the part of the skeleton lateral to and including the hip joint. (Do not confuse coxa [hip] with coccyx [tailbone].) The most common adult problems of the hip are osteoarthritis, other arthropathies, and avascular necrosis. These are defined in the sections dealing with bone, cartilage, and joint disease.

acetabular rim syndrome: pain and impaired function that precede osteoarthritis in hips that are congenitally dysplastic or have superior lateral trauma to the limbus and/or bony rim.

arthrokatadysis: deep hip socket formed as a part of degenerative arthritis.

coxa breva: short hip with a small femoral head caused by premature closure of the epiphysis.

coxa magna: enlarged femoral head.

coxa plana: flat femoral head (osteochondrosis) of the capitular epiphysis of the femur; *Legg-Perthes d.*

coxa saltans (snapping hip): snapping of the hip due to tightness of the iliotibial tract over the greater trochanter, snapping of the musculotendinous iliopsoas overstructures deep to it, or lesions within the hip joint, such as a labral tear.

coxa senilis: degenerative hip disease concomitant with old age; **malum coxae senilis.** (archaic)

coxa valga: hip deformity in which the angle of axis of the head and neck of the femur and the axis of its shaft (neck shaft angle) is increased.

coxa vara: reduced neck shaft angle, usually caused by failure of normal bone growth; **coxa adducta.**

coxa vara luxans: fissure of neck of femur, with dislocation of the head. (archaic)

coxalgia: hip pain. (archaic)

coxarthrocace: fungal disease of the hip joint. (archaic)

coxarthropathy: any hip joint disease.

coxarthrosis: degenerative joint disease or osteoarthritis of the hip joint.

coxitis: inflammation of the hip joint; **coxarthria, coxarthritis.** (archaic)

coxotuberculosis: tuberculosis of the hip joint. (archaic)

developmental dysplasia of the hip (DDH): spectrum of disorders of the hip associated with deficient development of the acetabulum. This is usually apparent at birth and may start as or progress to subluxation or dislocation of the hip. This term is now replacing the older terms **congenital hip disease, congenital hip dysplasia,** and **congenital hip dislocation.**

Crowe Classification (for Percent of Subluxation)
Grade I: < 50%.
Grade II: 50%–75%.
Grade III: 75%–100%.
Grade IV: more than 100%.

Meyer dysplasia: developmental anomaly that simulates Perthes d. of the hip but presents at an earlier age and does not have the progression of hip changes seen with Perthes d.; **dysplasia epiphysealis capitis femoris.**

Namaqualand hip dysplasia: autosomal dominant condition seen in African children from 3 to 20 years of age. There is a failure of growth in the femoral epiphysis, resulting in pain associated with an early degenerative arthritis of the hip.

observation hip: group of symptoms referred to the hip that includes a limp, pain, and limited motion of the hip joint with normal radiographs. The condition is a diagnostic dilemma in that it may be due to toxic synovitis, infection, or an early avascular necrosis.

protrusio acetabuli: arthritic development of hip socket into a deep, egg-shaped appearance.

proximal focal femoral deficiency (PFFD): failure of normal formation of the thigh side of the hip; varies in severity. The new term for this condition is **longitudinal deficiency of the femur, partial (LDFP).**

windswept hips: condition seen in individuals with cerebral palsy with pelvic obliquity, scoliosis, and one hip held in adduction and the opposite hip in abduction.

Deficiencies of the Acetabulum and Femur

The Committee on the Hip, American Academy of Orthopaedic Surgeons, has developed the following classification for congenital deficiencies of the acetabulum and femur:

Acetabular Classification

1. Segmental.
 • Peripheral (rim).
  a. Anterior.
  b. Posterior.
  c. Superior.
 • Central.
2. Cavitary.
  a. Anterior.
  b. Posterior.
  c. Superior.
  d. Medial (protrusion with intact medial wall).
3. Combined segmental and cavitary.
  a. Superior segmental, superior cavitary.
  b. Medial segmental, medial cavitary (protrusion with deficient medial wall).
  c. Posterior segmental, posterior cavitary.
4. Pelvic discontinuity.
5. Fusion.

Femoral Classification

segmental defect: any loss of bone in the outer cortical shell of the femur.

cavitary defect: excavation of cancellous and/or cortical bone from within, the outer cortical shell remaining unviolated.

ectasia: dilatation and/or expansion of the outer cortical shell without perforation.

intercalary: segmental defect with intact bone above and below (cortical window).

Level of Defect

Level I: proximal to the lesser inferior trochanter.

Level II: inferior lesser trochanter to 10 cm distal.

Level III: below level II.

Knee Disorders

Genu is a Latin term for knee (pl. *genua*). It is also a general term denoting any anatomic structure that is bent like a knee. Specifically, it is the site of articulation between the femur and tibia. Knee-related problems are divided into three sections:

1. Old genu descriptive terms.
2. Joint injury.
3. Other terms specifically related to the knee but not to a specific injury.

Genu Terms

genu recurvatum: ability of the knee to bend backward; caused by trauma or general joint laxity; *back-knee.*

genu valgum: deformity in which knees are close together, with ankle space increased; *knock-knee.*

genu varum: deformity in which knees are bowed out and ankles are close in; may be associated with internal tibial torsion (ITT).

Outcome of Joint Injury

The knee is an unusual joint because it contains *ligaments* within the joint. There are also medial and lateral *menisci* (crescent-shaped cartilages) that can be damaged. Finally, the normal motions of the knee are very complex, including two planes of rotation; therefore it is very common to see multiple injuries.

A sprained knee is often a benign injury involving only mild damage to the ligament. However, a tear of the meniscus can occur in association with a sprain (Fig. 2-7). A **meniscus tear** or **torn meniscus** is commonly described by its appearance, such as a **parrot-beak tear** or a **bucket-handle tear.** In the young person, a tear is usually vertical and longitudinal to the diameter of the meniscus. In degenerative tears that appear in older people, the tear is horizontal and may not be apparent on the superior surface of the meniscus. When the meniscus becomes fragmented, the condition is often termed a **degenerate tear** of the meniscus. The location of tears may be used to define a specific meniscus injury, for example, *posterior horn* or *anterior horn.* Meniscus injury commonly occurs as a result of a rotational injury. *Rotational instability* (rotatory or angular) is produced by rupture of specific anatomic structures. A meniscal rim can regenerate from the margin of a completely, or nearly completely, resected meniscus resulting in what is referred to as a **regenerated meniscus.** The normal up-and-down gliding mechanism of a patella may be disrupted, and the patella has a tendency to move out of its groove laterally (*subluxing patella*). A subluxing patella need not be caused by injury but does commonly occur with rotational injury. All these disorders can result in a chronic reaction in the knee, similar to the eyes' response to a foreign body. The lining of the knee becomes inflamed and may allow fluid (*effusion*) to collect. If the effusion is persistent, a *pouch,* called a *Baker cyst,* may form behind the knee.

Another outcome of knee injury is the formation of loose fragments (*loose bodies*) of meniscal cartilage or other tissue, causing inflammation (*synovitis* or *meniscitis*). The cartilage of the kneecap may become frayed (*chondromalacia patellae*). However, not all cases of chondromalacia result from injury. If the inflammation persists long enough, the patient will

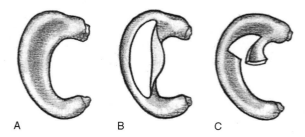

A   B   C

FIG 2-7 A, Normal meniscus. **B,** Longitudinal, or "bucket-handle," tear **C,** Tear of the posterior horn. (From Mercier LR: *Practical Orthopaedics,* ed 5, St Louis, Mosby, 2000.)

eventually develop *degenerative arthritis*. Often the examiner is not sure of the exact problem of the knee but suspects that something is functionally incorrect. The general term then used is *internal derangement of the knee* (IDK).

A surgically excised meniscus sometimes grows back in part (*regenerated medial meniscus*), or a portion may be left behind (*retained posterior horn*).

Other Conditions of the Knee

anterolateral rotatory instability (ALRI): the most common instability of the knee characterized by abnormal anterior displacement or subluxation of the lateral tibial plateau. It results from a tear of the anterior cruciate ligament and/or the mid-third of the lateral capsular ligament, and is determined by the Lachman test, anterior drawer sign, and flexion-rotation drawer test.

Baker cyst: sac of usually clear fluid specifically in the popliteal fossa of the knee. In the adult, it is a synovial fluid cystic extension due to intraarticular disease that results in a new synovial-lined sac in the popliteal fossa. In a child, the cyst is usually a ganglion arising from one of the tendons in the popliteal area.

bipartite patella: patella that has bony maturation occurring from two centers rather than one center, usually congenital, causing no symptoms, but may be mistaken for a fracture.

congenital dislocation: progressive anterior dislocation of the tibia caused by abnormal tissue remodeling; seen in infancy.

discoid meniscus: meniscus that is less crescentic and more D shaped. Often leads to symptoms in young adult life.

Watanabe Classification

Type I: complete, extending across entire lateral tibial plateau.

Type II: meniscus wider than normal but some articular cartilage exposed.

Type III (Wrisberg-ligament type): deficiency of posterior tibial meniscal attachment that allows meniscus to move abnormally back and forth in joint.

---

flexion contracture: formation of fibrous bands that prevent complete extension of the knee.

focal fibrocartilaginous dysplasia: rare cause of unilateral genu varum (bowleg), which appears before 18 months with a cortical lucency in the proximal tibia and surrounding sclerosis. Condition is usually self-limited and resolves by age 4.

hamstrung knee: tight hamstrings during growth resulting in a slight knee flexion gait with subsequent synovitis and chondromalacia.

housemaid's knee: prepatellar bursitis: inflammation of the bursa in front of the patella.

jockey cap patella: chronic subluxating patella resulting in lateral spurring deformity.

jumper's knee: tenderness in the area of the inferior pole of the patella; usually seen in volleyball and basketball players.

megahorn meniscus: a congenitally enlarged part of either the anterior or posterior portion of the meniscus of the knee, usually the lateral side, usually associated with a variety of discoid menisci.

meniscal flounce: a normal wavy or folded pattern of the meniscus seen during arthroscopic inspection.

patella alta: a patella that is located more superior than expected, usually considered by the ratio of the length of the patella tendon to the height of the patella being greater than 1.25; **high-riding patella.**

patella baja: low-riding patella with a relatively shortened patellar tendon, usually associated with knee pain.

patella clunk syndrome: a patellar snap that occurs in total joint replacement (knees) when going from flexion to extension; due to the catching of scar tissue immediately above the patella.

patellofemoral syndrome: patellar and peripatellar pain often ascribed to chondromalacia patellae, but which may be due to other disorders such as patellar malalignment.

plica syndrome: pain and/or snapping in knee due to inflammation or enlargement of a band of tissue that is present at birth and may become symptomatic in association with other conditions. There are four common plicas:

ligamentum mucosum: in front of the anterior cruciate ligament.

suprapatellar plica: in the suprapatellar area.

medial shelf/medial plica: from the infrapatellar fat pad to the medial wall of the knee.

lateral plica: from the lateral infrapatellar fat pad to the lateral synovium of the knee.

popliteal cyst: any ganglion or synovial cyst behind the knee. In adults, this is usually an outpouching of the posterior knee joint area and is a sign of chronic inflammation in the knee. In children and young adults, this may be a ganglion cyst arising from one of the tendons around the knee. Not to be confused with popliteal arterial cyst.

popliteal pterygium syndrome: severe flexion of the knee and equinus deformity of the foot associated with popliteal web extending from the ischium to the heel. Other concurrent deformities include toenail dysplasia and oral cavity abnormalities such as cleft palate or lip pits.

rhizomelic: short proximal end of a limb, such as seen in achondroplastic dwarfism.

small-patella syndrome: autosomal disorder with small patellae, pelvic girdle hypoplasia, and other skeletal anomalies.

snapping knee syndrome: the combination of dramatic popping and often intermittent locking is most commonly associated with discoid meniscus, but may also be due to other intraarticular abnormalities of the knee such as meniscal tears and enlarged bands of tissue.

snowstorm knee: formation of hundreds of brilliant, white loose bodies within the knee, usually following an earlier traumatic event.

squinting patella: patella that appears to point inward when the person is standing or walking forward. Usually a sign of femoral anteversion.

tethered patellar tendon syndrome: condition seen after total knee replacement. A large fibrous band develops behind the patella, causes pain, and interferes with joint motion.

Type I: band oriented medial to lateral in suprapatellar region.

Type II: band oriented vertically.

Type III: band oriented from anterior fat pad to posterior notch.

thigh atrophy: loss of muscle tone of the quadriceps, causing dynamic instability.

Congenital Limb Absences

The International Organization for Standardization adopted a limb absence classification system designed to eliminate terms such as ectromelia, peromelia, and dysmelia. This system has two basic categories, transverse losses in which all structures for that segment are absent and longitudinal in which only a part of the longitudinal part of the segment is absent. This is based on radiologic appearance as opposed to specific reference to embryology, etiology, or epidemiology.* It is presented first. However, given the variance in practice throughout the orthopaedic world, two systems are in this edition. A former standard classification divided congenital deficiency based on the end of a limb (terminal) or somewhere in the middle (intercalary). In addition, transverse or longitudinal deficiencies were defined the same way.[†]

International Organization for Standardization (IOS)

For both transverse and longitudinal absences.

1. Name the bone(s) affected from proximal to distal. Any bone not named is presumed normal (this defines "intercalary" defects).
2. State if each affected bone is totally or partially absent.
3. If partial, state the fraction and position of the absent part.
4. For the rays in hands and feet, the number of the digit starting from the radial or tibial side is stated.
5. The term ray (first ray, second ray, etc.) may be used.

*From International Organization for Standardization: IOS 8548-1: Prosthetics and orthotics-Limb deficiencies, Part 1: Method of describing limb deficiencies present at birth, Geneva, Switzerland, International Organization for Standardization, 1989.
[†]From Frantz CH, O'Rahilly R: Congenital limb deficiencies, *J Bone Joint Surg* 43:1202-1224, 1961.

Terminal Transverse

acheiria: absence of the hand (carpals, metacarpals, phalanges).

acheiropodia: an extremely rare congenital absence of forearms, hands, and feet.

adactylia: absence of all five rays (metacarpals and phalanges).

amelia: complete absence of a limb.

apodia: absence of the foot.

complete aphalangia: absence of one or more phalanges from all five digits.

ectromelia: severe form of hypoplasia or actual absence of one or more long bones involving one or more limbs. This term generally includes amelia, hemimelia, and phocomelia.

hemimelia: absence of the forearm and hand or leg and foot portion of a limb.

partial hemimelia: absence of part of the forearm or leg.

Terminal Longitudinal

complete paraxial hemimelia: lengthwise loss of one side or the other of the forearm and hand or leg and foot.

incomplete paraxial hemimelia: similar to hemimelia, but a portion of affected bone remains, for example, complete absence of the ulna with a portion of the diameter of the radius intact.

partial adactylia: absence of one to four rays (phalanges and metacarpals).

partial aphalangia: absence of one or more of the three phalanges from one to four digits.

Intercalary Transverse

complete phocomelia: presence of only a hand or foot.

distal phocomelia: hand directly attached to upper arm; or foot directly attached to thigh.

proximal phocomelia: presence of hand and forearm or leg and foot.

Intercalary Longitudinal

complete paraxial hemimelia: absence of radius or ulna with intact hand or absence of tibia or fibula with intact foot.

incomplete paraxial hemimelia: similar to complete hemimelia, except a portion of affected bone remains intact.

partial adactylia: absence of all or part of the first through fifth rays.

partial aphalangia: absence of the proximal or middle phalanx from one or more digits, one through five. A common deformity is a complete loss of the radius with the rest of the arm and hand being intact—intercalary complete paraxial hemimelia. Proximal focal femoral deficiency (PFFD) is an absence of a portion of the hip and/or proximal femur.

Miscellaneous Congenital Deficiencies

amniotic band syndrome: congenital presence of constricting bands that may affect trunk, limbs, and cranium; partial amputations may result.

arachnodactyly: unusually long "spidery" fingers and toes characteristically seen in patients with Marfan syndrome.

dolichostenomelia: increased length of the limb compared with that of the trunk.

fragile-X syndrome: familial form of mental retardation associated with flat feet and excessive joint laxity.

Larsen syndrome: associated skeletal abnormalities seen in infancy: dislocation of the elbows and hips, equinovarus deformities of the feet, long cylindrical fingers and shortened metacarpals, wide-spaced eyes, prominent forehead, and depressed nasal bridge.

Prader-Willi syndrome: spontaneous genetic mutation resulting in uncommon infantile disorder characterized by hypotonia, hypogonadism, obesity due to overeating, diabetes mellitus, delayed psychomotor development, mental deficiency, short stature, small hands and feet, hypermobile joints, and kyphosis.

rhizomelic: short proximal end of a limb, such as seen in achondroplastic dwarfism.

tibial dysplasia: rare congenital deformity. Must be distinguished from more common fibular dysplasia. **Three types:** Type I—total absence of tibia; Type II—distal tibial aplasia; Type III—distal dysplasia with tibiofibular diastasis.

Specific Regional Classification Systems for Congenital Limb Absences

Achterman and Kalamchi: For Fibular Hemimelia

Type 1: fibula present.

Type 1a: physis physids of proximal fibula distal to proximal tibial physis. Distal fibular physis proximal to dome of talus.

Type Ib: only partial fibula present.

Type II: fibula absent.

Aitken: For Longitudinal Deficiency of the Femur, Partial

A: portion of the femoral head distal to the femoral head is deficient.
B: a larger portion is deficient or absent.

C: the femoral head is absent, the femur is short, and the acetabulum is dysplastic.

D: the femoral head is absent, the femur is very short, and the acetabulum is very dysplastic.

Bayne: For Radial Bone Deficiencies

Type 0: hypoplasia of the radial carpus (scaphoid); radius of normal length.

Type I: radius slightly shorter than normal; physis evident both proximal and distal.

Type II: "radius in miniature": normally shaped but smaller radius with both proximal and distal physis.

Type III: partial aplasia of the radius; absence of the distal part of the radius, including the distal epiphysis.

Type IV: absence of radius.

Bayne: For Longitudinal Ulnar Deficiencies

Type I: hypoplasia, distal epiphysis intact.

Type II: partial hypoplasia distal epiphysis absent.

Type III: total aplasia.

Type IV: radiohumeral synostosis with total ulna hypoplasia.

Birch: For Fibular Deficiencies

Type I: functional foot.

A: 0%–5% predicted leg-length inequality at maturity.

B: 6%–10% predicted leg-length inequality.

C: 11%–30% predicted leg-length inequality.

D: > 30% predicted leg-length inequality.

Type II: nonfunctional foot.

A: functional upper extremity.

B: nonfunctional upper extremity.

Cole and Manske: For the First Distal Ray Absence with Ulnar Deficiency

Type A: normal thumb and first web space.

Type B: milod first web and thumb deficiency.

Type C: moderate to severe first web and thumb deficiency (loss of opposition, malrotation, thumb index syndactyly, absent extrinsic tendon function).

Type D: thumb absent.

Gillespie: For Longitudinal Deficiency of the Femur, Partial

Group I: the femur is 40%–60% shorter than normal and the hip and knee can be made functional.

Group II: the femur is shorter and the hip and knee cannot be made functional.

Jones, Barnes, and Lloyd-Roberts

1a: tibia not seen, hypoplastic lower femoral epiphysis.

1b: tibia not seen, normal lower femoral epiphysis.

2: distal tibia not seen.

3: proximal tibia not seen.

4: diastasis.

Kalamchi and Dawe

Type I: complete absence of the tibia.

Type II: presence of proximal tibia.

Type III: severe diastasis at ankle.

Kummel: For Longitudinal Ulnar Deficiency at Elbow Joint

Type A: normal radiohumeral joint.

Type B: radiohumeral synostosis.

Type C: dislocation of the radiohumeral joint.

Letts: For Fibular Deficiencies

Type A: affected side less than 10% shorter than opposite side, discrepancy projected to be less than 6 cm at maturity, foot nearly normal, minimal femoral shortening.

Specific Regional Classification Systems for Congenital Limb Absences—cont'd

Type B: affected side 10%–20% shorter than opposite side, discrepancy projected to be 6 to 10 cm at maturity, minimal foot deformities, minimal femoral shortening.

Type C: affected side greater than 30% shorter than opposite side, discrepancy projected to be greater than 10 cm at maturity, severe foot deformity, severe femoral shortening.

Type D: bilateral fibular deficiency or partial longitudinal deficiency of the femur.

Ogden: For Ulnar Longitudinal Deficiency

Type I: hypoplasia of otherwise normal ulna with a distal epiphysis.

Type II: partial aplasia (absence of distal part of ulna, including the distal epiphysis).

Type III: total, aplasia.

Stanistski and Stanitski: For Fibular Hemimelia

Type I: fibula nearly normal.

Type II: small or miniature fibula with, regardless of its portion in the limb.

Type III: total absence of fibula.

Tibiotalar Joint and Distal Tibial Morphology

H: horizontal

V: valgus (triangular distal tibial epiphysis.

S: spherical (ball and socket ankle)

Presence of a tarsal coalition denoted with lower case "c"

Number of foot rays medial to lateral (denoted 1–5)

Wassel: For Thumb Polydactyly

Type I: split distal tuft.

Type II: split distal phalanx.

Type III: split distal middle phalanx and distal phalanx.

Type IV: split middle and distal phalanx.

Type V: split distal metacarpal and distal phalanges.

Type VI: split distal metacarpal and distal phalanges.

Type VII: split distal phalanx with ulnar ray having three phalanges.

Symbols

The following symbols are used for congenital limb absences:

-: transverse.

/: longitudinal.

I: intercalary.

T: terminal.

1, 2, 3, 4, 5: denotes ray involved.

-: when line is used above a letter, indicates the lower extremity.

-: when line is used below a letter, indicates the upper extremity.

TI: tibia, complete.

ti: tibia, incomplete.

FI: fibula, complete.

fi: fibula, incomplete.

R: radius, complete.

r: radius, incomplete.

U: ulna, complete.

u: ulna, incomplete.

Associated Disease Terminology

Diseases of the musculoskeletal system are often described by other terms relating to the disease process or some qualitative nature of the disease. These associated defined terms are given in alphabetic order.

abrasion: any superficial scraping of skin tissue or mucous membrane mechanically or through injury.

abscess: localized collection of pus in a cavity, which may form in any tissue.

acute: describes symptoms, conditions, or diseases of recent onset or recurrence that are severe or of short duration. Acute refers to the initial stage, short stage, or most severe stage of disease (e.g., acute low back strain may take a protracted course, becoming chronic, or may occur a number of times as part of a long-term chronic low back syndrome).

adenopathy: glandular swelling of the lymph nodes with morbid pathologic condition.

adhesions: tissue structures normally separated that adhere together because of inflammation or injury.

adventitious: acquired, not congenital; found out of normal place.

afebrile: without fever.

aggravated: made worse, more serious, or severe.

-agra (suffix): violent pain or seizure of acute pain.

-algia (suffix): painful.

allergy: hypersensitive state manifested by specific tissue changes after repeated exposure to particular allergens; an antibody-antigen reaction.

analgesia: loss of sensitivity to pain.

analgia: absence of pain.

anastomosis: connection of two distinct parts of cavities forming a passageway; the results of trauma or surgery. An example is the reattachment of a ruptured blood vessel after the injured portion has been removed.

anesthesia: loss of feeling or sensation of pain with or without loss of consciousness.

anomaly: malformation; a deviation from normal, usually referring to a congenital or hereditary defect.

anteflexion: the abnormal forward bending of an organ or part, not commonly used for skeletal disorders.

anteversion: forward rotation, as commonly seen in the femoral neck.

aphasia: either partial or complete, transient or permanent inability to understand or speak the spoken word as a result of a central neurologic occurrence such as stroke or injury.

aseptic: free of bacterial or fungal contamination.

asphyxia: lack of oxygen.

aspiration: withdrawal of fluids from a joint cavity, such as a bloody effusion in the knee. Also the inhalation of a liquid or solid such as the aspiration of vomit in an unconscious patient.

asthenia: lack of strength and energy.

asymmetry: dissimilarity between two corresponding parts of the body.

asymptomatic: absence of symptoms.

asynergia: disturbance of coordination.

ataxia: lack of muscle coordination with voluntary movement. Various types.

athetosis: involuntary writhing motions of the body (usually upper extremities).

atonia: lack of normal muscle tone; **atony.**

atrophy: wasting away of tissue, usually refers to muscle tissue.

atypical: irregular; appearing abnormal.

avascular: absence of adequate blood supply.

avulsion: tearing away of a part or structure from its attachment.

benign: not causing destruction of life or limb; when used in reference to tumors, denotes the absence of metastasis.

bifurcation: site at which any given structure divides in two.

bipartite: having two parts where only one is expected, for example, a bipartite patella.

bossing: rounded prominence of bone that is abnormally visible under the skin.

bruit (pronounced *bru-ee*): abnormal sound heard on auscultation of a blood vessel or the heart.

cachexia: systemic symptoms of malnutrition, malfunction, or debility that accompanies ill health or tissue breakdown.

café-au-lait: brown spots on surface of skin, often symptomatic of a systemic disease. Smooth borders "coast of California" are associated with neurofibromatosis and irregular borders "coast of Maine" are associated with McCune-Albright syndrome.

calcification: deposition of calcium salts either in normal bone or abnormally in soft tissue.

callosity: hardening of the epidermis because of persistent pressure.

callus: formation of new bone around a fracture site.

caries: decay and death of bone from bacterial action.

caries sicca: dry form of infection (i.e., less fluid associated with purulent material), characteristic of tuberculosis.

cellulitis: swelling and inflammation of soft tissues; may be caused by bacteria or chemical irritation.

chronic: describes symptoms, conditions, or diseases of long duration, as opposed to acute.

chylothorax: chyle (lymph duct fluid) that accumulates in the chest cavity that may occur after thoracic spine surgery with inadvertent transsection of lymph duct.

cicatrix: scar, may be formed by healing of any wound or tissue injury.

clonus: the uncontrolled spasmodic muscle jerking seen in conditions such as epilepsy or cerebral palsy. This term can refer to the spasmodic contraction of a reflex such as the ankle reflex that once elicited, continues indefinitely. When there are only several jerks in the muscle reflex, the term **unsustained clonus** is used.

-coele (suffix): indicates a sac or cavity; *-cele*.

comatose: semiconscious state; in a coma.

congenital: present at birth.

contagious: refers to a disease or condition that can be transmitted from one person to another; communicable.

contractions: jerky movements; spasms of musculature.

contracture: permanent shortening of muscle tissue due to paralysis or spasm; loss of motion of a joint due to fibrosis of tissue around the joint.

contrecoup: a blow to one side of the body that causes damage on the other, as often seen in head injuries.

contusion: bruise of any tissue but without disruption.

convalescence: any given period of recovery.

conversion disorder: a response to psychological conflict or need manifested by unintentionally produced signs of a physical disorder in which there is no known identifiable cause.

convulsion: violent involuntary contractions of voluntary muscles; paroxysm, seizure.

cramp: painful muscle spasm affecting the nerve supply to that muscle due to overexertion. Recumbency cramps are often felt in the legs and feet and occur at rest. Tonic muscle contractions can be anywhere and are associated with job-related activity. A "true" cramp is a motor unit hyperactivity that occurs at rest in the lower limbs. It is associated with motor neuron disease, fluid and electrolyte disorders, drug therapy, alcohol ingestion, or heat exposure.

crepitus: any crackling or grating sound with sensation on movement of surfaces at the joint; may indicate wearing away of cartilage.

cyanosis (adj. cyanotic): bluish discoloration of skin resulting from abnormally low levels of oxygen in blood; the actual cause is an excessive concentration of reduced hemoglobin.

cyst: any sac, normal or abnormal, containing liquid or semisolid material.

debridement: removal of foreign material or devitalized tissue from a wound.

decalcification: loss of calcium salts from bone or soft tissue.

defervescence: period of abatement of fever.

degenerative: deterioration of quality of tissue; rarely refers to dead tissue; usually describes a state of abnormal remodeling or replacement of tissue, sometimes making it less functional.

dehiscence: splitting or separation of a part or all of a closed wound.

deossification: loss or removal of bone of osseous tissue.

derangement: displacement of position of any given anatomic part; commonly used in reference to joints.

diagnosis: identifying a disease process or the agent responsible by means of cultures, tests, surgery, or intuition (recognizing patterns of disease).

diffuse: widely distributed; used in association with symptoms or disease terms.

diverticulum: in orthopaedics, usually refers to outpouching of a joint or tendon sheath.

dowager's hump: round upper back deformity.

-dynia (suffix): denotes pain.

dys- (prefix): denotes defective, difficult, or painful.

dysesthesia: pinprick or other abnormal sensations; painful touch perception.

dysfunction: impairment of function.

dysplasia: abnormal development or replacement of tissue.

dystonia: simultaneous contraction of agonist and antagonist muscles.

dystrophy: failure of normal replacement of tissue; see osteo-, chondro-, and muscular dystrophies.

eburnation: in degenerative joint disease, changes in subchondral bone render its substance dense, smooth, and ivory-like. The bone surface becomes exposed due to complete loss of cartilage surface.

ecchymosis: extravasation of blood under the skin, as seen in a bruise.

edema: excessive accumulations of fluid in soft tissues causing swelling; may be the result of heart failure, venous insufficiency, kidney failure, or malnutrition. More specifically, in inflammation, an increase in postcapillary intraluminal pressure causes a shift in equilibrium so that fluid return is impeded and accumulates in tissues, which results in edema.

effusion: collection of fluid in a cavity such as the joint space.

emaciation: wasted condition of the body; malnutrition.

enucleation: removal, either surgically or traumatically, of a tissue, organ, or foreign body.

erosion: uneven wearing away of a surface, as seen on radiographs of diseased bones.

erythema: redness of skin, as seen in sunburn; caused by an increased blood supply (capillary congestion).

eschar: term usually restricted to skin; refers to full-thickness skin graft with the formation of a hard, black, leathery, contracted material that, if removed, would reveal living tissue underneath.

esthesia: perception, feeling, sensation.

etiology: the study of all possible causes of a condition or disease, separated or related, based on what is presently known about that disease process.

exacerbation: aggravation of symptoms or increased severity of disease.

exudate: escape of fluid, cells, or cellular debris that escapes from blood vessels and deposits into soft tissues, cavities, or wounds as a result of inflammation. An exudate, in contrast to a transudate, is characterized by a high content of protein cells or solid materials derived from cells.

factitious injury: unconscious production of symptoms or actual physical injury for purposes of secondary gain, that is, attention or preferential treatment.

Fanconi anemia: radial clubhand deformity associated with dwarfism, brownish pigmentation of the skin, anomalies of the thumb, and then at 5 to 10 years of age a diminished number of all blood cells develops; **congenital pancytopenia, idiopathic refractory anemia.**

febrile: with fever.

fibrillation: involuntary contraction of small groups of muscle fibers as occurs with nerve root irritation; the fraying of a tissue such as seen in degenerative cartilage.

fissures: groove or natural division in tissue; also, ulcer-like sore.

flaccid: lacking muscle tone, whether voluntary or involuntary muscle.

flail: absence of motor control, as seen in a flail joint, may connote an abnormal mobility associated with loss of normal control such as flail chest, which is a chest crush injury.

foreign body: anything within a tissue that may lead to infection, inflammation, or scarring, requiring removal.

fretting: mechanical abrasion from relative micromotion between two surfaces. For orthopaedic appliances, this is between metal and bone or metal and cement. Microscopic particles are produced, initiating an inflammatory process that produces more loosening.

friable: tissue that is easily crumbled or separated.

fusiform: spindle shaped, tapered at ends.

gangrene: death of tissue caused by loss of blood supply (ischemia), bacterial infection, or both.

glycocalyx: extracellular polysaccharide elaborated by some bacteria that provides a binding material to internal prosthetic and fixation devices resulting in resistance to antibiotics.

granulation: reddish, moist, new tissue along edges of a healing wound.

hemorrhage: abnormal bleeding into soft tissues or a cavity; should this process form a discrete pocket of blood, it is called a hematoma; if the blood is evenly distributed in the tissue, it may appear as petechiae (very small), purpura (up to 1 cm), or ecchymosis (larger than 1 cm).

hereditary: familial or genetic transmission of a quality or trait from parent to offspring by a gene. When the gene is inherited from the chromosome associated with the sex of the offspring, it is said to be **sex linked.** When the characteristic is inherited from the other chromosomes, it is called **autosomal.** If both chromosomes need the same gene to have the characteristic expressed, the condition is said to be **recessive.** If only one chromosome must carry the affected gene, the condition is called **dominant.**

herniation: abnormal protrusion of a body structure beyond its normal limits, such as disk herniation.

hibernoma: a rare, benign soft tissue tumor originating from brown fat and named for the brown appearance of fat seen in hibernating animals.

Holt-Oram syndrome: atrial septal defect or other cardiac abnormality associated with a radial clubhand deformity.

hypalgesia: diminished sensitivity to pain; hypoesthesia.

hyperalgesia: increased sensitivity to pain; hyperesthesia.

hyperextension: excessive extension of joint.

hyperglycemia: abnormally high blood glucose level increasing risk of infection.

hyperplasia: excessive increase in the number of normal cells in tissue, producing an increase in size.

hypertension: high blood pressure.

hypertonia: excessive tension of muscle or arteries.

hypertrophy: increase in size of a structure due to a functional activity such as in muscle hypertrophy.

hypoglycemia: abnormally low blood glucose level.

hypoplasia: defective or incomplete development of tissue or an organ (e.g., hypoplastic labrum; an abnormally small rim of cartilage in the shoulder joint can lead to a laxity of that joint).

hypotension: low blood pressure.

iatrogenic: adverse effects of medical or surgical treatment that could have been avoided under proper care.

idiopathic: disease process with an unknown cause.

impingement: pressure transmitted from one tissue to the next, such as nerve impingement.

induration: firmness of soft tissue caused by extravasation of fluids and/or cells from blood vessels.

infarct: local area tissue death resulting from reduced or completely obliterated blood supply.

infection: an invasion into tissue of any microorganisms (endoparasites) with an immune response by the host to the viable irritant. The terms *infection* and *inflammation* are not interchangeable. The distinction is important in that inflammation is a vascular response that may not specifically or necessarily be due to infection.

inflammation: localized increase in blood supply, resulting in small vessel dilatation and/or migration of white blood cells into the tissue. Inflammation is the normal response of living tissue to an injury with tissue alteration. The inflammatory process mobilizes the body's defense mechanism to initiate the healing process and react against any microbes that may be introduced at the site of injury with resultant heat, pain, swelling, and loss of function. Inflammation involves two basic sequences that develop separately: vascular alteration and cellular phenomena. Examples are bursitis, arthritis, and tennis elbow.

insidious: undetectable development of symptoms or disease, usually gradual in onset.

intractable: resistant to therapy, relief, cure, or control.

ischemia: insufficient blood supply to a tissue or organ.

laceration: a cut, any wound made by a sharp or blunt object.

lesion: circumscribed area of tissue altered by structural or functional disease. The word lesion describes a wound, injury, or pathologic change in tissue. A gross lesion is visible to the naked eye.

line of demarcation: zone of inflammatory reaction separating a gangrenous area from healthy tissue.

lipping: development of excess bone at the margins of a joint, as seen in arthritis.

loxoscelism: condition caused by a bite from a brown recluse spider. A local rash progresses to full-thickness skin death. Small hemorrhage or blister may form, surrounded by blanched skin due to ischemia. A classic description is a nonhealing ulcer with red, white, and blue phenomenon.

lytic: denoting dissolution of tissue; used to refer to radiographic appearance of bone that has been displaced by some pathologic process.

maceration: softening or loss of surface tissue caused by constant exposure to moisture.

malaise: subjective feeling of being ill.

malignant: applied to neoplasms and implies the properties of anaplasia, invasion, and metastasis. A disease resistant to treatment, resulting in eventual destruction of tissue; in tumors, implies that the tumor spreads by seeding itself in distant regions of the body or by local uncontrolled invasion.

malingering: a rare situation in which an individual intentionally pretends to be ill only when being observed. This differs from **secondary gain,** in which the person derives an emotional gain from believing that he or she is ill.

meliodosis: an infectious disease caused by *Pseudomonas pseudomallei,* which, when it affects the skeleton, may mimic tuberculosis or tumors.

mesenchymoma: neoplastic tumors in which there are at least two cells of mesenchymal derivation other than fibrous tissue; for example, chrondrolipoangioma (cartilage, fat, and blood vessel).

metastasis: spread of malignant cells to other organs or tissues—a malignant tumor is said to metastasize.

microgeodic d.: transient phalangeal osteolysis that presents with pain and swelling and is followed by spontaneous resolution.

morbid: the disease state; however, the term may denote ready visibility, such as "morbid anatomy."

morbidity: condition of being diseased with untoward results; could be congenital, acquired, or iatrogenic.

mucopurulent: denotes an exudate containing mucus and pus.

mucosanguineous: denotes an exudate containing mucus and blood.

myxedema: dry, waxy type of swelling associated with abnormal deposits of mucin in the skin; *nonpitting edema.*

necrosis: death of tissue or group of cells in tissue from trauma or disease.

neoplasm: abnormal new growth of tissue, either benign or malignant.

nevus: mole or birthmark.

nidus: place or source of infection or reaction.

node: confined tissue swelling or mass that can be readily seen or palpated, for example, lymph node.

nodule: small node, usually hard.

nutritional index: minimum metabolic condition required for wound healing that includes a total serum protein of at least 6.2 g/dl, serum albumin of at least 3.5 g/dl, and a total lymphocyte count of 1500/mm^3.

obesity: abnormal accumulation of body fat.

occlusion: obstruction.

occult: hidden, not observable unless closely examined.

-odynia (suffix): pain.

onco- (prefix): combining form denoting relationship to swelling, mass, or tumor.

-orrhagia (suffix): hemorrhage.

-orrhea (suffix): discharge.

-orrhexis (suffix): rupture.

-osis (suffix): abnormal condition.

pectus carinatum: pigeon chest.

pectus excavatum: central depression of breast bone.

petechiae: tiny hemorrhages into the tissue; when seen in the skin, they appear as little violet dots.

phantom limb syndrome: sensations of an amputated part still being present. The perception of the phantom limb gradually shrinks to localization of sensation appropriate to the level of the stump.

-phyma (suffix): swelling produced by exudate to subcutaneous tissue.

pleomorphic: taking on a shape that lacks description such as round, square, angular, and so forth. The term is often used to describe the shape of cells.

plexiform: taking on a tortuous or multiple form shape. Often used to describe the shape of a tumor.

polyps: protruding growths from mucous membranes.

procurvatum: angulation of a bone or joint that is convexed anteriorly.

prognosis: prediction of the outcome of disease or surgery.

prophylaxis: prevention of disease.

proprioception: sensibility to position, whether conscious or unconscious.

purpura: hemorrhage into the skin or other area with extravasation of blood into a congested area that is eventually resorbed.

purulent: pus-forming.

pyoderma gangrenosum: rare, destructive cutaneous lesion that starts as a painful, rapidly enlarging ulcer leading to a chronic, draining wound. Often associated with other diseases.

pyogenic: having the ability to produce pus.

pyrexia: fever.

quiescence: discontinuation of symptoms or a disease, the connotation being an expectation of the return of symptoms or disease.

rarefaction: decrease in density, usually used to refer to appearance of bone on radiograph.

recrudescence: relapse or recurrence of symptoms.

recurvatum: angulation of bone or joint that is convexed posteriorly.

regressive remodeling: removal and replacement of bone such that the replacement occurs progressively away from the original maximal border of bone, for example, codfish vertebrae.

rigidus: stiffness.

rubor: redness of the skin.

rudimentary: insufficient development of a part or the development of an extra part such that no function is served by its presence; a rudimentary limb is so deficient that it serves no function, and a thirteenth rib similarly serves no function and is rudimentary.

rupture: discontinuity of tissue, usually referring to muscles and tendons.

sanguineous: bloody, as in a wound. This is in contrast to serosanguineous fluid, which is serous fluid containing some red cells.

saponification: calcification that occurs with the breakdown of fatty acids in the avascular area of aseptic necrosis.

sarcoidosis: granulomatous disorder of unknown cause affecting mostly the skin, lungs, and eyes. The condition usually is seen in the third and fourth decade of life. When bone is involved, the disorder usually affects the hands and feet.

sebaceous: secreting a greasy substance, as in oily skin or sebaceous cyst.

sepsis: denotes the presence of infection caused by bacteria.

septicemia: bacteria in the blood. It should be noted that blood poisoning often refers to the red streaks seen in a limb that has an infection; however, this condition is more accurately a lymphangitis.

sequela (pl. sequelae): sequel that follows, that is, a morbid condition that follows the consequence of disease, meaning one pathologic condition leads to another discrete pathologic condition; for example, muscle spasticity is a sequela of cerebral palsy.

seropurulent: denotes an exudate containing both pus and serous material.

serosanguineous: denotes an exudate containing both blood and serous material.

serous: denotes an exudate that is usually yellow, fairly fluid, and possibly blood-tinged.

slough: spontaneous separation of devitalized tissue from living tissue.

somatization disorder: in some patients with chronic pain, there are recurrent somatic complaints without an apparent significant physical disorder. Physical symptoms are related to anxiety, and the patient may seek medical attention over a period of years.

spasm: sudden or violent involuntary contractions of muscle.

spastic: characterized by spasm.

splaying: to spread out, as in flatfoot deformity.

spurs: abnormal projection of bone at the margin or joints or strong ligamentous or tendinous attachments.

stenosis: stricture or narrowing of a canal or opening.

stigma: physical mark that aids in the identification of an abnormal process.

subliminal: below the threshold of sensation; weak; no muscle contractions.

supernumerary: excess number of anatomic parts, for example, six fingers on one hand.

suppurative: producing pus.

syncope: fainting.

TAR syndrome: *t*hrombocytopenia *a*genesis *r*adius; the coincidental findings of bilateral failure of formation of the radius associated with petechiae, black stools, and other signs of thrombocytopenia resulting from a failure of normal formation of platelets. This autosomal recessive disorder improves with proper support, leaving the skeletal deformity as the primary problem.

tardy: denotes delayed onset or appearance of a disease process (e.g., tardy ulnar nerve palsy, which may occur years after an elbow fracture).

tetany: symptom of a biochemical disturbance or imbalance in the body characterized by hyperactivity of sensory and motor units and marked by spasms and twitching of muscles of the hands and feet and possibly spinal muscles. Most common causes are hypocalcemia, hypokalemia, hypoparathyroidism (rare), hyperventilation, or lack of vitamin D. (Not to be confused with tetanus, an infection.)

tonus: involuntary continued contraction of a muscle after the patient has attempted voluntary relaxation.

torticollis: postural neck deformity associated with a turning and/or bending of the head and neck. May be due to congenital muscle tightness or disorders such as birth injury, psychogenic spasm, or spasm due to trauma. The term *wry-neck* is sometimes said of this condition.

toxic: poisonous.

transudate: fluid passage through a normal membrane due to imbalance in osmotic and hydrostatic forces.

trauma: any injury to tissue or psyche; can result from chemical, physical, or temporal events.

tumefaction: swelling, puffiness, edema.

tumor: a swelling, in the most generalized sense. However, the term connotes a neoplasm, that is, a new uncontrolled growth of tissue.

turgid: swollen or congested, describing a physical finding on palpation.

ulcer: penetrating disruption of mucous membrane of skin. There are two classification systems for ulcers:

Wagner
Grade 0: no open lesions.
Grade 1: superficial ulcer.
Grade 2: deep ulcer.
Grade 3: localized osteomyelitis or abscess.
Grade 4: forefoot gangrene.
Grade 5: gangrene of entire foot.

Depth-Ischemia
Depth
Grade 0: at risk foot, no ulcer.
Grade 1: superficial ulcer, no infection.
Grade 2: deep ulceration.
Grade 3: extensive ulceration with exposed bone and deep infection.
Ischemia
Grade A: not ischemic.
Grade B: ischemia without gangrene.
Grade C: partial forefoot gangrene.
Grade D: complete forefoot gangrene.

VATER association: acronym for a nonrandom group of occurrences that include *v*ertebral segmentation disorders and fusion, *a*nal atresia, *t*racheoesophageal fistula, *e*sophageal atresia, and *r*adial ray defects. Other defects may occur.

vestigial: remnants of a structure that functioned in a previous stage of species or individual development.

wound: any disruption of normal tissue. A break in the skin is usually implied, but the term can be applied to a traumatic injury in which deep tissue is injured but the skin has not been broken. The International Committee of the Red Cross (ICRC) has the following classification directed at war wounds:

X Exit wound
  X (cm): maximum diameter of exit wound.
E Entry wound
  E (cm): maximum diameter of entry wound.
C Size of cavity within limb
  C0: cavity will not admit two fingers at surgery.
  C1: cavity will admit two fingers at surgery.
F Fracture
  F0: no fracture.
  F1: simple hole in bone or insignificant comminution.
  F2: clinically significant comminution.
V Involvement of vital structure such as viscera or major vessel.
  V0: no vital structure involved.
  V1: at least one vital structure involved.
M Metallic bodies
  M0: no bullet or fragments.
  M1: one metallic body.
  M2: multiple metallic bodies.
Grading System
  Grade 1: Sum of E+X is less than 10 with scores C0 and F0 or F1.
  Grade 2: Sum of E+X is less than 10 with scores C1 or F2.
  Grade 3: Sum of E+X is 10 or greater with scores C1 or F2.

wryneck: torticollis; stiff condition of the neck caused by spastic muscle contractions.

Imaging Techniques

3

Computerized diagnostic imaging techniques have expanded the field of radiology. Computer technology applied to radiology has contributed to diagnosing diseases more than any other method in medicine. Thus, the computer has become an indispensable tool for managing information and for recording programs from various scanning devices, which can be retrieved and read out by a central computer bank. This technology, with computer graphics and anatomic color images, gives medical specialists a more accurate diagnostic picture, has changed diagnostic procedures, and saves considerable time.

The standard radiographic technique depicts a body part as a simple two-dimensional shadow portrayed on a negative film. The new imaging technology creates two- and three-dimensional views from any angle. The types of diagnostic imaging are as follows:

- *Nuclear medicine studies*—Invasive (require an injection) tests that utilize radioisotopes; examples are positron emission tomography (PET) and bone scan (scintigraphy) (Fig. 3-1).
- *Magnetic resonance imaging (MRI)*—Noninvasive technology that combines radiowaves and a strong magnetic field with the hydrogen atoms in the body to produce images of soft tissue structures.
- *Ultrasound (sonography, ultrasonography), digital color Doppler, pulsed Doppler, or power Doppler*—Noninvasive forms of imaging that use a small transducer (transmitter/receiver) that is in contact with the area being examined to produce high-frequency sound waves that penetrate the area involved and reflect back to the receiver.
- *Computed axial tomography (CAT) scanning* and *radioisotope imaging (RII)*—This may be an invasive (requiring intravenous injection of a radiopaque solution) or a noninvasive technique. Scans can now be obtained in a continuous helical motion and not just by a single slice at a time. These and other radiographic techniques are updated and defined in this edition.

Radiography has been an integral part of the orthopaedic examination, and the new diagnostic imaging techniques enable the orthopaedic surgeon not only to identify the anatomic site but to evaluate the physiologic conditions within and surrounding this site. Specifically, bone density, pathologic changes (necrosis of bone tissue, tumors, infections), spur formation, joint space narrowing, synovial inflammation, nerve impingements, and soft tissue changes can be evaluated. A computer compiles vast amounts of digital data during an examination, and these data are turned into picture form. Physicians compare the many views, which can ultimately be made into a single video image. The most important contribution of imaging technology is that it enables physicians to see detailed views of the body without surgery.

The radiologist, a board-certified physician and specialist in radiology, is often consulted by the orthopaedist and other physicians to give interpretations of imaging technology and of more complicated

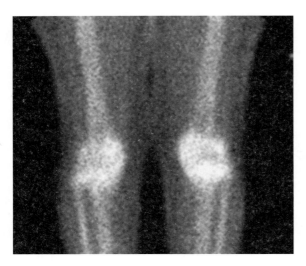

FIG 3-1 Bone scan image with areas of more active bone formation brighter at knee joint with arthritis.

pathologic conditions. The radiologist is assisted by qualified technologists who have learned the fundamentals of working with the radiographic and imaging equipment, developing film, and positioning patients. These specialists are challenged to meet the ever-changing technologic demands in their field to capably assist all branches of medicine.

This chapter presents the specialized terminology of radiology, new imaging technology, and its application to orthopaedics.

General Radiologic Terms

baseline radiograph: radiograph taken at time of first examination and compared with those taken later.

catheter: a thin plastic tube inserted through the skin and into an artery or vein for the injection of contrast material in a vascular arteriography procedure; see also **femoral arteriography.**

cathode ray tube: vacuum tube that with a high enough voltage will produce x-rays.

contrast: a radiopaque medium that appears white on x-ray and can be given intravenously, intra-arterially, intrathecally, orally, rectally, or into a joint to aid visualization of internal structures; **contrast**

radiography, contrast study. New **nonionic contrast agents** have been developed. Advantages over standard ionic agents are that there are fewer serious allergic reactions, meaning in patients at risk for allergic reactions, nonionic agents should be used.

echogenic: in ultrasound, giving rise to echoes of ultrasound waves. Examples are bone, metal, and air; produces white areas on the ultrasound images.

oscilloscope: instrument that displays computer data of electrical variations on the fluorescent screen of a cathode-ray tube.

Pantopaque: trade name for an iodinated oil (radiopaque contrast medium) used in a contrast radiographic procedure (i.e., myelography).

rad: measure of *r*adiation *a*bsorbed *d*ose, 100 erg/g (energy per gram).

radiograph: image produced on a film by means of ionizing radiation. **X-ray,** as in a "chest x-ray," is a commonly used synonym.

radiology: the specialized branch of medicine concerned with the diagnosis of disease utilizing ionizing (e.g., x-rays) and nonionizing (e.g., ultrasound and MRI) radiation; **roentgenology.** A **radiologist** is a specialized doctor who interprets the radiology studies.

radiolucent: permitting free passage of ionizing energy (x-ray) through an area, with dark appearance on exposed film.

radiopaque: preventing passage of ionizing energy (x-ray), thus allowing the representative area to appear light or white on exposed film; **opaque.**

roentgen (R): unit of x- or gamma radiation exposure; 1 **gray** = 100 roentgen; 1 **centigray** = 1 roentgen.

roentgenography: the use of x-irradiation to produce either positive or negative film images or fluoroscopic images of objects; **radiography.**

scout film: general term for a radiograph prior to the injection of contrast. The purpose is to check the radiographic technique and to look for abnormalities that may be obscured once contrast is given; **scout radiograph.**

translucent: allowing some light to pass through but not clearly transparent; for example, soft tissue appears as a light shadow on a radiograph when compared with bone.

wet reading: as implied. Today, films are dried automatically and are read dry. In the past, if an immediate interpretation of the film was required, it was read while still wet. Thus, a request for an immediate interpretation is still called *wet reading.*

x-ray: electromagnetic radiation generally greater than 10 Kev in energy and less than 1 nanometer in wavelength, capable of penetrating tissue; **roentgen ray.**

Orthopaedic Radiographic Techniques and Procedures

arthrography: x-ray procedure showing interior outline of a joint after radiopaque medium and/or air has been injected intra-articularly; tendon, ligament, or meniscal tears can be detected in this manner; **arthrogram.**

bone densitometry: procedure for determining the relative density of bone by using several different radiographic techniques. A density gradient plate can be placed on the film at the same time radiography of the part is being performed. From this plate, a comparative density of the bone can be made, usually of the spine. Photons from a single emitting source can be used to directly measure the density of bone, such as that of the distal radius and lumbar spine. These studies can then be compared with age-matched normal values. This procedure is called **photon densitometry.**

> *dual photon densitometry (DPD), dual photon absorptiometry (DPA):* the use of two different emitting sources to help correct for soft tissue density.

> *dual x-ray absorptiometry (DEXA):* the use of two different x-ray voltages to correct for soft tissue density.

> *quantitative computed tomography (QCT):* another method of measuring bone density by using computerized tomographic images through lumbar vertebral bodies and comparing the measured density with age-matched normal values.

bone marrow pressure (BMP): measurement taken to detect bone necrosis. The pressure is taken while *intraosseous venography* and *core decompression* are performed to aid in diagnosis of ischemic necrosis

of the femoral head (INFH), forming an early basis for treatment.

bursography: injection of radiopaque dye to show a bursa such as a retrocalcaneal bursa.

diskography: visualization of the cervical and lumbar intervertebral disks after direct injection of a radiopaque contrast medium into the disk; diskogram.

femoral arteriography: radiographic examination in which the femoral artery of the groin is catheterized. Through the femoral artery, the catheter can be directed to arteries throughout the body including the brain, chest, abdomen, and legs. Contrast is injected through the catheter to identify abnormalities in the arterial system or can be useful in outlining extent of a tumor; **arteriogram.** In some cases, a vascular abnormality can be treated through the catheter (e.g., by angioplasty).

fluoroscopy: direct visual radiographic procedure with the use of x-ray tube, fluoroscopic screen, and television monitor for intensification, that is, continuous monitoring showing organ function that can be videotaped; used in gastrointestinal studies, arthrography, and angiography.

Isovue (lopamidol) myelography: This and Omnipaque (lohexol) are newer water-soluble contrast agents used for myelography after injection of an iodine-based water-soluble contrast medium. The material does not have to be withdrawn after completion of the study, giving some advantages over the oil-based material that must be withdrawn.

KUB (kidneys, ureters, bladder): generally not an orthopaedic radiographic procedure but taken occasionally to study the abdominal wall and/or suspected masses.

lymphangiography: radiographic examination after introduction of radiopaque contrast medium into peripheral lymphatic vessels to determine presence of blockage or tumor in proximal lymphatic vessels.

myelography: radiographic examination with contrast medium injected into the subarachnoid space under fluoroscopy to examine the spinal cord and canal for possible disk protrusions or lesions; **myelogram.**

orthoroentgenography: for measuring limb-length disparity; three separate exposures are taken of the hip (or shoulder), knee (or elbow), and the ankle (or wrist) to produce an image of the entire limb; **orthoroentgenogram.**

pneumoarthrography: injection of air into a joint before radiographic examination to determine internal outline, as in meniscal tear or other injuries and abnormalities; **pneumoarthrogram.**

roentgen stereophotogrammetry: simultaneous anterior-posterior and lateral radiographic examination performed with the examined part in a calibration cage. Radiographs can be obtained serially over time to study the progression of bony changes. Computer-driven calculations allow for the identification of three-dimensional changes as small as 2 mm. The technique is particularly useful in the study of prosthetic wear and migration over time.

scanography: for measuring leg-length discrepancy, a film is moved beneath the patient for three successive exposures of the three pairs of joints, and a radiopaque scale is placed beneath the limbs so that measurements may be made from the scale of the film. A film 43 cm in length may be used rather than a film two to three times longer; **scanogram.**

sinography: radiographic examination for sinus tract infection in bone, performed after injection of water-soluble contrast medium, after saline cleanser, to determine the course of a deep draining wound; **sinogram.**

teleroentgenography: for measuring limb-length disparity; radiographic examination performed with the x-ray tube 2 to 3 m (6 to 7.5 feet) from the plate to obtain a more parallel roentgenogram. The entire bone is visualized, but the degree of magnification (about 10%) is difficult to assess; **teleroentgenogram.**

tomography: used to show detailed images of structures lying in a predetermined plane of tissue, while blurring or eliminating details of images of structures in other planes as in polytomography, planography, or zonography. It is used with radiographic magnification to detect abnormalities of the spine (laminography) or joints and in malunion fractures; **tomogram.**

Routine Radiographic Views

The number of views varies and is determined by the history and physical examination. For instance, an anteroposterior (AP) view may be unremarkable, but a lateral view may reveal a fracture or dislocation, depending on the angle of view taken. A complaint of knee pain often arises from a hip disorder, making radiographic (x-ray) views of the knee and/or hip important in diagnostic evaluation. Asymmetry of two identical bones (comparing femur to femur) can also exhibit an underlying abnormality. More than one view is usually required to diagnose the chief complaint. The terms are defined first and then given in abbreviated form by anatomic region.

Alexander v.: lateral view of scapula with shoulders protracted forward.

AP v.: anteroposterior view (x-ray beam passes from front to back).

apical v.: apex, tip, or point of subject radiographed.

apical lordotic v.: usually of the chest for the apices of the lungs, but for the clavicle if a patient's symptoms suggest an orthopaedic problem.

axillary lateral v.: for the shoulder, lateral view through axilla.

Breuerton v.: special view of the hand to search for early joint changes in rheumatoid arthritis.

Broden v.: for injuries affecting subtalar joint; lateral view of foot with a 45-degree rotation and various tilts.

Bura v.: for ulnar side of wrist; a supinated oblique view taken as an AP with 35 degrees supination.

Burnham v.: AP hyperextended view of thumb with dorsum on cassette and 15-degree cephalic tilt.

Canale v.: for the talus; an AP view with 75-degree cephalic tilt and 15-degree pronation.

carpal tunnel v.: for hook-of-hamate fracture; tangential view of volar wrist taken with wrist in dorsiflexion.

Carter-Rowe v.: view of the hip taken at a 45-degree oblique angle to determine size of bone fragment in a posterior acetabular hip fracture or other abnormality of the pelvis.

clenched fist v.: to demonstrate scapholunate instability; an AP view is taken with the fist clenched.

coned-down v.: close-up of a particular area, with radiation shielded from the rest of the patient's body.

cross-table lateral v.: for hip fracture; lateral view obtained with opposite hip in flexion.

false profile view: standing lateral x-ray of pelvis with person turned with the hip furthest from the cassette slightly posterior.

frog-leg lateral v.: AP view of hip in abduction and external rotation.

Garth v.: for acromioclavicular joint injury; apical oblique with 45-degree caudal and AP tilt.

Grashey v.: for shoulder impingement by acromion; scapular lateral with a 10-degree caudal tilt; **supraspinatus outlet v.**

Harris v.: for calcaneus; AP standing with 45-degree tilt.

Hobb v.: for sternoclavicular joint; while standing, the patient bends over end of x-ray table and cassette with hands on head, neck parallel to table, and chest about 45 degrees to table. The x-ray beam is vertical to the cassette.

Hughston v.: knee is flexed to 60 degrees, and view is obtained at a 55-degree angle to show a cartilage-osseous fracture of the femoral condyle or subluxing patella.

inlet v.: for pelvic injury; 45- to 50-degree caudad AP.

inversion ankle stress: AP view of the ankle, which is stressed in inversion to test the integrity of the lateral collateral ankle ligaments.

lateral v.: view taken side to side, left or right.

lateral monopodal stance v.: for anterior cruciate deficiency; lateral x-ray to detect posterior shift of femur on tibia.

Lowenstein v.: a frog-leg lateral.

lumbosacral series: multiple views of the lumbosacral spine to include AP, lateral, and oblique views.

Merchant v.: tangential superior to inferior patellar view taken with the knee flexed at 45 degrees; **Knuttson v.**

mortise v.: view of the ankle rotated internally until medial and lateral malleoli are parallel to film; demonstrates the talus, tibia, and fibula without superimposition; used for comparison with normal AP view and to detect joint abnormalities.

Neer transscapular v. (Neer lateral v.): posterior oblique scapular projection to help obtain a lateral view of the shoulder in trauma.

notch v.: prone view of knee with 45-degree caudal from vertical.

oblique v.: any view that is off angle from AP, posteroanterior (PA), or lateral.

odontoid v.: specific for the odontoid process of C2 vertebra; AP view obtained with mouth open; **open-mouth v.**

outlet v.: for pelvic injury; 45-degree cephalad AP view.

PA: posteroanterior view (from back to front).

plantar axial v. of foot: offers visualization of the plantar aspect of the metatarsal heads.

prayer v.: for wrist instabilities; lateral view of both wrists at same time with palms pressed together to bring about maximum wrist extension.

push-pull ankle stress: lateral view of the ankle, which is stressed in an attempt to evaluate the anterior talofibular ligament.

Robert v.: AP hyperextended view of thumb with dorsum on cassette.

Rosenberg v.: for osteoarthrosis knee; weight-bearing PA with knee at 45-degree flexion.

serendipity v.: for sternoclavicular dislocation or proximal-third fracture of the clavicle; AP view taken with patient supine and tube angled upward 40 degrees from the vertical position.

Slomann v.: for tarsal coalition; a 45-degree oblique view of the foot.

Stryker notch v.: for scapular notch; view taken with patient supine, hand on head, and camera with 10-degree cephalic tilt.

sunset v.: view of patella with knee bent at 120 degrees to permit a profile view; used for examination of patella and adjacent femoral surfaces; **sunrise v., tangential v.**

swimmer's v.: for lower cervical spine injuries; lateral view obtained with one arm held overhead while other arm is pulled down.

transthoracic lateral v.: for proximal humeral fracture or dislocation; view obtained with one arm held overhead and x-ray beam directed through chest.

trauma v.: for shoulder injuries; true AP, 45-degree oblique, and Y scapular (tangential) views.

true lateral v.: perfectly positioned lateral projection without rotation.

tunnel v.: view of tibia, fibula, and femur only with patella out of the way; a knee notch or intercondylar view; the radiographic examination is done with the tibia and fibula straight and the femur at a 45-degree angle.

von Rosen v.: view of the hips in abduction and internal rotation for determining dislocation of the hip(s) in developmental dysplasia.

West Point v.: for shoulder (glenoid) injuries; prone axillary lateral view with 25-degree lateral and posterior tilt to camera.

Y scapular v.: lateral view of scapula taken at an angle to view scapular blade such that it appears as stem of Y with coracoid and spine as the branches of the "Y."

Zanca v.: for distal-third clavicle fractures or acromioclavicular joint, a 10-degree cephalad view.

Radiographic Views by Anatomic Region
Thoracic Region
chest: PA, lateral.

clavicle: AP, apical lordotic, tangential.

ribs:
  anterior: PA, obliques.
  posterior: AP, obliques.

scapula: AP, oblique, lateral.

shoulder: AP, internal rotation; AP, external rotation; axillary lateral; transthoracic lateral.

sternum: right anterior oblique, lateral.

Upper Limbs
elbow: AP, lateral, oblique.

hands/fingers: AP, lateral, oblique.

humerus: AP, lateral, transthoracic lateral.

radius/ulna: AP, lateral.

wrist: AP, lateral, oblique, AP with ulnar and radial deviation (for scaphoid fracture), carpal tunnel.

Spinal Region
C-spine: AP, lateral, both obliques, open-mouth odontoid.

coccyx: AP, lateral.

L-spine: AP, lateral, both obliques, coned-down L-5 to S-1 lateral.

pelvis: AP, inlet, outlet.

SI joints: AP, both obliques.

sacrum: AP, lateral.

T-spine: AP, lateral.

Lower Limbs
ankle: AP, lateral, and mortise oblique.

femur: AP, lateral.

foot/toes: AP, lateral, oblique.

hip: AP, frog-leg, and/or cross-table lateral.

knee: AP, lateral, tunnel, Hughston.

patella: tunnel, sunset, lateral, PA, merchant.

tibia/fibula: AP, lateral.

calcaneus: lateral, plantodorsal, axial.

Additional views requested may be views in flexion and extension, special views of the skull, "push-pull" films of hips for piston sign, and cine (movies) of x-ray images.

Radiographic Angles, Lines, Signs, and Methods

Angles
The anatomic description is taken directly from points using the intersection of two straight lines to form the angle.

acetabular angle: angle created by the intersection of a line from the inferior margin to the superior margin of the acetabulum and a line horizontal to the pelvis (connecting two inferior acetabuli; Fig. 3-2).

acetabular index: angle created by intersection of line horizontal to pelvis with line of the superior subchondral bone of the acetabulum (**Tonnis angle**).

acromial a.: angle between clavicle and head of humerus.

anatomic femorotibial a. (FTA): angle created by the intersection of lines through shaft of the tibia and shaft of the femur.

Baumann a.: angle created by intersection of two lines drawn on an AP view of a child; one line is drawn from the medial margin of the distal humeral physeal line to the lateral margin of the lateral condylar epiphysis; and the other line is drawn in the line of the lateral condylar epiphysis. This angle is usually 11 degrees.

bimalleolar angle: angle drawn by bisection of line horizontal to ankle joint with line crossing medial and lateral malleolar tips. This angle is typically 23 degrees.

Böhler a.: angle formed by intersection of a line drawn from the cephalic aspect of the anterior calcaneal tuberosity to the superior point of the posterior facet with a line drawn from the superior point of

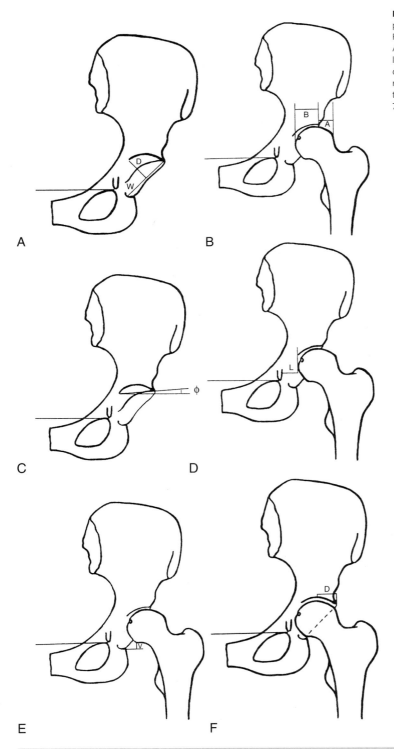

FIG 3-2 Radiographic measurements for hip dysplasia. **A,** Acetabular index of depth to width. **B,** Femoral head extrusion index (A / [A + B]) × 100. **C,** Acetabular index expressed as angle φ. **D,** Lateral luxation expressed as distance L. **E,** Superior (vertical) subluxation expressed as distance v from inferior tip acetabulum to inferior femoral head. **F,** Peak to edge distance D. (From *J Bone Joint Surg* 77A:985, 1995.)

the posterior facet to the superior posterior calcaneus, normally 20 to 40 degrees.

carrying a.: for the AP angle of the extended elbow, that is, the angle of the forearm when arm is extended.

CE (center edge) a. (Wiberg): created by two lines drawn from the center of the femoral capital epiphysis, one line being vertical and the other extending to the acetabular edge.

Codman a.: discrete angle at edge of the bone cortex produced by periosteal elevation and reactive bone in the area of a tumor; **Codman triangle.**

condylar-plateau a. (CPA): angle created by the intersection of a line parallel to the tibial plateau surfaces and the distal femoral condyles.

congruence a.: bisecting angle of the patella intersecting with vertical angle from trochlea (Fig. 3-3).

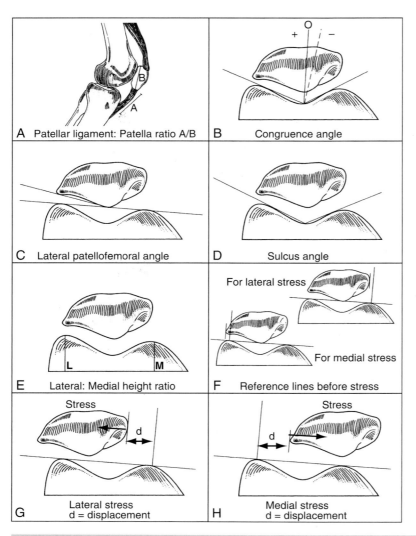

FIG 3-3 Radiographic measurements to evaluate patellar instability. **A,** Insall-Salveti ratio, *A-B,* normally 0.8 to 1.2. **B,** Merchant congruence angle, normally −6 degrees (medial) and is pathologic if 16 or more degrees. **C,** Lateral patellofemoral angle open 97% of the time in asymptomatic individuals and medially or 0 degrees in recent subluxation. **D,** Sulcus angle normally 142 degrees. **E,** Lateral height: medial height normally 1.65. **F-H,** Reference lines for patella margins before and after medial and lateral stress, measuring distance *d.* (From *J Bone Joint Surg* 78A:194, 1996.)

A Patellar ligament: Patella ratio A/B

B Congruence angle

C Lateral patellofemoral angle

D Sulcus angle

E Lateral: Medial height ratio

For lateral stress

For medial stress

F Reference lines before stress

Stress

G Lateral stress
d = displacement

Stress

H Medial stress
d = displacement

costophrenic angle: angle formed at the junction of the costal and diaphragmatic parietal pleura.

costovertebral angle: angle made between the 12th thoracic rib and the T12 vertebra at the posterior inferior margin of the thoracic cage on each side.

crucial angle of Gissane: seen on lateral radiograph of foot, angle created by posterior facet of calcaneus and the superior anterolateral surface of the calcaneus.

femoral tibial a.: angle created by anatomic axis of the femur and tibia (line drawn from midpoint of proximal and distal shaft). Average is 6 degrees of valgus.

Ferguson's angle (sacral base angle): represents the angle of the lumbosacral junction as measured by the inclination of the superior surface of the first sacral vertebra to the horizontal (usually measured from a standing lateral film).

Fick angle: standing foot angle or Fick's angle represents the amount of toeing in (**decreased foot angle**) or toeing out (**increased foot angle**) observed during stance.

Fowler-Phillip a.: to measure degree of "pump bump"; angle created by intersection of a line from the posterior surface and the plantar surface of the calcaneus.

hallux valgus a.: angle created by intersection of a longitudinal line through shaft of first metatarsal and the shaft of the proximal first phalanx.

head-shaft angle (Southwick a.): for slipped capital femoral epiphysis; angle of femoral head physis to vertical line drawn through the femoral shaft seen on frog-leg projection.

Hibb a.: two angles created by intersection of a longitudinal line of first metatarsal and the line of the plantar surface of the calcaneus.

Hilgenreiner a.: angle of the acetabular slope to the Y-line (horizontal line drawn through both acetabular centers); **acetabular index a.**

Hilgenreiner epiphyseal a.: for coxa vara or slipped epiphysis angle of intersection of Y-line with line drawn through femoral physis.

Kager triangle: triangular space anterior to the Achilles tendon normally visible on radiographs as a radiolucent area.

Konstram a.: for gibbus deformity; the obtuse angle created by the intersection of the two lines drawn parallel to the surface of the superior vertebral body above and inferior surface of vertebral body below the deformed segment(s).

lateral distal femoral a.: angle of a line from the femoral head to the tibial spine to a line across the two femoral condylar surfaces; measured from lateral to vertical.

Laquesna and Deseze a.: for acetabular coverage of femoral head in developmental hip dysplasia; using a lateral x-ray view, the angle between a line seen in the shaft of the femur and from the center of the femoral head to the anterior acetabular rim; **ventral inclination a. (VCA).**

Laurin (lateral patellofemoral a.): acute angle created by intersection of line drawn from medial to lateral condylar points and a line parallel to the lateral undersurface of the patella. The angle is positive when it opens laterally.

Levine Drennan a.: angle that lies between a line drawn through the most distal points of the medial and lateral beaks of the metaphysis and a line perpendicular to the lateral cortex of the tibia; **metaphyseal-diaphyseal a.**

lumbosacral angle: angle between the inferior plate of L5 to line of superior plate of sacrum. Typically the sacrum is inclined such that the sacral line opens anteriorly in reference to the lumbar line.

Meary angle: angle formed between the long axis of the talus and the first metatarsal on a lateral weight-bearing view. This line is used as a measurement collapse of the longitudinal arch. An angle that is greater than 4 degrees convex downward is considered pes planus.

mechanical axis: line created between the center of the femoral head and the center of the talus. In a normal knee, this axis passes close to the center of the joint; **Maquet l.**

medial proximal tibial a.: for tibial plateau slope; the angle created by a vertical tibial shaft line and a line across the tibial plateaus; measured to the medial plateau.

Merchant a.: created by intersection of two lines drawn from intracondylar apex of patella to center and a line perpendicular to plane of condyles.

Mikulicz a.: of declination formed by the neck of the femoral epiphysis and diaphysis center lines.

neck shaft a.: created by intersection of a line drawn through the femoral shaft and a line through the femoral head and neck.

Pauwels a.: of a femoral neck fracture in reference to the horizontal line of a standing patient.

pelvic femoral a.: of inclination formed by the pelvis with line of femoral shaft.

physeal a. (physeal slope): for Legg-Calvé-Perthes disease; the angle created by intersection of a line drawn vertically though the femoral shaft and the line of femoral head physis.

pitch angle: (**calcaneal inclination angle**) a line is drawn from the plantar-most surface of the calcaneus to the inferior border of the distal articular surface. The angle made between this line and the transverse plane of the floor is the calcaneal pitch angle. A decreased pitch is consistent with pes planus.

Q angle: made by intersection of lines drawn from anterosuperior iliac spine (ASIS) to midpatella and from midpatella to anterior tibial tuberosity.

radial inclination angle: measured by drawing a perpendicular line to the radial axis through the distal sigmoid notch and by drawing another line joining the tip of the radial styloid and the distal sigmoid notch. These two lines form the radial inclination angle (normal angle 21–25 degrees).

sacrovertebral a.: obtained by junction of lines through lateral projection of sacrum and lumbar spine.

Sharp a.: defined by intersection of lines from inferior acetabulum (bottom of teardrop) to superolateral acetabulum and a horizontal line.

slip a.: angle of the line of the inferior body of L5 to the line of the superior body of S1. As L5 slips forward on S1 this angle reverses.

sternal angle: angle formed by the junction of the manubrium and the body of the sternum. This is also called the **angle of Louis.**

sulcus a.: on Merchant view, lines drawn from apex of medial and lateral condyles to lowest point in groove to create this obtuse angle.

talocrural a.: angle created by intersection of lines, one drawn parallel to the tibial plafond, the other across the tips of the medial and lateral malleoli; normally 8 to 15 degrees.

Ward triangle: relatively radiolucent area of bone in the intertrochanteric area of the femur.

Lines, Indices, and Ratios

A *line* is defined as that seen or drawn directly on the film to help in the interpretation of the radiograph or an anatomic line of reference.

acetabular coverage: may be expressed as distance from lateral lip of acetabulum to lateral edge of the femoral head; or as a ratio of the width of the femoral head divided into distance from the lateral lip of acetabulum to the lateral edge of the femoral head.

acetabular depth: depth of the longest possible vertical line drawn perpendicular to a line crossing the superior and inferior acetabular margins.

acetabular head quotient: for hip dysplasia; the ratio of the radius of the femoral head divided by the distance from the femoral head center to a vertical line drawn from the acetabular lip.

acetabular l.: line drawn from superolateral tip of both acetabuli for measuring femoral head or prosthetic migration.

anteversion: descriptive of axial rotation. For example, the normal relationship of femoral head is 20 degrees anterior to axis of femur.

Blackburne ratio: for a patella alta; with the knee flexed at 30 degrees, the ratio is measured A:B. *A* is the distance from the point parallel to the tibial condylar surface to the inferior weight-bearing surface of the patella. *B* is the height of the weight-bearing portion of the patella. The noncartilaginous inferior pole portion of the patella is eliminated from the measurement.

Blumensaat l.: line parallel to superior part of intercondylar notch as seen on lateral radiographs; used to judge the relative height of the patella.

canal-to-calcar isthmus ratio: for proximal femoral canal cylindrical configuration; two vertical lines are drawn from points on the inner cortex, one 10 cm from the mid-lesser trochanter and the other 3 cm from the mid-lesser trochanter. The ratio is the width of the space between these two lines at the mid-lesser trochanter divided by the width of the canal 10 cm distal to that point.

carpal height ratio: for capitate instability in the wrist; the ratio of the length of the third metacarpal to the length of the wrist from the base of the third metacarpal to the distal radius. The **revised carpal height ratio** is the width of the wrist from the base of the third metacarpal divided by the length of the capitate.

central sacral line: the vertical line on a frontal radiograph that passes through the center of the sacrum.

cervico-obturator line (Shenton line): a curve that can be drawn on an AP view of the pelvis. This line continues from the inferior border of the femoral neck to the inferior border of the pubic ramus. If there is any interruption in the line, this is suggestive of an abnormal position of the femoral head.

Chamberlain l.: for developmental basilar skull impression onto cervical spine; a line drawn from the posterior edge of the foramen magnum to the posterior edge of the hard palate.

demarcation (demarcation line): zone between normal and abnormal tissue, most commonly used to denote area or line of normal-appearing tissue next to gangrenous tissue in a devitalized limb. This term is also used in describing radiographic evidence of disease that shows a clear line or zone of activity.

Dorr ratio: for proximal femoral canal cylindrical configuration; width of the canal at the mid-lesser trochanter divided by the width of the canal 10 cm distal to that point.

epiphyseal line: line of fusion of the physeal growth plate.

Feiss line: a line drawn on standing subject or standing lateral radiograph between the tip of the medial malleolus and the base of the first metatarsal phalangeal joint. The position of the navicular tuberosity is noted. The Feiss line is used in evaluation of pes planus.

femoral cortical index: ratio of the femoral diameter of the outer cortex to the inner cortex 10 cm distal to the mid-lesser trochanter.

femoral offset: perpendicular distance from the center line of the femoral shaft to the center of the femoral head.

femoral shaft l.: line drawn from mid point of proximal and distal shaft, also called the **anatomic femoral axis.**

fracture l.: any line thought to be the result of a fracture.

Frankel l.: a white line around the outer margins of the bony epiphysis, which can be seen on a bone radiograph in a patient with scurvy.

growth-arrest l.: line of bony density seen on radiograph of a long bone. This may represent a growth-arrest scar from the growth plate as a result of stress (fracture or an illness) during a period of growth; **Harris l, Harris-Park.**

herniation pit: not a true herniation, but a point of wear in the femoral neck where a misshaped femoral head or acetabulum leads to impingement on the anterior acetabulum.

Hilgenreiner's line: a horizontal line drawn between the two triradiate cartilage centers of the hips defines a horizontal plane and an approximation to the flexion axis of the hips.

Hueter l.: line drawn horizontal to the medial epicondyle of the humerus, passing tip of olecranon when elbow is extended.

Insall ratio: for patella alta; with the knee flexed at 30 degrees, the ratio is the length of the patella tendon to the height of the patella. A number greater than 1.3 indicates patella alta; **Insall-Salvati ratio.**

Klein's line: a line tangenital to the superior femoral neck on an AP view of the pelvis. Normally, a portion of the femoral head is above this line. In patients with a slipped capital femoral epiphysis, the femoral head is below this line or a smaller portion of the femoral head is above this line when compared with the contralateral view.

Kohler l.: slanted line drawn from the acetabular "teardrop" to the most lateral tangent of the pelvic ring.

lead line: radiopaque (white) thin line in the metaphysis (end region) of bones in a patient with lead poisoning.

Maquet l.: line drawn from center of femoral head to midtalus, normally passes through middle of knee.

McGregor l.: for developmental basilar skull impression onto cervical spine; line drawn from base of occiput to posterior edge of hard palate.

McRae l.: for developmental basilar skull impression onto cervical spine; a line drawn from anterior to posterior edge of the foramen magnum.

medialization ratio: percentage of the horizontal radius of the cartilaginous femoral head medial to vertical line drawn from lateral tip of acetabulum, as seen on an arthrogram with the hip in the position of reduction.

Nélaton l.: drawn from the anterosuperior iliac spine to the ischial tuberosity; normally goes through the head of the greater trochanter forming one side of Bryant triangle.

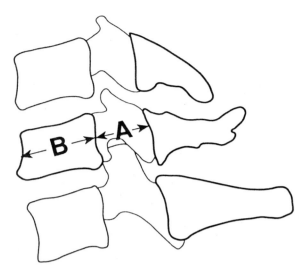

FIG 3-4 Pavlov ratio used to determine relative narrowness of cervical spinal canal, A:B, where a value 1.0 is normal and less than 0.8 indicates a developmentally narrow canal. (From *J Bone Joint Surg* 76A:1422, 1994.)

obturator/brim l.: drawn from inner pelvic brim to mid-obturator foramen. It is used in determining the degree of femoral head or prosthetic migration.

Ogston l.: drawn from adduction tubercle to intercondylar notch; used as a guide for transection of condyle in osteotomy for knock-knee deformity.

patella subluxation ratio: for patellar subluxation; ratio created by the distance of medial femoral condylar margin to apex of patella divided by the depth of the patella groove.

Pavlov ratio: for spinal cord space in cervical spine; ratio of vertebral body width to spinal canal diameter (Fig. 3-4).

Perkin l.: a line drawn perpendicular to the horizontal Hilgenreiner's line through the most lateral edge of the ossified acetabular cartilage. In normal newborns and infants, the medial aspect of the femoral neck or the ossified capital femoral epiphysis falls in the lower inner quadrant. The appearance of either of these structures in the lower outer or upper outer quadrant indicates subluxation or dislocation of the hip; **Ombrédanne.**

retroversion: descriptive of axial rotation. For example, in hip dysplasia, the femoral head is posterior to the axis of the femur.

sacroiliac l.: line drawn from both inferior sacroiliac joints, used in measuring proximal migration of femoral head or prosthesis.

sacroiliac/symphysis l.: horizontal line drawn from midpoint between superior symphysis pubis and sacroiliac line, used in measuring proximal migration of femoral head or prosthesis.

Shenton l.: curved line seen on radiographs of a normal hip joint, formed by the top of the obturator foramen and medial femoral neck to lesser trochanter.

Sourcil: eyebrow-shaped area of dense bone on the superior acetabulum seen on AP radiograph of hip.

Spontorno index: for proximal femoral canal cylindrical configuration; outer cortical diameter at the mid-lesser trochanter divided by the width of the canal 7 cm distal to that point.

teardrop: the appearance of a teardrop found on the AP radiograph of the acetabular joint. The outer border of the teardrop is the inner border of the acetabulum. The inner border of the "drop" is the outer wall of the pelvis next to the inferior acetabulum. In grading acetabular dysplasia, the position of the teardrop is graded as A, open, when the medial line is lateral to the ilioischial line; B, when it overlaps that line; C, when it is medial to that line; and D, when the lateral border of the teardrop is medial to the ilioischial line.

trough line: a vertical or arch-like line of cortical bone projecting parallel and lateral to the articular cortical surface of the humeral head. It is seen on a conventional AP radiograph of the shoulder. The trough line represents an anteromedial impaction fracture of the humeral head secondary to posterior dislocation of the shoulder.

Ullmann l.: line of displacement in spondylolisthesis.

Winberger l.: infraction (appearing as a radiolucent line) in the metaphysis, as seen in syphilis. (Not to be confused with Wimberger sign seen in scurvy.)

Y-line: line drawn through both triradiate cartilages at the acetabular center; Hilgenreiner l.

Radiographic Signs

anteater nose s.: seen in tarsal coalition; anterosuperior calcaneus has appearance of anteater nose seen on lateral radiograph.

anterior hiatal s.: seen in posterior ligament ankle instability; a lateral radiograph shows a wedge-shaped opening at the anterior dome of the talus when the foot is flexed and pushed backward.

Ashhurst s.: seen in ankle diastasis; a widening of the normal overlap of the distal anterior tubercle and fibula at the ankle joint.

bamboo spine: bamboo appearance of spine seen in ankylosing spondylitis.

cement-wedge s.: wedge-shaped area of radiographic lucency seen under tibial component, implying motion of the component.

chalk-stick fracture: appearance on a radiograph of a fracture through bone in a patient with Paget disease of bone.

choppy sea sign: an apparent but not real tear of a meniscus seen on arthrogram.

codfish vertebrae: radiographic appearance of vertebrae severely involved with osteoporosis, in which the central portion is depressed secondary to collapse.

crescent s.: radiographic finding in avascular necrosis in which there is a space between the subchondral plate and impacted bone of the femoral head, leaving a crescent-shaped area that is radiolucent (relatively black) on a radiograph.

cross-over s: in acetabular retroversion, the margin of the anterior acetabulum crosses over the posterior margin when seen on an AP radiograph of the pelvis.

double density s.: for os acromiale, overlap of two transversely elongated radiographic cortical densities seen in the AP projection of the shoulder.

Gage s.: seen in Legg-Calvé-Perthes disease; a small osteoporotic segment forms a translucent "V" on the lateral side of the femoral head epiphysis; seen on AP view.

geyser sign: seen on shoulder arthrogram, shoulder ultrasound, or MRI. Characterized by leakage of contrast material from the glenohumeral joint into the subdeltoid bursa, and then through the AC joint. It normally indicates a large full thickness tear of the rotator cuff.

Hawkins s.: seen in avascular necrosis of the talus; zone of radiographic translucency beneath the subchondral plate of the dome of the talus.

Matev s.: seen in median nerve entrapment; a gap in the fracture callus of the medial epicondyle of the humerus.

posterior hiatal s.: anterior ligament ankle instability; a lateral radiograph with the foot pulled forward shows a wedge-shaped opening at the posterior dome of the talus.

Reimers index (migration index): for lateral acetabular deficiency; the lateral border of the femoral head to Perkin line (vertical line from lateral tip of acetabulum) divided by the width of the femoral head parallel to Hilgenreiner line (line drawn through the inferior points of both acetabuli) and multiplied by 100.

ring s.: secondary to scaphoid ligament disruption, which causes rotation of the scaphoid, giving it a ring appearance on a radiograph.

Risser s.: for skeletal maturity, the degree of capping of the iliac apophysis from beginning (grade 1) to completion (grade 4).

rugger jersey spine: the appearance of alternate white and black zones seen on spine radiographs, frequently in patients with hyperparathyroidism or renal osteodystrophy.

Scotty dog (Scotch terrier) s.: seen in spondylolysis; the oblique radiograph reveals what looks like a Scotty dog. The "eye" is a pedicle seen end on; the nose, the transverse process; the collar, the lysis (fracture of the pars interarticularis); the body, the lamina; the tail, the posterior spinous process; the ears, the superior facet; and the forefoot, the inferior facet.

spur: a bony protrusion or lip at the edge of a joint, usually related to degenerative disease or osteoarthritis; **lipping, osteophyte.**

Thurston-Holland s. (corner s.): small fragment of bone seen at margin of metaphysis just proximal to epiphysis that indicates a type II Salter fracture.

Waldenström s.: apparent lateral displacement of - femoral head seen in early Legg-Calvé-Perthes disease.

Wimberger sign: relatively dense margin representing the provisional zone of calcification surrounding an osteopenic epiphysis seen in scurvy, not to be confused with Winberger line seen in syphilis.

windshield wiper s.: radiographic view outlines the shadow of a prosthesis with the appearance of a windshield wiper; with a loose internal prosthesis, there is bone absorption and formation secondary to a to-and-fro motion of the stem of the prosthesis in the shaft of the bone.

Methods

acromial profile: for impingement in the shoulder due to an anterolateral hook that develops in adults on the inferior surface of the acromion.

Type I: flat acromial profile.

Type II: curved acromial profile.

Type III: hooked acromial profile.

Ahlback changes: grading system for degenerative arthritic changes seen on anteroposterior knee radiographs.

Grade 0: normal joint space.

Grade I: joint space narrowing.

Grade II: joint space obliteration.

Grade III: minor bone attrition.

Grade IV: moderate bone attrition.

Grade V: severe bone attrition.

Grade VI: subluxation.

Bertol method: for dysplastic hips in newborn infants; the ratio of two lines, one being the distance from the top of the femoral physis to central acetabular horizontal line and the other being the distance from the medial acetabular wall and superior medial femoral shaft. A ratio of 2 or greater is normal, and progressive instability produces a line ratio that progresses to 1.

bone age: in pediatric orthopaedics and radiology, refers to the predictable skeletal changes of bone that take place from infancy to adulthood. Bone age studies observe the size of bone, development of ossification centers, and outline of bones in the hand and wrist. Comparison with radiographs of normal patients at specific ages allows determination if a patient's bones are growing too rapidly or too slowly. Standard sets of radiographs are found in Greulich and Pyle (1959).

Catterall hip score: for pediatric avascular necrosis of the femoral head or Legg-Calvé-Perthes disease (Fig. 3-5).

I: no finding on AP, compression on frog-leg lateral.

II: central compression on both AP and frog-leg lateral.

III: lateral femoral head compression seen on AP, not covered by acetabulum, and medial femoral head is intact.

IV: entire femoral head involved.

Cobb method: for measuring degree of curvature in scoliosis; a line is drawn across the superior vertebral plate of the superior vertebra with the greatest tilt and the inferior plate of the inferior vertebra with the greatest tilt. The intersection of these two lines creates the angle.

Edinburgh method: for dysplastic hip; radiograph obtained with a newborn's legs held parallel with slight traction and no rotation. Proximal migration is measured by distance from superior femoral shaft to a line through the central acetabulum (inferior ilium). The gap from the lateral ischium to the most medial part of the femoral metaphysis is the index of dislocation. This gap is normally 4 mm, suspicious if more than 5 mm, and diagnostic if 6 mm or more.

Fairbanks changes: a grading scale for the changes seen on the AP radiographs of osteoarthritic knees, originally used in postmeniscectomy patients seen in long-term follow-up.

Grade 0: normal.

Grade I: ridge from margin of femoral condyles.

Grade II: joint-space narrowing on side of meniscectomy.

Grade III: flattening of femoral condyle.

Fergusson method: for measuring angle of degree of curvature in scoliosis, using vertical lines through spinous processes.

Ficat-Arlet: for avascular necrosis of the femoral head, two similar grading scale systems are currently used.

Arlet Ficat	Marcus	
I	I	Mottled densities, may be obscure, anterosuperior weight-bearing area of femoral head
II	II	Well-demarcated infarction, rim of increased density of bone at base of area of infarction
III	III	Subtle flattening of femoral head or subchondral radiolucent crescent.
	IV	Pronounced collapse of avascular segment
IV	V	Degenerative arthritis with loss of cartilage space.
	VI	Marked degenerative changes

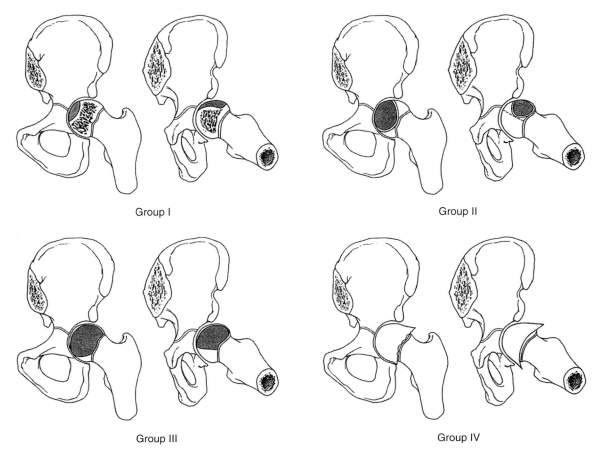

Group I

Group II

Group III

Group IV

FIG 3-5 Catterall classification of Legg-Calvé-Perthes disease. I: anterior head only involved, no collapse; II: only anterior head with sequestrum, III: only a small part of epiphysis not involved, IV: total head involvement. (1996 American Academy of Orthopaedic Surgeons. Reprinted from the *Journal of the American Academy of Orthopaedic Surgeons: A Comprehensive Review* 4(1):9-16, 1996, with permission.)

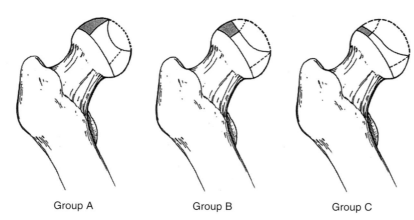

FIG 3-6 Herring classification of Legg-Calvé-Perthes disease. **A,** Lateral pillar retains its height, no collapse. **B,** Lateral pillar shows density changes with height loss. **C,** Lateral pillar loses more than 50% of its height. (1996 American Academy of Orthopaedic Surgeons. Reprinted from the *Journal of the American Academy of Orthopaedic Surgeons: A Comprehensive Review* 4(1):9-16, 1996, with permission.)

Group A   Group B   Group C

Gruen zones: for loosening of a femoral prosthetic component; lateral three zones are numbered from proximal to distal 1 to 3, zone 4 is at prosthetic tip, and zones 5 to 7 are from distal to proximal on the medial side, with zone 7 at the medial femoral neck.

Herring lateral pillar classification: for prognosis in Legg-Perthes disease (Fig. 3-6).

Group A: height of pillar (lateral head above physis) normal.

Group B: height of pillar 50% to 100% of original height.

Group C: height of pillar < 50% of original height.

Ishihara cervical spine curve index: for spondylolytic changes in the neck; a vertical line is drawn from the base of C2 to the base of C7. The sum of the distance of the posterior vertebral bodies of C3-C6 to that vertical line is divided by that vertical line and multiplied by 100 to get the percent value.

Kellgren osteoarthritis grade:

Grade 1: one or more osteophytes without joint-space narrowing.

Grade 2: sclerosis of the acetabulum and joint-space narrowing; may be accompanied by small osteophytes.

Grade 3: clear formation of osteophytes and narrowing of the joint space.

Grade 4: deformation of the femoral head with distinctive joint-space narrowing; cyst formation in femoral head and acetabulum; both bones sclerosed. This scoring method is also used for degenerative disk in the spine.

Knee Society total-knee arthroplasty roentgenographic evaluation and scoring system: a system of angles and absorption at specific numerical points of prosthetic fixation to bone.*

Mose concentric rings: for avascular necrosis of femoral head in children; a system using concentric rings with 2-mm separations.

Good: both hips perfect circles.

Fair: deviation is ≤ 2 mm.

Poor: deviation > 2 mm.

Perdriolle torsimeter: for measuring spinal rotation in scoliosis; a transparent celluloid overlay is placed on radiographs to help estimate the rotation.

Salter-Thompson classification: for dividing Legg-Calvé-Perthes d. into two groups of expected outcome.

Group A: bone underlying fracture presumed to be necrotic and any bone lateral presumed to be

*From Ewald FC: Knee Society total knee arthroplasty roentgenographic evaluation and scoring system, *Clin Orthop* 248:9–13, 1989.

viable; involves approximately one-half of the femoral head; similar to Catterall groups I and II.

Group B: no evidence of an intact, visible lateral margin seen on AP radiograph; subchondral fracture extends to most lateral extent of epiphysis; similar to Catterall groups III and IV.

Sauvegrain skeletal age: method of assessment of age base on elbow radiographs.

Severin hip dysplasia scale: for staging severity of hip deformity that may lead to dysplastic dislocation.

Group I: normal hips.

A: CE angle of > 19 degrees for ages 6 to 13 years; CE angle of > 25 degrees for ages 14 years and older.

B: CE angle of 15 to 19 degrees for ages 3 to 13 years; CE angle 20 to 25 degrees for ages 14 years and older.

Group II: moderate deformity of femoral head, neck, or acetabulum; otherwise normal joint. A and B—same as group I.

Group III: dysplastic hip without subluxation; CE angles < 15 degrees for ages 6 to 13 years and < 20 degrees for ages 14 years and older.

Group IV: subluxation.

A: moderate, CE angle positive or equal to 0 degrees.

B: severe, CE angle negative.

Group V: head articulating with secondary acetabulum in the upper part of original acetabulum.

Group VI: redislocation.

Singh index: an index of osteoporosis accomplished by a grading system using the three major trabecular patterns in the femoral intertrochanteric and head region; Grades I through VI, with lowest grade being the most osteoporotic.

Stahl index: for staging lunate necrosis in wrist, uses ratio of height to width.

Stage I: index of $\geq$ 45%.

Stage II: index 30%–44%.

Stage III: index < 30%.

Steinberg: for aseptic necrosis of the femur, Steinberg's stage II and IV are equivalent to Ficat stage III; and stage V and VI are equivalent to Ficat stage IV.

Stage 0: normal radiograph and bone scan.

Stage I: normal radiograph and abnormal bone scan.

Stage II: sclerosis and/or cyst in femoral head.

A: mild (<**B:** moderate (20%-40%).

C: severe (> 40%).

Stage III: subchondral collapse (crescent sign) with collapse.

A: mild (< 15%).

B: moderate (15%-30%).

C: severe (> 30%).

Stage IV: head flattening with joint narrowing or acetabular change.

A: mild (< 15% surface and 2-mm depression).

B: moderate (15%-30% surface or 2- to 4-mm depression).

C: severe (> 30% surface or > 4-mm depression).

Stage V: flattening of head with joint narrowing and/or acetabular changes.

A: mild.

B: moderate.

C: severe.

Stulberg method: system for measuring concentricity of femoral heads in Perthes disease.

Tönnis system: for hip dysplasia as seen on radiograph.

Grade 1: dysplasia of the hip and mild subluxation.

Grade 2: center of ossification of femoral head displaced laterally, inferior to superolateral corner of the true acetabulum.

Grade 3: center of ossification at level of superolateral corner of acetabulum.

Grade 4: center of ossification proximal to the superolateral corner of acetabulum.

Waldenström: stage of healing in Legg-Calvé-Perthes disease.

Stage A: formation stage.

1: initial stage; epiphysis is denser, patchy, more distal, and uneven at the margins.

2: fragmentation stage; epiphysis in pieces, can be further divided into a mass of small granules.

Stage B: healing period; the epiphysis becomes homogeneous, evidence of diffuse and extensive revascularization.

Stage C: period of growth; normal growth and ossification of deformed femoral head.

Invasive and Noninvasive Techniques

bone scan: a commonly employed nuclear medicine study in orthopaedics. A radioactive material (radio-isotope) is attached chemically to a substance that is taken up by active bone cells. The radioisotope is then injected into a vein, and the radioactivity emitted from the bones goes to bone collagen and can be detected by a gamma camera. Usefulness of the study includes detection of infection, fractures, and metastatic lesions. A bone scan demonstrates where bone is actively being produced or destroyed, whereas a radiograph shows only where bone is present; **bone scintigraphy.**

   three-phase bone scan: a modification of the routine bone scan, and applied when osteomyelitis is suspected. This scan examines the perfusion, immediate soft tissue blood pool, and delayed bone uptake; whereas a routine bone scan examines only the delayed bone uptake phase. The advantages of a **three-phase bone scan** is that it improves the specificity of the examination for osteomyelitis. A normal perfusion phase excludes an active inflammatory process.

calcium 47: for bone formation; an in vivo total body accretion test.

cinefluoroscopy: recorded fluoroscopic study for relative motion of bones in a joint, for example, to detect carpal instability; **videofluoroscopy, cineroentgenogram, cineradiography.**

computed tomography (CT): a computer generates a two-dimensional, cross-sectional image from a series of x-ray beams that rotate in a circular and forward motion around the patient. CT images show detailed anatomy and allow detection of differences in tissue density and shape. In orthopaedics, CT is especially useful for analyzing complicated fractures and may be performed after arthrography to aid visualization of joint pathology. With CT, bone structures are clearly defined, non-invasively; tumors are located with precision; tissue is recognized as normal or abnormal; and blockages in blood vessels can be sought, invasively. The advantages of this technique are that it can be

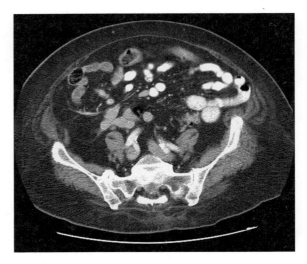

FIG 3-7 Computed tomography scan "slice" showing arthritis in left anterior sacroiliac joint.

invasive or noninvasive, and it provides a sharp, detailed image. This method is best for patients who cannot tolerate rigorous radiographic examinations. **CT scan, computed axial tomography (CAT), CAT scan** (Fig. 3-7).

   spiral (helical) CT: the latest development in CT, it allows scanning of a volume of tissue during a single breathhold by continuous scanning as the patient is moved through the gantry. Advantages over the conventional CT are that it eliminates motion artifacts and shortens examination time. The trade-off is some loss of resolution. It is not used where high resolution is important, for example, bone detail.

dual photon densitometry: to estimate bone density, the part being measured is exposed to two beams of photons of different intensity. A two-dimensional picture of bone density is obtained with calculated subtraction of soft tissue density. The results are expressed in grams of bone mineral per square centimeter.

fat saturation (fat sat, fat suppression): a technique used in MRI to suppress the signal from fat, causing it to appear black on the MR images. This technique allows pathology to be more easily identified.

gadolinium-enhanced MRI: the element gadolinium (Gd) has paramagnetic properties and is used to enhance magnetic resonance imaging. Gadolinium is especially useful in distinguishing scar tissue from disk herniation in cases of prior spine surgery. It is also useful in tumor imaging and in evaluating the blood supply to bone to exclude avascular necrosis.

gadopentetate dimeglumine: gadolinium. See **gadolinium-enhanced MRI.**

gallium scan (^{67}Ga): radioactive gallium-67 is introduced intravenously and localizes in areas of concentrated granulocytes; used to detect hidden infections, such as osteomyelitis.

gamma camera: instrument used for nuclear medicine studies. The camera contains many radiation detectors, which detect the radiation emitted from a radioisotope inside the patient's body. The gamma camera generates an image of the whole body or of a specific area of interest (e.g., see bone scan).

indium scan (indium leukocyte scan): radioactive indium-111 is incubated with white blood cells (WBCs) taken from the patient. The indium-111 is taken up inside the WBCs, which are then injected back into the bloodstream and localized in areas of acute osteomyelitis (infection).

integrated-shape imaging system (ISIS): for scoliosis; computer analysis of spinal and rib contours, may replace need for repeated radiographic evaluations.

LeukoScan: commercial term used for the method to localize infection in bone or soft tissue. Technetium-99m is attached to a monoclonal antibody that attaches to a specific cell surface protein seen only on neutrophils, the type of white cells that localize to areas of infection. It is then injected into the bloodstream.

magnetic resonance imaging (MRI): A radiographic technique in which the patient is exposed to a magnetic field. The movement of photons (water molecules) is usually random and is aligned by the magnetic field. Radiowaves are then used to change the alignment of the protons. When the radiowaves are turned off, the protons emit a weak signal. The signals are detected and transformed into cross-sectional images. The signal decay curves of the protons as they return to their relaxed state are

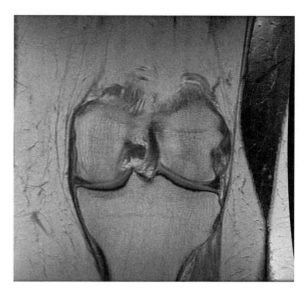

FIG 3-8 T1-weighted image of knee highlights fat in the bone marrow and subcutaneous tissue; cortical bone appears black.

dependent on two factors: **T1** (spin-lattice) longitudinal relaxation is dependent on the relationship between protons and their surrounding environment, and **T2** (spin-spin) transverse relaxation is the effect of spinning protons on each other. By adjusting certain imaging parameters, images can be more influenced by T1 or T2 (i.e., **T1-** or **T2-weighted images**) (Figs. 3-8 and 3-9).

In orthopaedics, MRI is especially useful for diagnosing injuries to ligaments, meniscal tears, tumors, avascular necrosis, and infection. It is also useful for diagnosing fractures that are difficult to see on radiographs, such as nondisplaced fractures of the hip in the elderly. An MRI is also helpful in diagnosing diabetic feet and growth plate injuries. New methods allow for the detection of cartilage changes in osteoarthritis.

This technology has a terminology unique to the system (Fig. 3-10).

magnetic resonance spectroscopy: technique using magnetic resonance to determine the relative amounts of specific chemicals in an anatomic part. One such study is the evaluation of chemical

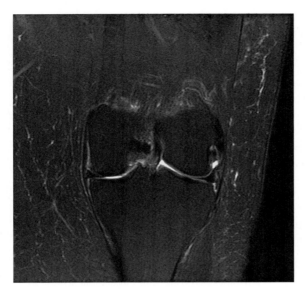

FIG 3-9 Matched fat suppressed T2-weighted image of the knee highlights water; cortical bone appears black as does the suppressed subcutaneous fat and bone marrow.

reactions involving phosphate in the muscle. This type of evaluation helps to determine the metabolic adequacy of the muscle.

neutron radiography: technique helpful in visualizing bony tissue. A narrow beam of neutrons is passed through tissue from a nuclear reactor.

proton density: an MRI study in which the image is strongly affected by the differences in the density of protons in the tissue. Such images are usually produced with a spin-echo pulse sequence having repetition time (TR) > 600 msec and an echo time (TE) < 80 msec.

SPECT (single photon emission computerized tomography): use of a single beam emission source

to make two-dimensional images revealing relative areas of bone abnormality. It may be used to diagnose avascular necrosis, fractures, and infection.

SPGR (spoiled grass): image obtained with lower flip angle, giving a fat suppressed image that makes articular cartilage appear white on a magnetic resonance image.

STIR (short tau inversion recovery): imaging signal acquisition that helps enhance image to detect fractures that are difficult to see on x-ray, particularly useful in occult hip fractures.

strontium-85 resorption rate: a nuclear medicine in vivo study to determine bone absorption rate.

T1-weighted image: an MRI study in which the image is strongly affected by the longitudinal magnetic relaxation time, T1. Such images are usually produced with a spin-echo pulse sequence generally having repetition time (TR) < 600 msec and an echo time (TE) < 20 msec.

T2-weighted image: an MRI study in which the image is strongly affected by the transverse magnetic relaxation time, T2. Such images are usually produced with a spin-echo pulse sequence having repetition time (TR) ≥ 2000 msec and echo time (TE) ≥ 80 msec.

technetium-99m: $Tc^{99}m$ is a radioactive substance that can be chemically attached to a variety of substances for nuclear medicine imaging studies. For example, $Tc^{99}m$ can be attached to diphosphonate for imaging of bones, attached to white blood cells (WBCs) for imaging of infection or attached to red blood cells for detection of a pulmonary embolus (blood clot to the lung); **technetium scan.**

technetium scan: see technetium-99m.

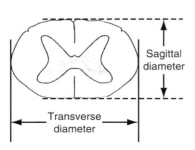

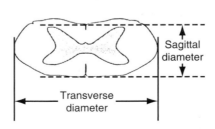

FIG 3-10 Cervical spinal cord as would be seen on magnetic resonance imaging (MRI) or computed axial tomography (CAT) scan with myelography. The ratio of the transverse diameter to the sagittal diameter greater than 0.4 is a sign of good recovery prognosis after surgical decompression. (From *J Bone Joint Surg* 76A:1422, 1994.)

thermography: to differentiate nerve irritation, vascular disorders, and increased muscle tone; a temperature-sensitive plate displaying color gradients reveals differences in skin surface temperature.

tomosynthesis: computer-driven radiographic techniques that allow for a 5-second radiation exposure, equivalent to a standard radiograph, and less than computer-assisted tomography.

ultrasound (ultrasound study, ultrasonography, sonography): the use of mechanical radiant energy having a 1 to 10 million MHz (megahertz = 1 million cycles per second) frequency to obtain images. The ultrahigh frequency sound (well beyond the upper limits of human hearing, which is 20,000 Hertz) is emitted, reflects off tissue surfaces, and is received and processed by a computer to form an image. In orthopaedics, this imaging technique is used to evaluate fluid collections, tendon and tissue abnormalities, tumors, cysts, and hemorrhages and infant hip disorders.

Vascular Diagnostic Studies

After the history and physical examination is complete, other tests may be required to diagnose abnormalities in the peripheral circulation to the limbs. These specific tests are often made in conjunction with an orthopaedic problem. These studies fall into two categories: invasive and noninvasive tests. The invasive tests are performed at the direction of vascular surgeons by radiologists.

Invasive Tests

To perform an invasive test, radiographic contrast is injected through a catheter placed into an artery or vein, and a computer-guided radiographic machine obtains an image as the iodinated contrast material courses through the vessel network. This contrast material enables visualization of any degree of narrowing (blockage) and the extent of blood flow around a blockage. Other abnormalities of vessels can also be detected. New computer technology allows vessel procedures to be performed in a short time.

angioplasty: can be performed following arteriography in which an area of narrowing has been identified. A special catheter with an inflatable balloon is placed at the area of narrowing. The balloon is inflated to open the narrowing. This procedure can treat areas of arterial narrowing that otherwise would require surgery.

arteriography: a radiographic examination in which an artery is catheterized and contrast injected to study the blood supply to an area or detect blockages of arteries. May be performed following an ultrasound study that indicates the presence of vascular compromise or in a patient with symptoms of blockage of blood vessels in the extremities. In some cases, a blockage or narrowing of an artery can be treated through the catheter (e.g., angioplasty); **arteriogram, angiogram, angiography.**

digital subtraction angiography (DSA): two-step imaging technique where radiograph is obtained of the area of interest before adding contrast medium. This first image is stored in the computer. Contrast medium that is opaque to x-ray is injected, and a second image is obtained. The opacity creates a shadow that allows visualization of blood flow. The computer subtracts the first image from the second image to produce a clear view of flowing blood and its blockages by narrowed vessels, ruptured vessels, or abnormal tissue.

phlebography: invasive radiographic procedure in which radiopaque material is injected into a vein to visualize possible blockage or other abnormalities; **phlebogram, venography, venogram.**

sclerotherapy: a procedure whereby a chemical (sclerosing agent) is injected into a blood vessel to scar the vessel shut. Usually done electively for veins but can also be used for small bleeding arteries.

venogram: a diagnostic procedure in which a contrast medium is injected into a vein and an x-ray is used to visualize venous anatomy and pathology, for example, a blockage, clots, or chronic changes; **venography, phlebography, phlebogram.**

Noninvasive Tests

These tests apply external techniques, and the body is not entered. These methods frequently provide dynamic information.

angioscopy: tiny cameras are used to visualize the inside of blood vessels and bypass grafts, and assess the lining and, in some cases, facilitate repair from within the vessel.

ankle-brachial index (ABI): comparison of pressure measured by blood pressure cuff and B-mode Doppler signal between arms and legs (e.g., normal −1.0, moderate decrease −0.75, severe decrease −0.35). Test principle relies on compressibility of blood vessels and results are often affected by diabetes. **Ankle-arm index.**

Doppler ultrasound (duplex or pulsed Doppler): Low intensity sound waves are reflected off blood vessels or other organs or moving blood and passed through a computer to produce sound (B-mode) or pictures. Detailed information of anatomy and pathology (clots, narrowing, dilatations, obstructions). Combining with duplex techniques provides physiologic information as well.

> **color Doppler:** assigns colors (usually red and blue) to blood flowing in specific directions and can be used to analyze blood flow. A **power Doppler** is an ultrasound technique that is more sensitive in detecting the presence of blood flow; however, it does not assess the direction of blood flow. Doppler studies are commonly used to detect narrowing of the carotid arteries and blood clots in the veins of the legs.

> **duplex ultrasound:** provides both a two-dimensional image of the vessel and the velocity of flow. There are many uses including carotid artery stenosis and venous blood flow to test blood clots. Duplex imaging for clots in leg veins is less invasive than venography and is the first imaging test of choice for this common clinical problem.

electrocardiogram: graphic recording of electrical activity of the heart.

plethysmography: noninvasive procedure that measures volume changes in an organ or extremity. Principle is applied in various forms to include volume displacement (air or water), strain gauge, mechanical, photoelectric, or impedance.

> *impedance plethysmography:* instrument to measure changes in electrical impedance in a limb, which indicates changes in blood content and limb volume.

> *oculoplethysmography (OPG):* noninvasive diagnostic procedure measuring carotid artery pressure indirectly by measuring blood pressure in the eyes. The medium of measurement may either be air (oculopneumoplethysmography) or water (oculohydroplethysmography).

> *photoplethysmography (PPG):* noninvasive procedure with an instrument that uses light to measure blood flow to skin and thereby measure blood in larger vessels that may be occluded by arteriosclerosis.

pulse volume recorder (PVR): segmental air plethysmograph to determine change in limb blood flow by change in cuff pressure.

transcutaneous oximetry (TcPO$_2$): produces local measurement of skin oxygen tension and can give measures of capillary perfusion and predict wound healing.

Radiation Therapy

Ionizing radiation causes molecules to split when the radiation particle or wave hits the molecule. This event can cause injury to cells, particularly those that are dividing rapidly such as in tumors, the blood, and normal gastrointestinal lining.

As a result, ionizing radiation for diagnostic purposes is kept to a minimum, and treatment is made focal by a variety of techniques. The terminology listed here is restricted to techniques commonly applied to orthopaedic conditions and to some dosimetry terms.

rad (roentgen absorbed dose): the actual energy absorbed by the local tissue, measured in ergs per gram. This is not a whole body count of absorbed dose but a number that looks at each tissue system or organ.

rem (roentgen-equivalent-man): biologic effectiveness of radiation in a human subject. For diagnostic purposes, rad is equal to rem.

roentgen: measure of the change resulting from the exposure of air to radiation.

strontium-89 (Metastron): treatment for metastatic bone pain. A beta-emitting radioactive material is injected intravenously. The isotope is taken up in bone and delivers the radiation to the affected areas. The effect lasts for several months.

Orthopaedic Tests, Signs, and Maneuvers

4

Tests, signs, and maneuvers provide some of the most frequently used terms in orthopaedics. Unfortunately, the terms possess the greatest possibility for confusion because of similar names or meanings. Thus, newcomers to orthopaedics meet a challenge at the very onset of their careers.

Eponyms for certain examinations vary regionally or among institutions within the same area. Such variations are a reflection of the training center's influence, in which the names of prominent local physicians are frequently used for these examinations. Occasionally, the same test is given two or more names, or the name can apply to more than one test or sign. In a problem-oriented situation, eponyms are routinely used in the physical evaluation process. Familiarity with the terms and techniques enables physicians and their assistants to record and clarify an orthopaedic examination.

The physical examination is performed by using direct visual observation, noting the way a patient walks (gait), or the manner in which the upper and lower limbs are used; or on auditory findings such as auscultation of pulses; or on palpation, which is the use of hands in determining firmness, shape, and motion of a part. All of these can stand alone or be combined to aid in diagnosis.

A **test** may be part of the physical examination in which direct contact with the patient is made, or it may be a chemical test, radiographic examination, or other study. All tests described in this chapter relate to the physical examination only.

A **sign** may be elucidated by a test, maneuver, or simply a visual observation, for example, a "list." It is an indication of the existence of a problem as perceived by the examiner. The terms sign and test are often interchanged.

A **maneuver** is a complex motion or series of movements used as either a test or treatment. It is also referred to as a method or technique.

A **phenomenon** is any sign or objective symptom, any observable occurrence or fact.

This chapter presents the many categories of tests, signs, and maneuvers. The A-to-Z list of all of these is presented first to guide one to the appropriate section. The categories are neck, back, shoulder, upper limbs, hands, hips, lower limbs, knees, feet and ankles, neurologic, metabolic, general, gait, scales and rating, and other examinations. A table of knee examinations is included. Scales and ratings, as pertains to outcomes assessment as well as degree of impairment, are listed along with a grading system for spinal cord injury.

In addition to many new terms, a table has been included on knee instability tests, an area that receives much attention. Scales and ratings, as pertains to preoperative and postoperative assessment of joints and degree of functional impairment, have been expanded to include a neurologic assessment grading system for spinal cord injury.

Tests, Signs, and Maneuvers

Abbott method (back)
abduction sign (shoulder)

abduction external rotation test (shoulder)

Achilles bulge sign (feet, ankles)

Achilles squeeze test (lower limb)

Addis test (lower limbs)

adduction sign (shoulder)

Adson maneuver or test (neck)

Allen maneuver (neck)

Allen test (hands)

Allis maneuver (hips)

Allis sign (hips)

American Shoulder and Elbow Surgeons (scales and ratings)

Amoss sign (back)

André Thomas sign (hands)

Anghelescu sign (back)

ankle clonus test (neurologic)

Anstrom suspension test (back)

antecedent sign (general)

anterior drawer sign (feet, ankles)

anterior drawer test (knee)

anterior slide test (shoulder)

anterior tibial sign (lower limb)

anvil test (neck, hips)

Apley test and sign (knees)

Aply scratch test (shoulder)

apprehension test (shoulder)

arthrometer test (knees)

artifact (general)

axial compression test (hand)

Babinski sign and reflex (back, neurologic)

ballotment test (hands)

ballotable patella sign (knee)

Barlow test (hips)

bayonet sign (knees)

Beevor sign (neurologic)

Bekhterev test (back)

belly press test (shoulder)

bench test (back)

benediction attitude sign (hands)

benediction sign (hands)

Booth test (shoulder)

bounce home test (knees)

Bouvier maneuver (hands)

bowstring sign (lower limb)

Boyes test (hands)

Bozan maneuver (hips)

bracelet test (hands)

Bragard sign (back)

British test (knees)

Brudzinski sign (neck, neurologic)

Bryant sign (shoulders)

café-au-lait (general)

Callaway test (shoulders)

camelback sign (knees)

Carducci test (hands)

carpal compression test (hands)

Chaddock sign (neurologic)

Chapple test (hips)

Chicago (back)

Chiene test (hips)

Childress test (knee)

Chvostek sign (metabolic)

circumduction maneuver (hands)

circumduction test (shoulder)

claw hand sign (hands)

Cleeman sign (lower limb)

Codman sign (shoulders)

cogwheel phenomenon, sign (general)

Coleman lateral standing block test (feet, ankles)

commemorative sign (general)

Comolli sign (shoulders)

confrontational test (hands)

contralateral straight leg raising test (back)

Coopernail sign (back)

costoclavicular maneuver (neck)

Cozen test (back)

cram test (back)

crank test (shoulder)

cross-body abduction (shoulder)

cross-over test (knee)

Dawbarn sign (shoulders)

Dejerine sign (back)

Demianoff sign (back)

Desault sign (hips)

Destot sign (hips)

Deyerle maneuver (hip)

Deyerle sign (back)

Dial test (knee)

dimple sign (feet, ankle)

dimple sign (neurologic)

doll's eye sign; Cantelli sign (neurologic)

dropback phenomenon (knee)

double camelback sign (knees)

drawer sign (knees)

drawer sign (load and shift t.) (shoulder)

drop arm test (shoulder)

Dugas test (shoulders)

Duchenne sign (hands)

Dupuytren sign (general)

Earle sign (hips)

elbow flexion test (elbow)

Elson middle slip test (hands)

Ely test; femoral nerve stretch test (hips, neurologic)

Erichsen sign (back)

external rotation recurvatum test (knees)

extrinsic tightness test (hands)

FABERE test; Patrick, LaGuerre test (back)

FADIRE test (back)

Fairbank sign (knee)

fan sign (neurologic)

femoral nerve traction test (back)

Fick angle (angles)

finger to nose test (neurologic)

Finkelstein sign (hands)

flexion rotation drawer test (Noyes) (knees) (FRD)

foot slap (gait)

forced adduction test (shoulder)

Forestier (back)

Fouchet sign (knee)

Fournier test (neurologic)

Fowler maneuver (hands)

Fowler test (shoulder)

Fränkel sign (neurologic)

Froment sign (hands)

fulcrum test (shoulder)

Gaenslen sign (back)

Galeazzi sign (hips)

gear-stick sign (hips)

Gilliat tourniquet test (hand)

Godfrey test (knee)

Goldthwait sign (back)

Gordon reflex sign (neurologic)

Gower sign (general)

gravity stress test (elbow)

grimace test (knees)

grip strength test (hands)

Guilland sign (neurologic)

Halstead test (neck)

Hamilton test (shoulders)

Harris-Beath footprinting mat (feet)

Hawkins impingement sign (shoulder)

heel height difference (knee)

heel-to-buttocks difference (knee)

Helbing sign (feet, ankles)

Helft test (knee)

hemodynamic test (general)

Hirschberg sign (neurologic)

Hoffmann sign (neurologic)

Homan's sign (lower limbs)

Hoover test (back)

hop test (one-legged hop t.) (knee)

Hueter sign and line (general)

Hughston jerk test (knee)

Huntington sign (neurologic)

Hutchinson sign (hands)

hyperabduction test (neck)

impingement sign (shoulder)

International Classification for Surgery of the Hand in Tetraplegia (hands)

intrinsic tightness test (hands)

inverted radial reflex (back)

Jansen test (hips)

Jeanne test (hands)

Jendrassik maneuver (neurologic)

jerk test (shoulder)

Jobe test (shoulder)

Kanavel sign (hands)

Kapandji thumb opposition score (hand)

Keen sign (feet, ankles)

Kernig sign (neurologic)

Kerr sign (neurologic)

Kleinman shear test (hands)

Klippel-Feil sign

knee instability tests (knees)

King maneuver (hips)

Kocher maneuver (shoulders)

Lachman test (knees)

Langer line (general)

Langoria sign (hips)

Lasègue sign (back)

Laugier sign (upper limbs)

Leadbetter maneuver (hips)

lead line; Burton sign (metabolic)
Leichtenstern sign (neurologic)
Léri sign (neurologic)
Lhermitte sign (neurologic)
Lichtman test (hands)
lift-off test (shoulder)
Linder sign (back)
list (back)
load-and-shift test (shoulder)
long finger extension test
long tract sign (neurologic)
Losse test (knee)
Lorenz sign (back)
Lovett test (hands)
Ludington sign (shoulder)
Ludloff sign (hips)
McBride test (foot)
McElvenny maneuver (hips)
McMurray test; circumduction maneuver (knees)
Magnuson test (back)
Maisonneuve sign (hands)
Marie-Foix sign (feet, ankles)
Marvel test (shoulder)
masses sign (hands)
Mendel-Bekhterev sign (neurologic)
Mennell sign (back)
Merke sign (knee)
Meryon sign (metabolic)
Meyn and Quigley maneuver (upper limbs)
Michele buckling sign (back)
Michele flip sign (back)
Milch maneuver (shoulder)
Milgram test (back)
military brace maneuver (back)
Mills test (upper limbs)
Mimori test (shoulder)
Minor sign (back)
Moro reflex sign (neurologic)
Morquio sign (neurologic)
Morton test (feet, ankles)
MRC sensory grade (neurologic)
Mulder sign (feet)
Murphy sign (feet, ankles, hand)
Nachlas (back)

Naffziger sign (back)
Napoleon test (shoulder)
Neer impingement test (shoulder)
Nélaton line (hips)
Neri bowing sign (back)
Neviaser test (shoulder)
no touch rule (lower limbs)
nuchocephalic reflex (neurologic)
O'Brien test (shoulder)
O'Connell test (back)
Ober test (hips)
objective sign (general)
obturator sign (hips)
Oppenheim sign (neurologic)
Ortolani test (hips)
Oshsner clasping test (hand)
overhead exercise test (neck)
paratonia (neurologic)
Parvin maneuver (upper limbs)
patellar glide test (knee)
patellar grind test (knee)
patellar retraction test (knees)
Payr sign (lower limbs)
pelvic rock test (back)
Phalen test and maneuver (hands)
piano key sign (hands)
Piotrowski sign (neurologic)
piston sign; Dupuytren sign (hips)
pivot-shift test (MacIntosh) (knees)
Pitres-Testut sign (hand)
Pollock sign (hands)
Popeye deformity (shoulder)
posterior drawer test (knees)
posterolateral instability, rotatory instability test
  (elbow)
postural fixation (back)
pronation sign (neurologic)
prone external rotation test (knees)
prone hanging test (knees)
pseudo-Babinski sign (neurologic)
pseudostability test (hand)
push-pull test (shoulder)
Putti sign (shoulder)
quadriceps test (general)

quadriceps active test (knees)
Queckenstedt sign (neurologic)
radialis sign; Strümpell sign (neurologic)
Raimiste sign (neurologic)
Raynaud phenomenon (general)
release test (shoulder)
relocation test (shoulder)
reverse Bigelow maneuver (hips)
reverse pivot-shift (Jacob) (knees)
Romberg test and sign (neurologic)
Roos test (neck)
Roux sign (hip)
Rust sign (neck)
sag sign (knee)
sagittal stress test (feet, ankles)
Sarbo sign (neurologic)
scaphoid test (hands)
scapular sign of Putti (shoulder)
scapular winging sign (shoulder)
Schlesinger sign (lower limbs)
Schreiber maneuver (neurologic)
screw-home mechanism (knee)
Seimon sign (neck)
Semm and Weinstein monofilament test (hands)
Sharp-Purser Test (neck)
Silfreskiold test
Slocum test (knees)
Smith maneuver (hips)
Smith and Ross test (hand)
Smith-Peterson test (back)
somatic sign (general)
Soto-Hall sign (back)
speed test (shoulder)
spilled teacup sign (hands)
spine sign (back)
sponge test (back)
Spurling test (neck)
stairs sign (neurologic)
standing apprehension test (knees)
station test (neurologic)
Steinmann test (knee)
Stimson maneuver (hips)
stoop test (back)
straight leg raising test (back)
Strunsky sign (feet, ankles)

succinylcholine test (neurologic)
sulcus sign (shoulder)
supraspinatus isolation test (shoulder)
swallow-tail sign (shoulder)
table top test (hand)
talar tilt test (feet, ankles)
tendon reflexes (neurologic)
tenodesis test (hands)
Tensilon test (metabolic)
Terri-Thomas sign (hand)
Thomas sign (hips, neurologic)
Thomas squeeze test (leg)
Thompson (Simmonds) test (lower limbs)
thumbnail test (knees)
thumb-to-forearm test (neurologic)
tibialis sign (neurologic)
Tinel sign; distal tingling on percussion sign (neurologic)
toe spread sign (feet, ankles)
too many toes sign (feet, ankles)
tourniquet test (lower limbs)
Trendelenburg gait (hips)
Trendelenburg test (hips)
Trotter bulge sign (knee)
tuck sign (hands)
Turyn sign (back)
two-point discrimination test (hands)
valgus stress test (elbow) (knee)
valgus thrust ((knee)
Valsalva maneuver (back)
Vanzetti sign (back)
varus recurvatum test (knee)
varus stress test (elbow) (knee)
varus thrust (knee)
Waddell (back)
Walker-Mureloch wrist sign (metabolic)
Wartenberg sign (hands)
Watson test (hands)
Wellmerling maneuver (hips)
wet leather sign (hands)
Whitman maneuver (hips)
Wilson sign (knees)
Wright maneuver (neck)
wrinkle test (neurologic)
Wu sole opposition test (feet, ankles)

Yergason test (shoulders)

Zachary or MRC sensory grade (neurologic)

Neck (Fig. 4-1)

Adson maneuver (test): for scalenus anticus (thoracic outlet) syndrome, noted on obliteration of radial pulse; upper limb to be tested is held in dependent position while head is rotated to the ipsilateral shoulder while inhaling.

Allen maneuver: for same diagnosis as *Adson m.,* except the forearm is flexed at right angle with the arm extended horizontally and rotated externally at the shoulder, with the head rotated to the contralateral shoulder.

anvil test: for vertebral disorders; a closed fist striking blow on top of the head elicits pain in the vertebra(e).

costoclavicular maneuver: for thoracic outlet syndrome; pulling shoulders and chin back at the same time reduces the radial pulse when arm is by side; **military brace maneuver.**

Halstead test: for thoracic outlet; the standing patient keeps arm by side while pulse is taken, extending neck and turning head to opposite side obliterates pulse.

hyperextension test: for thoracic outlet; both arms are fully abducted after confirming radial pulse with

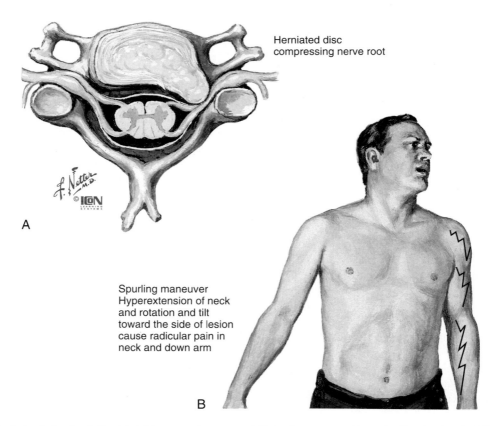

Herniated disc compressing nerve root

A

Spurling maneuver Hyperextension of neck and rotation and tilt toward the side of lesion cause radicular pain in neck and down arm

B

FIG 4-1 Cervical radiculopathy. **A,** Herniated disk compressing nerve root. **B,** Spurling maneuver. Hyperextension of neck and rotation and tilt toward the side of lesion cause radicular pain in neck and down arm. (Reprinted from Netter Anatomy Illustration Collection, © Elsevier Inc.)

arms at side. The pulse is obliterated on the affected side.

overhead exercise test: for thoracic outlet syndrome; the hand is held overhead and making repeated fists results in immediate soreness in the forearm muscles; **Roos test.**

Rust sign: for osteomyelitis or malignant disease of the spine; the patient supports head with hands while moving body.

Seimon s.: for fractured odontoid in small child; child cries if sat upright without support to head and neck.

Sharp-Purser test: for chronic subluxation of the first on second cervical vertebra; with the patient sitting, the head is tilted forward and then backward with the examining finger on the first cervical spinous process to detect slippage.

Spurling test: for cervical spine and foraminal nerve encroachment; compression on the head with extension of the neck causes radicular pain into the upper extremities.

Wright maneuver: in thoracic outlet syndrome, downward pressure on shoulder with shoulder being pulled back obstructs the radial pulse (**costoclavicular maneuver**).

Back

Abbott method: for scoliosis of the spine; traction is applied to produce overcorrection, followed by casting.

Amoss sign: for painful flexure of the spine; pain is produced when the patient places hands far behind body in bed and tries rising from supine position to sitting position.

Anghelescu sign: for testing tuberculosis of the vertebrae or other destructive processes of the spine; in the supine position the patient places weight on head and heels while lifting body upward; inability to bend the spine indicates an ongoing disease process.

Anstrom suspension test: for sciatica; while tapping on the affected area of the lumbar spine the patient will have pain while standing but not if suspending weight using arms to hold the spine in suspension.

Bekhterev test: for nerve root irritability in sciatica; while sitting up in bed, the patient is asked to stretch out both legs; with sciatica, patient cannot sit up in bed this way but can only stretch out each leg in turn.

bench test: for nonorganic back pain; in normal hip motion, the patient should be able to bend over and touch the floor kneeling on a 12-inch high bench; not being able to implies a nonorganic (or psychologic) back pain; **Burns test.**

bowstring sign: with leg raised with knee bent in same position, pain is felt in the back of the limb pressing on the central popliteal fossa. Increased pain is sign of nerve irritability; depending on position of the patient, test also known as **cram test, Forestier test, Deyerle test.**

Bragard sign: for nerve or muscular involvement; with the knee stiff, the lower extremity is flexed at the hip until the patient experiences pain; the foot is then dorsiflexed. Increase in pain points to nerve involvement; no increase in pain indicates muscular involvement.

Chicago test: to distinguish between back strain with muscle spasm and disk disease without spasm, the patient kneels on a chair and attempts to touch the floor. With muscle spasm the patient has difficulty (**Bench Burn disease**). Note: this same test is also used to study the way the patient returns to a more erect position. Slow movement implies an emotional component.

contralateral straight leg raising test: for sciatica; when the leg is flexed, the hip can also be flexed, but not when the leg is held straight. Flexing the sound thigh with the leg held straight causes pain on the affected side. **Fajersztajn crossed sciatic sign.**

Coopernail sign: for fracture of pelvis; ecchymosis of the perineum, scrotum, or labia indicates a pelvic fracture.

Cozen test: to distinguish sciatica from muscle spasm; the supine patient is assisted in sitting up with the knees out straight. An inability to do this without flexing the knee implies nerve irritation or muscle spasm in the lower limb.

Dejerine sign: for herniated intervertebral disk causing radiating limb symptoms; a Valsalva maneuver, such as coughing, sneezing, or straining at stool, accentuates the symptoms.

Demianoff sign: for differentiation of pain originating in the lumbosacral muscle from lumbar pain of any other origin; the pain is caused by stretching of the lumbosacral muscle.

Erichsen sign: for sacroiliac disease; when the iliac bones are sharply pressed toward each other, pain is felt in the sacroiliac area.

FABERE test: for testing lower back or sacroiliac joint disorder by using a forced position of the hip, the patient crosses the leg with the foot of the affected side resting on the opposite knee, then in extension by pressing down on the knee. Acronym for *f*lexion *ab*duction *e*xternal *r*otation in *e*xtension; **Patrick test, figure of 4 test, LaGuerre test.**

FADIRE test: forced position of the hip causing pain. Acronym for *f*lexion *ad*duction *i*nternal *r*otation in *e*xtension; **Patrick test, fadire sign.**

femoral nerve traction test: for radiculopathy of the second through fourth lumbar nerves; with patient prone, the knee is flexed, causing back or thigh pain; **Ely test.**

Gaenslen sign: for sacroiliac disease; pressure on hyperextended thigh with the opposite hip held in flexion elicits pain on the affected side over edge of bed, indicating a sacroiliac problem.

Goldthwait sign: for distinguishing lumbosacral from sacroiliac (SI) pain; with the patient supine, the leg is raised with one hand, while the examiner's other hand is placed under the patient's lower back; leverage is then applied to the side of the pelvis. If pain is felt by the patient before the lumbar spine is moved, the lesion is a sprain of the SI joint; if pain is not felt until after the lumbar spine is moved, the lesion is in the SI or lumbosacral articulation.

Hoover test: for a supposed malingering back disorder; while lying supine, the patient is asked to raise one leg with the knee straight and with the examiner holding the opposite heel. Any active effort to do this will result in pressure of the opposite heel against the examiner's hand. The lack of such effort implies malingering. Excessive pressure of the heel against the examiner's hand implies abdominal muscle weakness.

inverted radial reflex: for cervical spondylotic myelopathy (cord compression); there is spontaneous flexion of the digits when the brachialis reflex is being tested.

Jasndrassik maneuver: to help distract the patient or to help determine present or absence of a weak reflex; patient is asked to push hands together or lock fingers and pull hands apart while reflex is tested; **reinforcement maneuver.**

Lasègue sign: for sciatica; flexion of thigh on hips is painless, and when the knee is bent, such flexion is easily made. If painless, there is no hip joint disease. If test produces pain when the knee is straightened, nerve root irritation or lower back disorder may be present. See **straight leg raising test.**

Linder sign: for sciatica; with the patient sitting or recumbent with outstretched legs, passive flexion of the head will cause pain in the leg or lumbar region.

list: said of a patient who leans to one side or another when standing or walking; most commonly seen in lumbar disk disease.

Lorenz sign: for ankylosing spondylitis (*Marie-Strümpell disease*); ankylotic rigidity of the spinal column, especially thoracic and lumbar segments.

Magnuson test: for malingering; put an x mark on spot where patient reports pain. At a later time in the examination, test for tender points by palpation. The patient indicating pain not including that mark implies malingering.

Mennell sign: for spinal problems; examiner's thumb is taken over the posterosuperior spine of sacrum outward and inward for noting tenderness, which may be caused by sensitive deposits in gluteal aspect of posterosuperior spine; ligamentous strain and sensitivity.

Michele sign: for sciatica; the continued straight leg past the point of nerve irritation will cause the patient to flex the knee if he or she has true sciatica.

Michele flip sign: for sciatica; the sitting patient who has the flexed knees passively extended will lean backward if true sciatica exists.

Milgram test: for a lesion within the dural sac; while lying supine, the patient flexes both hips so that the knees are straight and both feet are lifted by only several inches. If the patient is able to hold this position without pain for 30 seconds, there is no problem within the dural sac. However, a positive test may occur for both intrathecal and extrathecal disorders.

Minor sign: for sciatica; patient rises from sitting position; supporting body on healthy side, placing hand on back, and bending affected leg, revealing pain.

Naffziger test: for sciatica or herniated nucleus pulposus; nerve root irritation is produced by external jugular venous compression by examiner.

Neri bowing sign: for sciatica; the standing patient with knees extended is asked to bend forward. Knee flexion implies sciatica.

O'Connell test: for lumbar nerve irritability; with knee extended both lower limbs are raised to maximum hip flexion to the point of pain, lowering the unaffected limb will exacerbate pain in sciatica.

pelvic rock test: for sacroiliac joint disorder; forcible compression of the iliac crest toward the midline will produce pain.

postural fixation: a sign noted on range of motion of the back; any postural deformity (stiffness) noted does not reverse with range of motion.

Smith-Peterson test: for sacroiliac joint origin of pain; with one hand under the spine the opposite hand raises the leg. If the hamstrings are tight, apply posterior leverage to the pelvis. Pain prior to lumbar movement can be present in both lumbar and sacroiliac joint disorders. If this occurs at the same level for both legs, sacroiliac disease is implied.

Soto-Hall sign: for lesions in back abnormalities; with the patient supine, flexion of the spine beginning at the neck and going downward will elicit pain in the area of the lesion.

spine sign: for poliomyelitis; the patient is unable to flex the spine anteriorly because of pain.

sponge test: for detecting lesions of the spine; the examiner passes a hot sponge up and down the spine, and the patient feels pain over the lesion.

stoop test: for spinal stenosis; with persistent walking the patient will begin to stoop forward to reverse lumbar lordosis and improve spinal space. Likewise, in a sitting position the patient will lean forward.

straight leg raising (SLR) test: for determining nerve root irritation; the supine patient elevates the leg straight until there is back or ipsilateral extremity pain or until the pain is increased with dorsiflexion of the foot; **Lasègue sign.**

Turyn sign: for sciatica; when examiner bends the patient's great toe dorsally, pain is felt in the gluteal region.

Valsalva maneuver: for determining nerve root irritability within the spinal canal. This maneuver is also used for many other unrelated reasons. The patient takes a deep breath and then on bearing down, such as one does when lifting a heavy object, feels pain.

Vanzetti sign: for sciatica; the pelvis is horizontal in the presence of scoliosis. In other scoliotic conditions, the pelvis is inclined as part of the deformity.

Waddell sign: for non-physical origin back pain; pressure on "tender" area results in jump away pain that is in excess of that expected for level of disease, implying a strong emotional component. The term Waddell has commonly been used on other areas to reflect the same implications.

Shoulder

abduction external rotation test: abduct shoulder to 90 degrees with elbow at 90 degrees. On external rotation, pain without apprehension implies rotator cuff disorder. Apprehension implies anterior instability.

abduction sign: for subacromial impingement; the examiner places the shoulder in 90 degrees abduction and 30 degrees flexion and then internally rotates arm, producing pain.

adduction sign: for acromioclavicular joint disease; the shoulder is abducted 90 degrees, brought horizontally forward 90 degrees, and then flexed maximally forward, producing pain at the acromioclavicular joint.

anterior slide test: while patient is sitting, humeral head is translated anteriorly with examiner's hand resulting in increase translation if anterior capsular laxity exits.

Apley scratch test: the patient is asked to put hand behind the back and elevate the hand as far as possible as in trying to scratch the mid-back. A measurement of shoulder extension combined with internal rotation is measured by the thoracic level at which the finger can reach, typically T7.

apprehension test: for anterior subluxing or dislocating shoulder; the arm is held abducted and extended while in external rotation. The patient is apprehensive in a positive examination.

belly press test: for ruptured subscapularis; patient is unable to hold hand on abdomen when hand is forcibly being pulled away (**lift-off test, Napoleon test**).

Booth test: for transverse humeral ligament rupture; with pressure on biceps groove, the arm is abducted and externally rotated. A snap indicates subluxation of the biceps tendon due to ligament insufficiency (**Marvel test**).

Bryant sign: for dislocation of the shoulder with lowering of the axillary folds, as noted on visual examination.

Callaway test: for dislocation of the humerus; the circumference of the affected shoulder measured over the acromion and through the axilla is greater than that on the opposite, unaffected side.

circumduction test: for posterior shoulder instability; to bring the shoulder passively from an abducted and extended position to anterior adduction position results in subluxation in the provocative anterior position. Not to be confused with circumduction maneuver for the knee to determine torn meniscus.

Codman sign: for rupture of the supraspinatus tendon; the arm can be passively abducted without pain, but when support of the arm is removed and the deltoid muscle contracts suddenly, pain occurs again.

Comolli sign: for scapular fracture; shortly after injury, there is triangular swelling, reproducing the shape of the body of the scapula.

crank test: for anterior shoulder instability; the supine patient has the shoulder abducted and externally rotated. On full external rotation there is apprehension and resistance.

cross chest test: for acromioclavicular joint arthritis; passively or actively bringing the affected arm across the chest causes pain in the acromioclavicular joint region.

Dawbarn sign: for acute subacromial bursitis; with arm hanging by side, palpation over the bursa causes pain; when the arm is abducted, pain disappears.

drawer test (load and shift test): for shoulder instability; the patient may be sitting or lying. The scapula and clavicle are held securely in one hand, the head of the humerus in the other, the humeral head is pushed forward and backward to compare the two sides for crepitus and ligamentous stability.

drop arm test: for rotator cuff tear; the patient is unable to actively control bringing the arm down from a full abducted position past 90 degrees. The arm drops at 90 degrees. This test is best performed with a local anesthetic injected into the subacromial space.

Dugas test: for dislocation of the shoulder; placing hand of affected side on opposite shoulder and bringing elbow to side of chest, a dislocation may be present if the patient's elbow will not touch side of the chest; **Dugas s.**

forced adduction test: for acromioclavicular joint arthritis; the arm is forcefully adducted across the upper chest, eliciting pain in the acromioclavicular joint.

Fowler test: for anterior shoulder instability; patient lies supine, the shoulder is held in an abducted and externally rotated position using the edge of the examining surface as a fulcrum. Posterior force is then applied to the humerus. Relief of apprehension is a sign of anterior instability; **push-pull test.**

fulcrum test: for anterior-inferior shoulder instability; patient lies supine, the shoulder is held in an abducted and externally rotated position. The arm is then further abducted and extended using the edge of the examining surface as a fulcrum.

Hamilton test: for luxated shoulder; a rod applied to the humerus can be made to touch the lateral condyle and acromion at the same time to determine a dislocation.

Hawkins impingement sign: for rotator cuff disorder; forward flexion of humerus to 90 degrees followed by horizontal adduction and internal rotation produces pain.

impingement sign: the examiner forces the shoulder into flexion and internal rotation with downward pressure on the acromion produced by the other hand. Pain is a positive sign of impingement. Subacromial injection of local anesthetic transiently relieves shoulder symptoms and eliminates impingement sign.

jerk test: for posterior shoulder instability; the supine patient has the shoulder flexed to 90 degrees with the elbow at 90 degrees, pressure in a posterior direction causes a jerk or jump with subluxation.

Jobe test: for supraspinatus pathology; standing patient is asked to actively abduct the shoulder to 90 degrees and forward flex 30 degrees with thumbs down. Pain occurs if patient is asked to push arm toward the ceiling (**supraspinatus isolation test**).

Kocher maneuver: for reducing anterior dislocations of the shoulder; done by abducting the arm, externally rotating, adducting, and then internally rotating.

lift-off test: for rupture of subscapularis muscle; weakness of internal rotation is demonstrated by inability of patient to lift hand from back.

load-and-shift test: with the patient supine and the shoulder slightly abducted on the edge of the examining table, the humeral head is shifted anteriorly and posteriorly while the forearm or scapula is stabilized by the examiner's opposite hand.

Ludington sign: for integrity of the long head of the biceps tendon; patient interlocks hands overhead and then presses hands together. Failure of biceps contraction implies long head rupture.

Milch maneuver: for anterior shoulder dislocation reduction; with one hand on the acromion to support thumb pressure on humeral head, the arm is abducted and externally rotated followed by pressure on humeral head to reduce over glenoid rim.

Mimori test: for superior labral tears; the sitting patient has the shoulder abducted to 90 to 100 degrees, externally rotated with the elbow at 90 degrees, and the forearm supinated. If there is an increase in pain with forearm pronation, the test is positive for a tear.

Neer impingement sign: for rotator cuff disorder; examiner passively flexes humerus to maximal forward flexion with one hand while depressing the scapula with the other to produce pain.

Neer impingement test: injection of the subacromial bursa eliminates pain elicited with Neer sign. The terms Neer test and Neer sign are often used without discrimination.

Neviaser test: for proximal triceps tendonitis; with shoulder fully adducted, tenderness over origin of triceps is increased with subsequent active elbow extension against force.

O'Brien test: for acromioclavicular joint arthritis or labral tear; the patient is asked to flex shoulder to 90 degrees with an extended elbow and then bring the arm across the chest. Pain indicates one of these two conditions.

push-pull test: for anterior shoulder instability. See Fowler test.

release test: for anterior instability of the shoulder; supine patient with arm abducted at 90 degrees and maximally externally rotated with posterior direct pressure on humeral head is comfortable. Release of humeral head pressure causes apprehension or subluxation.

relocation test: for occult anterior shoulder subluxation in throwers; patient lies supine, the shoulder is held in abducted and externally rotated position using the edge of the examining surface. Posterior force is then applied to the humerus with relief of pain.

scapular sign of Putti: for contractures about the scapula; when the arm is forcibly drawn into the chest and externally rotated the superior lateral side of the scapula wings out; **Putti sign.**

speed test: for proximal long head of biceps tendonitis; anterior proximal humeral pain created with humerus forward flexed against force while elbow is in full extension.

sulcus sign: for inferior shoulder instability; a downward longitudinal force is applied to the humerus of a resting arm. The thumb of the opposite hand can press into the lateral subacromial area, indicating a developing sulcus.

swallow-tail sign: for deltoid muscle function; extension of both arms posteriorly results in a lag on the side that has axillary nerve palsy.

Yergason test: for subluxation of the long head of the biceps tendon; while pulling distally on the elbow, the patient holds it flexed at 90 degrees with supination and forced external rotation of the shoulder against resistance by the examiner. Painful subluxation of the tendon can be palpated.

Upper Limbs and Elbow

elbow flexion test: for cubital tunnel syndrome (ulna nerve compression at elbow); the examiner holds the elbow in passive maximal flexion. Production of tingling in the ring and little finger is positive for ulnar nerve irritation.

gravity stress test: for medial instability; the supine patient has the externally rotated arm out over the edged of the bed. With elbow at 20 degrees, the weight of the forearm reveals the laxity.

Laugier sign: for a displaced distal radial fracture; condition in which the styloid process of radius and ulna are on same level.

Meyn and Quigley maneuver: for dislocation of the elbow; the patient lies prone with the arm resting on the examining table and the elbow flexed at 90 degrees. The forearm is pulled distally while the opposite hand guides the olecranon.

Mills test: for tennis elbow; with wrist and fingers fully flexed and the forearm pronated, complete extension of the elbow is painful.

Parvin maneuver: for dislocated elbow; the patient lies prone with the arms and forearm over the edge of the examining table. Traction is applied on the wrist in a distal direction while the opposite hand pushes on the anterior distal arm in a posterior direction.

posterolateral instability (pivot shift of elbow): for lateral ulnar collateral ligament laxity; with patient supine, shoulder flexed to 90 degrees, elbow extended, and forearm supinated, examiner the forearm is supinated with a concurrent valgus stress. The instability will increase at 40 degrees of elbow flexion.

Hands

Allen test: for occlusion of radial or ulnar artery; a method of determining if radial and ulnar arteries communicate through the two palmar arches. Both arteries are occluded digitally. First one artery is released, then the other, to observe pattern of capillary refill in the hand. This can be performed with a Doppler placed on the digits during test. The test is valuable prior to an invasive procedure on the arteries at the wrist.

André Thomas sign: in low ulnar nerve palsy; in an effort to extend the fingers, flexing the wrist using the tenodesis effect will increase the claw.

axial compression test: for thumb carpometacarpal joint arthritis; thumb is compressed with rotation causing pain in that joint.

Ballotment test: assesses triquetrolunate dissociation; stabilize the lunate with one hand, the triquetrum with the other. Displace one from the other dorsally and volarly. If there is crepitus, pain, and extreme laxity, the test is positive.

benediction attitude (sign): for paralysis of the anterior interosseous branch of the median nerve; in the resting hand the index finger and thumb are held in full extension.

benediction sign: in low ulnar nerve palsy; there is metacarpophalangeal hyperextension, proximal and distal interphalangeal joint flexion in the fourth and fifth digits, and the index and middle fingers are relatively spared.

Bouvier maneuver: in low ulnar nerve palsy; passively preventing metacarpophalangeal hyperextension will allow proximal and distal interphalangeal extension.

Boyes test: for boutonnière deformity; with full extension of the proximal interphalangeal (PIP) joint of the finger, there is decreased distal interphalangeal (DIP) flexion compared with the contralateral finger.

bracelet test: for early rheumatoid arthritis involving the distal radioulnar joint; compression of the lower ends of the ulna and radius elicits moderate lateral pain.

Carducci test: for boutonnière deformity; with full metaphalangeal (MP) and wrist flexion there is 15- to 20-degree loss of proximal interphalangeal (PIP) extension compared with the contralateral finger.

carpal compression test: compression of the carpal tunnel for as long as 30 seconds will produce or exacerbate symptoms of carpal tunnel syndrome. A sphygmomanometer bulb can gauge the proper pressure, about 150 mm Hg.

circumduction maneuver: for the thumb; any general test or motion involving a rotation action of a group of joints; a range of motion examination.

claw hand sign: in lower ulnar nerve palsy, there is metacarpophalangeal hyperextension with proximal and distal interphalangeal flexion, and intrinsic minus posture in all palmar digits. These may be static or dynamic.

confrontational test: for hand intrinsic muscle weakness; the strength of specific muscle or muscle groups is compared by pressing the thumb or finger against opposite thumb or finger in a fashion to produce resistance against those muscles. Weakness is indicated by an inability to oppose the compared digits with equal strength (i.e., one side gives out).

Duchenne sign: in low ulnar nerve palsy with extrinsic muscles intact; the ring and little fingers will claw with metacarpophalangeal hyperextension and flexion of the middle and distal phalanges.

Elson middle slip test: for ruptured central extensor tendon slip of the PIP joint; the finger is flexed to 90 degrees. If the central slip is intact, the patient can extend the PIP joint, but the DIP joint is flail. Otherwise, the PIP joint will not have extension power, and the DIP joint will extend while in that position.

extrinsic tightness test: to assess extrinsic extensor tendon adherence or foreshortening; passive metacarpophalangeal (MCP) joint flexion will cause MCP joint hyperextension. MCP flexion will force the PIP joint into extension.

Finkelstein sign: bending the thumb into the palm to determine synovitis of the abductor pollicis longus tendon to wrist. Passively flexing and ulnar deviating the wrist with the thumb in full opposition will elicit pain over the first dorsal extensor compartment in de Quervain disease.

Fowler maneuver: for testing rheumatoid arthritis; tight intrinsic muscles in ulnar deviation of the digits and a heavy, taut ulnar band are demonstrated when the digit is held in its normal axial relationship.

Froment sign: for ulnar nerve loss; there is paralysis of the adductor pollicis and first dorsal interosseous and second palmar interosseous. The flexor pollicis longus flexes the interphalangeal joint up to 90 degrees to effect power pinch.

Gilliat tourniquet test: to diagnose carpal tunnel syndrome; a tourniquet is placed on the upper arm of affected limb. Inflate cuff to a point above the systolic pressure to 220 mmHg. Arm pain normally occurs within 2 to 3 minutes. Tingling in the median nerve distribution of thumb, index, and long finger will occur in 30 to 60 seconds in carpal tunnel syndrome.

grip strength test: to measure the strength of coordination of intrinsic and extrinsic finger/thumb flexors; a grip dynamometer is used.

Hutchinson s.: seen in malignant melanoma; lesion under a fingernail or toenail in which the pigment extends into the proximal nail fold.

International Classification for Surgery of the Hand in Tetraplegia: to determine extent of muscle capacity for intrinsic and extrinsic muscle and tendon transfers that improve hand function.

Motor Group

0: no muscle below elbow available.

1: brachioradialis (BR) > 4+.

2: BR and extensor carpi radialis longus (ECRL) > 4+.

3: BR, ECRL, and extensor carpi radialis brevis (ECRB) > 4+.

4: BR, ECRL, ECRB, and pronator teres (PT) > 4+.

5: BR, ECRL, ECRB, PT, and flexor carpi radialis (FCR) > 4+.

6: BR, ECRL, ECRB, PT, FCR, and finger extensors > 4+.

7: BR, ECRL, ECRB, PT, FCR, finger extensors, and thumb extensors > 4+.

8: BR, ECRL, ECRB, PT, FCR, finger and thumb extensors, and partial digital flexors > 4+.

9: lacks only intrinsic muscle function.

X: exceptions.

Sensation

O: two-point discrimination in the thumb > 10 mm.

Ocu: two-point discrimination in the thumb < 10 mm.

intrinsic tightness test: to assess adherence or contracture of intrinsic muscles with metacarpophalangeal joint passively extended. Active or passive proximal interphalangeal flexion is limited.

Jeanne test: in ulnar nerve palsy; with adduction, pollicis dysfunction with metacarpophalangeal hyperextension will result with key pinch or gross grip.

Kanavel sign: for infection of a tendon sheath; there is a point of maximum tenderness in the palm 1 inch proximal to the base of the little finger. In pyogenic tenosynovitis, the four signs are a flexed position of the finger, symmetric fusiform enlargement of the fingers, marked tendon sheath tenderness, and pain on passive digital extension.

Kapandji thumb opposition score: for ability to oppose thumb; with fingers extended, increasing ability to oppose from base of index to the finger tip, graded 1 to 3; 4, opposition to long finger tip; 5, opposition to ring finger tip; 6 to 8, opposition from tip of little finger to base; 9, opposition to palm distal to flexion crease; 10, opposition to palm proximal to flexion crease.

key pinch: the strength in the ability to grasp, as in holding a key; lateral pinch.

Kleinman shear test: to assess triquetrolunate disability. Stabilize the lunate with a thumb placed on the dorsum of the lunate. If the test is positive, the pisotriquetral joint is pushed dorsally from the volar side with pain, crepitus, and increased motion.

Lichtman test: in nondissociative midcarpal instability; a painful clunk is elicited with passive (and sometimes active) ulnar deviation of the wrist. The clunk occurs as the hamate reduces on the triquetrum and the entire proximal row rotates rapidly from its flexed to an extended position.

long finger extension test: for radial (supinator) tunnel compression; the patient holds wrist at 30 degrees extension while extending all fingers. The examiner attempts to press on the dorsum of the long finger to produce the dorsal forearm symptoms.

Lovett test: for boutonnière deformity; with full MP and wrist flexion there is decrease in PIP extension strength compared with the contralateral finger.

Maisonneuve sign: for Colles fracture; there is marked hyperextensibility of the hand.

masses sign: in ulnar nerve palsy; there is flattening of the metacarpal arch and hypothenar atrophy due to intrinsic dysfunction with loss of metacarpophalangeal flexion of the fifth digit.

Murphy sign: for scaphoid fracture or lunate dislocation; tapping on the index metacarpal head causes pain with navicular fracture and tapping long finger metacarpal head causes pain with lunate dislocation.

Oshsner clasping test: for high median nerve paralysis; the index finger will not flex when clasped hand are brought together.

Phalen test and maneuver: for carpal tunnel syndrome; irritation of the median nerve is determined by holding the wrist flexed or extended for 30 to 60 seconds, reproducing symptoms.

piano key sign: test for distal radioulnar joint instability; the wrist is pronated, the radius and ulna are grasped in examiner's hands, and moving each bone up and down relative to the other, a painful movement indicates instability.

Pitres-Testut sign: for ulnar nerve paralysis; the patient is unable to make a cone shape with the hand and fingers due to intrinsic muscle weakness.

Pollock sign: in high ulnar nerve palsy; inability to flex the distal interphalangeal joints of the fourth and fifth digits with paralysis of the flexor digitorum profundus to fourth and fifth digits.

prehension: the ability to grasp with the fingers and thumb.

pseudostability test: for carpal bone stability; in the normal wrist, if the hand is held in one hand and the distal forearm in the other, there is a normal anterior posterior translation. This translation is lost in carpal bone instability.

pulp pinch: the strength in the position one would use to pick up a piece of paper.

scaphoid test: for dynamic scapholunate instability; the examiner places his or her thumb under the scaphoid tubercle, moving wrist from ulnar to radial deviation. The scaphoid flexes against the thumbs in an upward push causing a painful clunk at the scapholunate articulation; **Watson test.**

Semm and Weinstein monofilament test: an array of nylon filaments are used to quantitate the cutaneous sensory pressure threshold. They are arranged in increasing thickness on a logarithmic scale. They will access the slowly adapting fiber receptor system. A 5.07 filament is commonly used to test foot sensitivity for neuropathy such as diabetes.

Smith and Ross test: for boutonnière deformity; with passive MP joint and wrist flexion, there is passive PIP extension if the central slip is intact, and a greater than 20-degree lag if there is central slip rupture.

spilled teacup sign: in perilunate dislocation; the lunate will assume a volar flexed posture as seen on lateral radiographs. A spectrum exists from normal lunate position to complete volar dislocation of the lunate.

table top test: for timing of surgery in Dupuytren's contracture; the patient has limitation putting hand flat on table top.

tenodesis test: to check structure integrity of the extrinsic extensors; extreme wrist flexion will passively extend the metacarpophalangeal joints, whereas wrist extension will allow passive digital proximal and distal interphalangeal flexion. This is due to resting tension of extrinsic extensor and flexor groups, respectively.

Terri-Thomas sign: in scapholunate dissociation; there is an apparent gap between the scaphoid and lunate seen on a neutral anteroposterior wrist radiograph.

tuck sign: the puckering seen just proximal to a mass of chronically inflamed dorsal tenosynovium. This is accentuated by digital extension and commonly seen in rheumatoid arthritis.

two-point discrimination test: measures innervation density under the skin. Static two-point discrimination t. is for *slowly* adapting fibers; moving two-point discrimination t. is for *rapidly* adapting fibers. It is the ability to distinguish one point and two points with eyes closed. (Normal range is 1–5 mm.)

Wartenberg sign: for intrinsic muscle weakness of the hand; while the fingers are extended there is an inability to bring together the ring and little finger. In ulnar nerve palsy with interosseous paralysis, there is an inability to adduct the extended fifth digit to fourth digit (**oriental prayer sign**).

Watson test: for scapholunate instability; the examiner can elicit a painful wrist click by compressing the scaphoid while the patient moves the wrist (**rotary click test**).

wet leather sign: subcutaneous palpable crepitus or squeaking with movement of tendons affected by tenosynovitis.

Hips

Allis maneuver: for reduction of anterior hip dislocation; the supine patient has the knee flexed, hip slightly flexed with longitudinal traction, and an assistant stabilizes the pelvis while applying a lateral traction force to the medial thigh. The surgeon then adducts and internally rotates the femur.

Allis sign: for femoral neck fracture or congenital dislocation hip; there is relaxation of the fascia between the crest of the ilium and the greater trochanter.

anvil test: for early hip joint disease or diseased vertebrae; a closed fist striking a blow to the sole of the foot with leg extended produces pain in the hip or vertebrae.

Barlow test: for dysplastic hip in infants; holding the symphysis pubis to sacrum with one hand, the opposite hip is flexed and an attempt is made to dislocate the hip. Pulling the hip back up or abducting the hip should produce a perceptible reduction.

Bozan maneuver: for reducing femoral neck fractures; a large swathe is placed around the crest of the ilium of the affected limb and a small swathe in the inguinal fold; traction, abduction, and internal rotation forces are then applied.

Chapple test: for infant congenital hip dislocation, the hips cannot be abducted past 45 degrees while in flexion.

Chiene test: for determining fracture of the neck of the femur by use of a tape measure.

Desault sign: for intracapsular fracture of the hip; alternation of the arc described by rotation of the greater trochanter, which normally describes the segment of a circle, but in this fracture, rotates only as the apex of the femur rotates about its own axis.

Destot sign: in a pelvic fracture; there is the formation of a large superficial hematoma beneath the inguinal ligament and in the scrotum.

Deyerle maneuver: for femoral neck fracture reduction; patient placed in traction with over-distraction and external rotation. The leg is then internally rotated with some traction release and inward pressure on the greater trochanter to reduce and impact fracture site.

Earle sign: for pelvic fracture; bony prominence or hematoma associated with tenderness on rectal examination.

Ely test: for determining tightness of the rectus femoris, contracture of the lateral fascia of the thigh, or femoral nerve irritation; with patient in prone position, flexion of the leg on the thigh causes buttocks to arch away and leg to abduct at the hip joint **(Nachlas knee flexion test)**.

Galeazzi sign: for congenital dislocation of the hip; the dislocated side is shorter when both thighs are flexed to 90 degrees, as demonstrated in infants; in an older patient, a curvature of the spine is produced by shortened leg.

gear-stick sign: for femoral head deformity of dysplastic hip or Legg-Calvé-Perthes disease; thigh abduction is full in flexion, but as the hip is extended with the hip abducted, there is impingement between the greater trochanter and ilium.

Jansen test: for osteoarthritis deformans of the hip; the patient is asked to cross the legs with a point just above the ankle resting on the opposite knee. If significant disease exists, this test and motion are impossible.

King maneuver: for femoral neck fracture reduction; on fracture table, the affected leg is in traction with pressure placed on the posterior thigh with internal rotation. Lateral traction with a groin sling may be added.

Langoria sign: for symptoms of intracapsular fracture of the femur; relaxation of the extensor muscles of the thigh is present.

Leadbetter maneuver: for slipped capital femoral epiphysis or femoral head fracture; injured hip is flexed to 90 degrees and manual traction applied to axis of the flexed thigh with adduction. The leg is then circumducted slowly to abduction maintaining internal rotation, and then the thigh and leg are brought down to the horizontal level.

Ludloff sign: for traumatic separation of the epiphysis of the lesser trochanter; swelling and ecchymosis are present at the base of Scarpa triangle, together with inability to raise the thigh when in a sitting position.

McElvenny maneuver: for femoral neck fracture reduction; with 36- to 45-kg traction the hip is abducted and internally rotated. Medial to inferior force is produced over the greater trochanter, and then the hip is adducted.

Nélaton line (radiographic and physical examinations): for detecting dislocation of the hip; there is a line from the anterosuperior iliac spine to the ischial tuberosity, which normally passes through the greater trochanter.

Ober test: for tight tensor fascia lata; with patient lying on side with hip and knee flexed, the opposite hip is extended while the knee is flexed. Inability to place the knee being tested on the table surface indicates a tight fascia lata.

obturator s.: inward rotation of the hip so that the obturator internus muscle is stretched. Results may be positive in acute appendicitis.

Ortolani test: for congenitally dislocated hip; an audible click is heard when the hip goes into the socket as noted in infancy. If the sign is elicited, the dislocation should be corrected at that time to avoid hip dysfunction later; **Ortolani click.**

piston sign: for congenital dislocation of the head of the femur; if positive, there is up-and-down movement of the head of the femur; **Dupuytren sign.**

reverse Bigelow maneuver: for anterior dislocation of the hip; two maneuvers are done, both starting in hip flexion and abduction: In the first maneuver, while lifting the lower leg of the supine patient, there is a quick jerk on the flexed thigh; the second maneuver involves traction in the line of deformity with the hip then being adducted, sharply internally rotated, and extended.

Roux sign: in a pelvic lateral compression fracture, there is a distance between the greater trochanter and pubic spine on the affected side.

Smith maneuver: for reduction of femoral neck fractures; thigh is externally rotated and placed in traction, then fully abducted, internally rotated, and subsequently adducted.

Stimson maneuver: for posterior hip dislocation; the patient is placed prone on a table with the involved hip flexed and the opposite hip extended. With the involved knee flexed downward, pressure is applied to the calf, resulting in reduction of the dislocation.

Thomas sign: for hip joint flexion contracture; when the patient is walking, the fixed flexion of the hip can be compensated by lumbar lordosis. With the patient supine and flexing the opposite hip, the affected thigh raises off the table; **Strümpell sign, Thomas test.**

Trendelenburg test: for muscular weakness in poliomyelitis, ununited fracture of the femoral neck, rheumatoid arthritis, coxa vara, and congenital dislocations. With the patient standing, weight is removed from one extremity. If gluteal fold drops on that side, it signifies muscular weakness of the opposite weight-bearing hip; **Trendelenburg sign.**

Wellmerling maneuver: for femoral neck fracture reduction; the affected hip is overdistracted by 0.64 cm (¼ inch) in external rotation, and the foot is then internally rotated and traction released.

Whitman maneuver: for femoral neck fracture reduction; the hip is flexed and then extended with traction being applied and the normal hip abducted. The affected side is then abducted and a spica cast applied.

Lower Limbs

Achilles squeeze test: for Achilles tendon rupture; squeezing the calf muscle fails to produce plantar flexion of the ankle joint.

Addis test: for determination of leg-length discrepancy; with patient in prone position, flexing the knees to 90 degrees reveals the potential discrepancies of both tibial and femoral lengths.

anterior tibial sign: for spastic paraplegia; involuntary extension of the tibialis anterior muscle when thigh is actively flexed on the abdomen.

Cleeman sign: for distal fracture of femur with overriding of the fragments; shows creasing of the skin just above the patella.

Homan's sign: pain in calf on dorsiflexion of foot (active or passive). Once considered a reliable test in diagnosing deep vein thrombophlebitis but no longer considered valid.

Payr sign: early sign of impending postoperative thrombosis, indicated by tenderness when pressure is placed over the inner side of the foot.

Schlesinger sign: for extensor spasm at the knee joint; with patient's leg held at the knee joint and flexed strongly at the hip joint, there will follow an extensor spasm at the knee joint with extreme supination of the foot.

Thompson test: compression of calf muscle with foot at rest results in ankle flexion if Achilles tendon is intact; **Simmons test, Achilles squeeze test.**

tourniquet test: for phlebitis of the leg; tourniquet is applied to the thigh and pressure gradually increased until the patient complains of pain in the calf; result is compared with the effect on the opposite leg.

Knees (Table 4-1)

anterior cruciate instability test: with the knee flexed, a supine patient extends the knee slowly with the foot against the table surface; there is a sudden anterior shift of the tibia.

Apley test: for differentiating ligament from meniscal injury; tibial rotation on femur with traction or compression with the patient prone and knee flexed; **Apley s., grind test.**

arthrometer test: mechanical testing device for measuring anteroposterior ligament stability of the knee. The arthrometer is most often used in a physician's office to document the outcome of anterior cruciate ligament replacement surgery.

ballotable patella test: for knee effusion; with knee extension, pushing patella onto distal femoral surface results in rebound due to swelling.

bayonet sign: lateral placement of infrapatellar tendon with a valgus knee produces a bayonet appearance in the quadriceps patellar tendon complex.

Bounce home test: for bucket handle tear meniscus; passive pressure past maximum active extension results in a bounce back to more flexion.

British test: for knee pain and/or injury; compression of patella during active quadriceps contraction as knee is extended elicits pain.

camelback sign: an unusually prominent infrapatellar fat pad of the knee and hypertrophy of the vastus lateralis.

Childress test: for torn meniscus; when duck walking the supporting leg will have pain on the side of the torn meniscus.

cross-over test: for anterior cruciate ligament laxity; with patient's permission, the examiner stands on the foot of the affected side of standing patient. When the patient attempts to cross the opposite

TABLE 4-1 Knee Instability Tests

Instability	Positive Test	Deficient Structure
Medial	Valgus stress at 30 degrees	Medial collateral ligament
Lateral	Varus stress at 30 degrees	Minor lateral complex tear
Anterior	Anterior drawer at 90 degrees, neutral rotation	Anterior cruciate and partial medial and lateral collateral ligaments
Posterior	Posterior drawer at 90 degrees	Posterior cruciate, arcuate complex, posterior oblique ligaments
Anteromedial	Slocum at 30 degrees external rotation accented	Medial capsular, tibial collateral, posterior oblique, anterior cruciate ligaments
Anterolateral	Slocum at 15 degrees internal rotation accented	Lateral capsular ligament
	Jerk test	Arcuate complex
	Lateral pivot shift	Anterior cruciate ligament
Posterolateral	Reverse pivot shift	Arcuate complex Lateral capsular ligament, popliteus tendon, some posterior cruciate ligament
Posteromedial (controversial)	Medial tibial plateau shifts posterior on stress	Tibial collateral, medial capsular, posterior oblique, semimembranosus, anterior cruciate ligaments

leg over the knee there is a sense of the knee wanting to go out of place.

dial test: for posterolateral corner and posterior cruciate instability; isolated posterior cruciate instability will allow 15 degree plus increased passive external rotation of the foot and ankle when the knee is flexed at 90 degrees. Posterolateral corner instability will have 15 degree or greater increased external rotation of the foot and ankle at 30 degrees.

double camelback sign: prominence of a high riding patella and infrapatellar fat pad, producing the appearance of a camelback.

drawer sign: for ligamentous instability or ruptured cruciate ligaments; with the patient supine and knee flexed to 90 degrees, the sign is positive if knee is not displaced abnormally in a posterior direction with knee pulled forward. Also called an **anterior drawer sign,** meaning the anterior cruciate is lax or ruptured.

drop back phenomenon: for posterior cruciate rupture; posterior sag of tibia in relationship to distal femur when knee is flexed and patient is at rest (**sag sign**).

extension lag: a sign of patella tendon rupture; there is an injury-related change in the ability of the patient to actively extend the knee.

external rotation recurvatum test: with the patient supine, the knee is brought from 10 degrees of flexion to maximum extension while palpating for external rotation of the tibia.

Fairbank sign: for subluxating patella; with the affected knee in extension the examiner pushes the patella in a lateral direction causing apprehension.

flexion rotation drawer test (Noyes): with the knee extended and the thigh relaxed, there is anterolateral tibial subluxation. The knee is gradually flexed with reduction of the subluxation occurring at about 30 degrees of flexion.

Godfrey test: for posterior cruciate ligament laxity; with patient supine and the knee and hip flexed at 90 degrees and the examiner supporting heel, the proximal tibia is more posterior on the affected side.

grimace test: for knee pain or crepitus; if compression of the patella elicits pain or crepitus is noted, the patient will grimace.

heel height difference: for knee flexion contracture; prone patient in knee extension has different level of heels (**prone hanging test**).

heel to buttocks difference: for swelling or obstruction of flexion; the heel is further from the buttocks in flexion compared with the unaffected side.

Helft test: for proximal tibio-fibular instability, the standing patient is asked to gradually flex the involved knee. If laxity exists the person will cross the opposite leg and foot behind the affected knee to stabilize it.

hop test (one-legged hop test): for anterior cruciate examination; patient hops forward on affected knee. Ability to do this is one sign of adequate anterior cruciate stability.

Hughston jerk test: for anterolateral instability of the knee; noted by starting at 90 degrees flexion with tibia internally rotated and applying valgus force while rotating fibula medially. There is a jerk at about 20 degrees from full extension.

Lachman test: with the patient supine and the knee flexed to 20 degrees, the tibia is pulled anteriorly. A "give" reaction or mushy end point indicates a torn anterior cruciate ligament.

Losse test: for posterolateral laxity; the supine patient has the affected knee held at 30 degrees flexion with the distal leg on the examiner's chest and the examiner's opposite thumb behind the head of the fibula and fingers on the patella. As the thumb pulls the fibular head forward the knee is gradually extended and a shift should occur as the plateau subluxes anteriorly.

McMurray circumduction maneuver: for noting joint menisci tears or tags; there is cartilage clicking medially or laterally on manipulation of the knee; **McMurray s.**

medial subluxation test: for tight lateral patellar retinaculum; the patella is pressed in a medial direction with the knee at full extension and then at 30 degrees of flexion. More that 15 mm of medial displacement in flexion implies that the patella tracks laterally due to a tight retinaculum.

Merke sign: for meniscal tear; the standing patient will have a meniscal tear on the medial side if there is pain on internal rotation, and a tear on the lateral side if there is pain on external rotation.

"no touch" test: for checking patellar stability after total knee joint replacement, also for anterior cruciate instability; with the patient supine and the knee flexed, there is a sudden anterior shift of the tibia when the patient extends the knee slowly with the foot on the surface.

patellar glide test: for maltracking of the patella; the sitting patient is asked to extend the knee and the tracking of the patella is observed. Maltracking is typically in a lateral direction.

patellar grind test: described as being for chondromalacia patella; this is a nonspecific test in which the patella is pressed into the trochlea on active or passive knee extension from flexion. Pain may be from the patella or from regional synovium (**Fouchet sign**).

patellar retraction test: for synovitis; compression of patella causes pain when the patient attempts to set the quadriceps muscles with the knee in full extension.

pivot-shift test (MacIntosh): with the knee extended, the examiner internally rotates the leg and with a valgus stress gradually flexes the knee. There is a shift at 30 degrees to 40 degrees.

Popeye deformity: physical appearance of the bunched up lateral biceps due to a rupture of the long head of the biceps.

posterior drawer test: with the hips at 45 degrees and the knees flexed at 90 degrees the examiner sits on the foot and pushes the tibia backward; also with the hips and knees flexed at 90 degrees the heels are held together and the two knees observed for comparison of relative posterior sag of the tibia.

prone external rotation test: for posterior cruciate knee rupture; with the patient prone and knees flexed at 30 degrees, the test is considered positive for rupture if the foot externally rotates more than 10 degrees compared with the normal side.

quadriceps active test: with the patient supine the involved knee is flexed at 90 degrees and the foot rests on the table. With one hand, the examiner supports the thigh and palpates the relaxed quadriceps muscle; the other hand stabilizes the foot. When the patient is asked to slide the foot down the table, the proximal leg is pulled forward by the patellar tendon, indicating a posterior cruciate tear with resulting posterior sagging of the leg.

reverse pivot-shift (Jacob, jerk): with the patient supine, the lateral tibial plateau shifts from posterior subluxation to reduction as the knee is brought from flexion to extension.

screw-home mechanism: the small degree of external rotation that occurs as the knee is brought to the last few degrees of extension.

Slocum test: for rotary instability of the knee; the examiner pulls on the upper calf of a supine patient with the knees flexed 90 degrees. Then, while sitting on the patient's foot, the examiner pulls anteriorly, comparing the amount of give with the foot turned in 15 degrees neutral and turned out 30 degrees.

standing apprehension test: for anterior cruciate laxity; with patient standing and knee slightly flexed, examiner's hand holds the knee firmly with the thumb pushing the lateral femoral condyle medially, resulting in motion.

Steinmann test: for medial meniscal tear; on the supine patient the knee is held flexed at 90 degrees, the calf held firmly, and the tibia rotated internally and externally. Sharp medial pain implies a meniscal tear.

thumbnail test: for patellar fracture; fracture is felt as a sharp crevice when the examiner's thumbnail is passed over the subcutaneous surface of the patella.

Trotter bulge test: for knee swelling; massaging pressure on medial side of knee may make swelling move superiorly so that pressure from above may make fluid more apparent on return to medial side.

valgus stress test: although this term is commonly applied to the knee, the test may also be done on the elbow. The upper part of the limb is supported while a laterally directed force is produced on the distal limb. If knee laxity is found in full extension, both the anterior cruciate and medial collateral ligaments are compromised. If there is laxity at only 30 degrees, there is an isolated medial collateral ligament tear.

varus stress test: although this term is commonly applied to the knee, the test may also be done on the elbow. The upper part of the limb is supported while a medially directed force is produced on the distal limb. If knee laxity is found in full extension, both the anterior cruciate and lateral collateral ligaments are compromised. If there is laxity at only 30 degrees, an isolated medial collateral ligament tear or posterolateral corner injury is likely.

Wilson sign: with knee extended from 30 degrees with valgus stress and internal rotation of the foot, a click is heard in cases of osteochondritis dissecans.

Feet, Ankles

Achilles bulge sign: seen in ankle instability; a bulging Achilles tendon occurs when the foot is pulled forward while the leg is pushed backward with the knee flexed; **heel-cord sign.**

anterior drawer sign: for ankle instability; the heel is pulled forward with the leg being restrained by the opposite hand. A precise lateral radiograph is obtained with the patient supine and both the popliteal area and heel supported and 5 kg applied to the ankle.

Coleman lateral standing block test: to detect flexibility of cavovarus deformity of foot; lateral side of foot and full heel are placed on a 1-inch block, and loss of varus deformity implies flexibility.

dimple sign: for ruptured lateral collateral ligament of ankle; an anterior force is directed on the heel while a posterior force is directed on the distal leg. In the case of a ruptured ligament, a dimple will appear.

drawer sign: for lateral collateral ligament injury in the ankle; with the foot and ankle at rest and the knee flexed and the ankle flexed at 10- to 15-degree plantar flexion, the heel is pulled forward. The center of rotation is the deltoid ligament.

Harris-Beath footprinting mat: a pressure sensitive mat used to reflect the various pressure points under the foot.

Helbing sign: for hyperpronation of foot; medialward curving of the Achilles tendon as viewed from behind.

Keen sign: for Pott fracture of the fibula; if fracture exists, there is increased diameter around the malleoli area of the ankle.

Marie-Foix sign: for central nervous system disorder; withdrawal of the lower leg on transverse pressure of the tarsus or forced flexion of toes, even when the leg is incapable of voluntary movement.

McBride test: for contracture of lateral capsule metatarsal phalangeal joint of the big toe or tight adductor; an ability to passively put toe in neutral position.

Morton test: for metatarsalgia or neuroma; transverse pressure across heads of the metatarsals causes sharp pain in the forefoot.

Mulder sign: for interdigital neuroma in the foot; a palpable click can be heard on motion of the metatarsal heads.

Murphy sign: for Achilles tendon bursitis at the heel; dorsiflexion of the foot produces pain.

sagittal stress test: for ankle instability; with the knee flexed to at least 45 degrees, the foot is pulled forward while the leg is pushed backward. If the usual concavity of the Achilles tendon is flattened or reversed, the sign is positive for an instability of the anterior fibular collateral ligament.

Silfreskiold test: for ankle equines contracture; test passive restriction of ankle dorsiflexion with knee in flexion and extension. Contracture that is due to soleus alone will not change with knee flexion. That due to gastrocnemius will have better ankle dorsiflexion when knee is flexed.

Strunsky sign: for detecting lesions of the anterior arch of the foot; sudden flexing of the toes is painless in a normal foot, but painful if inflammation exists in the anterior arch.

talar tilt test: with the ankle in neutral position the heel is grasped in one hand and the ankle in the other. The ankle is then supinated with maximum force. An anteroposterior radiograph may be obtained to define the talar tilt.

Thomas squeeze test: for Achilles tendon rupture; the prone patient with knee flexed at 90 degrees has calf squeezed. Failure of foot flexion indicated Achilles rupture.

toe spread sign: for Morton neuroma; disproportional spreading of the toes, comparing one foot with the other.

too many toes sign: increased hindfoot, valgus, pronation, and abduction of forefoot. On clinical observation, refers to the excessive number of toes that appear laterally when foot is viewed from behind. Often indicates collapse of the medial arch and flatfoot deformity.

Wu sole opposition test: for posterior tendon rupture; a visual test that shows a defect as both feet are opposed to each other.

Neurologic Examination

ankle clonus test: implies a central nervous system condition of cord or brain, sudden forced dorsiflexion of the ankles results in repeated flexion. **Sustained clonus** does not stop as long as dorsiflexion pressure is applied to the foot.

Babinski reflex: for loss of brain control over lower extremities; scraping the soles causes toes to pull up; **toe sign.**

Babinski sign: for testing of first sacral nerve root pathology; an absent Achilles tendon reflex or diminished reflex as compared with the other side.

Beevor sign: for segmental nerve disease involving T5–T12 or L1 nerve roots; the patient does an active sit-up with the arms held behind the head. In a positive examination, the umbilicus moves toward the segment that is weak.

Brudzinski sign: for meningitis; flexion of the neck forward results in flexion of the hip and knee; when passive flexion of the lower limb on one side is made, a similar movement will be seen in the opposite limb; **neck sign, contralateral sign.**

Chaddock sign: for upper motor neuron loss (brain); the big toe extends when irritating the skin in the external malleolar region; indicates lesions of the corticospinal paths; **external malleolus sign, Chaddock reflex.**

doll's eye sign: for testing normal or abnormal brain function; the normal coordinated eye motions seen when passively turning the head of an unconscious patient; **Cantelli sign.**

Ely test: for L3 and L4 nerve root irritation; flexing thigh with patient prone causes back and/or thigh pain; **femoral nerve stretch test, Ely sign.**

fan sign: for central nerve problems; stroking the sole of the foot with a needle causes toes to spread; part of Babinski reflex examination.

finger to nose test: for cerebellar disease; patient attempts to put a finger on nose and then on the examiner's finger, back and forth rapidly, any incoordination indicates positive test; **coordination extremity test.**

Fournier test: for determining ataxic gait; it is noted with the patient moving about abruptly in walking, starting, and stopping.

Fränkel sign: for tabes dorsalis; noted by diminished tonicity of muscles about the hip joint.

Gordon reflex: for loss of brain control; percussion on lateral thigh causes toes to go up rather than the normal downward motion.

Guilland sign: for meningeal irritation; when the contralateral quadriceps muscle group is pinched, there is brisk flexion at the hip and knee joint.

Heel-bisector method: used for assessing metatarsus adductus. The heel-bisector line passes through the longitudinal axis of the heel. When the foot is held in the simulated weight-bearing position, the line should pass through the second toe. Metatarsus, adductus is mild if the line passes through the third toe, moderate if through the fourth toe, and severe if through the fifth toe.

Hirschberg sign: for pyramidal tract disease; internal rotation and adduction of foot on rubbing inner lateral side.

Hoffmann sign: for testing digital reflex; nipping of three fingernails (index, middle, ring) produces flexion of terminal phalanx of thumb and second and third phalanx of some other finger; digital reflex.

Huntington sign: for lesions of the pyramidal tract; patient is supine, with legs hanging over the examining table, and is asked to cough; if coughing produces flexion of the thigh and extension of the leg in the paralyzed limb, a lesion is indicated.

Jendrassik maneuver: to enhance a patellar reflex; the reflex is tested when the patient hooks hands together with flexed fingers and pulls apart as hard as possible.

Kernig sign: for meningitis; in dorsal decubitus, the patient can easily and completely extend the leg; when sitting or lying down with thigh flexed on the abdomen, the leg cannot be completely extended.

Kerr sign: for spinal cord lesions; alteration of the texture of the skin below the somatic level is used to locate level of lesions.

Klippel-Feil sign: for pyramidal track disorders; passive flexion and extension of index finger causes thumb flexion and adduction.

Leichtenstern sign: for cerebrospinal meningitis; tapping lightly on any bone of the extremities causes patient to wince suddenly.

Leri sign: for hemiplegia; passive flexion of the hand and wrist of the affected side shows no normal flexion at the elbow.

Lhermitte sign: for cervical cord injuries or unstable cervical spine; transient dysesthesia and weakness are noted in all four limbs when the patient flexes the head forward.

long tract sign: any sign that one would see in affection of either sensory or motor tracts in the spinal cord. For example, **Babinski reflex, Romberg test.**

Mendel-Bekhterev reflex: for organic hemiplegia; using a percussion hammer, the examiner notes flexion of the small toes if the dorsal surface of the cuboid bone is struck.

Moro reflex: for testing normal early neurologic development or the failure to progress neurologically; the infant is placed on a table, then the table is forcibly struck from either side, causing the infant's arms to be thrown out as in an embrace; should disappear as infancy progresses.

Morquio sign: for epidemic poliomyelitis; the supine patient resists attempts to raise trunk to a sitting position until the legs are passively flexed.

MRC (Medical Research Council) or Zachary sensory grade: for assessment of sensation of peripheral nerve after injury and/or repair.

S 0: absence of any sensory recovery.

S 1: recovery of deep cutaneous pain sensibility.

S 2: return of some superficial pain and tactile sensibility.

S 2+: recovery of touch and pain sensibility throughout the autonomous zone, but with persistent overreaction.

S 3: return of superficial pain and tactile sensibility throughout the autonomous zone with disappearance of overreaction.

S 3+: as S 3 but with good localization and some return of two-point discrimination.

S 4: return of sensibility as in S 3, with recovery of two-point discrimination.

nuchocephalic reflex: for diffuse cerebral dysfunction as in senility; when the shoulders are turned to the left or right, there is a failure of the head to turn in that direction within 0.5 second.

Oppenheim sign: for pyramidal tract disease; dorsal extension of the big toe is present when the medial side of the tibia is stroked in a downward direction.

paratonia: for diffuse cerebral dysfunction as in senility; the patient is asked to relax with the elbow passively flexed and extended. Intermittent opposition is abnormal.

Piotrowski sign: for organic disease of the central nervous system; percussion of tibialis muscle produces dorsiflexion and supination; **anticus sign** or **reflex.**

pronation sign: for central nervous disorders; there is a strong tendency for the forearm to pronate; **Strümpell sign.**

pseudo-Babinski sign: in poliomyelitis; the Babinski reflex is modified so only the big toe is extended, because all foot muscles except dorsiflexors of the big toe are paralyzed.

Queckenstedt sign: for detecting a block in the vertebral canal; compression of veins in the neck on one or both sides produces rapid rise in pressure of cerebrospinal fluid of a healthy person and quickly disappears. In a patient with blockage in vertebral canal, pressure of cerebrospinal fluid is little or not at all affected.

radialis sign: for nerve impairment; inability to close the fist without marked dorsal extension of the wrist; **Strümpell sign.**

Raimiste sign: for paretic condition; patient's hand and arm are held upright by examiner; a sound hand remains upright on being released, but a paretic hand flexes abruptly at the wrist.

Romberg test: for differentiation between peripheral and cerebellar ataxia; increase in clumsiness in movements and in width and uncertainty of gait when patient's eyes are closed indicate peripheral ataxia; no change indicates cerebellar type. (NOTE: Romberg sign is similar in testing but used for noting tabes dorsalis.)

Sarbó sign: for locomotor ataxia; analgesia of peroneal nerve is noted.

Schreiber maneuver: for patellar reflex testing; rubbing the inner side of the upper part of thigh enhances the reflex.

stairs sign: in locomotor ataxia; there is difficulty or failure of ability to descend stairs.

station test: for coordination disturbance; feet are planted firmly together; if the body sways, lack of coordination is indicated.

Strumpell confusion test: for dyskinesia as seen in cerebral palsy; the sitting patient is asked to flex hips while knee is bent. Ankle dorsiflexion will occur with dyskinesia.

tendon reflexes: for testing continuity of normal muscle to spinal cord to muscle reflex arc. Any tendon may be so tested, but the most common are the deep tendon reflexes (DTRs):

Achilles r.: ankle jerk.

quadriceps r.: patellar tendon or knee jerk.

biceps r.: elbow jerk.

triceps r.: elbow jerk.

mental r.: jaw jerk or reflex.

Thomas sign: for cord lesions; pinching of the trapezius muscle causes goose bumps above the level of the cord lesion.

tibialis sign: for spastic paralysis of the lower limb; there is dorsiflexion of the foot when the thigh is drawn toward the body; **tibial phenomenon.**

Tinel sign: for noting a partial lesion or beginning regeneration of a nerve; tingling sensation of the distal end of a limb when percussion is made over the site of divided nerve as in carpal tunnel impingement on the median nerve of the hand; **formication sign, distal tingling on percussion (DTP) sign.**

Metabolic Tests

Chvostek sign: for determining low serum calcium leading to tetany; tapping the cheek near the facial nerves causes the muscles to twitch or go into spasm; **Chvostek test, Chvostek-Weiss sign, Weiss sign, Schultze-Chvostek sign.**

lead line: a blue line seen in the gums of a patient with lead poisoning; **Burton sign.**

Tensilon test: for myasthenia gravis; a chemical test for denoting muscle strength or weakness; injection of edrophonium chloride (Tensilon) will reverse the symptoms in patients whose muscle weakness is caused by myasthenia gravis.

Walker-Mureloch wrist sign: for Marfan syndrome; ability of patient to grasp opposite wrist with fingers and thumb such that the little finger overlaps with thumb due to narrow wrists and long digits characteristic of that condition.

wrinkle test: for sensory nerve loss; skin of part that is denervated will not wrinkle like normal skin on prolonged immersion.

General Observations

antecedent sign: any precursory indication of a malady.

artifact: a feature of a *test* that stimulates pathology or interference with the correct results of the test.

café-au-lait: flat, hyperpigmented areas of skin with rugged "coast of Maine" borders or smooth borders. The presence of four or more café-au-lait spots with "coast of Maine" borders is seen often in von Recklinghausen disease.

cogwheel phenomenon: jerky motions produced on testing a muscle's strength; the jerks are neither rhythmic nor equal and represent malingering or protection from pain; **cogwheel sign.**

commemorative sign: any sign of a previous disease.

dimple sign: for a variety of joint dislocations; in the shoulder, when there is an anterior dislocation, there is a dimple in the deltoid below the acromion; in a posterolateral dislocation of the knee where the medial femoral condyle buttonholes, the anteromedial capsule, the skin is furrowed.

Dupuytren sign: for determining sarcomatous bone; a crackling sensation on compression of that area is noted.

Gower sign: for progressive muscular dystrophy or congenital myopathy; the patient must use hands to press on leg and then thighs to stand up.

hemodynamic test: to determine the relationship of blood flow in normal as compared with diseased anatomic structures.

Hueter sign: for indication of fracture; absence of the transmission of osseous vibration in fractures as heard by a stethoscope, where the fibrous material is interposed between the fragments.

Langer line: the normal tension lines of skin commonly used to define direction of scar, as to how the scar runs with or across those lines.

Meryon sign: for muscular dystrophy; lifting child up by underarms the child will slide through due to shoulder muscle weakness.

objective sign: one that can be seen, heard, measured, or felt by the diagnostician to confirm or deny an ongoing symptom; **physical sign.**

quadriceps test: for hyperthyroidism or debilitating condition; while standing, the patient is asked to hold leg up and straight out; a disease is present if patient cannot maintain this position for 1 minute.

Raynaud phenomenon: pallor or blueness of fingers, toes, or nose brought about by exposure to cold and less commonly by other stresses.

somatic sign: any sign presented by trunk or limbs rather than sensory apparatus.

succinylcholine test: for differentiation of muscle power loss due to nerve injury or tendon rupture; injection of succinylcholine will produce contractions lasting several minutes when there is denervation.

thumb-to-forearm test: an index of generalized joint laxity; the examiner places the tip of the thumb on the forearm while flexing the wrist.

Gaits

A patient's walking pattern (gait) is very important in the evaluation of disorders, particularly those affecting the lower limbs. A limp is more apparent in the stance phase of walking. Of the various gait patterns, some have very specific characteristics, such as the following:

ambling gait: for observing a patient's gait, both upper and lower limbs on the same side advance at the same time.

antalgic gait: due to pain in the stance phase (while walking through on the foot), the time spent on the affected side is shortened compared with that on the normal side.

ataxic gait: usually due to cerebellar or cord disease, uncoordinated gait with legs lifted high and whole sole of foot strikes at once **(cerebellar gait)**.

circumduction gait: typically with spastic hemiplegia or cerebral palsy, lower limb is swung forward in a circumduction manner.

Fick angle: a measure of toe in and toe out during normal gait; the angle formed by the axis of the foot and the direction of the gait.

foot slap gait: seen in peroneal nerve palsy and other source of ankle dorsiflexor weakness, forefoot comes down hard on the ground after heel strike; **drop foot gait, equine gait.**

gluteus maximus gait: due to weak or nonfunctioning hip extensor muscles, the patient thrusts the thorax posteriorly to maintain hip extension **(gluteal gait)**.

gluteus medius gait (abductor lurch): due to weak or nonfunctioning hip abductor muscles, the patient lurches toward the weak side to place the center of gravity over the hip; **gluteal lurch.**

scissors gait: in paraplegia or spastic diplegia, thighs cross on ambulation due to overpowering hip adductors. Often the hips are internally rotated with knees and ankles flexed.

shuffling gait: seen in Parkinson disease, walking with feet barely leaving the ground and with short steps.

slap foot (drop foot) gait: due to weak or nonfunctioning ankle dorsiflexor muscles, the foot slaps down after heel strike.

spastic gait: variety of gaits associated with central nervous system disease in which patient walks with abrupt uncoordinated motion.

Trendelenburg gait: lateral bending of trunk when in stance. This can reflect hip disease with pain, muscle weakness of abductors, or lumbar nerve insufficiency.

WOMAC: specific scales designed at the Western Ontario and MacMasters Universities for hip, knee, and other disorders.

Scales and Ratings

To have a reproducible presentation of the preoperative and postoperative condition of certain joints, various scales and rating systems have been developed. The scales and ratings are usually based on pain and the degree of functional impairment.

American Shoulder and Elbow Surgeons system: a five-point grading system for level of pain and four-point system for lowest to highest level of function in activities of daily living, work, and sports.

Charnley hip scale: for evaluating hip disease and postoperative results; scale uses pain, range of motion, and function for scoring.

Frankel neurological assessment: for spinal cord injury.

complete (A): no motor power below the level of the lesion.

sensory (B): no motor power but some sensation below the level of the lesion.

motor useless (C): some motor power below the level of the lesion, but of no functional use to the patient.

motor useful (D): motor power of functional use below the level of the lesion; the patient is able to walk with or without aids.

recovery (E): full motor power, normal sensation, and no sphincter disturbance, although reflexes may be abnormal.

Harris hip scale: 100-point scale with 40 points for function and 60 points for pain in the hip.

Iowa hip scale: for evaluating hip disease and postoperative results; scale uses pain, range of motion, and function for scoring.

Knee Society clinical rating system: the Knee Society presented this rating system as a uniform system for research. It uses pain and physical examination for a maximum of 100 points. Function is scored by walking and use of stairs for a maximum total of 100 points.

Lynholm knee-scoring scale: knee scale incorporating pain, swelling, function, and stability.

Marshall knee-scoring scale: knee scale including symptoms, function, and examination references.

Mazur ankle rating: grading system for the ankle using pain and function as a basis for the rating.

Merle d'Aubigne and Postel hip scale: for evaluating hip disease and postoperative result; scale uses pain, range of motion, and function for scoring.

total hip arthroplasty outcome evaluation*: designed by the American Academy of Orthopaedic Surgeons for universal definition of outcome of total hip arthroplasty. Includes function, satisfaction, physical examination, complications, and radiographic examination. This form also takes into account preoperative factors.

Other Physical Examinations

The portions of a physical examination that are not described as a test, sign, or maneuver include tests for ranges of motion, muscle strength and sensation, and sensory examinations. These tests are found in Chapter 12 and Appendix B.

---

*Liang MH, et al: The total hip arthroplasty form of the American Academy of Orthopaedic Surgeons, *J Bone Joint Surg Am* 73:639-645, 1991.

Laboratory Evaluations

5

Laboratory medicine, or clinical pathology as it is also called, is the field of science and medicine that tests and examines tissue samples from the human body significant to the diagnosis, prognosis, and treatment of diseases. The studies and tests are made in the areas of biochemistry, bacteriology, hematology, histology, cytology, and serology and are performed by physicians and lab technicians.

This chapter discusses the examination of blood and its components, synovial fluid, and urine. The first section deals with those tests commonly performed as part of the routine evaluation of outpatients or preoperative patients. The next section discusses the laboratory findings of specific diseases as related to orthopaedics, taking into account that some generalized diseases result in orthopaedic problems. The definitions are designed to be comprehensive. According to accreditation and regulation, normal ranges of laboratory values must be reported with each laboratory result.

Because normal values are dependent on the geographic area, patient population, test methodology, and laboratory standardization, such values are not considered useful when published in textbooks because they are likely to be misleading. Therefore, normal values have been deleted and the initial statement or sentence in either section should be an adequate overview for those not concerned with the complete nature of the study.

Care must be exercised when using laboratory terminology, decimal points, significant figures in laboratory data, and other specific information. Forms are provided for most tests requested. Laboratory results should never be given over the telephone except in emergency situations. Requests may be emergency (stat), urgent, or routine.

A blood test may examine the quantity and type of cells, the level of chemicals in the serum, and (rarely) the chemical composition of the blood cell. For each laboratory test, the definition states what portion of blood is tested. For example, if it is a test on both cells and fluid of the blood, the phrase "whole blood" is used. The preferred unit of volume is the liter (L).

The third and final section gives a list of laboratory abbreviations and annotation of units.

Routine Evaluations

Complete Blood Count (CBC)

The CBC is a series of whole blood tests to determine the quantity and other characteristics of blood cells. Some physicians prefer only a hemoglobin, hematocrit, and white count. Most laboratories use automated instruments to provide all the parameters as a part of a standard report, and a limited study such as an "H&H" is not cost-effective. The comprehensive CBC may include the following tests.

Hgb (Hb, hemoglobin): the iron-carrying protein in the blood. Normal values depend on age and gender (g/dl).

Hct, PCV (hematocrit, packed cell volume): the proportion of the red cells in whole blood expressed as a percentage.

H&H (hematocrit and hemoglobin): determination of hematocrit and hemoglobin levels only.

RBC (red blood count): the number of red cells per unit volume of whole blood (million cells/μl) (# cells × 10^{12}/L).

MCV (mean corpuscular volume): average volume of a red cell. May not be reliable if red cells are abnormal (i.e., sickle cell disease) (fl).

MCH (mean corpuscular hemoglobin): the average amount of hemoglobin in each red cell (pg).

MCHC (mean corpuscular hemoglobin concentration): the average concentration of hemoglobin in the red cells (g Hb/dl red cells).

WBC (white blood count): number of white blood cells per unit volume of whole blood (thousand cells/μl) (× 10^9/L).

> **differential WBC (diff):** percentage of different white cell types: neutrophils (segmented [mature] and/or precursors [immature]), lymphocytes, monocytes, eosinophils, basophils, and occasionally other forms. With present laboratory technology, the differential count is usually performed automatically and may not indicate the maturity of the neutrophils. In the unusual cases in which segmented neutrophils must be distinguished from more immature forms, the test may be performed by microscopic examination of the stained blood smear (× 10^9/L).

platelets (Plt): a blood test measuring the number of platelets (thrombocytes) per volume of whole blood. Platelet counts are routinely done by automated instruments. Platelets play an important role in hemostasis (× 10^9/L).

bone marrow biopsy: laboratory test performed on bone marrow from a medullary cavity, such as the posterior iliac crest, to determine, by microscopic examination, the adequacy and morphology of hematopoietic cells.

Basic Chemistry Profiles

Many hospitals offer groups of chemistry tests (called profiles or panels) because these tests are frequently ordered together (e.g., serum electrolytes, hepatitis panel, renal panel). The basic components of these panels are listed here.

albumin: serum concentration of the major osmotically active component of blood. May be decreased in acute or chronic inflammation, liver disease, severe burns, or fever (mg/dl).

ALP (serum alkaline phosphatase): enzyme present in bone, liver, and other organs. Marked elevation over adult normal values may be seen in healthy adolescents (U/dl, U/L).

ALT (alanine aminotransferase): enzyme present in several organs but generally used to assess liver disease (U/L); **SGPT.**

AST (aspartate aminotransferase): enzyme present in many organs, particularly muscle and liver. Increased values may indicate damage to the organ (U/L); **SGOT.**

BUN (blood urea nitrogen): a metabolic waste product usually cleared by the kidney. When increased, may indicate kidney disease (mg/dl).

Ca, P: calcium and phosphorus (the latter as phosphate), in general, constitute the two main bone ions. The blood levels of these two ions do not necessarily denote bone problems (mg/dl).

cholesterol: a steroid-based compound that has been associated with predisposition to coronary artery disease. The level of cholesterol is dependent on both genetic and dietary factors. Cholesterol is usually bound to a carrier lipoprotein, which comes in two primary densities: high and low. High-density lipoprotein (HDL) cholesterol appears to vary inversely with coronary artery disease—the higher the level, the lower the disease frequency. On the other hand, low-density lipoprotein (LDL) cholesterol appears to vary directly with coronary artery disease (mg/dl).

Cr (creatinine): a metabolic byproduct usually cleared by the kidney. Increased levels may indicate kidney disease (mg/dl).

gamma GT (gamma-glutamyltransferase, gamma-glutamyltranspeptidase, GGTP): serum enzyme that is frequently increased in liver disease caused by obstruction of the bile duct(s) (U/L).

LDH (lactate dehydrogenase): enzyme present in many organs. Increased values may indicate liver disease, red blood cell destruction within blood vessels, or recent heart attack (within 24-36 hours) (U/L).

total bilirubin: metabolic byproduct of liver metabolism of hemoglobin. Usually an indicator of liver function (mg/dl).

total serum protein: concentration of all proteins in the serum (g/dl).

UA (uric acid): metabolic byproduct usually elevated in cases of chronic gout. Elevated levels of uric acid are not necessarily correlated with acute attacks of gout (mg/dl).

Urinalysis (UA; Routine and Microscopic [R&M])

The routine urinalysis includes a notation of the color turbidity (appearance), specific gravity (density with respect to that of water—tells how concentrated the urine is), pH (acidity or alkalinity), and the presence or absence of glucose, protein, bilirubin, ketone bodies, urobilinogen, and occult blood. A microscopic examination may be done on the urinary sediment, and the material seen may be described as white cells, red cells, epithelial cells, and a variety of crystals and casts (microscopic debris usually from diseased kidneys). The quantity of cells and crystals is expressed in the number of observed objects per high-power field (HPF) of the microscope, whereas the quantity of casts is expressed in the number of observed objects per low-power field (LPF).

General Blood and Serum Tests

The general orthopaedic and related laboratory examinations and results found in this section are grouped according to similar disease processes, such as arthritis, infection, metabolic disturbances, and hematologic disorders, and also for assessment of spinal fluid and liver function.

However, these categories are not used as unit headings because the tests are often used to study a variety of problems, depending on the clinical circumstance. The orthopaedic laboratory work-up may include any or all of the following.

acid phosphatase (AcP): a serum assay test for acid phosphatase activity. Elevations are usually associated with disease of the prostate, particularly cancer. *Prostate-specific antigen (PSA)* may be increased in prostatic disease, particularly in prostatic cancer. High PSA values (> 20 ng/ml) have been shown to correlate with metastatic disease. The % free PSA also correlates with disease. In general, lower % free PSA correlates with higher risk of disease. Greater than 30% free PSA has a lower probability of prostate cancer. Serial PSA levels are of value in following patients with prostate cancer after surgery or radiation (ng/ml).

activated partial thromboplastin time (APTT, PTT): a test that measures the clotting factors in the *in*trinsic coagulation system. It is the test of choice in monitoring patients receiving heparin to retard blood clotting.

alanine aminotransferase (ALT): an enzyme present in several organs but generally used to assess liver disease (U/L).

ALP (alkaline phosphatase, alk PO4 tase): test to determine the level of this enzyme. The most common sources of high values are rapid growth or fracture healing. In any growth spurt the value may be as high as three times normal. Other bone disorders causing an increase in alkaline phosphatase include Paget disease, primary bone tumors, some metastatic diseases, and osteomalacia. Because elevations in alkaline phosphatase can result from liver disorders, two additional tests may be performed: (1) heating the enzyme will destroy it if it comes from the liver and (2) abnormally high values of serum gamma glutamyltranspeptidase (gamma GT) and alanine aminotransferase (ALT) indicate liver disease. Isoenzymes of alkaline phosphatase can be measured by indicating the organ of origin (U/L).

anti-double-stranded (native) DNA: test for antibodies against the genetic chemical information in the cell. High values are highly suggestive of systemic lupus erythematosus (IU/ml).

antinuclear antibody (ANA): an immunologic screening test that reveals the presence of serum antibodies against cellular nuclear material (DNA);

usually reported as positive or negative. Elevations of ANA, especially when accompanied by the "peripheral rim" pattern of fluorescence, are associated with lupus erythematosus.

ASO (antistreptolysin O) titer: this test is done mostly on children with joint complaints who are suspected of having rheumatic fever. The most meaningful finding for this test is an increase in the values over a period of a week. Values greater than 100 IU/ml in children and greater than 200 IU/ml in adults are associated with strep throat infection.

blood gases: a measurement of the amount of oxygen (O_2) and carbon dioxide (CO_2) in the blood. The oxygen is usually presented with a percent saturation value, which is normally above 90%. The pH (acidity) of the blood is simultaneously determined.

C-reactive protein (CRP): a plasma protein not affected by the presence of circulating hormones or anti-inflammatory drugs. Good indicator of inflammation and/or trauma. Correlates well with ESR (see later), but elevations appear and disappear before changes in ESR (mg/L or µg/L).

creatine kinase (CK; creatine phosphokinase [CPK]): an enzyme contained in many organs, principally skeletal muscle, heart muscle, and brain. In muscle disorders, particularly muscular dystrophy, it is elevated. In cases of suspected acute myocardial infarction, isoenzyme determinations help distinguish the organ of origin of the elevated enzyme level (U/L).

creatinine: byproduct of metabolism that is cleared by the kidney. A 2-hour *creatinine clearance (Ccr)* indicates how effectively the kidney is functioning as a blood filter (mg/dl).

erythrocyte sedimentation rate (sed. rate, sedimentation rate, ESR):

modified Westergren method: test performed on anticoagulated whole blood to determine the speed of settling of cells in 1 hour. Three stages of sedimentation occur: initial aggregation and rouleaux formation, quick settling, and packing. The test is nonspecific, similar to determination of temperature or pulse, and a normal value is perfectly consistent with many disease states. An increased sedimentation rate may indicate certain conditions, particularly inflammation. Therefore, this test is often used in evaluating bone and joint infections and other inflammatory diseases (mm/hr).

FBS (fasting blood sugar): test done to detect diabetes. Blood sample must be obtained at least 12 hours after the last meal. In the past, a *glucose tolerance test (GTT)* was a 2- to 5-hour study of both the blood and urine obtained from a patient who had taken 75 g of sugar after fasting. The most efficient GTT is a fasting and 2-hour postprandial (after eating) blood glucose. If these values are sufficiently abnormal according to the expected values for that particular laboratory, diabetes mellitus can be diagnosed.

Three different sets of criteria are available for interpreting the plasma glucose levels in the GTT. These include the National Diabetes Data Group (NDDG), the World Health Organization (WHO) criteria, and age-related expected values for glucose criteria. Those values are available on request from your laboratory. There is usually little value in performing a 3- to 5-hour GTT (mg/dl).

hemoglobin electrophoresis: a test to determine types of red cell hemoglobin. Abnormalities are present in sickle cell disease, thalassemia, and other red cell disorders. The results of this test are reported as normal or described by the specific abnormality.

HLA-B27: an antigen on the surface of cells frequently present in patients with ankylosing spondylitis.

INR (international normalized ratio): ratio of value of patient's prothrombin time to the mean of normal raised to the power of the international standard index.

prothrombin time (pro time, PT): a test that measures the clotting factors in the *ex*trinsic coagulation system, commonly done to monitor patients taking blood thinners as warfarin sodium (Coumadin).

reticulocyte count: a blood cell test to determine the erythropoietic activity, thereby helping in the classification of anemia. When observed under the microscope, only 1 of 100 red cells will normally take up a stain, indicating it is less than 24 hours old. Finding an increased number of reticulocytes means probable increased red blood cell production, usually in response to anemia. However, the percentage of reticulocytes is relative to the total red cell count, so that mathematical correction of the percent reticulocytes is necessary for proper interpretation. Some centers have moved to reporting *absolute* reticulocyte counts (reference range, 25,000-75,000 cells/μl or 25-75 × 10^9/L).

rheumatoid factor (RF): a serologic test to determine the presence of certain antibodies frequently seen in autoimmune diseases. The antibodies may be detected by several methods; some are more sensitive than others. The individual laboratory will interpret the importance of positive, negative, or numeric results.

salicylates: a test can be done on the blood to determine the specific levels of salicylates or on the urine as a screening test for the presence of aspirin. This can be done to follow the treatment of arthritis or in the event of an accidental overdose. Salicylate is also present in oil of wintergreen, which some people use topically for relief of muscle pain, so elevated levels do not always indicate aspirin therapy or overdose (μg/ml).

serum lead: in cases of lead poisoning, the serum can be tested for that element specifically. Because lead is a heavy metal, a heavy metal screening test is frequently used to determine the presence of lead poisoning. Elevated lead levels can also be indirectly tested for by measuring the free red cell protoporphyrin or zinc protoporphyrin levels (μg/dl).

serum protein electrophoresis (SPE, SPEP): a test to determine the presence and amount of particular types of serum proteins; used to detect multiple myeloma—a malignancy of the cells that produces immunoglobulin (Ig). A report of a high immunoglobulin or monoclonal pattern may indicate myeloma. An *immunoelectrophoresis* is a similar test reporting the concentrations of various immunoglobulins (IgG, IgA, and IgM) in the serum.

T3 (triiodothyronine), T4 (thyroxine), and TSH (thyroid-stimulating hormone): measures of the levels of thyroid active hormones and the pituitary hormone controlling thyroid function. There are various methods for determining these levels to help recognize hyperthyroidism and hypothyroidism.

A caution in interpreting such values should be made in chronically ill patients (ng/dl, μg/dl, μU/ml).

troponin: screen for evidence of myocardial infarction.

Serum and Urine Tests for Metabolic Disease

The following tests, as well as some urine excretion tests, are done to assess bone metabolism (i.e., bone formation and resorption). These tests are used most often for diagnosing and following therapeutic response in patients with osteoporosis, Paget's disease, hyperparathyroidism, and other metabolic bone diseases. In Paget disease, patients can have either evidence of decreased bone formation or increased bone resorption. These studies are often ordered by an endocrinologist but have interest to the orthopaedist.

Serum Tests for General Bone Turnover Markers

calcidiol (25[OH]D): measurement of 25(OH)D, a liver metabolite of vitamin D, in the serum is a good index for determining vitamin D deficiency and intoxication and aids in diagnosis of patients with metabolic bone diseases. It is measured by radioimmunoassay or competition binding protein assay (ng/ml).

calcitonin: serum calcitonin is most frequently used for the diagnosis and management of medullary thyroid carcinoma. It is measured by either radioimmunoassay or the concentration technique (pg/ml).

calcitriol 1,25(OH)2D: measurement of 1,25(OH)2D is used in the management of hypocalcemic and hypercalcemic disorders; specifically, the following bone diseases: parathyroid gland disorders, renal failure, sarcoidosis, and for therapeutic management of treatment. It is measured by radioreceptor assay (pg/ml).

parathyroid hormone (PTH): measured in serum for the evaluation and differentiation of disorders of calcium metabolism. Intact PTH is measured by either immunoradiometric or immunochemiluminescent assay (pg/dl, pmol/L).

serum calcium (Ca): measures serum calcium concentration. Serum calcium levels are increased in hyperparathyroidism, while there is a concurrent decrease in serum phosphorus (PO_4). The phosphorus determination in parathyroid disease is dependent on renal function. Determination of calcium and phosphorus levels is commonly done as a screening measure. Many diseases affect the blood levels of these two chemicals (mg/dl).

Serum Tests for Bone Formation

bone specific alkaline phosphatase (BAP, BSAP): determined by alkaline phosphatase isoenzyme electrophoresis; can be a useful marker for the rate of bone formation. It is usually elevated in Paget disease, and its determination can help in monitoring Paget disease patients being treated with antiresorptive therapy (U/L, IU/L).

osteocalcin or "bone Gla protein" (OC, ON, BGP): a serum marker for assessment of bone formation; most abundant noncollagenous protein in bone. The method of the test is radioimmunoassay or immunoradiometric assay (ng/ml).

procollagen propeptide: serum marker of osteoblastic activity measured in two chemical forms: the **carboxyterminal propeptide (c-PCP, PICP)** and the **aminoterminal propeptide (N-PCP).**

Serum Test for Bone Resorption

tartrate-resistant acid phosphatase (TRAP): a serum test to measure bone resorption and to determine the metabolic activity of osteoclasts; specific acid phosphatase seen from active metabolic osteoclastic activity.

Urine Chemical Tests

Some minerals and other chemicals measured in blood are also measured in urine. These include calcium, phosphorus, creatinine, and uric acid. The following are indicators of bone resorption, with the exception of the mucopolysaccharides, which are an index of proteoglycan metabolic abnormalities.

hydroxyproline (HYP): urine test that measures the degradation products of bone matrix; total fasting urinary hydroxyproline-creatinine ratio is used traditionally as a marker of bone resorption. It is markedly increased in Paget's disease. It is used to monitor treatment with antiresorptive drugs.

mucopolysaccharides: test done on the urine to determine the excretion of abnormal amounts of specific mucopolysaccharides that are seen in diseases causing dwarfism, gargoylism, mental retardation, and other congenital problems.

pyridinoline collagen cross-links (PYD) and pyridinium collagen cross-links (PYD): these two names refer to the same urine tests used to measure cross-linked fragments of collagen that result from bone degradation.

C-telopeptide (cross-links, C-tx): enzyme-linked immunosorbent assay is used to measure Type I collagen degradation products in urine as a bone resorption marker. It is reported as cross-links NMOL/mmol creatinine. It is used for research applications such as to monitor effectiveness of different antiresorptive therapies.

N-telopeptide (NTx): quantitative measure of excretion of cross-linked N-telopeptides of Type I collagen (NTx) is done by enzyme-linked immunosorbent assay (ELISA) as a resorption marker. NTx is reported as bone collagen equivalents/creatinine. Measurement of NTx is intended for use in predicting skeletal response to hormonal antiresorptive therapy in postmenopausal women and therapeutic monitoring of other antiresorptive therapies (ng/ml).

free pyridinium cross-links: for bone resorption; these are the cross-links of Type I collagen, which constitutes 90% of the organic bone matrix. **Pyridinoline (PYD)** and **deoxypyridinoline (Dpd, DPYD)** are excreted in the urine and not affected by diet. Deoxypyridinoline (Dpd) is more specific for bone metabolism. It is a useful marker to monitor therapies for metabolic bone diseases.

Bacteriologic Studies

acid-fast bacillus (AFB): refers to the bright red appearance of mycobacteria when stained by a special technique and observed under a microscope. A more efficient method involving fluorescence microscopy is presently used.

anaerobic culture: bacterial culture grown in the absence of oxygen (obligate anaerobes) or minimal free oxygen (facultative anaerobes). Certain organisms require this environment for growth in contrast to the standard aerobic cultures grown in the presence of normal oxygen. Anaerobic bacteria, like their aerobic counterparts, can be pathogenic or nonpathogenic.

C&S (culture and sensitivity): bacteria from a wound, urine, blood, joint fluid, throat, or any other source are grown in tubes or on plates. The bacteria are identified by combinations of biochemical reactions that they can or cannot carry out. The results of bacterial cultures are usually listed by individual organism along with its antimicrobial sensitivity.

typical bacterial species reports: the following bacterial species are frequently encountered in laboratory studies; they are listed for spelling purposes, without definitions. The terms "common flora" and "normal flora" denote the presence of normal, nonpathogenic bacteria.

Acinetobacter baumannii
Escherichia coli (E. coli)
Klebsiella pneumoniae
Mycobacterium avium
Mycobacterium marinum
Mycobacterium tuberculosis
Neisseria gonorrhoeae (cause of gonorrhea)
Pseudomonas aeruginosa
Salmonella organisms
Staphylococcus aureus (Staph. aureus)
Streptococcus organisms

Common fungal organisms are:
Actinomyces
Aspergillus
Blastomyces
Candida
Coccidioides
Cryptococcus
Histoplasma

colony count (CC): the placement of a known amount of urine on culture media; the report is usually given in number of bacterial colonies per milliliter of urine.

fluorescent treponemal antibody (FTA): a highly specific treponemal serologic test for syphilis; usually interpreted as positive or negative. Nontreponemal screening tests commonly used are the VDRL (Venereal Disease Research Laboratories) and RPR (rapid plasma reagin). These are essentially the same test, with VDRL used on cerebrospinal fluid (CSF) and RPR used on serum.

Gram stain: a general stain used on microscopic slide specimens to aid in seeing various organisms and estimating their numbers. Depending on their color after the processing, they will be described as gram positive or gram negative. This aids in the initial selection of antibiotics that are likely to be useful. Also, white blood cells should be noted in sputum and wound specimens to indicate whether one is dealing with colonization (if white cells are not present) or actual infection (if they are).

polymerase chain reaction (PCR): used as a rapid identification for microorganisms of DNA, bacteria, human virus, anthrax, and in bioterrorism.

Other Special Studies

cerebrospinal fluid (CSF): a study that includes the following:

protein: normally 45 mg/dl.

glucose: normally two thirds that of the serum glucose; decreased in bacterial infections.

white blood cells: normally 0 to $3/mm^3$; when an increased number of cells are present, they are divided into polys and lymphs.

culture: some fluid is placed on a growth medium to see if any organisms are present; occasionally, a slide is made from a smear of the fluid and a Gram stain done directly to determine the presence of bacteria.

bacterial antigen assay: used predominantly on pediatric population for rapid screening of bacterial surface antigens.

TABLE 5-1 Classification of Synovial Effusions*

			Routine Laboratory Examination			
Gross Examination	Normal	Noninflammatory (Group I)	Inflammatory (Group II)	Septic (Group III)	Crystal (Group IV)	Hemorrhagic (Group IV)
WBC (mm³)	<200	200–2000	2000–75,000	Often > 100,000	2000–75,000	50–10,000
PMN leukocytes (%)	<25	<25	>50 often	>75	>50 often	>50
Crystals present	No	No	No	No	Yes	No
Glucose (am fasting)	Nearly equal to blood	Nearly equal to blood	<50 mg% lower than blood	> 50 mg% lower than blood	>50 mg% lower than blood	Nearly equal to blood

Adapted from Schumacher HR: Synovial fluid analysis and synovial biopsy. In Kelley WN, Harris ED, Ruddy S, Sledge CB, editors: Textbook of rheumatology, ed 3, Philadelphia, 1989, WB Saunders.
PMN, Polymorphonuclear; WBC, white blood cell.
*In septic arthritis, the leukocyte count is almost always greater than 50,000 cells/μl. Occasionally, however, a patient with gout, pseudogout, or rheumatoid arthritis may have counts in this range. Noninflammatory synovial findings reveal a white count of up to 5000 with less than 30% polymorphonuclear leukocytes. In inflammatory synovitis, a 2000 to 200,000 white count be anticipated with greater than 50% polys. In infectious or septic arthritis, greater than 90% polymorphonuclear leukocytes can be expected. In crystal-induced arthritis, the synovial cell count can be 500 to 200,000 with less than 90% polymorphonuclear leukocytes. In hemorrhagic arthritis, 50 to 10,000 white cells may be present, but fewer than 50% are polymorphonuclear leukocytes.

cryptococcus latex antigen test: a rapid latex agglutination test for the qualitative and semi-quantitative detection of the capsular polysaccharide antigens of *Cryptococcus neoformans.*

flow cytometry: for evaluation of tumors. A stream of single-file tumor cells is passed by the path of a laser that is able to measure the relative amounts of DNA. This may help in the relative grading of the tumor cells. Also, after staining with certain antibodies, which have been linked to fluorescent chemicals, lymphocytes from patients with the acquired immunodeficiency syndrome (AIDS) can be counted by flow cytometry to determine the concentration of helper T lymphocytes—an indication of response to therapy.

synovial fluid evaluation (Table 5-1): evaluation of synovial fluid for the type and quantity of cells in the fluid. The normal white count of synovial fluid is considered to be less than 200 cells/μl or mm³. The leukocyte count is performed in a standard hemocytometer.

Gram stains are routinely performed for the detection of infectious arthritis, and, under certain circumstances, bacterial, fungal, and mycobacterial cultures are done. Viscosity may be useful; inflammation is associated with decreased viscosity. If crystals are seen, **polarized light microscopy** may be used to distinguish the two types of crystal-induced arthritis, gout and pseudogout, allowing the distinction between uric acid crystals seen in gout and calcium pyrophosphate crystals in pseudogout.

Blood Bank Procedures and Products*

Procedures and Terms

autologous donor: a patient who donates his or her own blood that is labeled and tagged specifically for use by the same patient. Donations typically occur once a week during the weeks prior to surgery; however, the final unit must be collected more than 72 hours prior to the anticipated surgery or transfusion. There is controversy regarding the use of autologous blood. Many feel it is a safer product because the donor and patient are one and the same. However, risks associated with patient misidentification, and bacterial contamination of the blood products still exist. Patients who provide their own blood may also be more likely to require a blood transfusion due to lower presurgical hemoglobin and hematocrit levels caused by the autologous donations.

---

*Prepared by Corey Jenkins, MS, MT(ASCP) SBB, Blood Bank Officer, National Naval Medical Center, Bethesda, MD.

directed donor: blood from a certain donor targeted specifically for use by a particular patient. Blood products supplied are subject to the same testing requirements as allogeneic donors. Controversy exists as to the use of directed donors due to the "peer pressure" often felt by these donors to provide blood for a friend or family member when in reality these donors may not be the best choice for blood donation.

intraoperative autologous transfusion (IAT): the intraoperative recovery of red cells for reinfusion during the course of surgery. The efficiency of this system has been improved with a *hemodilution* technique.

irradiation: American Association of Blood Bank Standards state that cellular blood products should be irradiated prior to issue when the patient is at risk for developing transfusion associated graft versus host disease, when the donor is a blood relative of the recipient, or when the donor is selected for HLA compatibility. Irradiation is accomplished by delivering at least 25 Gy of irradiation to the center plane of the blood product. Radiation sources are usually cesium-137, cobalt-60, or x-ray.

leukocyte reduction: a process that removes a majority of the leukocytes in cellular blood products ($< 5.0 \times 10^6$ leukocytes/unit for random and single donor platelets). The process usually involves filtration either at the bedside, in the laboratory prior to issue, or shortly after collection (prestorage). Leukocyte reduced products are indicated for patients who experience repeated febrile reactions from blood transfusions and to prevent alloimmunization to human leukocyte antigen (HLA) antigens. Leukocyte reduced products have been shown to be as effective as cytomegalovirus (CMV)–negative products in preventing transmission of CMV.

maximum surgical blood order schedule (MSBOS): a preoperative blood ordering guideline established by many institutions based on past surgical blood use. The MSBOS provides a list of common surgical procedures along with the recommended blood use for each procedure (e.g., hip arthroplasty = T&C 2 units RBCs; ORIF ankle = T&S).

type and cross-match (T&C): the potential blood recipient's ABO and Rh type is determined through antigen/antibody testing. In addition, the recipient's serum/plasma is screened for unexpected antibodies. Compatible donor units are then selected based on the results of the recipient's blood type and antibody screen. Cells from segments attached to these units are then cross-matched against the recipient's serum to determine true compatibility. Some facilities perform a computer cross-match provided certain regulatory agency requirements are met.

type and screen (T&S): the potential blood recipient's ABO and Rh type is determined through antigen/antibody testing. In addition, the recipients' serum/plasma is screened for unexpected antibodies. Antibodies detected in the antibody screen are identified through additional testing. For patients with a positive antibody screen, many facilities will antigen type ABO/Rh compatible donor units to find products that are antigen negative for the corresponding antibody(s) in case red cell transfusions are needed.

Blood Products

whole blood: approximately 500 ml of blood. After 24 hours, platelets and granulocytes are not viable. The labile clotting factors (V and VIII) also decrease with prolonged storage. Whole blood is seldom used. Instead, component therapy is usually indicated, providing the patient with the specific component needed. Whole blood may be useful when oxygen carrying capacity and volume replacement are both required.

red blood cells (RBCs): RBCs are made by removing most of the plasma from whole blood. RBCs contain the same oxygen-carrying capacity as whole blood with less risk of volume overload. Depending on the anticoagulant solution used, RBCs can be stored at $1°–6°C$ for up to 42 days. One unit of RBCs is expected to increase the average adult hemoglobin by 1 g/dl or the hematocrit by 3%. RBCs can be leukocyte reduced, irradiated, and/or washed.

platelets: platelets can be prepared from whole blood via centrifugation and then pooled or collected from a single donor via apheresis. One single donor platelet is equivalent to approximately five or six random pooled platelets. Platelet transfusions are indicated in cases of thrombocytopenia and/or abnormal functioning platelets. One unit of apheresis platelets is expected to increase the platelet count by 30,000 to 60,000/µl in an average adult. Platelets are stored at room temperature with gentle agitation and expire 5 days after collection. Platelets can be leukoreduced and/or irradiated.

fresh frozen plasma (FFP): the plasma portion of whole blood is separated within 8 hours of collection, frozen, and stored at less than −18°C for up to 1 year. Once thawed, FFP is good for 24 hours and contains one unit of coagulation factor per ml of FFP.

thawed plasma: thawed plasma is FFP that has been thawed for more than 24 hours. This product is good for 4 additional days but has decreased amounts of the labile clotting factors (V and VIII).

cryoprecipitate (Cryo): cryo is the cold-insoluble portion of FFP that been prepared by thawing FFP at 1°-6°C, removing the plasma, and then refreezing the precipitated portion of the FFP, along with a small volume of plasma, for up to 1 year at less than −18°C. Cryo contains fibrinogen, factor VIII (VIII:C and VIII:vWF) and factor XIII. Each unit of Cryo contains at least 80 units of factor VIII and 150 mg of fibrinogen.

Blood Bank Immunology Tests

alloantibodies: circulating atypical antibodies that are the result of prior antigenic stimulation from previous transfusion of blood products, pregnancy, or some other event. The presence of these antibodies may cause a delay in locating compatible blood products.

anti-HCV: test performed on donor blood to detect the presence of the antibody to hepatitis C antigen. This is also necessary in preventing transmission of hepatitis to a blood recipient. Its presence is detectable in certain patients who currently have, or have previously had, clinical or subclinical hepatitis C. This test may be negative in patients with hepatitis A, hepatitis B, or hepatitis E. Positive results are confirmed with a RIBA Recombinant Immunoblot Assay test. HCV genotyping is done to identify genotypes responsive to medication.

anti-human immunodeficiency virus antibodies (anti-HIV): test for antibodies to the viruses causing autoimmune deficiency syndrome (AIDS)—human immunodeficiency virus 1 and 2 (HIV-1 and HIV-2). It is performed routinely on every donated unit of blood to prevent the transmission of this disease to blood recipients. In patients, it is used to detect those who are suspected of having AIDS, although a positive test (i.e., having the antibody) is not necessarily the same as having AIDS. The screening methodology for this antibody can give falsely positive results, so each positive must be confirmed by the *Western blot* technique.

direct Coombs test (direct anti-human globulin test [DAT]): performed on patient's red blood cells to detect the presence of antibodies or complement components attached to the red cells. The red cells with attached antibodies or complement components usually have a shortened life.

factor VIII and factor IX: blood coagulation factors that may be absent or substantially reduced in hemophilia A (factor VIII) or hemophilia B (factor IX). These factors and certain specially prepared blood products are available for replacement in acquired disorders of the labile coagulant system.

HB$_s$Ag: test performed on donor blood to detect the hepatitis B surface antigen. This is also necessary in preventing transmission of hepatitis to a blood recipient. Its presence is detectable in certain patients who currently have, or have previously had, clinical or subclinical hepatitis B. This test may be negative in patients with hepatitis A, hepatitis C, or hepatitis E.

human immunodeficiency virus-1 antigen (HIV-1 antigen): test for the actual HIV-1 virus itself. This test measures a specific molecular portion (antigen) of the virus and is used in addition to anti-HIV-1 for screening blood and blood products. Reported as positive or negative.

human immunodeficiency virus, viral load test (HIV, viral load): quantitative test for determining the actual number of HIV particles within a patient's blood. The test uses polymerase chain reactive methodology to detect and measure levels of HIV RNA. The test is used to determine when to initiate drug therapy and to monitor response to therapy.

immune serum globulins: various immunoglobulins produced from sensitized individuals whose serum contains these antibodies; used for disease prophylaxis or attenuation, for example, $Rh_o(D)$. Immune globulin is given to $RH_o(D)$-negative women to prevent the sensitization to the Rh antigen and the resulting potential for Rh hemolytic disease of the newborn.

indirect Coombs test (indirect anti-human globulin test): performed on patient's serum to detect abnormal circulating antibodies. Presence of these atypical antibodies may cause a transfusion reaction. If present in women of childbearing age, these antibodies may cause hemolytic disease of the newborn (erythroblastosis fetalis).

isoantibodies: circulating, naturally occurring antibodies, which are usually of the IgM classification of immunoglobulins. Group O individuals usually have isoantibodies A and B in their plasma, group AB usually have neither, group A usually have anti-B, and group B usually have anti-A.

Routine Physiologic Parameters

ECG (electrocardiogram): recorded measurement of the spontaneous electrical activity of the heart, using multiple leads to assess the heart from a variety of directions. This study is commonly obtained before surgery to give a baseline in the event of operative or postoperative complications, such as pulmonary embolus or cardiac arrest.

EEG (electroencephalogram): recorded measurement of the spontaneous electrical activity of the brain using multiple leads placed on the head and ears. This study is obtained to detect certain seizures and brain disorders and the lack of activity when there has been severe damage leading to brain death.

height and weight: taken into consideration in an orthopaedic work-up because many back problems are related to being overweight and the stress that is placed on the vertebrae.

vital signs: the easily measurable sustaining functions include temperature, pulse, respiration rate, and blood pressure. A fifth vital sign, pain, has been

added and is graded on a scale from 0 (no pain) to 10 (most severe pain imaginable). These vital signs have been and will continue to be the major index of a patient's general progress.

Laboratory Abbreviations

Blood Components and Clotting

CBC: complete blood count.

Hct: hematocrit.

Hgb, Hb: hemoglobin.

H&H: hemoglobin and hematocrit.

WBC: white blood cell count.

wbc: white blood cell.

diff: differential white blood cell count.

> *polys:* polymorphonuclear leukocytes.
>
> *segs:* segmented neutrophils.
>
> *nonsegs:* bands, stabs, metamyelocytes, myelocytes, promyelocytes, myeloblasts.
>
> *lymphs:* lymphocytes.
>
> *monos:* monocytes.
>
> *basos:* basophils, basophilic granulocytes.
>
> *eos:* eosinophils, eosinophilic granulocytes.
>
> *blasts:* extremely immature blood cells.

RBC: red blood cell count.

rbc: red blood cell.

MCV: mean corpuscular volume.

MCH: mean corpuscular hemoglobin.

MCHC: mean corpuscular hemoglobin concentration.

Plt: platelet (thrombocyte).

T&C: type and crossmatch.

T&S: type and screen.

Rh: rhesus factor ($Rh_o[D]$).

ABO: blood group system comprising A, B, AB, and O blood.

FFP: fresh frozen plasma.

IAT: intraoperative autologous transfusion.

MSBOS: maximum surgical blood order schedule.

ESR: erythrocyte sedimentation rate.

PTT: partial thromboplastin time; (activated) **APTT.**

PT: prothrombin time.

INR: international normalized ratio.

Serum Chemistries

Ca: calcium, serum calcium.

BAP, BSAP: bone specific alkaline phosphatase.
OC, BGP: osteocalcin or bone Gla protein.
PTH: parathyroid hormone.
TRAP: tartrate-resistant acid phosphatase.
1,25(OH)2D: calcitriol, 1,25OH Vitamin D.
25(OH)D: calcidiol, 25OH Vitamin D.
Na: sodium.
Cl: chloride.
K: potassium.
CO2: carbon dioxide (bicarbonate).
BUN: blood urea nitrogen.
FBS: fasting blood sugar.
GTT: glucose tolerance test.
PO$_4$: phosphorus, phosphate.
Chol: cholesterol.
HDL: high-density lipoprotein.
LDL: low-density lipoprotein.
VLDL: very low-density lipoprotein.
UA: urinalysis, uric acid.
Cr: creatinine.
Alb: albumin.
AcP: acid phosphatase.
PSA: prostate-specific antigen.
PAP: prostatic acid phosphatase.
ALP: alkaline phosphatase.
Alk Ø: alkaline phosphatase.
GGTP: gamma-glutamyltranspeptidase.
AST: aspartate aminotransferase (SGOT).
ALT: alanine aminotransferase (SGPT).
SGOT: serum glutamic oxaloacetic transaminase (obsolete).
SGPT: serum glutamic pyruvic transaminase (obsolete).
LDH: lactate dehydrogenase.
T. Bili: total bilirubin.
CRP: c-reactive protein.
CPK: creatine phosphokinase (same as CK).
CK: creatine kinase.
SPE, SPEP: serum protein electrophoresis.
Ig: immunoglobulin. There are five classes: IgA, IgD, IgE, IgG, and IgM.

Serology
DAT: direct anti-human globulin test.
HLF: human leukocyte antigen.
HIV: human immunodeficiency virus.

RF: rheumatoid factor assay.
ASO: anti-streptolysin O titer.
ANA: anti-nuclear antibody.
anti-DNA: anti-double-stranded (native) DNA antibody.
FTA (ABS): fluorescent treponemal antibody (absorbed).
VDRL: Venereal Disease Research Laboratory.
STS: serologic test for syphilis.
HbC: hepatitis C antigen.
HB$_s$Ag: hepatitis B surface antigen.
HB$_e$Ag: hepatitis B e antigen.
HB$_s$Ab: hepatitis B surface antibody.
HB$_c$Ab: hepatitis B core antibody.
HB$_e$Ab: hepatitis B e antibody.
Anti-HIV-1: anti-human immunodeficiency virus 1 antibody.
Anti-HIV-2: anti-human immunodeficiency virus 2 antibody.
ELISA: enzyme-linked immunosorbent assay.
EMIT: enzyme-multiplied immunoassay technique.

Urine
c-PCP, PICP: carboxyterminal propeptide.
C-Tx: cross-links: C-telopeptide.
DPYD, Dpd: deoxypyridinoline.
PYD: pyridinoline and pyridinium collagen cross-links.
HYP: hydroxyproline.
NTx: N-telopeptide.
PYD: pyridin*oline* collagen cross-links.
PYD: pyridin*ium* collagen cross-links.
UA: urinalysis.
R&M: routine and microscopic examinations.
Ccr: creatinine clearance.
pH: concentration of hydrogen ions; solution to measure acidity and alkalinity.
Glu: glucose.
Ace: acetone.
KB: ketone bodies.
Prot: protein.
BHB: beta-hydroxybutyrate.
s.g.: specific gravity.
spec grav: specific gravity.
spgr: specific gravity.
HPF: high-power field.
LPF: low-power field.

Other

PPD: purified protein derivative (tuberculosis skin test).
C&S: culture and sensitivity.
CC: colony count.
T_3: L-triiodothyronine.
T_4: L-tetraiodothyronine (thyroxine).
TSH: thyroid-stimulating hormone (also called thyrotropin).
EKG: electrocardiogram.
ECG: electrocardiogram.
AFB: acid-fast bacteria.
spec: specimen.
CSF: cerebrospinal fluid.

Annotation of Units

Weight

pg: picogram = 1/1,000,000,000,000 gram.
ng: nanogram = 1/1,000,000,000 gram.
μg: microgram = 1/1,000,000 gram.
mg: milligram = 1/1000 gram.
g: gram (454 gram = 1 pound).
kg: kilogram = 1000 gram = 2.2 pounds.

Volume

fl: femtoliter = 1/1,000,000,000,000,000 liter.
μl: microliter = 1/1,000,000 liter.
ml: milliliter = 1/1000 liter.
dl: deciliter = 1/10 liter.
L: liter = 0.943 quarts (1 quart = 1.06 liter).

Length

μm: micrometer = 1/1,000,000 meter.
μ: micron = micrometer (obsolete).
mm: millimeter = 1/1000 meter.
cm: centimeter = 1/100 meter (= 0.39 inch; 2.54 cm = 1 inch).
m: meter (= 39.37 inch).

Other

mEq: milliequivalent; 1/1000 equivalent weight.
Eq: equivalent; 6.023×10^{23} ionic charges.

Important Lab Notes

In an attempt to standardize the way medical (and other scientific) units are reported, Le Système Internationale d'Unités was developed. Among others, it makes the following specifications:

1. Omit periods in abbreviations (kg, mm, ml, mg).
2. Omit plurals (70 kg, not 70 kgs).
3. Avoid commas as a spacer in expressing large numbers. (In some countries, the comma is used as a decimal point.)
4. Compound prefixes should not be used (10^{-9} meter = nanometer, not millimicrometer [mμm]).
5. Omit the degree sign for the Kelvin temperature scale (310 K, not 310° K).
6. Multiples and submultiples are used in steps of 10^3 or 10^{-3} as follows:

Multiplier	Prefix	Abbreviation
10^3	kilo-	k
10^6	mega-	M
10^9	giga-	G
10^{12}	tera-	T
10^{-1}	deci-	d
10^{-2}	centi-	c
10^{-3}	milli-	m
10^{-6}	micro-	μ
10^{-9}	nano-	n
10^{-12}	pico-	p
10^{-15}	femto-	f
10^{-18}	atto-	a

7. Only one solidus (/) may be used when indicated "per" or a denominator: acceleration = velocity per second = m/s^2, not m/s/s.
8. When the compound unit is derived from the multiplication of two base units, a point (·) is used to so indicate. A unit of torque is the Newton-meter, written N·m not Nm.
9. Preferred spellings are meter not metre, liter not litre, kilogram not kilogramme.

Casts, Splints, Dressings, and Traction

This chapter defines the materials applied and prescribed by an orthopaedist or assigned individual in the direct care of patients with fractures, dislocations, and conditions of the musculoskeletal system. The types of cast immobilization materials are described, as are the traction devices and weights designed for hospital or home care. Some emergency stabilization devices are included at the end of the chapter.

The techniques of cast immobilization, splints, dressings, and traction devices are designed to provide an external means of support or protective covering while healing proceeds under optimal conditions. Casts are generally applied in fracture reduction and immobilization, but they are also helpful in the correction of pediatric deformities, dysplastic hip disease, scoliosis, and foot deformities such as club foot, with the goal being to maintain or obtain a correction of deformity, promote alignment following surgery, and give support to damaged soft tissues in the healing process of fractures, dislocations, and sprains.

Because the care of the orthopaedic patient is a team approach, orthopaedists in private or group practice and in hospital settings are assisted by qualified orthopaedic nurses and technologists who are also involved in patient care. The orthopaedic nurse may choose to work in a doctor's office or an outpatient clinic of a hospital or become directly involved with inpatient management by assuming diverse responsibilities for a plan of quality care from admission to discharge. This requires not only the specialized knowledge of orthopaedic nursing but also skills in

the use of traction equipment and appliances and the ability to manage patients with this armamentarium.

Depending on educational background, training, and hospital policies, qualified nurses and technologists "scrub in" on orthopaedic surgical procedures in the operating room, clinic, or physician's office.

The National Association of Orthopaedic Nurses (NAON), founded in 1980, is the professional organization that offers a certification program to orthopaedic nurses who wish to further develop their skills in the management and care of orthopaedic patients. The NAON provides support and educational opportunities through its sponsored activities to promote continued professional development.

There are numerous organizations that support orthopaedic technicians in professional growth. One is the National Board for Certification of Orthopaedic Technologists (NBCOT), founded in 1982, that offers a certifying examination and an ongoing program of education and training to promote skills in the practice of orthopaedic technology. In 1999, the American Society of Orthopaedic Professionals (ASOP), an Internet organization, was formed to include all allied professionals working within orthopaedics, such as the orthopaedic, radiologic, and surgical technicians; physician assistants; paramedics; emergency room technicians; and orthopaedic product representatives. Under this organization is the certified Orthopaedic Allied Professionals (OAP(C)) and the Registered Orthopaedic Technologists (ROT), a designation that will become recognized as the standard of orthopaedic knowledge required by allied professionals who are actively upgrading their skills.

With appropriate orders the technologist assists in setting up traction appliances, Circ-O-Lectric beds, and similar devices of care and has the shared responsibility of proper application of traction, weights, and equipment required for patient rehabilitation. Administrative tasks involve ordering supplies and equipment for the plaster rooms, examining rooms, wings, and clinics and conferring with medical suppliers on catalogue items and supplies.

The orthopaedic technologist, with training and practice, becomes skilled in the art and science of cast application and the many types needed for specific injuries and conditions. Under a physician's directions, technologists instruct patients on cast care and prevention of complications. In addition, they may assist patients in gait training (crutch-walking, ascending and descending stairs) and various home exercises after immobilization. Technologists also maintain and prepare the plaster room for specific procedures, as well as assume the clean-up duties that follow. In some orthopaedic offices, the technologist is skilled in basic orthopaedic radiographic techniques—skills that clearly enhance the team approach.

The orthopaedic specialty is so diversified that opportunities for continuing medical education for nurses and technologists are offered through the AAOS instructional courses across the country and within the specialty organizations of orthopaedics. Corporate-sponsored activities have also been instrumental in updating product designs and state-of-the-art equipment. Together, these groups seek to promote the highest standards of quality care in cooperation with orthopaedic surgeons and other members of the health care team.

The basic tools of the trade are as follows.

A **cast** is a circumferentially wrapped plaster of Paris-impregnated bandage or encasement applied to a portion of the body. Additional materials, such as fiberglass and plastics, are also used instead of plaster of Paris.

A **splint** is a rigid or semirigid, noncircumferential material used to reinforce a soft dressing or to provide additional support for or immobilization of the body part being treated. The splint may be made of plaster of Paris, metal, wood, plastic, or, in an emergency, newspapers or magazines.

A **dressing** involves those materials used to cover a wound or surgical incision, a fabric with or without accessory medications or self-adhesive properties.

A **bandage** is a nonrigid, usually cotton material that holds a dressing in place or acts as the dressing by itself. It may be applied to provide padding over a body prominence under a cast. An elastic bandage provides support for a joint or soft tissue to control swelling.

Traction devices are any adjustable external appliances used in early treatment of fractures that suspend or deliver pull to any given part of the body. Traction is also used for temporary treatment of specific spinal conditions.

Cast Materials

Casting materials have improved considerably over the years; however, plaster of Paris casts are still widely used and familiar to all practitioners. These rolled crinoline bandages are impregnated with gypsum powder (calcium salt) that, when exposed to water, crystallizes. The reaction then slows to a maturation process (hardening) that takes approximately 24 hours to dry. The heat felt by the patient is the crystallization process that takes place within the cast material. To fabricate and mold plaster of Paris bandages is considered an art, and the technician soon learns the numerous techniques of application.

Fiberglass and thermoplast casts have become a popular form of treatment. They are lightweight, are radiolucent, are easier to apply, can tolerate moisture, and harden within 5 minutes, allowing for immediate weight-bearing. This rolled type consists of fiberglass and resin, fiberglass and plastic polymer, and polyurethane that also crystallize on exposure to water. Most fiberglass casts are long-wearing.

cast cutter: electrical circular oscillating saw for splitting and/or removing a cast. Long-handled cast-cutting instruments are also designed to remove small plaster casts from children.

cast padding: soft cotton wrap or synthetic wrap-around material used with a plaster or fiberglass cast.

cotton roll: material made from cotton that can be rolled as a bandage and acts as a buffer between the skin and plaster material; **Webril.**

felt padding: thick felt or felt-like material added to the undersurface of a cast to relieve pressure on local areas of bony prominences or pressure areas; **Reston.**

fiberglass cast: lightweight fiberglass wrap material that is impregnated with resin or another substance that polymerizes when exposed to water.

moleskin: adhesive, thin, velvet-like material used to smooth edges of casts or to buffer areas of excessive skin wear.

plaster rolls: gauze roll impregnated with plaster of Paris, which, when dipped in warm water, can be applied, rolled smoothly, and molded, becoming hard within minutes.

sheet wadding: strong, cotton material that clings to part being applied and molded to contour of that part.

stockinet: cloth stocking roll used initially in cast applications; comes in many sizes; can be covered by padding followed by firm cast material. Bias-cut and tubular are two different varieties.

Cast Immobilization

Cast immobilization involves the following anatomic areas: upper and lower limbs, cervical to chest region, and chest to lower spine. The various types are described later.

Body Casts

A body cast is a circumferential cast enclosing the trunk of the body and may extend from the head or upper chest to the groin or thigh. This type of cast immobilization is used in treating disorders of the cervical, thoracic, and lumbar spine such as fractures and scoliosis, or it may be applied following some types of surgery on the spine. There are several types of body casts.

extension body c.: chest-groin cast in which the patient is positioned so that the trunk is extended backward; applied for specific fractures.

flexion body c.: chest-groin cast in which the patient is positioned so that the trunk is flexed forward; for treatment of painful lower back conditions.

halo c.: for cervical fractures; a thoracic to pelvic level cast incorporating the necessary extensions used to support the posts that are attached to a metal halo skeletally affixed to the head.

Minerva jacket: cast immobilization extending along the side and in back of the head and neck, chest to hip area, incorporating a plaster of Paris headband; for fractures of the neck and in certain scoliosis problems.

scoliosis c.: special modification of the body cast for preoperative and postoperative treatment of scoliosis (curvature of the spine). These casts have in large part been replaced by operative fixation and prefabricated braces. Modifications of this type are as follows:

> ***Cotrel c.:*** modified scoliosis cast applied following Cotrel traction.

> ***turnbuckle c.:*** special modification to allow changes in angle by use of turnbuckles on either side of the cast.

> ***Risser localizer:*** specialized body cast with localizer pressing over convex side of curve.

Spica Casts

A spica cast immobilizes an appendage by incorporating a part of the body proximal to that appendage. The most common spica casts are hip, thumb, and shoulder spicas. They are listed by anatomic region in the following sections.

Limb Casts
Upper Limb Casts

arm cylinder c.: long-arm cast with the elbow flexed and the wrist free.

Dehne c. (three-finger spica): cast incorporating the thumb with a separate extension incorporating the index and middle fingers; for fractures of the navicular.

drop out cast: for elbow contracture, a modification of the long-arm cast with posterior portion above elbow, cut out to allow arms extension due to gravity on forearm.

gauntlet c.: short cast extending from slightly above or proximal to the wrist to some point in the palm; usually has some outrigger to control one or more digits; for metacarpal and phalangeal fractures or dislocations.

hanging arm c.: long-arm cast that, through suspension from a sling around the neck, brings about traction of fracture fragments of the distal humerus.

long-arm c. (LAC): extends from the palm and wrist to the axilla, with the elbow at 90 degrees and the wrist at neutral, preventing movement at the elbow; for treatment of fractures of the forearm, elbow, and humerus.

> *cotton-loader position c.:* rarely used long-arm cast applied with the wrist in full pronation, flexion, and ulnar deviation; for distal radial fractures.

Munster c.: cast that comes above condyles to prevent pronation and supination but allows some flexion/ extension of the elbow; **supracondylar c.**

short-arm c. (SAC): any of a number of casts extending from the elbow to the palm or digits; commonly used for distal forearm and wrist fractures.

shoulder spica (airplane c.): cast that incorporates the upper torso and envelops a part or all of the limb in a position of abduction; for proximal humeral fractures.

thumb spica: short- or long-arm cast that incorporates the thumb; for treatment of navicular fractures (**navicula c., scaphoid c.**).

Lower Limb Casts

cylinder c.: cast from proximal thigh to just above the ankle; for injuries of the knee.

Delbert c.: a short-leg cast that is trimmed away from the anterior and posterior portions of the ankle and from the heel. This allows dorsiflexion and plantar flexion while maintaining lateral stability.

gel c.: semirigid paste cast, usually applied to the lower leg and foot for ankle injuries or swelling; **Unna boot.**

hip spica: cast incorporating the lower torso and extending to one or both lower limbs.

> *Batchelor plaster:* hip spica cast that holds the hip in internal rotation but allows motion in other planes; for dysplastic hip in an infant.

> *double hip spica:* cast incorporating both the lower torso and lower limbs, usually because of bilateral fractures of the hips, femur, and/or tibia. If only the thighs are incorporated leaving the knees and leg free, called a **panty c.**

> *1½ hip spica:* cast that incorporates the lower torso, the entire affected limb, and the opposite limb to just above the knee; for proximal femoral fractures and some pelvic fractures.

> *Petrie spica c. (broom-stick):* specially applied cast for abduction to assist in ambulation for Legg-Calvé-Perthes disease.

> *single hip spica:* cast incorporating the lower torso and entire position of only one leg; for femoral fractures.

long-leg c. (LLC): non-weight-bearing cast extending from the upper thigh to the toes; for fractures of the tibia and fibula or ligament injuries of the knee.

> *long-leg walking c. (LLWC):* a cast from the upper thigh to the toes, with a cast shoe or with an attached rubber sole device called a walker.

Quengle c.: for flexion contracture of the knee, a two-part cast hinged at the knee level, with the lower end of the cast ending at the ankle or foot, and the above-knee portion ending at the upper thigh.

short-leg c. (SLC): non-weight-bearing cast extending from just below the knee to the toes; for injuries of the lower limb, ankle, and foot.

> *short-leg walking c. (SLWC):* reinforced to accept a cast shoe or with an attached rubber walker; for ankle and foot injuries.

> *patellar tendon weight-bearing cast (PTB):* also known as a **Sarmiento cast;** for distal one third or lower tibial fractures, a short leg walking cast with special molding at the patellar tendon, condyles, and calf in order to reduce rotation and provide hydraulic forces on ambulation.

slipper c.: incorporating the foot up to the ankle; a rigid postoperative dressing following forefoot procedures.

toe spica: cast specifically designed to incorporate all of the great toe and a portion or all of the foot; usually after bunion surgery.

well-leg c.: casts applied to both lower limbs and then attached together; used in some rare instances for treatment of femoral fractures.

Other Cast-Related Terms

air cast: term use for a wide variety of items. Most commonly used for ankle stirrups, which have air bags on both sides. However, the term is often used for larger devices such as a high tide boot with air bladders.

ankle stirrup: for ankle sprains and some fractures; a hard plastic that covers the lateral and medial ankle and lower part of the leg, held in place with Velcro straps and has air bladders.

bivalve c.: cast that is split in half (shelled) by cuts made on opposite sides of the cast to release pressure or allow removal and reapplication of the cast such as would be needed for wound care and physical therapy treatments.

> **Boston bivalve:** cast split in half with a step cut rather than a straight line; most often done when the cast is going to be removed, often for physical therapy, and then reapplied.

> **univalve c.:** cast split on one side to relieve pressure.

cast boot: any of a variety of commercially available strap-on boots that can often serve the function of a short-leg cast. These devices may have free motion ankles and are called **CAM walkers.** Some of these commercially available boots have adjustable air-filled bags and are referred to as an air cast walker; **high tide walker, low tide walker, tibial gaiter.**

collar and cuff: sling with a soft portion wrapped around the neck and a cuff-like device wrapped around to support the distal forearm, sometimes with the additional support of a waist band; for humeral fractures.

corrective c.: made to correct a deformity by nonsurgical technique; commonly applied to clubfeet.

fenestrate: to cut an opening (window) in a dressing or cast to allow inspection of a part.

petaling edges: to eliminate abrasion from the edge of a cast, small vertical slits are made at the edges of the cast, and then the edges (petals) are folded out and held in place by adhesive tape, moleskin, or other material.

serial c.: any sequence of casts applied in the progressive correction of deformity.

wedge: circumferential cutting of the cast and reapplication of plaster over the same cast after a manipulation has been performed to change bone position.

> **closing wedge:** removal of a segment of plaster, with closing of that wedge by manipulation and reapplication of plaster.

> **opening wedge:** circular cut cast that is opened by manipulation and then covered with a new layer of plaster.

window: removal of a piece of cast, usually square or rectangular, to allow inspection of a wound or relieve pressure at a specific point. Also said to "fenestrate."

Devices Applied to Casts

abduction bar: to help maintain hip abduction; any bar placed between two long-leg casts.

cast brace: modifications of standard casts often applied to facilitate early motion. The cast brace is designed with normal physiology in mind while still protecting the fracture site; it is molded in the manner of prosthetic-type devices. In addition, it is usually hinged at the joints to allow some free motion of joints and to improve muscle recovery.

cast protectors: waterproof covers for a limb cast, allowing patient to shower or bathe.

cast shoe: for the most part replaces walking heels, a Velcro strap-on shoe to protect the bottom of the cast from weight bearing.

walker (walking heel): hard rubber wedge directly incorporated into the sole of a cast to allow walking or resting the leg.

Cast Complications

Generally, a neurovascular and neuromuscular examination is made before, during, and after cast immobilization. However, even with close attention to treatment, the following complications can occur.

burns: applying cast material with water temperature too warm, which, when added to the crystallization process that produces heat, can produce skin burns.

constrictive edema: disruption of normal venous drainage with resulting fluid accumulation in soft tissue and swelling distal to the point of constriction caused by circulatory impairment. Severe swelling may lead to neurovascular involvement to include compartment syndrome.

decubitus ulcer: an area of breakdown of skin and/or subcutaneous tissue as a result of unrelieved pressure on a bony prominence or portion of the body resting on a firm surface for a long time. The lesions are staged as follows:

Stage I: only the dermis is involved.

Stage II: dermis and subcutaneous fat are involved.

Stage III: ulcer involves some deep fascia or muscle; bone not uncovered.

Stage IV: bone is exposed.

dropfoot: when referring to a complication of cast treatment, applies to paralysis of the peroneal nerve resulting from pressure over the fibular head leading to inability to dorsiflex the ankle.

muscle atrophy: loss of muscle tissue due to protracted disuse secondary to joint immobilization.

pin tract infection: direct bacterial contamination of area where pins have been used for external traction or skeletal fixation; could potentially lead to osteomyelitis.

pressure sore: breakdown of skin and/or subcutaneous tissue because of direct pressure of displaced or bunched cotton padding under cast, creating pressure lasting usually in excess of 4 hours; often caused by patient inserting object in cast to reach an area that is itching from plaster dust in cast; **decubitus ulcer.**

superior mesenteric artery syndrome: disruption of circulation to the bowel, occurs after application of body cast, results in abdominal pain, diarrhea, and, if unrecognized, severe problems; **cast syndrome.**

Splints and Accessories

This section is restricted to those splints applied in the early treatment of injury or management of postoperative conditions and their accessories.

Splints

airplane s.: removable cast or prefabricated device used to hold the arm in abduction.

aluminum foam s.: straight, metallic foam, padded splint of various widths from ½ to 2 inches; can be used separately or in association with casts for hand and finger injuries.

baseball s.: prefabricated metallic splint applied to the volar forearm and hand; the palm portion of the splint positions the hand as if it were holding a baseball.

Bohler s.: for spiral phalangeal fractures of the fingers; a device designed to maintain proper position and continuous traction.

coaptation s.: two slabs of plaster that are placed on either side of the limb and held together by some outer dressing; for limb injuries.

dynamic s.: any splint device that incorporates springs, elastic bands, and other materials that produce a constant active force to help reduce a deformity or counteract deforming forces.

frog s.: aluminum foam splint for finger injuries; before application the splint has a frog-shaped appearance.

gutter s.: semicircular or U-shaped splint fashioned around the injured part, usually in metacarpal and phalangeal fractures of the ulnar side of the hand.

hairpin s.: spring-assisted splint to help gain extension in a finger injury affecting the joint.

half shell: usually refers to spica casts; the section of cast that remains after it has been bivalved and a portion removed.

laced splint: for ankle sprains, a laced canvas ankle and proximal foot wrap that is held in place by laces; **Swede-o.** Some have side pockets for insertion of more rigid plastic inserts.

long-arm s.: splint applied from the axilla to wrist or distal palm posteriorly; holds the elbow and wrist in any given position.

long-leg s.: splint extending from the thigh to the lower calf or distally to the toes.

night s.: any splint or similar device used only at night. Commonly refers to a volar splint for treatment of carpal tunnel syndrome and leg splints for ankle dorsiflexion.

pneumatic compression boot or sleeve: provides periodic compression to a limb to help prevent venous thrombosis and is often used on an uninjured limb. This is in contrast to the sequential type of pump used in lymphedema. The pneumatic sequential compression boot is another type used after knee replacement and is effective against deep vein thrombosis after lower limb surgery.

short-arm s.: splint extending from distal elbow to palm; used for nondisplaced fractures or after advanced fracture healing.

short-leg s.: splint extending from the upper calf to toes for initial immobilization.

sugar tong s.: long slab of plaster applied to the affected limb in the fashion of a sugar tong and held together with outer dressing; for wrist fractures and injuries to the shoulder, arm, and forearm; sugar tong cast.

universal gutter s.: wire mesh splint for lower extremity fractures.

Velcro s.: commercial name becoming generic referring to splints that have straps or surfaces that adhere to each other; these surfaces may be approximated and separated as many times as needed, and there is no loss of the original strength of the adhesion of the two surfaces; can be used for any part of the body.

Velpeau s.: for shoulder dislocation, humeral fracture, and other condition of the upper limb; soft dressing that surrounds the shoulder and arm with arm held close to chest and typically elbow flexed more that 90 degrees. Commercially available devices have an adjustable waist belt and shoulder immobilizer. **Sling and swathe, Velpeau dressing.**

volar s.: specifies a splint applied to the anterior forearm.

wraparound s.: various commercially available splints that can be wrapped around a limb but are easily removable for physical therapy or wound care.

Accessories

In the area of casts, splints, and dressings, the following important aids to patient management are provided.

canes: for a painful hip; the patient is instructed to hold cane in hand opposite affected hip to transmit load through cane at the same moment that weight-bearing takes place on affected extremity.

crutches: when a three-point gait is needed to relieve weight-bearing on affected side; used in fractures, sprains, and after surgery. A three-point gait is when both crutches are placed on the ground simultaneously with the affected limb, decreasing body weight from three to one.

spring-loaded crutches: new type of crutch assist that absorbs peak stress, reduces shock, and reduces fatigue in upper limbs. The down directed weight is borne by the crutches that have energy-storing ability on weight-bearing.

walkers: assistive lightweight metallic devices (usually four legged) that allow patient to apply weight-bearing bilaterally when there is instability in walking. New variations in these devices include the option for a pair or quartet of wheels, hand brakes, and baskets for carrying items.

Dressings

The term *dressing* may apply to any material used to cover a wound; however, when there is considerable swelling without a wound, a dressing is used to apply pressure.

General Types of Dressings

Adaptic d.: nonadhesive mesh dressing for the direct covering of wounds.

Betadine d.: any dressing that has been impregnated with povidone-iodine (Betadine) and then applied directly to the wound.

compression d.: any dressing intended to apply pressure to reduce or prevent swelling or bleeding.

dry d.: dressing that has not been impregnated with any solution.

figure eight d.: dressing applied in the shape of an 8, as is often done for clavicular fractures; commercially prefabricated dressings, referred to as **clavicle straps,** are available.

gauze d.: any dressing made of cheesecloth-type material, for example, Kling, Kerlix, 4 × 4.

iodoform d.: narrow gauze strip impregnated with an iodine compound; for the treatment of open wounds.

Kerlix d.: broad elastic gauze dressing often a part of a compression dressing.

Kling d.: narrow gauze elastic bandage for compression.

Koch-Mason d.: warm occlusive saline dressing placed over a limb with cellulitis.

occlusive d.: any dressing that protects a wound from outside contamination.

packing: describes that portion of a dressing that is placed inside an open wound.

pressure d.: dressing designed to apply pressure to a specific location.

protective d.: any dressing that protects a wound from trauma.

saline d.: any dressing impregnated with normal saline; for treatment of open wounds.

Telfa d.: sterile nonadherent dressing, often applied on fresh wounds or incisions.

transparent dressing: a class of transparent, occlusive dressings that are weatherproof and allow direct observation of the wound. Brand name terms include **Op Site** and **Tegaderm**.

vacuum assisted dressing (V.A.C.): commercially available dressing that is applied directly to an open wound. Vacuum pressure is felt to help speed wound healing.

wet-to-dry d.: dressing that is impregnated with normal saline and allowed to dry; used as a part of open wound treatment.

Xeroform d.: nonadherent mesh dressing applied to fresh wounds or incisions.

Other Dressing Materials

Ace bandage: nonadhesive, elastic material that is a direct compressive wrap or holds other dressings or splints in place. The trade name is now used generically.

adhesive tape: sticky nonpermeable tape used to secure local dressing.

bandage adhesive: sticky material applied to the skin to help in the application of various forms of tape; commonly used adhesive is *tincture of benzoin*.

pads: variety of bulky materials (rectangular or square) that cover large wounds; often referred to as ABD (abdominal) pads.

Specialized Dressings

Esmarch bandage: special rubber, rolled bandages used to expel blood from a limb before surgery; **Martin bandage.**

Gibney bandage: strips of adhesive tape applied in alternate directions about the ankle; for ligament and other injuries.

high Dye dressing: method of noncircumferential ankle taping designed to support the ankle after an inversion injury.

Kenny-Howard splint (A/C harness): for acromioclavicular separations, a sling that supports wrist and elbow with a counterforce strap to push the clavicle down and a chest strap to hold the device in place.

low Dye dressing: taping technique for plantar fasciitis.

Robert Jones bandage: layered bulk dressing applied to the lower limbs for a variety of injuries but specifically following knee surgery or injury; **Shands dressing.**

Shands d.: composed of two layers of cast padding and two layers of elastic bandage applied to the leg and foot; for ankle sprains and nondisplaced fractures of the metatarsals.

universal hand d.: for compression or extensive injuries involving the hand and fingers; a bulky, even-pressured hand dressing composed of cotton or gauze fluffs and wrapped with gauze or other circular dressing material, leaving the fingertips exposed. Over this dressing, a cock-up splint is applied to hold the wrist in 15-degree extension. Some of these dressings are incorporated into a stockinet sling for elevation.

Velpeau d.: bandage applied to the arm and torso such that the elbow is at the side in flexion and the hand is pressed against the upper chest.

Suspensions, Tractions, and Frames

Suspension, traction, and frames are adjustable appliances used with pulleys, bars, weights, and other supports in the treatment of fractures with casts or splints, for scoliosis, and in the care of patients before and after surgery. This method of treatment is offered to ensure proper alignment in healing and to provide suspension or deliver pull, directly or indirectly, to bone, muscle, skin, and fascia.

Many of the parts of various suspensions and traction devices are known by the originator's name. Devices are listed by placement, each with its component. New techniques and methods of traction can be found in suppliers' catalogs, but the user should find this section helpful in deciphering why such devices are used in the care of patients. The various types of traction equipment are defined, followed by some emergency stabilization equipment.

Suspension

Suspension is the means by which a limb or part is held suspended by some external device. Traction often accompanies the suspension.

balanced suspension (Fig. 6-1): suspension device that allows the patient to move the affected limb without changing the fracture position of that limb;

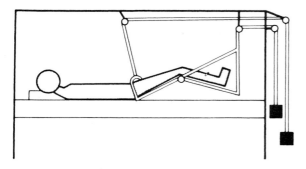

FIG 6-1 Balanced suspension. (Used with permission of Carol L. Willis.)

preferred for treatment of long bone injuries. There are two components:

Arizona universal leg support: for lower limb fracture; a balanced suspension device with adjustable anterior thigh pad and suspension support by two parallel lines from the knee and foot.

Thomas splint: originally designed to help splint fresh fractures; composed of a full ring around the thigh and two metal rods that extend down either side of the limb and are joined distally to the foot. The **half-ring Thomas splint** is the most commonly used. Most are adjustable for length and are thus called **adjustable Thomas splints.**

Pearson attachment: attached to a Thomas splint; consists of two metal rods joined distally, allowing flexion of the knee.

overhead suspension: the forearm is suspended overhead with the elbow bent; used in treatment of forearm and elbow fractures.

Traction (Fig. 6-2)

In general, traction is the pull on a limb or a part thereof. Skin traction (indirect traction) is applied by using a bandage to pull on the skin and fascia when light traction is required. Skeletal traction (direct traction), however, uses pins or wires inserted through bone and is attached to weights, pulleys, and ropes. This is applied when a longer period is needed in traction. External fixators can be attached to the traction apparatus to help in the healing process. Internal and external fixation techniques have mostly replaced the devices. The following devices are applied:

Barton tongs: skull tongs for cervical skeletal traction.

Böhler-Braun frame: metallic adjustable frame for support of the thigh and leg; for leg elevation and often in severe ankle fractures in which os calcis traction is applied.

Bryant t. (Fig. 6-3): for infants only; an overhead suspension of leg and thigh such that the knees are extended and the thighs flexed to 90 degrees.

Buck t.: originally designed as skin traction incorporating the entire lower limb but now describes skin

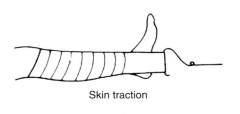

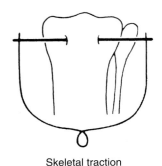

FIG 6-2 Traction. (Used with permission of Carol L. Willis.)

Skin traction

Skeletal traction

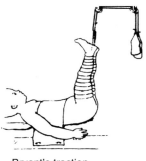

Bryant's traction

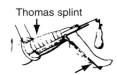

Thomas splint

Pearson attachment

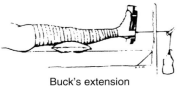

Buck's extension

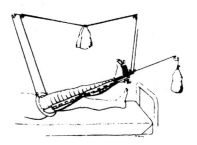

Suspended or floating traction

FIG 6-3 Various traction devices. (From the American Orthopaedic Association: *Manual of orthopaedic surgery*, ed 5, Chicago, 1979, American Orthopaedic Association.)

traction of the leg only; generally used in knee injuries but also a temporary measure applied in hip fractures.

cervical halter t.: a cloth, halter-like sling for traction of the neck; applied when patient is sitting or lying down, continuously or intermittently; head halter traction.

Charnley t.: for femoral fractures; wire or pin through proximal tibia, incorporated into a short-leg cast that has a flanged extension at heel to prevent leg rotation.

constant passive motion (CPM): for early knee or hip motion following injury or surgery; frames that support calf and thigh with electric motor-driven continuous flexion and extension of knee.

Cotrel t.: combination of a sling cervical and pelvic traction used in scoliosis before surgery or casting to help straighten the back.

Crutchfield tongs: type of cranial skeletal tongs used for traction of the cervical spine.

Dunlop t.: commonly used for elbow fractures; the arm is held suspended by skin or a combination of skin and skeletal traction, with a weight applied to the lower arm.

Gardner-Wells tongs: device for immobilization of cervical spine injuries in which two sharp metal pins are screwed into the superficial layer of the skull. They are then connected to hanging weights or other traction devices for stabilization of the spine. They may also be used for definitive treatment of spine injuries.

halo-femoral t.: bed-type traction using a ring-shaped device directly affixed to the bone of the skull in conjunction with femoral skeletal traction; used in scoliosis or injury distraction.

halo-pelvic t.: ambulatory-type traction for cervical spine injuries that uses a ring-shaped device directly affixed to the bone of the skull in conjunction with pelvic skeletal pins. These are interconnected to hold the spine rigid when the patient is ambulatory.

Kirschner wire (K-wire): skeletal t. in which small wires are placed across bone(s) so that a traction device can be placed externally; applied to some pediatric and hand fractures. May be threaded or nonthreaded.

Lyman-Smith t.: use of olecranon pin and overhead traction for supracondylar (elbow) fractures.

Neufeld roller t.: for fractured femur; a cast for the calf and thigh is hinged at the knee and suspended by a line to the anterior midthigh looped around a pulley and to a spring attached to the anterior midleg. The pulley for this loop is then supported by an overhead suspension with weight and a second pulley.

pelvic sling: sling encircling the hip and pelvic region in treatment of pelvic injuries; sling is suspended overhead.

pelvic t.: cloth, girdle-type device with traction directed at the foot of the bed; for lower back disorders such as herniated disks.

Quigley t.: for lateral malleolar and trimalleolar fractures; a stockinet is placed around the leg and ankle, with the ankle being suspended by the stockinet attached to an overhead frame.

Russell t.: skin traction on the lower limb from thigh to ankle or knee to ankle, attached to a sling that suspends the distal thigh. This may be done with a continuous rope and a number of pulleys (simple) or with two different weights, one for the leg and the other for thigh suspension portion (split). Russell traction is often used in the elderly as a temporizing treatment for fractured hips or in the very young in treatment of femoral fractures (**Hamilton-Russell**).

semi-Fowler position: semisitting position with knees flexed; used in lower back and lumbar disk disorders.

skeletal t.: any traction using a pin through the bone to deliver traction; for the tibia, femur, olecranon, os calcis, and metacarpal.

Steinmann pin: wide-diameter pin for heavy skeletal traction such as in the tibia or femur. May be threaded or nonthreaded.

traction bow: U-shaped piece of metal for placement into a K-wire or Steinmann pin in skeletal traction.

Vinke tongs: special set of skeletal traction tongs used for skull traction in neck injuries.

well-leg t.: bilateral casting of lower limbs with an interconnecting metal bar that allows traction on one leg to be supported by the other; for femoral fractures, it has the advantage that a patient can be moved out of bed.

90–90 t.: for some femur fractures and low back disorders; the patient is placed supine, with hips and knees flexed to 90 degrees such that the calf is suspended; for femoral fractures.

Frames

Frames are specialty units for an entire bed or additions to a bed.

Balkan f.: upright metal bars based at the corners of a bed and connected by overhead metal bars that hold suspension and traction pulleys.

Bradford f.: canvas bed suspended from rectangular poles with opening for the buttocks; split Bradford.

claw-type basic f.: traction frame that is attached to the bed by a claw-like clamp device.

Foster f.: special bed composed of two stretcher-like parts that, when connected, hold the patient sandwiched firmly between them, allowing the patient to be completely turned without injury to the spine; used for tuberculosis and spinal fractures or for patients with scoliosis following a Harrington instrumentation and fusion. A **Stryker frame** is a similarly constructed device.

Heffington f.: device that attaches to a standard operating table to allow prone position of a patient for lumbar spine surgery. The table end is dropped 90 degrees with patient's hips flexed over the edge and the patient further flexed to reverse the lumbar lordosis.

IV-type basic f.: traction frame that is attached to the bed by a device similar to that used for holding intravenous (IV) poles.

Jones abduction f.: a special frame used on standard beds to assist in gaining hip abduction in tuberculosis, acute arthritis, and other diseases of the hip.

Watson-Jones f.: for holding tibial fractures in surgery; a semicircular posterior-inferior thigh cuff with an attached adjustable extension that runs posterior to the leg with the knee in 90-degrees flexion. Tibial traction is maintained with a Steinmann pin.

Whitman f.: specially constructed frame to assist in gaining spine extension; may be used when cast application is necessary.

Emergency Stabilization

The use of emergency measures in trauma situations has saved many lives and limbs. There are many new types of equipment made for stabilization of the injured. These "temporary" measures of tamponade, fracture immobilization, and tissue protection are generally performed by trained emergency medical technicians (EMTs) and paramedics acting under the guidance of emergency room physicians. The various types of air splints should be used only by those trained in their use. The following emergency equipment may be used before the patient reaches the hospital.

air pressure splints: double-walled plastic tubes that, in the deflated state, are placed around the injured limb and are then inflated (by mouth) to bring about even pressure and immobilization.

Hare traction: metallic splint with multiple straps and a special distal traction device for use in transporting unstable lower-limb-injured patients.

inflatable splint: sometimes referred to as an **air splint,** it is a first-aid device used at the onset of injury; when blown up, this balloon-like splint provides good immobilization with even pressure. It is usually applied to the lower leg and foot, but other inflatable splints incorporate the entire arm or entire lower limb.

MAST (medical antishock trousers): pneumatic sleeve for immediate stabilization of lower limbs in cases of trauma. MAST encompasses lower limbs and abdomen to provide sufficient pressure to force blood to the central portion of the body. This provides some stabilization of shock and provides stability for pelvic, hip, and femoral fractures and aids in preventing further tissue damage. In addition to tamponading sites of bleeding, this device sometimes acts by increasing pulse and blood pressure. Its use is controversial, and it should be used carefully and briefly (if at all) to avoid prolonged muscle ischemia and MACS (MAST-associated compartment syndrome). MAST is inflated by a foot-operated pump.

Neal-Robertson litter: modified spine board for transporting trauma patients with spinal injuries to the emergency room.

posterior splint: for emergency immobilization; rigid devices used for initial stabilization of upper and lower limb fractures.

Sager traction splint: for femoral fractures; emergency traction splint with a unit that measures the force of traction at the ankle. For children and adults; this device maintains fracture position and alignment without excessive pressure around the ankle or sciatic nerve injury.

spinal board: rigid board with multiple slots for straps used for head and thoracolumbar restraints; designed to transport patients in a relatively immobile state.

For further information on emergency stabilization measures, refer to Crosby LA, Lewallen DG, editors: *Emergency care and transportation of the sick and injured,* ed 6, Rosemont, IL, 1997, American Academy of Orthopaedic Surgeons.

Prosthetics and Orthotics

Prosthetists and orthotists are allied health professionals who measure, design, fabricate, and fit prostheses (artificial limbs) and orthoses (braces).

Prosthetics is the science that deals with functional and/or cosmetic restoration of all or part of a missing limb, following the directive of a physician's prescription.

Orthotics is the science that deals with orthoses designed to provide external control, correction, and support for the patient in need for nonoperative management of musculoskeletal disorders. Service in this area is also provided on a prescription basis.

The words *prosthetics* and *orthotics* may be used as nouns to describe the body of knowledge each pertains to, as in the preceding two paragraphs. The devices themselves are called protheses and orthoses. When referring to a specific device, the words *prosthetic* and *orthotic* are adjectives needing an appropriate noun.

Specialists in these areas are certified by the American Board for Certification (ABC) and titled certified prosthetist (CP) and certified orthotist (CO). A certified prosthetist-orthotist (CPO) has demonstrated proficiency in both fields during examinations by the board. Supportive personnel are assistants and technicians, with varying responsibilities and duties.

This chapter was contributed in part by Wilton H. Bunch, MD, PhD, formerly Dean, College of Medicine, Professor, Department of Orthopaedic Surgery, University of South Florida, Tampa, Florida, retired; and Stephen Kramer, CPO, President, Universal Orthopedic Laboratories, Chicago, Illinois.

Many major institutions have ongoing prosthetic and orthotic clinics or conferences that meet as often as patient need requires. Members of the clinic team consist of a chief physician, physical and occupational therapists, a prosthetist, an orthotist, a rehabilitation nurse, and a social worker. The clinic team approach is oriented toward management of the total patient, so although the rationale for prescription of an appropriate prosthetic or orthotic system is a prerequisite, the complete rehabilitation program is the long-range goal and responsibility of the team. Factors such as vocational retraining, if necessary, financial considerations of various phases of management, the necessity and duration of physical or occupational therapy, and a possible need for psychological counseling are all taken into account. Perhaps most important, the patient must be made to feel comfortable in the clinical setting and be assured that the result will be as satisfactory as it is realistic and attainable.

The prosthetist or orthotist is responsible for assisting with the prescription regarding components, elements of design, definitive and proper fitting of the system, and follow-up and adjustments as indicated at future visits to the clinic.

If prosthetic and orthotic practitioners are to serve patients at the highest professional level, they must maintain a program of further education to remain informed of new techniques, components, and concepts. Such programs are available through the American Academy of Orthotists and Prosthetists (AAOP). Other groups are the American Orthotics and Prosthetics

Association (AOPA) and the Children's Amputee Prosthetic Program (CAPP).

Prostheses

Prosthetic systems, or artificial limbs, are designed to replace function and/or cosmesis of a missing body part. Internal prostheses are surgically implanted devices, such as the artificial hip, and are described in Chapter 8.

Upper Limb Prostheses

An upper limb prosthesis is any external system designed for the amputee from the partial hand level distally to the interscapulothoracic forequarter level proximally.

partial hand amputation: distal to or through one or more of the phalanges or metacarpals or resection at any level of the thumb. Restore function with cosmetic individual finger replacements with fillers and/or opposition-type posts. Slightly more proximal amputation sites necessitate cosmetic gloves and wired finger fillers and/or more intricately designed opposition posts to restore function.

wrist disarticulation (WD): amputation through the wrist joint. Correct with wrist disarticulation prosthesis designed to fit over the sometimes bulbous distal end of the residual limb, retaining as much pronation and supination as possible; trimmed anteriorly to allow maximum flexion; used with cable and figure eight harness control, flexible elbow hinges, wrist unit, and terminal device.

below-elbow (BE) amputation: proximal to wrist but distal to elbow joint. Correct with below-elbow prosthesis designed to fit the residual limb, retaining pronation and supination in the longer levels and allowing maximum flexion; used with cable and figure eight harness control, flexible or rigid elbow hinges, wrist unit, and terminal device. **Münster** or **Hepp-Kuhn** prosthetic sockets make the system applicable for short to very short below-elbow amputations; they are carefully fitted proximal to the epicondyles at the elbow to provide adequate suspension without the aid of additional devices; sometimes limit forearm flexion because of restriction of tissue at cubital fold; used with cable and figure nine harness control, wrist unit, and terminal device.

elbow disarticulation (ED): amputation through the elbow joint. Correct with elbow disarticulation prosthesis with socket encompassing the residual limb and trimmed proximally at the shoulder to allow good range of motion; used with cable and figure eight harness control, external elbow hinges with lock, wrist unit, and terminal device.

above-elbow (AE) amputation: proximal to elbow joint but distal to shoulder. Correct with above-elbow prosthesis with socket extending over the acromion to support axial loading and carefully fitted at axilla; used with cable and figure eight harness, internal locking elbow, forearm lift assist, wrist unit, and terminal device.

shoulder disarticulation (SD): amputation through the glenohumeral joint. Correct with shoulder disarticulation prosthesis with larger socket extending from the spine posteriorly to near the xiphoid process anteriorly and fitted closely at the neck; used with cable and modified chest strap-type harness, shoulder joint or bulkhead (spacer) to allow passive positioning in abduction and adduction, passive positioning, and flexion and extension, internal locking elbow, forearm lift assist, wrist unit, and terminal device.

interscapulothoracic forequarter amputation: through the midsection, including resection of the scapula. Correct with cosmetic shoulder cap to restore normal appearance for clothing or forequarter prosthesis with socket similar to that used for shoulder disarticulations but differing in that an extension is usually used going around and over the sound shoulder to provide additional suspension; used with cable, modified chest strap, and waist belt-type harnessing, excursion amplifier, shoulder joint similar to that used in shoulder disarticulations, internal locking elbow, forearm lift assist, wrist unit, and terminal device.

Upper Limb Prosthetic Components

The components of an upper limb prosthesis include any device that is a supportive or integral part of the prosthesis, including terminal devices.

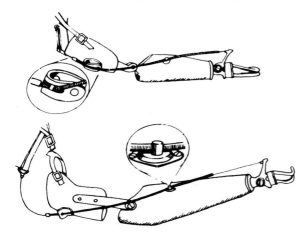

FIG 7-1 Control cable housing. (From *Below and Above Harness and Control System,* Evanston, IL, 1966, Northwestern University Prosthetic-Orthotic Center.)

Boston Digital Arm System: for electronically driven prosthetic elbow action.

Centri Electric hands: commercially available prehensile hands that include the CentriAB.

control cables: steel cable traveling inside housing to move and lock mechanical joints, for example, flexion and locking of the elbow joint; also provide prehension to the terminal device. The housing is sometimes lined with Teflon to reduce friction and thereby increase efficiency. Cable systems are generally lightweight, as for small children, with standard 1/8-inch or heavy-duty cable (e.g., Bowden single, dual, and triple control cables). Fig. 7-1 illustrates single control only.

elbow hinges: mechanical types of hinges to provide specific strength or allow controlled mobility. The following types are commonly used: single pivot providing mediolateral control, suspension polycentric, multiple action, sliding action step-up, and stump-activated locking. These are all designed to provide additional forearm flexion for the very short below-elbow amputee or the patient with flexion contracture.

electrical switch control: prosthesis for the patient with shoulder disarticulation or above-elbow or forequarter amputation; uses switches to control current from a battery that operates an electrical elbow and/or hand. The switches are placed in strategic positions within the harness system, and by opening these switches the patient is able to operate the electrical elbow and/or hand. This type of system is most feasible for patients with limited excursion from causes such as contractures, higher levels of amputation, or bilateral limbs, because each position in the switch is 1/16-inch excursion—considerably less than that required to operate the standard system.

excursion amplifier sleeve: pulley and cable system used to increase efficiency in patients with limited excursion; generally used in shoulder disarticulation and forequarter systems.

flexible hinges: hinges made of Dacron tape or metal spirals to provide suspension while allowing retention of available pronation and supination.

forearm lift assist: adjustable spring-loaded device attached to the elbow to provide initial forearm flexion; especially applicable for those with higher level amputations such as shorter above-elbow amputation and shoulder disarticulation.

Greifer prosthesis: electrically enhanced, strong-gripping hand component.

Hosmer NU-VA Synergistic Prehensor: an electric prehensor device that is not shaped like a hand and designed for strong prosthetic grasp.

Homer NY Electric Elbow: for electronically driven prosthetic elbow action.

Motion Control Hand: specific commercial brand of electronically driven prosthetic hand.

Motion Control Utah Arm: for electronically driven prosthetic elbow action.

myobock system: The *myo*electrical *b*uilding-bl*ock* system includes optimal cosmetic configuration, high-wearing comfort, functional value, and easier service.

myoelectric control: sophisticated prosthesis available for the patient with wrist disarticulation, below-elbow or above-elbow amputation: uses electrodes placed over the flexor and extensor muscle groups to pick up the milliamperes of electricity emitted by a muscle during contraction. This electrical stimulus is then used to operate a switch that controls a motor in a mechanical hand or other component. Prosthetic sockets are generally self-suspended, thereby eliminating the need for any harness.

nudge control: mechanical unit that can be pressed by the chin to lock or unlock one or more joints of the prosthesis; seen in forequarter systems.

Otto Bock Ergo Arm: various types of electronically driven prosthetic elbow action devices.

Otto Bock System: system of electric hands that include (DMC) **Dynamic Mode Control Plus Hand, Sensor Hand, Transcarpal Hand,** and **System Electric Hand.** Non-hand-like devices **System Electric Greifer.**

outside locking hinge: used on the elbow disarticulation system because of length of residual limb. Outside locking elbow and internal positive locking elbow hinges with multiple locking positions are used for above-elbow, shoulder disarticulation, and forequarter systems.

RSLSteeper Electric Elbow Lock: for electronically driven prosthetic elbow action.

RSLSteeper Electric Hand: commercially available electric prehensile grip hand that includes the **MultiControl Plus Electric Hand.**

shoulder harness, chest straps, and waist belts: an infinite variety of Dacron, cloth, and leather materials is used to fabricate these components, which provide suspension as well as control through their attachment to cables that operate locks for various joints and provide function for the terminal device. The figure eight ring harness is one of the most common and provides suspension and control of prosthesis. The figure nine harness supplies only control, as the Münster socket provides suspension (Fig. 7-2).

terminal devices: hooks or hands affixed to the wrist unit, affording function and/or cosmesis.

    hooks: lyre-shaped fingers that open in opposition to one another, achieved by forces exerted through the harness and cable systems, and close involuntarily by means of dynamic rubber bands or springs. Hooks are available in numerous sizes, generally in aluminium with plastisol covering for children, aluminium or stainless steel with neoprene lining, stainless steel with serrated inner surface such as the model 5X, and for heavy-duty tasks the 7 or 7LO types **(farmer's hook)**, designed to hold devices such as shovels or rakes. Although certain hooks differ, such as

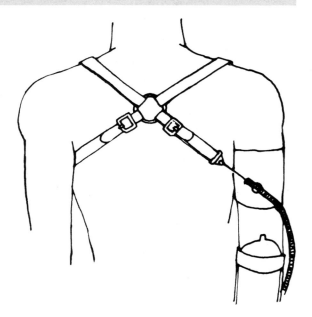

FIG 7-2 Cross point of harness connected by stainless steel ring. (From *Below and Above Elbow Harness and Control System,* Evanston, IL, 1966, Northwestern University Prosthetic-Orthotic Center.)

the Trautman Locktite and the APRL (Army Prosthetics Research Laboratory) types, most use rubber bands or springs to close, and prehension is directly proportional to the strength and number used. Other devices are Model 8x small adult, model 10 childrens, model 12P infants, mitts, and **N-Alber II** for task specific tool interchange.

    hands: there are a number of both functional and passive hands available. The mechanically functional hand provides prehension by means of springs attached to its internal parts; a cosmetic glove matched to the patient's skin color is applied externally. Passive hands, although nonfunctional, generally provide increased cosmesis. Some specific hands are **Dorrence** voluntary-opening, **Sierra** voluntary-opening hand, APRL voluntary-closing hand, soft voluntary-closing hand, Becker locking grip hand, and **CAPP** terminal device.

wrist flexion unit: allows prepositioning of terminal device closer to the midline of the body; generally used for the bilateral patient.

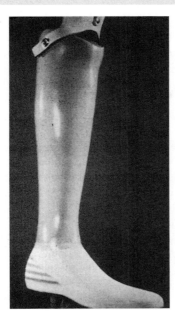

FIG 7-3 A patellar tendon-bearing (PTB) exoskeletal prosthesis with supracondylar cuff and solid ankle cushioned heel (SACH) foot.

wrist units: integral components at the distal end of the prosthesis that allow attachment, interchangeability, and pronation and supination of the terminal devices; types are standard constant friction and quick change; units are oval or round and available in different diameters.

Lower Limb Prostheses and Components (Fig. 7-3)

Lower limb prostheses are any external system designed for the amputee from the partial foot level distally to the hemipelvectomy level proximally. They are categorized as *exoskeletal* or *endoskeletal*. The exoskeletal prosthesis has a rigid outer shell that provides structural strength and cosmetic shape. The endoskeletal prosthesis has a tubular structure connecting the components and is covered by cosmetic foam. The primary components of the prosthesis are the socket, suspension system, foot, and knee unit.

Lisfranc: a disarticulation through the medial metatarsophalangeal joint or metatarsal-tarsal joints. Correct with extended steel shank in shoe to provide a place to push off and toe filler or foot plate with toe filler.

Chopart: distal to the ankle joint. Correct with distal weight-bearing socket with partial foot replacement.

Syme: through the ankle joint; results in a bulbous distal weight-bearing residual limb. Correct with a medial-opening or expandable-wall prosthesis, which facilitates application and removal. Weight-bearing is distributed between the distal end and the patellar tendon. The socket is self-suspending because of the reduced circumference above the distal limb.

transtibial: formerly called below knee (BK), it is proximal to the ankle but distal to the knee. Correct with patellar tendon-bearing (PTB) prosthesis, designed to bear weight through the patellar tendon, medial tibial flare, and other pressure tolerant areas; socket may be hard or have a soft liner. Suspension is with supracondylar cuff strap or without waist belt, sleeve, or suction. Self-suspending variations of the PTB prosthesis include the following:

joint and corset: for the patient with mediolateral instability of the knee, for a very short below-knee amputation, or for residual limb incapable of supporting total body weight because of conditions such as burns and skin adherent tissue. A typical prescription would be as follows: PTB type of socket, external mechanical knee joints, thigh corset, fork strap, waist belt, and prosthetic foot.

suction socket suspension: for below knee prosthesis, a new design of suspension that incorporates a valve or silicone liner and locks in position, or incorporates a sock with silicone ring. Differs from PTB type.

supracondylar (PTB-SC): PTB with supracondylar cuff incorporates higher medial and lateral walls that encompass the femoral condyles. A medial wedge, either movable or built into a soft liner, is placed firmly over the medial epicondyle.

supracondylar-suprapatellar (SC-SP): similar to supracondylar but also includes a high anterior wall that encompasses the patella. This provides increased suspension and limits hyperextension of the knee.

knee disarticulation (knee bearing, K/B): amputation through the knee joint. Correct with distal weight-bearing socket. The socket is self-suspending with either a medial opening or a soft liner to facilitate donning. A Silesian belt is worn as an auxiliary suspension. There is also a polycentric (four-bar linkage) knee unit and prosthetic foot. Still in use are end-bearing leather or plastic sockets with external hinges, fork straps, and waist belts.

stubbie: short lower limb prosthesis, typically for above knee amputations, designed to help with initial ambulation efforts in bilateral amputees.

transfemoral: formerly called above knee (AK), it is proximal to the knee joint but distal to the hip joint. Correct with quadrilateral or narrow medial-lateral ischial containment socket prosthesis.

>*CAD-CAM:* computer-assisted design/computer-assisted manufacturing refers to the contour of the socket and how it is modified. It is a hand-made computer-assisted method of providing a cosmetically accurate fit that can use any of the ischial containment sockets. Types are:

PTB	patellar tendon–bearing, with cuff suspension
PTBS	patellar tendon–bearing suspension
PTB-SC	patellar tendon–bearing supracondylar
PTB-SP	patellar tendon–bearing suprapatellar
SPC	suprapatellar cuff
PTS	patellar tendon socket

>*ischial containment sockets (narrow M/L= medial-lateral; CAT-CAM=contour adducted trochanteric, controlled alignment method):* an above-knee amputation socket design incorporating a narrow M/L shape, high lateral wall, and a slanted pocket for the ischium. Provides greater control of lateral forces during gait and a more even distribution of proximal weight-bearing areas.

>*quadrilateral ischial weight-bearing socket:* wooden or plastic socket designed with a shelf to transpose weight through the ischial tuberosity; suspension may be achieved by a hip joint with a pelvic band and control belt or with a suction socket with a mechanical knee and prosthetic foot.

hip disarticulation (HD): amputation at the hip level but with the ischial tuberosity intact. Correct with plastic socket designed to transpose weight through the ischial tuberosity and related gluteal musculature, mechanical hip and knee joints, and prosthetic foot.

hemipelvectomy: amputation at hip level with ablation of the ischial tuberosity. Correct with plastic socket designed to distribute weight using remaining musculature, rib margin, cosmetic socket build-up, mechanical hip and knee joints, and prosthetic foot.

Lower Limb Prosthetic Components

foot and ankle components: allow normal gait patterns.

>*C-Sprint running foot:* longitudinal bar spring that attaches directly to AK prosthesis pylon.

>*Cheetah running foot:* longitudinal bar spring that attaches directly to posterior.

>*dynamic response:* curve metal strip that brings about spring action to assist in toe-off.

>*energy storing feet:* incorporates a cushioned heel with a resilient toe lever that stores energy in stance phase and releases it at toe-off. Typically lighter than SACH foot. Varieties include **Seattle foot, Carbon Copy II and III foot, Quantum foot.**

>*flex foot (Springlight):* energy-storing foot for high activity levels. Top lever and pylon are one continuous carbon graphite spring, similar in appearance to a ski tip.

>*flexible keel:* designed to accommodate for variabilities such as small stones on the surface.

>*flex sprint foot:* for running; longitudinal bar spring that attaches directly to AK prosthesis pylon.

>*SACH foot: s*olid *a*nkle *c*ushioned *h*eel (wedge).

>*SAFE foot: s*tationary *a*ttachment *f*lexible *e*ndoskeletal.

>*single axis:* allows anteroposterior motion and controlled plantar flexion with dorsiflexion stop.

>*multiaxial:* allows plantar flexion and dorsiflexion, inversion and eversion. It is the traditional SACH foot with sides to flex. Types are **Greisinger** and **Endolite.**

Multi-flex foot: like the SACH foot but allows medial and lateral angulation.

knee components: designed to provide stability during early and middle stance phases and bend in late stance and swing phase, as well as in kneeling and sitting.

external: most common application in knee bearing; no controlled friction.

fluid controlled (hydraulic or pneumatic): provides swing phase control for a variable rate of gait, eliminating excessive heel rise and terminal impact. Varieties include **Dupaco, Dyneplex, Daw, Otto Bock, Mauch.**

four-bar linkage: a polycentric system that creates a moving center of rotation. Inherently very stable.

Henschke-Mauch S'n'S: hydraulic unit that provides stance as well as swing phase control; **Mauch S'n'S.**

hybrid knee: combined polycentric knee with pneumatic fluid-control cylinder component.

manual locking: knee automatically locks at full extension. Patient-controlled latch disengages lock for sitting.

Mauch S 'n' S: hydraulic swing phase with stance phase control.

Oklahoma cable system (OKC system): cable that harnesses hip flexion into extension control of artificial knee, allowing step-over-step running.

Otto Bock 3R55: a modular polycentric axis joint with hydraulic swing phase.

safety: weight-activated stance control. When knee is extended and weight-bearing, an adjustable braking mechanism is activated to resist flexion.

single axis: single point of rotation with constant friction to control swing phase.

below-knee suspension: used to support below-knee prostheses.

billet: connects supracondylar cuff to waist belt.

condylar cuff: mediolateral attachment to prosthesis with strap proximal to femoral condyles.

fork strap: anterolateral attachment to prosthesis connecting to waist belt.

suction: a silicone gel skin-tight liner worn directly over residual limb. Various devices are built into the liner that attach it directly to the prosthesis.

supracondylar cuff: tabs that attach mediolaterally to prosthesis with cuff strap going around knee proximally to femoral condyles.

waist belt: webbing wrapped circumferentially at pelvis with connection to billet or fork strap.

knee disarticulation suspension: fork strap and waist belt.

transfemoral suspension: used to support above-knee prostheses.

control belt: leather wrapped circumferentially at pelvis and attached to pelvic band.

hip joint: mechanical free-motion joint positioned anatomically on lateral wall of socket.

pelvic band: metal band contoured to pelvis and attached to upright of hip joint.

Silesian bandage or belt: webbing over hip on sound side with one lateral and two anterior socket attachments. Used in conjunction with a looser-fitting suction socket.

shoulder harness or suspenders: webbing straps traversing shoulders with roller and cord or various attachments to socket.

suction socket: worn against the skin with no intervening liners or socks.

hip disarticulation or hemipelvectomy suspension: webbing over shoulder on sound side with anteroposterior socket attachments.

Other Components, Materials, and Techniques

cast sock: used to take negative plaster impressions; sometimes used with or in place of stump socks; especially applicable for the new below-knee amputee during volume reduction of the residual limb.

check socket: a disposable clear plastic socket used to ensure integral fit before definitive fabrication.

distal pad: injection of Silastic or an equivalent foam into end of socket of below- or above-knee systems; provides total contact distally and reduces possibility of edema.

extension aid: to assist knee extension in the above-knee prosthesis.

Icelandic Roll-On Suction Socket (ICEROSS): suction-based elastic liner with tip that integrates with socket.

pylon: adjustable tubular section connecting socket and prosthetic foot (endoskeletal construction).

rigid dressing: plaster socket worn on residual limb to reduce volume.

rotator or torsion unit: component in the prosthesis designed to compensate for shear forces, thereby reducing torque and friction between the residual limb and interface of the socket.

sheath: nylon interface worn between residual limb and stump socks to reduce shear forces.

silicone gel socket insert: inner liner made of silicone gel designed to absorb shear forces. Often used for problem-fitting below-knee amputees. Also used for below-knee suction suspension.

sleeve: neoprene or latex sleeve worn over proximal portion of the prosthesis and extending onto the patient's thigh. Provides suction suspension.

socket: custom-designed receptacle into which the residual limb fits.

soft cosmetic cover: foam material covering endoskeletal components; shaped cosmetically.

soft socket insert: soft inner liner for PTB socket. Petite or silicone gel most common.

stockinette: tubular open-ended cotton or nylon material used to don suction socket, sometimes used with or in place of stump socks; especially applicable for the new above-knee amputee during volume reduction of the residual limb.

stump shrinker: elastic sleeve worn on residual limb to reduce volume.

stump sock: wool or cotton sock worn over residual limb to provide a cushion for friction between skin and socket interface. Available in various thicknesses called "plys."

total contact: intimacy between socket and residual limb, particularly at distal end, to control edema.

Specialized Systems

immediate postsurgical fitting (IPSF): procedure performed immediately after surgery; patient is fitted with plaster type of socket, adjustable pylon, and prosthetic foot. Advantages include early ambulation, more rapid stump maturity, and psychologic benefits.

intermediate (temporary): thermoplastic type of socket with adjustable pylon and prosthetic foot; intermediate phase of management used to expedite fitting, establish early ambulation, and reduce volume of residual limb prior to definitive fitting.

modular (endoskeletal): selectively applicable for below-knee or any level of proximal amputations; use socket according to prescription with adjustable pylon and foot and socket attachment plates; exterior surface is made of custom-shaped foam and covered with cosmetic material.

Orthoses

An orthosis is an externally applied system designed to provide control, correction, and support and check deformity. The brace can either resist or assist motion to control deformity, to unweight a body segment and reduce the load, and to provide corrective measures.

The Task Force on Standardization of Prosthetic-Orthotic Terminology of the Committee on Prosthetic-Orthotic Education (CPOE), National Research Council, and the American Orthotic and Prosthetic Association (AOPA) have been largely responsible for the implementation of the terminology generally in use today. In an effort to enhance communication between the prescribing physician and the orthotist, the following descriptive guideline has been adopted. The standardization is based on indicating those joints and regions that the orthosis is to encompass or control. The orthosis would control the named joint by allowing free, assisted, or resisted motion. Orthosis types are as follows:

AFO: ankle-foot.
AO: ankle.
BFO: balanced forearm.
CO: cervical.
CTLSO: cervicothoracolumbosacral.
CTO: cervicothoracic.
EO: elbow.
EWHO: elbow-wrist-hand.
FO: foot.
HKAFO: hip-knee-ankle-foot.
HdO: hand.
HpO: hip.
KAFO: knee-ankle-foot.

KO: knee.

LSO: lumbosacral.

PRO: passive prehension.

PTBO: patellar tendon bearing.

SEWHO: shoulder-elbow-wrist-hand.

SIO: sacroiliac.

SO: shoulder.

SOMI: sterno-occipital mandibular immobilizer.

TLSO: thoracolumbosacral.

TO: thoracic.

WAWHO: wrist-action, wrist-hand orthosis.

WDWHO: wrist-driven, wrist-hand orthosis.

WHO: wrist-hand.

Use of the foregoing terms leaves the materials, design, and components to the discretion of the orthotist unless otherwise indicated by prescription, as demonstrated in the following typical examples.

Prescription: AFO to provide dorsiflexion assist. (This simple prescription leaves orthotic management regarding materials for the system to be determined by the orthotist according to patient evaluation.)

Prescription: AFO to provide dorsiflexion assist; double uprights, Klenzac ankle, calf band, Velcro closure, and shoe attachments.

Prescription: AFO to provide dorsiflexion assist; thermoplastic fabrication.

As demonstrated this format provides the prescribing physician with various controls over the patient's management.*

Lower Limb Orthoses

Because all orthoses currently in use are too numerous to discuss, we confine our list to those most commonly prescribed.

Foot Orthoses

Denis-Browne bar: rarely used; consists of a rigid bar riveted or clamped to shoes at either end. The bar

*Those individuals in need of further information in the area of orthotics would benefit from American Academy of Orthopaedic Surgeons: *Atlas of orthotics, biomechanical principles and applications,* St Louis, 1975, Mosby.

provides hip abduction, with ratchet adjustments controlling rotation; generally prescribed for treatment of clubfoot, equinovarus, pes planus, or tibial torsion. The new system allows for more independent control and leg movement with infant able to crawl because of jointed bars.

Fillauer bar: clamp-on bar to place on feet to hold leg in internal or external rotation. Attaches to shoes by a clip-on device.

flexible o.: leather, foam, or equivalent, providing longitudinal arch and/or metatarsal support; orthosis is removable from shoe.

hallux valgus o.: designed for day and night use; reduces bunion pain by decreasing valgus deformity (pulls toe to midline of body).

rigid o.: carbon composite fiberglass, and stainless steel designed to provide arch support for pes planus or other related problem; orthosis is removable from shoe; *Whitman plate, Schaeffer type,* and modifications thereof.

UCB o.: (developed at the University of California, Berkeley) similar to the rigid type but fabricated of thermoplastic or thermoset resin.

Ankle Orthoses

Arizona brace: leather, canvas, or equivalent material provides substantial immobilization of the ankle to alleviate pain caused by motion.

elastic o.: provides minimal support; helps control swelling.

Ankle-Foot Orthoses

Charcot restraint orthotic walker (CROW): rigid orthotic with rocker bottom foot; inner aspect lined with foam with a double density custom insert for the foot portion.

double adjustable ankle joint (DAAJ, BiCAAL): ankle motion can be adjusted to lock for various flexion and dorsiflexion ranges of motion.

floor reaction orthosis: rear-entry plastic device that allows full plantar flexion but stops at 90 degrees and thus gives good push-off from the foot component that is in the wearer's shoe.

metal o.: fitted ¾-inch distal to head of fibula and is an integral part of the shoe; examples are single or double upright jointed ankle, free motion, limited motion, and dorsiflexion assist; used with calf band, buckle, or Velcro closure and stirrup with shoe attachments.

patellar tendon-bearing (PTB) o.: weight-bearing terminates just proximal to the patellar tendon and is fitted around the knee similar to the below-knee prosthetic socket; used with molded foot plate or ankle joints and stirrup with shoe attachments; designed to transmit body weight through the patellar tendon and medial femoral condyle to achieve controlled unloading of weight on the tibia and ankle-foot complex; anteroposteriorly sectioned proximally.

spring wire o.: medial and lateral spring wire uprights attached to calf band proximally and the shoe distally; designed to provide dynamic dorsiflexion assist.

thermoplastic o.: terminates at or near the apex of the gastrocnemius muscle proximally, with molded foot plate fitted into shoe distally; ambulatory, nocturnal, or combination of both; designed to control and correct specific problems of the foot-ankle complex.

Wheaton brace: for metatarsus adductus; a brace designed to help correct forefoot adductus in children while walking.

Knee Orthoses

dynamic o.: similar to static with the addition of external knee joints with or without locks to allow controlled motion.

elastic knee cage: elastic sleeve encompassing the knee; provides minimal support and stabilization. Variations are the following.

with medial and lateral contoured knee joints: similar, with the addition of joints providing some increased stabilization. Other options include medial and lateral condylar pads, adjustable anterior laces, and additional spiral control straps.

Swedish knee cage: metal and leather system allowing flexion but preventing hyperextension of the knee.

ligamentous control braces: commercially available custom-made braces designed to control special ligament deficiencies about the knee.

static o.: leather, thermoplastic, or equivalent; immobilizes knee in desired attitude of flexion or extension.

Knee-Ankle-Foot Orthoses

Legg-Perthes disease o.: the following are specialized systems designed for the treatment of Legg-Perthes disease.

A-frame o.: when this system is used with an extra-long bar to treat developmental dysplasia of the hips (DDH), an A-frame orthosis is sometimes incorporated to control the tendency for genu valgum (knock-knee), which may occur because of extensive hip abduction. The A-frame consists of a metal component fitted medially from the bar up both legs with calf and thigh bands and valgus control pads.

Atlanta brace: a hip abduction brace that allows ambulation without crutch assistance.

Newington o.: bilateral and similar in design to the Toronto o.; differs in that flat bars are used, and no joints are incorporated.

Salter sling: sling device that holds hip in abduction and internal rotation while the knee is held flexed.

Toronto o.: bilateral proximal high cuffs, center tubular column with universal multiaxial joints at base, outriggers with angled mounting blocks at either end to receive attachment of shoes; ambulatory system providing hip abduction and controlled rotation.

trilateral o. (Tachdjian): plastic quadrilateral socket fitted at the level of the ischium similar to that of the above-knee prosthetic socket; single upright with shoe attachments; designed to provide weight unloading, hip abduction, and internal rotation.

metal o.: fitted approximately 1½ inches inferior to the perineum and is an integral part of the shoe; single or double upright jointed ankle, free motion, limited motion, or dorsiflexion assist calf, distal and proximal thigh bands, buckle or Velcro closures, jointed knee with or without lock, stirrup, and shoe attachments.

reciprocating gait o. (RGO): provides support to lower limbs and trunk for paraplegic patients; an orthosis that has a gear box or cable system attached to bilateral knee-ankle-foot o. and lumbosacral o., allowing a lower-level paraplegic to have a reciprocating gait.

thermoplastic o.: similar to the standard orthosis but fabricated of plastic material with molded foot plate fitted into shoe distally. This type of system has found increased acceptance because of its lighter weight and total contact fitting capabilities.

Other specialized knee-ankle-foot orthoses include those designed to manage patients with neuromuscular conditions and fractures using plaster or plastic with polycentric knee joints and other sophisticated components.

Hip Orthoses

The following are specialized hip orthoses designed for treatment of developmental dysplasia of the hips (DDH) or Legg-Perthes disease.

abduction o. (Ilfeld splint): bilateral thigh cuffs of plastic, covered metal, or equivalent with adjustable bar to provide hip abduction and waist belt and/or thoracic section to maintain positioning. Some systems have additional adjustment for hip flexion control.

Barlow (Malmo) splint: for dysplastic hips in infants; an abduction, flexion, external rotation splint.

Ferrari o.: for spina bifida patient with high level weakness; a combined thoracic lumbar orthosis with full lower limb orthosis.

Louisiana State University reciprocating gait o.: for spinal cord injuries; a cable driven brace that allows for support while the flexion of one lower limb drives extension of the other.

Pavlik harness: a series of straps passing over the shoulders both anteriorly and posteriorly, transversing the chest and leading to the feet where they are attached to plastic booties; designed to provide hip flexion, abduction, and external rotation.

pillow (Frejka) o.: soft splint fitted between the thighs to provide hip abduction with straps over the shoulders to maintain positioning.

Scottish Rite o.: pelvic band, bilateral free-motion hip joints, proximal thigh cuffs, adjustable tubular spreader bar with universal joints at inferior medial aspect of cuffs; ambulatory system providing hip abduction for treatment of Legg-Perthes disease.

Steeper advanced reciprocating gait o.: for spinal cord injuries; a cable driven brace that allows for support while the flexion of one lower limb drives extension of the other.

thermoplastic/metal o.: custom-fabricated system designed to maintain the hips in degrees of flexion, abduction, and rotation, as prescribed.

Von Rosen o.: for developmental dysplasia of the hip in infants and very young children; passive motion restraint in abduction and flexion.

Hip-Knee-Ankle-Foot Orthoses

The following orthoses, except for the RGO and standing frame type, are described in a unilateral application, although they can be fitted bilaterally.

cable twister o.: rarely used; pelvic belt, free-motion hip and ankle joint, plastic-covered cable, connecting joints, stirrup, and shoe attachments; calf and thigh bands are incorporated as necessary; adjustable at hip and ankle to provide dynamic control of hip rotation and tibial torsion.

elastic twister o.: rarely used; pelvic belt with elastic straps wrapped around leg and attached to a hook in the shoe; provides dynamic control of hip rotation and tibial torsion.

parapodium: for paraplegia; allow for support in sitting, standing, and transfer from sitting to standing.

standard o.: standard, thermoplastic, metal, or combination of materials used in any of the knee-ankle-foot orthoses to which has been added a pelvic band that is static or with a mechanical hip joint for dynamic control of the pelvis.

standing frame (parapodium) orthosis: thoracic region reaches to floor, pelvic band, lateral uprights attached to platform base, which has cutouts to accept patient's shoes, uprights are generally overlapped to allow growth adjustment. Some type of control is used for knee extension. Joints are optional at hips and knees. This system is used to achieve standing and increase awareness in the child with afflictions such as spina bifida.

Components Applicable to Lower Limb Orthoses

ankle, knee, or hip joint: mechanical axis placed anatomically to allow or control motion.

Bail knee lock: posterior spring-loaded ring extending from medial to lateral knee joints with capability of automatic locking.

calf band: metal covered with leather or equivalent fitted to the calf area on ankle-foot or knee-ankle-foot orthoses.

dial lock: may be set in varying degrees of flexion or extension to accommodate and/or reduce contractures; other comparable types.

distal thigh band: lower thigh band on knee-ankle-foot orthoses.

double-action ankle joint: anterior and posterior compartments provide infinite adjustment for solid, limited, or dynamic assist.

drop-lock ring: fitted into place at knee joint to maintain extension; may be unlocked for sitting.

extended steel shank: inserted in sole of shoe to or past metatarsal heads to more effectively use floor reaction force.

floor reaction ankle foot o.: plastic mold orthosis with plantar flexed position and anterior upper leg bar that forces knee to extension on floor reaction force.

ischial weight-bearing ring or band: metal or equivalent component covered with soft material and fitted at the level of the ischial tuberosity; designed to unload weight from the lower limb; Thomas ring.

Klenzak orthosis: dorsiflexion or plantar flexion assist for ankle joint; spring-loaded dynamic assistive control of the foot.

lateral spring-loaded lock: spring-loaded ring lock with lever that dynamically locks at full extension.

limited- or free-motion ankle joint: permanently adjustable to allow motion as desired.

metal foot plate: similar to NYU insert but fabricated of stainless steel, Monel, or equivalent.

NYU (New York University) insert: metal o. using thermoplastic foot plate attached to ankle joint stirrups; provides correction of the foot and allows various shoes to be worn.

overlapped upright or growth extensions: uprights placed on top of one another to accommodate growth in children.

patellar pad: leather or equivalent; fits over patella with straps around uprights to maintain knee extension.

proximal thigh band: higher thigh band on knee-ankle-foot orthoses.

quadrilateral brim: similar to ischial weight-bearing ring but fabricated of plastic.

split stirrup: component mounted on various shoes to allow interchangeability of the orthosis.

spreader bar: attached medially to both stirrups of bilateral knee-ankle-foot orthoses to prevent uncontrolled abduction.

stirrup: attaches orthosis to upper shoe sections; has receptacles for ankle joints.

suprapatellar and infrapatellar straps: small straps above and below knee, continuing around uprights to maintain knee extension.

upright: metal, plastic, or equivalent used to connect various other components.

varus or valgus corrective ankle straps: soft, padded leather or equivalent components that wrap around the opposite side.

varus or valgus knee control pads: leather or equivalent components that wrap around an opposing upright to correct deformity.

Upper Limb Orthoses

Physiology in design considerations for hand and wrist-hand orthotic systems include the following:

1. Maintain thumb in opposition for prehension.
2. Allow for thumb abduction as may be required.
3. Maintain skeletal integrity.
4. Avoid restrictions in use of the orthosis.
5. Prevent or correct contractures.
6. Maintain wrist in the functional 25 to 35 degrees of dorsiflexion.

Because of infinite and intricate variety of systems, only a few common examples are given.

Wrist-Hand and Hand Orthoses

basic hand splint: for muscle weakness in the hand; a dorsal splint that wraps around the ulnar, distal, and volar side of the hand and held in place with a strap around the distal wrist.

cock-up splint: one plastic section providing wrist dorsiflexion with incorporation of a C bar for prehension or a soft Velcro brace with palmar bar to dorsiflex the wrist.

externally powered tenodesis o.: through activation of a microswitch, tenodesis graft is achieved using a mechanical muscle.

Galveston metacarpal brace: for distal metacarpal fractures; an adjustable brace that provides dorsally directed pressure on the distal component of the fracture with counter pressure on the middorsum of the hand.

long opponens o.: identical to short opponens with forearm extension for wrist control.

palmar wrist splint: easily removable volar wrist splint that has molded palmar extension that helps hold thumb in functional position.

ratchet flexor tenodesis splint: wrist-hand o. to passively lock hand in a grasp position for a partially paralyzed forearm and hand.

reciprocal finger prehension: for severe paralysis of forearm and hand; this orthosis allows patients to use their good hand to adjust and set the fixed position of fingers.

safety pin o.: fitted to individual fingers to dynamically influence flexion or extension of a joint; sometimes called *finger benders.*

short opponens o.: consists of radial extension, opponens bar, palmar arch, ulnar extension, and dorsal extension; fabricated of plastic or metal. Positions hand and thumb for opposition.

tenodesis o.: for nerve paralysis; wrist-hand orthosis with connected hinge at wrist and metacarpophalangeal joint located such that extension of wrist brings about finger flexion.

wrist-driven lateral prehension o.: similar to long opponens with jointed radial side and a rod or connection between hand and forearm sections and thumb post. Wrist dorsiflexion produces a lateral prehension pattern using the mechanical axis.

Elbow Orthoses

Elbow orthoses may be static with humeral and forearm sections for immobilization, as in hand orthoses, and external joints to allow motion. Some are designed with turnbuckles or the equivalent to reduce contracture and may be static or dynamic.

dynamic hinged elbow fracture brace: orthotic device to allow graded active range of motion with dynamic support to the fracture joint structure to promote healing (Fig. 7-4, *A*).

Santana elbow extension splint: designed to decrease flexion contractures of the elbow and to gain total maximum range of motion and strength (Fig. 7-4, *B*).

Elbow-Wrist-Hand Orthoses

These are static systems to provide immobilization. A torsion bar may be incorporated to assist in pronation or supination. They are useful to correct fractures of the forearm.

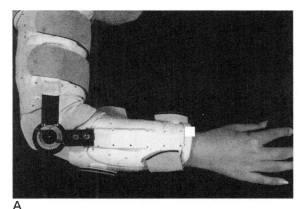

A

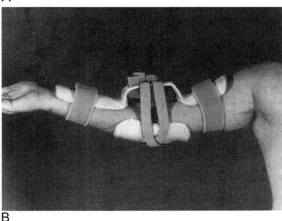

B

FIG 7-4 A, Elbow orthosis: dynamic hinged elbow fracture brace. **B,** Santana elbow extension splint. (Courtesy of EC Jeter, OTR, Occupational Therapy Department, National Naval Medical Center, Bethesda, MD.)

Shoulder Orthoses

Generally these are static or passive jointed systems used for positioning to correct chronic shoulder dislocation.

Shoulder-Elbow-Wrist-Hand Orthoses

airplane splint: jointed elbow and shoulder, allowing controlled flexion and rotation; glenohumeral joint permits controlled abduction; used for muscle injuries humeral fractures, dislocations, surgery involving the glenohumeral joint, and nerve injuries such as to the brachial plexus.

gunslinger o.: for shoulder injuries and surgery; a forearm trough mechanically anchored to a hemigirdle on the person's pelvis.

static orthosis: provides controlled positioning.

Components Applicable to Upper Limb Orthoses

C bar: component attached to or an integral part of the palmar arch, designed to maintain the web space between the thumb and hand.

first dorsal interosseous assist: principle similar to that of the spring swivel thumb; designed to hold the metacarpophalangeal (MP) joint of the index finger in abduction to provide opposition with the thumb.

flail-elbow hinge: used to overcome muscle deficit at the elbow. Spring assist provides flexion and locks in position for a chosen activity.

joint stabilizer: rigid component extending proximally and distally to a joint of a digit; provides stability or realignment for subluxation.

mobile arm support (MAS): arm trough device with attachment for resting arm on wheelchair.

opponens bars: exert a static holding force on saddle joint of thumb. Keep thumb in palmar abduction, an optimal position for opposition.

outrigger: MP, proximal interphalangeal (PIP), or distal interphalangeal (DIP) extension assist; MP stop (lumbrical bar) positioned just proximal to the IP joints; holds MP joints in approximately 15 degrees of flexion.

spring swivel thumb: wire spring attached to radial aspect of orthosis and in turn connected to thumb ring. Patient flexes against this dynamic resistance; in a relaxed state, the thumb is held in the open position.

thumb interphalangeal (IP) extension assist: principle similar to the first dorsal interosseous assist; designed to return IP of the thumb to neutral after flexion and during prehension.

thumb post: static control for prehension achieved by rigid member encompassing thumb.

turnbuckle: adjustable component used to reduce contractures.

Specialized Systems for Upper Limbs

For those patients with severe involvement, external power sources are at times used. Electrically powered or CO_2-operated artificial muscle systems are available.

Spine
Sacroiliac Orthoses

cloth binder: material encompassing appropriate region with Velcro closure.

sacroiliac belt: adjustable corset with posterior pad.

Lumbosacral Orthoses

Bennett o.: cloth lumbar corset with reinforced frame consisting of a pelvic and thoracic band with two paravertebral uprights.

chairback o. (sagittal control, sagittal-coronal control): posterior frame with lateral and posterior uprights and apron front anteriorly; control restrictions include anterior flexion, extension, and lateral flexion; used for lower back pathologic conditions, severe strain, arthritis.

lumbosacral corset: custom-fitted corset, generally having rigid paraspinal uprights.

Norton-Brown o.: rigid low-back postoperative brace. The lateral bars extend to cover the greater trochanter to help reduce lateral bending.

sacral belt: for low back pain; a semi-rigid or canvas device that is placed across the upper buttocks and fastens near the pubis, similar to a weightlifter's belt.

surgical corset: garment encasing the torso and hips and adjustable circumferentially. Adjustment may be made anteriorly, posteriorly, laterally, or in combination. In general, the following statements apply.

> *function:* serves as a reminder to restrict anteroposterior and mediolateral motions; minimal unweighting of vertebral bodies and disks; restricts some rotary and twisting motions; creates intracavitary pressure system, lending support to the spinal column.

> *materials:* nylon, cotton, canvas, elastic, or a combination.

> *fabrication:* single or multiple layers.

> *anterior height:* superior border 1 inch below xiphoid process or above lower ribs; inferior border ½ to 1 inch above symphysis pubis.

> *posterior height:* superior border 1 inch below inferior ankle of scapula; inferior border extends to the sacrococcygeal junction or approximately the gluteal fold.

> *modification possibilities:* posterior semirigid or rigid paraspinal uprights, posterior semirigid or rigid plate, posterior inflatable control pads, additional abdominal reinforcements with flexible stays, thoracic extension with shoulder straps and axillary loops, separate frame posteriorly, one-piece garment, special control pads for ptosis (prolapse of any organ), hernia pads, perineal straps, thigh skirt.

Williams o. (posterior and mediolateral control): posterior frame; lateral sliding uprights with apron front anteriorly; control restrictions; extension and lateral flexion; permits free anterior flexion; used for herniated disks, severe lordosis, and situations in which it is desirable to increase intervertebral space posteriorly.

Willner's instrument for spinal instrumentation (WISS): a TLSO designed to treat low back pain with adjustable pad to change relative lumbar flexion and extension.

Thoracic Orthoses

clavicle o.: figure eight harness under the axilla and over the shoulder, crossing posteriorly; control restrictions: glenohumeral flexion; used for clavicular fractures.

rib belt: foam padded or elastic with Velcro closure; minimal control, reducing muscle strain; used for fractures and costochondritis.

Thoracolumbosacral Orthoses (TLSOs)

flexion control (Jewett, hyperextension) o.: anterior frame with superior and inferior pads; three-point fixation provided by additional posterior pad; control restrictions: maintains hyperextension and tends to increase lumbar lordosis; used for spondylitis, compression fractures, osteoporosis (reduction in the quality of bone or skeletal atrophy; remaining bone is normally mineralized), arthritis, spinal fusion, adolescent epiphysitis, and osteochondritis.

sagittal-coronal control (Knight-Taylor) o.: chairback-Taylor combination; posterior and lateral uprights with corset front; control restrictions: anterior flexion, extension, and lateral flexion; used for high spinal fusion, lordosis, and osteoporosis.

sagittal control (Taylor) o.: posterior uprights with shoulder straps and apron front; control restrictions: anterior flexion and extension; used for kyphosis, fractures, arthritis, lordosis, carcinoma (any of the various types of malignant neoplasms derived from epithelial tissue), and after spinal surgery.

Arnold brace: brace primarily molded over the sacro-iliac area with posterior support and rigid scapular thoracic support harness.

body jacket: anteroposterior sectioned, posterior or anterior opening; thermoplastic fabrication; control restrictions: general immobilization and intra-cavitary pressure; may be designed to provide some distraction; used for conditions such as postsurgical management of fusion, spina bifida, muscular dystrophy, and scoliosis.

Boston brace: molded brace used in scoliosis and other special disorders, for example, osteoarthritis of the dorsal and lumbar spine.

CASH o.: *c*ruciform *a*nterior *s*pinal *h*yperextension o., a hyperextension TLSO or CTSO that allows more freedom of chest movement.

Charleston bending brace: for scoliosis, used only at night to hold the patient in maximum side bending correction.

dorsal lumbar corset: high corset with shoulder straps and paraspinal uprights; control restrictions: forward flexion, used for problems related to higher levels of amputation; see **thoracolumbosacral anterior control.**

Lexan jacket: for scoliosis treatment; a prefabricated TLSO.

lumbodorsal support: lumbar corset with thoracic extension of stays and straps that go over shoulder, pass under axilla, and attach to bottom of thoracic component of the posterior stay; **dorsal lumbar o.**

Lyonnaise o.: for treatment of thoracic curves with apices as high as T8.

Miami o.: the shortest of the TLSO group that allows for forward bending of the person without a check restraint.

Rosenberger o.: a TLSO that uses adjustable slings for curve correction.

New York orthopedic front-opening o.: for scoliosis treatment, a prefabricated TLSO.

Prenyl jacket: for scoliosis treatment, a prefabricated TLSO.

Rosenberger o.: custom-molded polyethylene orthosis for scoliosis, similar to Miami o. and Wilmington jacket.

triplanar control: thoracic band with supraclavicular extensions (cow horn projections), pelvic band, paraspinal bars, and lateral bars.

underarm o.: custom-fabricated or modular system; thermoplastic, generally with posterior opening; used for scoliosis. Application is most effective when apex of curve is inferior to T-10.

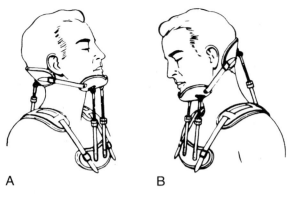

FIG 7-5 Cervical flexion-extension control orthosis (poster appliance). **A,** Cervical spine in slight extension with head erect. **B,** Cervical spine in flexion with chin depressed. (From American Academy of Orthopaedic Surgeons: *Atlas of Orthotics*, St Louis, 1975, Mosby.)

Wilmington jacket: used in scoliosis in circumstances in which control through the cervical spine is not essential.

Cervical Orthoses (Fig. 7-5)

Cervical orthoses are used when immobilization is necessary due to whiplash type of injuries, fractures, and surgical fusion. The following provide minimal restrictions.

four-poster o.: same as two-poster o., but uses two bars anteriorly and two posteriorly.

hard (plastic) collar (Mayo Thomas): overlapping plastic sections with Velcro closures; wraps around neck and contacts chin.

molded Thomas collar: custom-fabricated leather or plastic over modified cast.

Plastazote collar: unicellular foam, contoured to fit chin and make contact with occiput; Velcro closure. This configuration is often called a **Philadelphia** collar.

soft collar: foam with Velcro closure; wraps around neck.

halo extension: fitted bands at forehead and back of head in conjunction with a two- or four-poster device attached to a thoracolumbar or thoracolumbosacral orthosis.

halo traction: skeletal immobilization traction using a pelvic plaster cast or plastic girdle; outriggers to metal ring encircling head; pins are then inserted into skull and outriggers adjusted for distraction.

SOMI (sternal occiput mandibular immobilizer) o.: chin and occiput sections and sternal and posterior sections; may be fitted while patient is supine. The SOMI brace can be attached to a thermoplastic body jacket to allow control of the cervical, thoracic, and lumbar spine.

two- or four-poster o. with extension to waist: body length orthosis for greater neck stability and control.

two- or four-poster o. (Dennison brace) with thoracic extension: anterior and posterior bands incorporated into the cervical orthosis.

two-poster o. (Dennison brace): for fractures and postsurgical support, a cervical brace with chest and thoracic extension; one anterior bar with chin cup and chest plate, and one posterior post with thoracic and chest plates attached by shoulder harness (straps) that can be connected to a waist circular support. A thoracic extension can be added.

wire frame collar: rounded, rectangular ring that fits under chin and onto chest, held in place by two straps supported by expansion of material on posterior neck. When optimal control and restriction are required, the following are prescribed:

Cervicothoracolumbosacral Orthoses

Milwaukee o.: leather or thermoplastic pelvic girdle, throat mold, occiput pads, neck ring, and full, connecting superstructure with control pads as necessary; used for spinal scoliosis or kyphosis.

Components and Descriptions Applicable to Spinal Systems

Beaufort seating orthosis: for trunk control in a severely disabled, sitting patient; a large bean bag full of polystyrene beads is molded to patient and then air evacuated to make a firm support.

corset front: cloth anteriorly attached to lateral uprights of spinal orthosis.

matrix seating system: for severely disabled patients; a seating system constructed from interlocking plastic components.

Milwaukee cervicothoracolumbosacral orthoses
axillary sling: axillary pad with webbing used to maintain alignment of neck ring.

Friddle low profile neck rings: function predominantly by reducing the sway of the vertebral column and keeping the upper thoracic spine centered over the sacrum.

lumbar pad: firm foam or metal and leather incorporated into or attached near postero-superior edge of girdle on same side as thoracic curve.

neck ring: metal ring at neck that opens posteriorly for donning and doffing and serves as attachment for throat mold and occiput pads.

occiput pads: plastic or metal oblong disks fitted bilaterally to the inferior angle of the occiput bones of the head; aligned to provide slight distraction.

pelvic girdle: custom-fitted section serving as foundation for orthosis.

shoulder ring: component fitted to axilla and over acromion; attached to the orthosis and used to depress an elevated shoulder.

superstructure: two posterior and one anterior metal component connecting pelvic girdle and neck ring.

thoracic pad: floating pad attached to anterior and posterior uprights on same side as thoracic curve.

throat mold: plastic or equivalent material, attached to neck ring and fitted to within 0.5 cm of throat and just below chin; limits anteroposterior motion.

perineal loops: straps passing between legs to reduce migration of spinal orthosis superiorly.

rotary control: modification of rigid spinal orthosis with lateral extension or sternal plate fitted bilaterally into the deltopectoral grooves to restrict rotation.

sternal attachment: component fitted to chest.

thoracic extension: component parts attached to cervical orthosis and fitted to the chest and back regions to provide increased control.

uprights: see components and descriptions applicable to lower limb orthoses.

Shoe Modifications

Terms for the normal components of shoes are used frequently in describing modifications used in orthopaedic treatment.

counter, heel counter: toe helps hold the heel, firm cup incorporated into the rear of the shoe.

foxing: stripping that adds support to the medial and lateral side of the shoe.

last: three-dimensional model of which the shoe is made, taking the form of the sole of the foot.

shank: reinforcing material that bridges between the ball and heel area of the shoe.

toe box: stiff material that prevents collapse and protects the toes.

tongue: part that protects foot from pressure from the laces.

Shoe modifications are various alterations made in a shoe to complement the orthosis. On occasion, a shoe modification is prescribed by itself to correct a specific problem; for example, leg-length discrepancy is treated by a shoe elevation on the shorter side, and valgus ankles may be treated with medial sole and heel wedging or medially flared heel.

custom-molded shoes (space shoes): specially and individually constructed shoes designed to fit a patient with multiple foot deformities, as occur with rheumatoid arthritis.

orthopaedic oxford: a hard leather shoe with a leather or rubber sole; sometimes such a shoe has a steel shank (portion of shoe that lies between the floor of the shoe and the sole), with firmly constructed sides that support the foot in an upright position. This type of shoe is constructed uniformly, allowing for the addition of assistive devices.

surgical shoe or boot: a hard shoe that is constructed of thick walls, usually leather, with lacing designed to allow the shoe to be firmly tightened around the foot; generally used as part of an orthosis.

Devices for Flatfeet

ankle corset: a laced leather device that encompasses ankle and rear foot to support arch and subtalar joint.

combined arch support: an interchangeable arch support that has both a tarsal (arch) component and a forward pad to support the metatarsal arch.

extended counter: a piece of leather extending from the inner back side of the shoe to the level of the arch, giving arch support.

medial heel wedge: small wedge of extra leather or rubber placed on the arch side of the heel.

plantar arch support: an interchangeable pad that helps support the tarsal arch.

Plastazote: for a variety of prosthetic and orthotic needs, this is a closed-cell polyethylene foam that, with 280° F heating, can be molded in to a force distribution piece of foam.

scaphoid (navicular) pads: better known as *shoe cookies* or tarsal supports; inserted directly under the arch of the foot in the shoe.

Shaffer plate: arch support made of stainless steel; usually for adults.

Shoemaker's swan: for molding relief in pressure areas of a shoe, a long-handled device that has a ring on one arm and a ball on the other for stretching shoe material at points of pressure.

Thomas heel: a heel with a curved extension for the arch side of the foot.

Whitman plate: arch support made of stainless steel; for growing feet.

Metatarsal Supports

metatarsal bars: an extra piece of rubber applied externally to the sole, providing support proximal to the metatarsal heads; used in treatment of callosities on the ball of the foot and stiff great toes. Types of metatarsal bars include **Denver, Flush, Hauser,** and **Mayo** metatarsal bar.

metatarsal pads: pads permanently placed in shoe just proximal to the ball of the foot.

metatarsal supports: interchangeable supports that have raised areas just proximal to the ball of the foot.

Devices for Insensitive Feet (Devascularized or Diabetic Neuropathies)

controlled ankle walker: plastic device incorporating a calf wrap and rigid ankle and foot plate to unweight the foot; to allow healing of an ulcer.

custom-molded shoes: see space shoes.

Plastizote shoes: commercially available shoe(s) in which upper is lined with Plastizote as is the insole; to accommodate deformity or heel ulcers.

rocker sole modification: rigid sole attachment to reduce shear force of metatarsal heads and to prevent a healed ulcer from reulcerating.

Devices for Callosities

Budin splint: splint designed to relieve symptoms due to hammertoe deformity.

calcaneal spur pad: a heel with a special cutout center designed to redistribute the weight from a painful area of the heel.

heel pad: any soft pad inserted into the shoe to cushion the heel; used for tendonitis, heel spurs, Achilles bursitis, and similar conditions.

sole inserts: known by a variety of trade names, these inserts are made of foam rubber or other material and are designed to cushion the entire walking surface of the foot.

Special Shoes for Infants and Children

equinovarus outflare shoes: used in treatment of clubfoot condition.

inflare last shoes: used to maintain correction for overpronation.

normal last shoes: constructed with normal sole; term used to distinguish this from a reverse or straight last shoe.

reverse last (outflare last) shoes: look as if the left shoe were made for the right foot and vice versa; the side where the arch would normally be is curved out; used in treatment of clubfeet and metatarsus varus.

straight last shoes: look as if they could be worn on either foot, with a straight sole; used in treating mild forefoot problems such as metatarsus varus; incurring last.

tarsal pronator shoes: used in treatment of clubfoot condition.

torque heels: specially designed heels to make the foot turn in or out, depending on the direction of rubber slits that are arranged to cause torsion on weight-bearing.

Anatomy and Orthopaedic Surgery

Orthopaedic surgery is the branch of medicine concerned with the preservation of the musculoskeletal system. Therefore, the goal is to treat diseases and injuries, correct deformities, and make surgical repairs to bone, cartilage, muscles, tendons, ligaments, synovia, bursa, fascia, and nerves of the upper and lower limbs, shoulder, spine, and pelvis. A general list of the types of surgery performed on these tissues is presented in Table 8-1.

Orthopaedic surgery encompasses an overwhelming number of procedures in an attempt to alter normal or abnormal anatomic structures. The four-volume *Campbell's Operative Orthopedics* (Canale ST: *Campbell's Operative Orthopedics,* ed 10, St Louis, 2003, Mosby-Year Book) is one of the textbooks of this surgical specialty. Many of the new terms are briefly described in this chapter.

The anatomy of the musculoskeletal system is defined here to correlate with the surgery on specific tissue by anatomic area. Numerous figure illustrations are provided to enhance the understanding of anatomic structures. An associated surgical word list is included at the end of the chapter.

Osteo- (Bone)

Anatomy of Bone

Osseous tissue (bone) constitutes the majority of the skeletal framework. It is living, hard connective tissue composed of organic (cells and matrix) and inorganic (mineral) components with submicroscopic laminations of protein and crystal layers. The matrix contains a framework of collagenous fibers that are impregnated with the mineral components, mainly in the form of apatite crystals, which give the quality of rigidity to bone. Another quality is its hematopoietic ability, i.e., to create and develop blood in the bone marrow.

If all the mineral were removed from bone, the resulting structure would be firm and pliable and have the exact shape of the mineralized bone. The process of **calcification** is not restricted to bones; it may occur in an amorphous form in tendons, bursae, and other tissues. **Ossification** is actual formation of bone tissue, which then calcifies by addition of hydroxyapatite crystals composed of calcium, phosphate, and hydroxyl ions. The following terms relate to the shape, structure, and microanatomy of bone (Fig. 8-1).

apophysis: a tubercle of bone that contributes to its growth but is the point of strong tendon insertion rather than a part of the joint. It usually has a center of ossification.

articular cartilage: epiphyseal covering; thin layer of hyaline cartilage covering articular surface (ends) of bone to respond to shear forces.

bone marrow: an "organ" whose function is the manufacture (hematopoiesis) of the formed elements of blood, that is, red cells, white cells, and platelets, the most important material in the body. It is a network of connective tissue filled with blood vessels that form and develop blood corpuscles and is found

TABLE 8-1 Orthopaedic Procedures*

Prefixes/Roots: Tissue Types	Procedures[†]
Osteo- (bone)	2, 4, 5, 6, 7, 8
Myo- (muscle)	2, 3, 4, 5, 6, 7
Tendo- or teno- (tendon)	3, 4, 5, 6, 7, 10
Desmo- (ligament)	5
Syndesmo- (ligament)	6, 7
Fascio- or fascia- (fibrous bands)	4, 5, 6, 7, 9
Burs- (bursa, sac, pouch)	1, 4, 6, 9
Spondylo- (spine)	3, 6
Myelo- (spinal cord, meninges, bone marrow)	1, 5, 6, 9
Lamin- (lamina)	4, 6
Rachio- (spine)	1, 6
Neur- (nerves)	4, 5, 6, 7, 10
Arthro- (joint)	1, 2, 3, 4, 6, 7, 9, 10, 11
Chondro- (cartilage) (Fig. 8-2)	2, 4, 6
Synov-(synovium)	4
Capsul- (capsule)	3, 4, 5, 6, 7
Condyl- (condyle)	4, 6
Aponeur- (fascial bands)	4, 5, 6

*The left column (prefixes/roots) indicates the anatomy; corresponding numbers in the right column (procedures) describe the types of surgery performed on those tissues.

[†]1, **-centesis:** surgical puncture; perforation or tapping with aspirator, trocar, or needle; 2, **-clasis:** surgical fracture or refracture of bones and other tissue by crushing; refracture of bone in malposition; 3, **-desis:** binding, fixation by means of suture (tendon) or fusion (joints); not to include spine; 4, **-ectomy:** excision of organ or part; 5, **-orrhaphy:** to suture or sew; 6, **-otomy:** surgical incision into a part or organ; cut into; 7, **-plasty:** to form, mold, or shape; surgical shaping or formation; 8, **-synthesis:** putting together, composition, surgical fastening of ends of fractured bones by sutures, rings, plates, or other mechanical means; 9, **-gram:** injection of contrast media for x-ray examination; 10, **-lysis:** dissolution of tissue; decomposition, freeing of scar or adhesions; 11, **-oscopy:** to view by a scope.

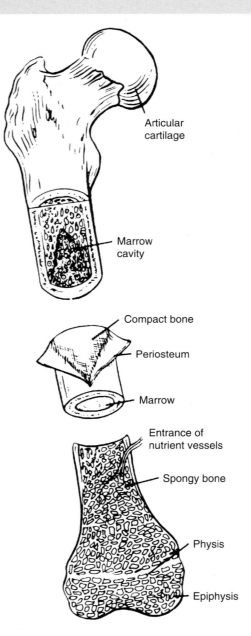

FIG 8-1 Composition of bone. (From Young CG, Barger JD: *Learning Medical Terminology Step by Step*, ed 3, St Louis, 1975, The CV Mosby.)

in the proximal epiphyses of the humeri and femora, ribs and sternum, and cancellous bone of vertebrae. Yellow bone marrow is found in the medullary cavity (in adults) and contains fatty marrow.

bone matrix: the intracellular substance of bone composed of osteocollagenous fibers embedded in an amorphous ground substance and inorganic salts.

calcium: a necessary mineral in combination with phosphorus to form calcium phosphate (apatite crystals), the dense, hard material of bones (and teeth); it is the most abundant mineral in the body and found in all organized tissues. Calcium is

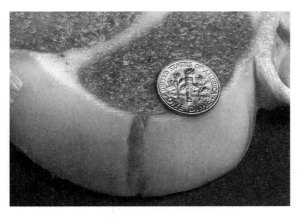

FIG 8-2 Cartilage on surface of soup bone. Dime for contrasts to strip or removed cartilage. Cartilage within bone is the growth plate cartilage.

important in the function of muscles, nerves, blood coagulation, and heartbeat. Bones are a storage center for calcium.

cambium layer: loose cellular inner layer of the periosteal tissue in the intramembranous ossification of bone.

canaliculus: communicating, narrow tubular channel between osteocytes in bone.

cancellous bone: spongy, porous, lattice-like tissue within midshaft of long bone.

condyle: prominence at the widened end of long bones and the attachment for ligaments, tendons, or muscles. Two examples are the femoral condyles, the inner and outer palpable prominences of the upper knee joint.

cortical (compact) bone: the thick outer portion of bone that surrounds the medullary (marrow) cavity.

cut-back zone: in growing bone, the zone just proximal to the epiphyseal growth plate, where the diameter of the bone is being cut back.

cutting cone: cone-appearing blood vessel as seen on longitudinal microscopic section; osteoclasts can be seen absorbing bone at the head of the cone.

diaphysis: the thick, compact, long mid-shaft of bone providing strong support.

enchondral bone: bone formed from cartilage, whether from the cartilage growth plate or from cartilage in fracture callus; **cartilage bone, substitution bone.**

endosteum: the lining of the trabecular and cortical bone that is within the medullary canal or cavity.

epiphysis: the bulbous growth end of a long bone, usually wider than the shaft and entirely cartilaginous or separated from the shaft by a cartilaginous disk. The epiphysis is a part of the bone formed from a secondary center of ossification at the ends of long bones, margins of flat bones, and at the tubercles and processes. During growth, the epiphyses are separated from the main portion of bone by cartilage, properly termed the **physis** or **epiphyseal plate.** There are two types of epiphyses:

pressure e.: a secondary center of ossification in the articular end of a long bone with articular elements subjected to pressure.

traction e.: a secondary center of ossification at the site of attachment of a tendon and subjected to traction. Contributes to bone shape (e.g., apophysis).

physis: the cartilage between the apophysis or epiphysis and the shaft of the bone. This cartilage is responsible for most of the longitudinal growth of the bone. Although the epiphyseal cartilage is called the growth plate, as in the previous definition, the term **epiphyseal cartilage** may also refer to the cartilage lining the joint; **growth plate, epiphyseal plate.**

hypertrophic zone: zone where cells become larger.

proliferating zone: zone of cell replication. Cells appear to be stacked like coins.

provisional calcification: calcium appears in matrix, and beyond this point, invading blood vessels appear with bone cells on surface of calcified cartilage.

resting zone: zone of cartilage cells with little metabolic activity and no cell division.

Other terms related to epiphyseal growth:

atavistic e.: a bone that fuses naturally to another bone as in the coracoid process of the scapula.

punctum ossificationis: point of ossification (center) where bone begins to form in a specific bone or part; **ossification center.**

primary center of ossification: the first site where bone begins to form in the shaft; in a long bone, the diaphysis; **punctum ossificationis primarium.**

secondary center of ossification: a center of bone formation that appears later, on the joint side of a growth plate where the center of ossification is a part of bone that has a strong muscle attachment outside of the diaphysis; **punctum ossificationis secundarium.**

facet: a flat, plate-like surface that acts as part of a joint; facets are seen in the vertebrae and in the subtalar joint of the ankle.

flat bones: bent or curved rather than flat, these bones protect viscera and other soft tissues and include the pelvis, ribs, and shoulder blade.

haversian canals: one of the minute canals running lengthwise in compact osteonal bone filled with blood vessels that are centrally enclosed and protected; part of an important system in transporting blood-borne material to widely separated bone cells. This transport system is comprised of the haversian canals, surrounding lamellae, connecting canaliculi, and lacunae. The lateral branches of these vessels are called **Volkmann canals.**

Howship lacuna: microscopic area of small depressions or grooves on the surface of bone where resorption of bone is occurring as a result of osteoclastic activity.

isthmus: narrow portion of the canal in the shaft of the bone.

lamellar bone: description of bone that, under a microscope, reveals a pattern of lamination.

line: a less prominent ridge on bone, for example, iliopectineal line; whereas, a crest is a ridge (iliac crest).

medullary canal: the canal in the center of a bone shaft containing soft, fatty marrow elements (in adults) and cancellous bone.

membranous bone: collagen model bone that is formed directly from the periosteum, without development of cartilage, and develops within a connective tissue membrane.

metaphysis: the wider portion of a long bone between the diaphysis, shaft, and the epiphysis. This portion of bone represents the most recently formed bone (growth zone) during the growth process. With closure of physis, it is continuous with the epiphysis.

ossification: process of forming bone (ossifying, adj.). Other related terms include the following:

osseous: general term referring to bony matter.

ossiferous: implies that bone is being produced.

ossific: refers to the presence of bone.

osteoid: the uncalcified bony matrix (young bone).

osteoblast: a bone-forming cell; cells that produce osteoid, which is the matrix that is predominantly type I collagen and a number of bone proteins that then normally calcify with apatite crystals (hydroxyapatite).

osteoclast: bone-removing cell; these are cells derived from monocellular precursors, which under the influence of parathyroid hormone and other systemic and local substances absorb bone in the form of multinucleated cells. The divot that is created in the bone is called a **Howship lacuna.**

osteocyte: bone cell; a living cell that has cell extensions called **canaliculi,** allowing the cell to affect the metabolism of the surrounding matrix. Osteocytes exist in both trabecular and cortical bone.

osteonal bone: a microscopic description of bone that is seen in mature adults and is composed of little tubes that look like stubby pieces of chalk, having an arteriole running down the middle. There are circular laminations of bone concentric with the artery. An **osteon** is a single unit and is barely visible to the eye.

periosteum: firm, thin, two-layered fibrous outer covering of bone; outer layer contains blood vessels; inner layer contains connective tissue cells and elastic fibers. The periosteum is important for circumferential bone growth and in bone repair because of its bone-forming cells and blood vessels that supply the osteogenic layer. The nerve endings in periosteum are responsible for the sensitivity of bone in trauma. The thin layer of multipotential cells that is immediately next to the bone is called the **cambium layer.**

sesamoid: denoting a small, round bone found in tendons (and some muscles), whose function is to increase movement in a joint by improving angle of approach of tendon into its insertion. The patella is the largest sesamoid bone in the body.

subchondral bone: bone directly under any cartilaginous surface.

trabecula: type of bone that is in small spicules, normally referred to as trabecular bone (**cancellous bone**); predominantly makes up the ends of long bones.

trabecular pattern: refers to the arrangement of the trabeculae of bone such that, when seen on radiographs or in cross-sections, there is a pattern of arches or other designs, like the spokes of a bicycle, providing the structural needs of the bone.

tubercle (small), tuberosity (large): rounded, elevated projection of bone giving attachment to a muscle or ligament; for example, ischial tuberosity or Lister's tubercle (dorsal, of radius).

Volkmann canals: found in osteonal bone; lateral passageways for transporting nutrients from the central haversian canals to bone cells (osteocytes).

woven bone: immature bone seen in very early growth and development, fracture healing, and some disease states. Also known as **wormian bone.**

coarse woven bone (burlap bone): rapidly developing woven bone with coarse-appearing matrix.

fine woven bone (linen bone): bone with smooth-appearing matrix but that is not lamellar.

General Surgery of Bone

bone marrow biopsy: surgical or local needle aspiration of bone marrow for microscopic inspection to determine the presence of disease affecting bone, that is, decreased cellular production or abnormal white blood cells (leukemia); usually drawn from superior iliac crest.

bone marrow transplant: a special procedure done (occasionally) in an effort to treat certain disease conditions of bone marrow. Diseased marrow is chemically destroyed and replaced (transfused) with healthy donor marrow of the same blood type. The transfused cells eventually matriculate to recipient's bone marrow where, if the transplant takes, they become established.

bone suture fixation: placement of a peg or screw device to affix a suture to bone for capsular, ligamentous, or tendon repair. There are numerous brands of permanent and absorbable devices.

callotasis: for lengthening a bone; production of fracture and then gradual distraction using an external fixator.

closed reduction: nonsurgical manipulation of the fractured part, with return to proper position (called apposition) and alignment.

condylectomy: excision of a condyle at the joint; more specifically, removal of the round bony prominence of the articular end of bone.

condylotomy: surgical incision or division of a condyle or condyles.

corticotomy: complete transection of the cortex of a bone without transection of the intramedullary structures. This procedure is basically an osteotomy with care taken to preserve the intramedullary vessels.

diaphysectomy: removal of the shaft of bone, leaving the distal and proximal ends of bone intact.

diaplasis: reduction of a fracture or dislocation.

distraction osteogenesis: lengthening of bone with an external fixator to produce gradual distraction across growth plate.

ebonation: removal of fragments of bone from a wound.

epiphysiodesis: fusion of an epiphysis to the metaphysis of a bone by disruption of the growth plate **(epiphyseolysis)** or by metallic fixation between the epiphysis and metaphysis of bone. An **epiphyseolysis** may also occur traumatically.

fenestration: cutting a window in bone to allow drainage or access to an object covered by the bone, such as a tumor or foreign body.

open reduction: surgical incision and correction of a bone fracture under anesthesia; may or may not include internal fixation.

ostectomy: removal of a portion of bone.

osteoarthrotomy: the excision of the articular end of bone.

osteoclasis: surgical fracture or refracture of bone to bring about a change in alignment in cases of nonunion.

osteoplasty: surgical correction by shaping or formation of bone (osteorrhaphy).

osteosynthesis: surgical fixation of bone by the use of any internal mechanical means; usually done in the treatment of fractures.

periosteotomy (periostomy): incision through the membranous covering of bone.

sequestrectomy: removal of a portion of dead bone.

synostosis: surgical fusion of any two or more bones that would otherwise be separated; may occur in a natural state as well.

Osteotomies

An osteotomy is a surgical procedure that changes the alignment of bone with or without removal of a portion of that bone. It may be considered for correction of a malaligned fracture, osteoarthritis, or other joint conditions. The following procedures are types of osteotomies.

Abbott and Gill: for bone growth asymmetry in lower limbs; a distal femoral and proximal tibial epiphysiodesis done through a medial approach. Also, proximal tibial and fibular epiphysiodesis through a lateral approach.

Amspacher and Messenbaugh: for cubitus varus with rotatory deformity of the elbow; correction of both deformities is with a distal humeral osteotomy.

Amstutz and Wilson: for congenital coxa vara.

Bailey and Dubow: for deformities of the femoral shaft; multiple osteotomies held by a telescoping intramedullary rod.

Baker and Hill: for heel valgus; lateral opening wedge osteotomy with bone allograft.

ball-and-socket o.: dome-shaped osteotomy.

Bellemore and Barrett (modified French): for varus deformity of elbow; lateral closing wedge osteotomy of distal humerus.

Bernese: for acetabular dysplasia, osteotomy of pubis and ischial-ilial part of acetabulum that allows for more anatomic rotation of entire acetabulum, held in place by internal fixation (**Ganz**).

Blount: for bone growth asymmetry in the lower limbs; epiphyseal growth is arrested using staples across the growth plate.

Blount displacement o.: for hip osteoarthritis.

Blundell Jones varus o.: varus osteotomy of the hip for paralysis.

Borden and Gearen: for aseptic necrosis of the hip; an extracapsular transtrochanteric osteotomy.

Borden, Spencer, and Herndon: for coxa vara.

Brackett o.: ball-and-socket type for the fused hip.

Brett: for proximal tibia for genu recurvatum.

closing wedge o.: wedge cut out of bone, the open space closed, leaving a straight line.

Cole: anterior tarsal wedge for cavus deformity.

Cotton: for correction of a distal tibial deformity.

Coventry: a proximal tibial osteotomy for varus or valgus knees.

Crego: for femoral anteversion.

cuneiform: a cuneiform-shaped wedge cut in bone allowing for correction of deformities in two planes.

derotation o.: correction of rotational misalignment of a long bone.

dial o.: dome- or circular-shaped osteotomy.

Dickson: for malunion of the femoral neck.

Dimon: for intertrochanteric fractures; medial displacement of the distal fragment (**Dimon and Hughston**).

Dwyer: for clubfoot and pes cavus deformities; a lateral closing wedge osteotomy that reduces both the cavus and heel varus deformities.

Ferguson-Thompson-King-Moore o.: for long-bone deformity such as malunion; a concave side resection of cortex with replacement after bone is made into chips, careful closure of the periosteum over the chips, and then closing wedge osteotomy on opposite side after sufficient callus formation has taken place.

Fish: for fixed slipped capital femoral epiphysis deformity; a cuneiform osteotomy at the base of the femoral head.

French: for cubitus varus (elbow); a closing wedge osteotomy.

Gant: open-wedge osteotomy for the fused hip.

Ganz o.: for adult acetabular dysplasia; a periacetabular osteotomy.

Ghormley: part of a hip fusion procedure.

Hass: for dislocation of the hip.

Ingram: for fusion of growth plate because of trauma; opening wedge osteotomy with concurrent insertion of fat at growth plate area.

innominate o.: of the pelvis for dislocation of the hip; two common types are **Pemberton** and **Salter.**

Irwin: for genu recurvatum; a posterior closing wedge osteotomy of the proximal tibia.

Kramer, Craig, and Noel: for fixed slipped capital femoral epiphysis deformity; osteotomy at base of femoral neck.

Langenskiöld: for fusion of growth plate; an excision of bony bridge across the epiphysis with insertion of fat. Also called coxa vara procedure.

Lorenz: for dislocation of the hip.

Lucas and Cottrell: notched rotation type of the proximal tibia.

Macewen and Shands: for congenital coxa vara.

Martin: for fixed slipped capital femoral epiphysis deformity; a closing wedge osteotomy at the base of femoral head and superior neck.

McKay: for stabilization of the hip in myelomeningocele; varus osteotomy of the proximal femur with transfer of adductors to the ischial tuberosity and external oblique muscles to the greater trochanter.

McMurray: for nonunion of the femoral neck.

Meyer-Burgdorff o.: for recurrent anterior dislocation of the shoulder; a proximal humeral osteotomy.

Moore: for long-bone deformity such as a malunion; a three-quarter width wedge resection with replacement after bone is made into chips, careful closure of the periosteum over the chips, and then closed manipulation after sufficient callus formation.

Müller: for osteoarthritis of the hip; an intertrochanteric varus osteotomy.

open-wedge o.: straight cut made across the bone, creating angulation, and leaving an open wedge-shaped gap.

Osgood: for correction of malrotation of the femur.

Pauwels: for nonunion fracture of the femoral neck.

Pauwels-Y: for congenital coxa vara.

Phemister: for bone growth asymmetry in the lower limbs; a block of bone is fashioned at the growth plate and then rotated 90 degrees.

Platou: for femoral anteversion.

Pott eversion o.: for correction of a distal tibial deformity.

redirection o.: term typically applied to acetabular osteotomy in which the acetabulum is redirected to give more appropriate orientation for the femoral head in cases of dysplasia and in some Legg-Perthes disease. Also known as **periacetabular osteotomy (PAO), Bernese, Ganz, triple, Steele, Wagner.**

Sarmiento: for intertrochanteric fractures; a wedge-shaped piece of bone is resected from the distal fragment to achieve a valgus osteotomy.

Sofield: multiple osteotomies of the tibia or femur for bowing deformities or nonunions.

Southwick: for slipped capital femoral epiphysis; a combination lateral and anterior trochanteric closing wedge osteotomy.

Speed: for malunion of the distal radius.

spike o.: creation of a bony spike in a long bone to help hold the fixation of position.

Sugiuka o.: for avascular necrosis of femoral head; the femoral head and neck are rotated to transpose the avascular area away from the weight-bearing portion of the joint.

Thompson telescoping V o.: used in distal femoral deformities.

Weber: internal rotation osteotomy of the proximal humerus for recurrent dislocation associated with large posterior humeral head defect.

Whitman: closing wedge procedure for the fused hip.

Y-osteotomy: for cavus deformity of the foot; also referred to as **Japas osteotomy.**

Bone Grafts*

Bone grafts are used several hundred thousand times annually in the United States to aid in repair or reconstruction of the skeleton. The scope of applications is associated with congenital (skeletal hypoplasia, pseudarthrosis), developmental (scoliosis), traumatic (fractures, segmental loss), degenerative (osteoarthritis), and neoplastic (benign, malignant) disorders. Most bone grafts are autogenous, and their advantages include maximal biologic potential, histocompatibility, and no potential of transfer of disease from donor to recipient.

In general, bone grafts are removed from one site and transferred to another without direct reestablishment of the blood supply. Consequently, osteogenic cells fail to survive unless they receive sufficient nutrition by diffusion, a circumstance met only by those cells very close to the bone surface. These few surviving cells play an important role in initiation or augmentation of the early phase of bone graft incorporation.

Bone graft repair depends on local factors at and emanating from the recipient site, including ingrowth of new blood vessels and both specialized and multipotential cells required for resorption and new bone

---

*Gary E. Friedlaender, MD, Professor and Chairman, Department of Orthopaedics and Rehabilitation. Yale University School of Medicine, New Haven, Connecticut.

formation. The exception to dependence on local tissues occurs with immediate reanastomosis of the blood supply to the graft, often requiring microvascular techniques.

Today, tissue banks have become research centers for bone marrow, stem cell, and growth factor studies. Because all types of blood cells are produced in the bone marrow, research experiments are limitless. Bone marrow collection (harvesting) is still an important part of tissue banking, as is storage and type-matching of bone, tissue, and blood products, but greater emphasis is now being placed on biomedical research of tissue and bone marrow.

General Terminology

histocompatibility: immunologic similarity or identity with respect to cell surface antigens determined by genes of the major histocompatibility complex. There can be varying degrees of histocompatibility, some consistent with successful transplantation and some incompatible with this approach unless accomplished with immunosuppression.

major histocompatibility complex: a sequence of genes that control expression of cell surface glycoproteins that are recognized as foreign when transferred into a genetically dissimilar host. Different terms are used to identify this gene complex, depending on the species, for example, human leukocyte antigen (HLA), histocompatibility-2 (H2) in mice, and rabbit leukocyte antigen (RLA).

immunosuppression: a term applied to any effort directed at lowering the body's natural immune response to foreign substances. Specifically, in transplant physiology, the use of specific chemicals to decrease the body's reaction to transplanted tissues from sources outside the body. Nonspecific immunosuppression reduces host responses to most or all antigens and is usually caused by a systemic drug or chemical agent. Total body (or lymphoid) irradiation is another approach to nonspecific immunosuppression, useful in conjunction with bone marrow transplantation in humans and for a variety of investigational approaches in laboratory animals. Specific immunosuppression is targeted at a specific antigen or small group of related antigens, leaving responsiveness to most other foreign proteins intact. The use of monoclonal antibodies or induction of tolerance is a form of this selective approach.

implant: a synthetic device or the act of transferring into a host a synthetic device. Some include implants to reflect biologic material without cell viability.

transplant: a tissue or organ transferred from one site to another or the act of accomplishing this transfer. Some use this term to denote the transfer of viable tissue only (versus implant), and others use it to refer to any biologic material.

Classification by Species Source

allograft (allogeneic, formerly homograft): a tissue or organ transferred between genetically dissimilar members of the same species.

autograft (autogenous, autochthonous): a tissue or organ removed from one site and placed in another within the same individual.

isograft (isogeneic): a tissue or organ transplanted between genetically identical members of the same species. Synonymous with *syngraft* (**syngeneic**).

xenograft (xenogeneic, formerly heterograft): a tissue or organ transferred between species, for example, cow to human, rat to dog.

Special Procedures for Preserving Bone Grafts

Most grafts are subject to some form of long-term preservation. The most common approaches to storage include deep-freezing, freeze-drying (lyophilization), chemosterilization, and chemical extraction of proteins, or combinations of these techniques. The methods applied to long-term preservation have some impact on biologic, immunologic, and biomechanical properties, but these changes are predictable and often compatible with clinical success. Storage permits time for careful assessment of the donor graft material for potentially harmful transmissible diseases. Processing procedures may vary from one tissue bank to another. Graft material should be obtained from tissue banks that use strict processing procedures for allograft processing and donor procurement, under the guidelines of the American Association of Tissue Banks (AATB).

Some bone recovery methods are as follows:

AAA bone: a chemosterilized, autolyzed antigen-extracted, and partially demineralized allogeneic preparation.

chemosterilized grafts: graft material rendered free of microbial organisms by exposure to a chemical, such as ethylene oxide, although thimerosal and alcohol have been used for bacteriostatic properties.

demineralized bone graft: one that has undergone extraction of minerals (superficially or completely) usually by exposure to hydrochloric acid.

freeze-dried grafts: the removal of water from tissue in a frozen state, the same as lyophilized. With respect to bone, usually reflects residual moisture being reduced to approximately 3% or less by weight. Tissues can be stored indefinitely at room temperature in evacuated, sealed containers until required for use. Moisture is then reconstituted by submerging the tissue in water (saline).

irradiation sterilized grafts: exposure of tissues to high-dose ionizing irradiation for the purpose of killing potential pathogens, requiring a dose between 1.5 and 5.0 megarad.

lyophilized grafts: same as freeze-dried grafts.

Revascularization of Grafts

The application of immediately revascularized *autografts* is limited by expendability of bone at the donor site, a discrete blood supply to the graft, vessels of sufficient caliber for repair (the fibula, ribs, and iliac crest represent the practical limitations), and microvascular expertise. This approach is especially well-suited for recipient sites compromised by prior irradiation or infection or when rapid repair is mandatory.

The incorporation of devitalized grafts occurs by a lengthy process analogous to "creeping substitution," in which the sequence of events includes revascularization of the bone, followed by resorption and new bone formation. Autografts transferred on a vascular pedicle or in which the blood flow is reestablished immediately by vascular anastomoses are incorporated rapidly by a process analogous to fracture repair.

In cases of bone *allografts,* immediate reanastomosis of blood supply is not clinically feasible because it engenders the same immunologic considerations encountered with viable solid organ transplantations, adding the requirement for substantial immunosuppression of the recipient. The following are related terms.

creeping substitution: the process by which a devascularized segment of bone *in situ* or a transferred bone without immediate reanastomosis of its blood supply undergoes repair, beginning with vascular invasion, followed by bone resorption and subsequent new bone formation (incorporation). This is a lengthy process that may take large cortical segments several years to incorporate, and even then, substantial portions of the graft may escape remodeling.

free-revascularized autograft: tissue transferred to a distant site along with its discrete blood supply such that direct reanastomosis of circulation can be accomplished immediately.

incorporation: a process by which recipient site factors grow into and remodel an initially devascularized bone graft. This includes invasion by blood vessels, resorption, and new bone formation. Often used interchangeably with creeping substitution with reference to grafts.

Classification of Grafts by Bone Type

cancellous g.: a bone transplant consisting of cancellous (or medullary) tissue as opposed to cortical bone.

composite g.: a transfer of more than one type of tissue simultaneously, such as bone and muscle transferred at the same time, or bone, muscle, and skin transferred simultaneously; must be accomplished in conjunction with reanastomosis of blood supply at the recipient site. This provides the potential advantage of repairing both bone and soft tissue defects simultaneously.

cortical g.: a transferred bone composed of the cortical (outer) tissue.

> **strut g.:** cortical bone graft used to give mechanical support in the area of a cancellous bone graft.

corticocancellous g.: transferred bony tissue with both cortical and cancellous elements.

free g.: a bone graft freed of its vascular supply and soft tissue that would encumber its transfer from one location to another. This includes free revascularized autografts as well as other bone graft preparations.

intercalary g.: a segment of transferred bone without an articular surface; usually a portion of diaphysis or diaphysis plus metaphysis, with bone intercalated into bone to reestablish continuity.

intramedullary g.: graft placed in medullary canal. Also called medullary graft.

osteoarticular g.: bone graft containing an articular surface.

osteochondral g.: a transplant composed of both bone and cartilage (articular surface).

osteoperiosteal g.: bone graft taken complete with periosteal membrane coverings.

pedicle g.: tissue transferred to another site while retaining (at least temporarily) its required blood supply at the donor site, consequently limiting the distance over which a pedicle can be transferred. The recipient site vascularity can be transected or interrupted following reestablishment of sufficient vascularity at the recipient site.

segmental g.: a portion of transferred tissue representing less than the entire anatomic part being replaced.

Classification by Shape and Bone Grafted

bone block: a bone graft that is inserted next to a joint to prevent a given direction of motion in that joint; also, a bone graft that is shaped in the form of a block and used for fusion of a joint.

chip g.: bone graft broken up into chips.

clothespin g.: coarsely shaped graft used in the spine; resembles a clothespin.

hemicylindric g.: graft cut into the shape of half a cylinder.

inlay g.: any graft that has been cut in a fusion procedure to fit the shape of the graft site.

diamond inlay: graft cut in a diamond shape with recipient site cut to receive that shape.

sliding inlay: a slot of bone cut and moved across the graft site, usually a fracture of a large bone.

massive sliding g.: large graft designed to slide when two portions of recipient bone are compressed.

morcellized g.: cortical and or cancellous bone graft that has been finely crushed before implanting.

onlay g.: graft laid directly onto the surface of recipient bone.

dual onlay g.: two strips of bone laid down on either side of the shaft.

peg g.: cylindric bone graft to be inserted into or through the medullary canal of a bone.

Eponymic Bone Graft Terms	
Albee	Hey-Grooves-Kirk
Banks	Hoaglund
Boyd	Huntington
Campbell	Inclan
Codivilla	McMaster
Flanagan and Burem	Nicoli
Gillies	Phemister
Haldeman	Ryerson
Henderson	Soto-Hall
Henry	Wilson

Osteosyntheses: Internal Fixation Devices for Fracture Healing

Osteosynthesis is a surgical procedure that uses internal fixation devices, especially in the treatment of fractures. This procedure is referred to in context as open reduction and internal fixation (ORIF). It cannot be overemphasized how the orthopaedic surgeon must apply the principles of engineering to biology. The surgeon must be adept in using metal plates, nails, rods, pins, bands, screws, bolts, and staples in the correction of skeletal defects (Fig. 8-3). Pegging, pistoning, reefing, shelving, shaving down, shucking, doweling, and saucerization are a few of the shaping and engineering procedures applied within biologic principles. The following internal fixation devices are used or have been used in the past in orthopaedic surgery.

AO: abbreviation for designer of a variety of implant devices. The letters stand for *Arbeitsge-meinschaft für Osteosynthesefragen.*

ASIF: abbreviation for group that studies internal fixation systems and engineering. The letters stand for *Association for the Study of Internal Fixation.*

Asnis screw: for hip cervical fractures; a cannulated screw with reverse cutting thread.

Badgley nail: for hip fractures; an uncannulated triflanged nail with beveled proximal end that can be attached and inserted through a special side plate.

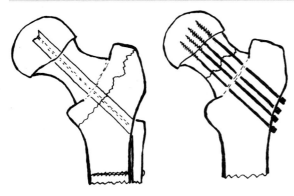

FIG 8-3 Two internal fixation devices for hip fractures.

Bailey-Dubow nail: for osteogenesis imperfecta; an extensible intramedullary nail used in osteotomies.

Basile screw: for hip cervical fractures; a drill point tip screw with pronged washer to be placed over trochanter for compression.

Benoit-Gerrard: for hip fractures; a spring-loaded sliding nail plate with a proximal outside thread, smooth shaft, and a side plate; provides continuous compression.

biodegradable fixation: a variety of screws, pins, plates, and other fixation devices made of material that will be absorbed by the body. Such materials include plastic made from single or combined glycolic acid, lactic acid, and other small organic acid capable of forming polymers.

blade plate: general class of plate fixation devices that has a right-angle or nearly right-angle flange.

Blount plate: for fixation of hip fractures and for reconstructive procedures about the hip; a blade plate that can be bent easily to adjust to the correct shape and angle.

Blount staple: type of staple used around the knee.

Bohler nail: for hip fractures; a triflanged nail with potential use of a side plate.

Bohlman pin: for hip fractures; a threaded pin with a sharp point and smooth proximal portion.

bollard: a short, flat-headed, nail-like device that is slotted along a portion of the shaft, used in fixation of ligaments into bone.

Boyd side plate: to help stabilize trochanteric portion of hip fracture; a plate that could be placed over plate of a Jewett nail.

Brooker-Willis nail: for unstable femoral fractures; a femoral nail with distal locking screws.

cable: typically a threaded wire that can be tightened around a piece of bone or the shaft of a bone to maintain apposition or prevent fracture propagation. Often used in association with hip prosthetic surgery.

Calandruccio device: a metallic device for pantalar fusions.

Calandruccio nail: for hip fractures; a sliding compression screw and plate associated with two to four smaller threaded pins through the plate and into the femoral head for extra fixation.

cancellous screw: used for trabecular problems near the joints, especially the hip.

cannulated nail/cannulated screw: general terms used for nails and screws that have a hole in the center. This hole can be used to direct the nail or screw over a guide wire.

Charnley screw: for intracapsular hip fractures and hip arthrodesis; a compression screw that slides into a barrel and attaches to a side plate.

cloverleaf nail: used in femoral shaft fractures.

cobra plate: plate that is shaped like the head of a cobra at the end of a plate used to hold the femur to the pelvis in hip fusion surgery.

Crawford-Adams pin: for hip fracture; use of small threaded pins.

cruciate screw: screw with cross-shaped head.

Delta nail: for femoral shaft fractures; a nearly triangular nail with interlocking screws.

Derby nail: for femoral shaft fracture; an intramedullary nail with wings that can be extended at the distal tip, and an antirotation washer at the proximal end.

Deyerle pin: for intracapsular hip fracture; thick, wide plate with multiple holes to permit the insertion of numerous pins parallel to one another.

dome plunger: device to facilitate injection of cement into femoral head for better fixation of sliding device.

Dooley nail: for intracapsular hip fractures; a modified Smith-Petersen nail that has an external groove around the base.

dynamic-compression plate (DCP): plate for fixation of long-bone fractures and osteotomies, with plate fixation designed to allow for compression from muscle and weight-bearing forces.

dynamic hip screw (DHS): for hip fractures; a sliding screw and plate device.

Eggers plate and screw: used in long-bone fractures.

elastic stable intramedullary nailing (ESIN): for fixation of femoral fractures in children; insertion of a highly elastic intramedullary nail that allows early protected weight-bearing.

Elliott plate: a type of blade plate used mostly in distal femoral procedures.

encerclage: wiring or banding of bony fragments in the shaft of a bone or for onlay grafts.

Ender nail: intramedullary nail that is curved and can be used to fix intertrochanteric hip fractures through a small incision just above the knee joint; used in a condylocephalic technique.

exchange nailing: use of a larger nail after failure of fixation or union with a smaller nail.

Gamma nail: for hip fractures; a sling screw and plate device.

Gaenslen spikes: for intracapsular hip fractures; smooth spikes driven from a small incision of greater trochanter.

Garden screws: for intracapsular hip fracture; large cannulated screws usually used in pairs and inserted at varus and valgus angles.

Giebel blade plate: blade plate with two screws for fixation of proximal tibial osteotomy.

Godoy-Moreira stud-bolt: for intracapsular hip fracture; an early model compression screw with external flange and bolt.

Gore AO screw: AO cortical bone screw modified to affix a ligament replacement implant.

Gouffon pin: pointed, threaded pin used in the fixation of cervical neck fractures of the hip.

grommet: a short, flat, hollow cylinder with a head. The device fits over a screw that is considerably narrower than the inner portion of the grommet. Used for fixation of ligaments into bone.

Gross-Kemph nail: for unstable femoral shaft fractures; an interlocking nail system.

GSH (Green-Seligson-Henry) nail: for supracondylar fractures; nail inserted through intercondylar notch.

GSU nail: for distal intra-articular fracture of femur; a retrograde nail inserted through joint with nail fixed by transcortical screw.

Haboush universal nail: for intracapsular hip fractures; a fenestrated plate with a shallow "H" cross section; inserted into head and neck of femur, and outside portion bent down over lateral side of femur.

Hagie pin: used for femoral neck fractures.

Hansen pin: for intracapsular hip fractures; use of nonthreaded, wide pins.

Hansen-Street nail: used for larger bone fractures.

Hardinge expansion bolt: for intracapsular hip fractures; a hollow screw with expandable tip and short side plate for femur.

Harrington rod: used in spinal fixation for scoliosis and some fractures.

Harris nail: intramedullary nail system for intertrochanteric fractures.

Henderson lag screw: used for hip fractures.

Herbert screw: for wrist scaphoid fixation; a short screw threaded at both ends; also used in fixation of other small bone fractures or osteotomies such as bunion surgery.

Hessel/Nystrom pins: threaded pin for internal fixation of femoral neck fractures.

hex screw: hexagon head screw.

Higley side plate: for hip fractures; a side plate that could be attached superiorly for screw fixation into greater trochanter.

Holt nail: for hip fractures; a one-piece nail-plate combination, with plate fixed by Barr nuts and bolts.

hook-pin fixation: for femoral neck fractures; a hollow nail has internal hooked pins that can be deployed into the femoral head after introduction of the nail.

Howmedica compression screw: for hip fractures; wide compression screw with side plate and hexagonal shape to cross-section of shaft and barrel to prevent rotation.

Hubbard side plate: for hip fractures; a wide, long femoral side plate designed to be used with triflanged nail.

Huckstep nail: for osteotomy of femur with limb lengthening; a nail with holes for cross-screw fixation.

intramedullary nail: class of nails placed in medullary canal of long bones for midshaft fractures; includes Hansen-Street, Küntscher, Lottes, and Schneider.

Inyo nail: for fractures of the distal fibula, a tapered V-shaped nail made of malleable stainless steel.

Jewett nail: nail plate used in hip fractures.

Johansson nail: for hip fractures; a triflanged nail that is cannulated and similar to a Smith-Petersen nail.

Ken nail: 135-degree sliding nail plate used for hip fractures.

Kirschner wire (K-wire): small wire used for fixation or traction.

Klemm nail: for femoral shaft fractures; a cloverleaf intramedullary nail with provision for proximal and distal screws.

Knowles pin: used for hip fractures.

Küntscher nail (rod): original form was a cloverleaf-shaped nail for simple shaft fractures of the femur. Subsequent modifications are a curved V-shaped nail for valgus reductions of intracapsular hip fractures; a self-locking "Y" device for hip fractures in which the hip nail has an open base for the passage of a cloverleaf intramedullary nail; and a device for unstable shaft fractures with interlocking proximal and distal screws.

Kurosaka screw: special screw designed for fixation of tendon attached to bone in ligament reconstruction.

lag screw: screw with threads at the tip only; used for compression.

Laing H-beam nail: for hip fractures; an H-shaped nail with an adjustable side angle plate.

Lane plate: plate for long-bone fixation.

Leinbach screw: long flexible screw; used often for olecranon fractures.

Lewis nail: intramedullary nail for metacarpal bone fixation.

limited-contact dynamic-compression plate (LC/DCP): plate for fixation of long-bone fractures and osteotomies in which there is only focal point of contact of the plate, with plate fixation designed to allow for compression from muscle and weight-bearing forces.

Lippman screw: for hip fractures; a threaded compression screw with a smooth shaft and threaded base with washer.

LISS plate: acronym for a *less invasive stabilization system* in which the screws are locked into the plate.

locked intramedullary osteosynthesis (LIFO): for unstable long-bone fractures; a set of flexible 4- or 5-mm diameter pins with a device for proximal interlocking and fixation of two of the pins.

Lorenzo screw: bone fixation screw.

Lottes nail: used for tibial fractures.

Luck nail: several different designs for hip fractures; triflanged nail in which the distal end has multiple perforations to cut off excess length, a proximal pointed nail that can accept a side plate, and a V-shaped nail-plate combination.

Lundholm screw: for hip fractures; compression screw with proximal washer and nut that could be used with or without side plate.

Mancini plate: for hip fractures; side plate with multiple-angled screw holes.

Martin screw: used in hip fractures.

Massie nail: 155-degree sliding nail used in hip fractures.

McLaughlin plate, screw: used in hip surgery.

Medoff sliding plate: for fixation of intertrochanteric and subtrochanteric femur fractures; plate is slotted to allow central portion to slide distally.

medullary rod: metallic device used in central shaft of bone.

Moe plate: for hip fractures; a long lateral plate over femoral shaft and greater trochanter fixed with multiple screws.

Moore plate (pin): used in hip surgery.

Morscher (AO-Morscher) plate: for anterior cervical fusion.

Müller plate: type of blade plate used in hip surgery.

Murphy nails: for early attempts at fixation of hip fractures; 8 to 12 penny nails inserted across fracture site.

Nancy nail: elastic stable intramedullary nails used for pediatric long-bone fractures.

nested nails: a general term for two nails placed side by side in the medullary canal of long bones.

Neufeld nail: for hip fractures in elderly; a V-shaped proximal end portion with short side plate.

Neufeld pin: for hip fractures; smooth rods with notches easily broken off to adjust length.

Ogden plate: for fixation of long-bone fractures associated with preexisting intramedullary devices such as rods or the stem of a prosthesis. Long metal plates have slots that are designed to accept encircling bands in locations where screws cannot be easily used.

olive wire: to help approximate a bone fragment in external skeletal fixation; a small olive-shaped expansion on a fixation wire can be pulled through the skin to the surface of the small fragment and brought against the main portion of bone.

Parham band: for oblique long-bone fractures; a metal band that can be tightened around the shaft of the bone to achieve fixation by compression.

Partridge band: for oblique long-bone fracture; a band with ribbed undersurface so that when band is tightened there might be less interference with periosteal and cortical blood flow.

PGP nail: a flexible nail used in intramedullary fixation of femoral fractures.

Phillips screw: any screw with a Phillips head.

Pidcock pin: for hip fractures; a small pin that could be passed through a hip nail and into the lateral cortex to prevent shortening.

Preston screw: for hip fractures; original screw and side plate device.

Pugh nail: 155-degree sliding nail used for hip fractures.

Putti screw: for hip fractures; a compression screw that can be attached to a flange and nut or to a Mancini plate.

Richard screw: for hip fractures; a sliding compression screw with side plate held by smaller screw to cortex.

Rush nail, rod, pin: used for major long-bone fractures.

Russell-Taylor nail: intramedullary nail for femur with slots for cross-screw fixation.

Rydell nails: for femoral neck fractures; a four-flanged spring-nail.

Sage rod: diamond-shaped rod used in forearm fractures.

Sarmiento nail: for hip fractures, an I-beam with side plate.

Schanz pins: for external skeletal fixators; screw fixation pins with proximal smooth surface for attachment to the fixation device.

Schneider nail, rod: used in femoral shaft fractures.

Seidel nail: for humeral fractures; a proximal and distal interlocking nail.

Sheffield rod: for osteogenesis imperfecta; an extensible intramedullary nail used for osteotomies.

Sherman plate: used for long-bone fractures.

slide plate: used for long-bone fractures.

Smillie nail: small pin used for attachment of the osteochondral fragments in the knee.

Smith-Petersen nail: flanged nail used in hip surgery.

Smyth pin: for hip fracture; attachment of two different sized, nonparallel screws through a plate over the greater trochanter.

Steinmann pin: used in skeletal traction; of larger caliber than a K-wire.

Street medullary pin: used for large long-bone fractures.

Street nail: split diamond nail for hip fixation.

Thompson nail: for nondisplaced intracapsular hip fractures; a Z-shaped nail.

Thornton nail: for femoral neck fractures; a three-flanged spring-nail.

tibial bolt: used for proximal and distal tibial fractures.

Tieman-Jewett nail: for hip fracture; a one-piece triflanged nail and side plate.

toggle: a small metallic cylinder with each end slightly larger than the center. Used by tying sutures around it to affix ligaments or tendons to bone.

Tronzo nail: triflanged nail used alone or with side plate.

True-Flex nail: for fixation of long-bone fractures; fluted intramedullary rods.

Uppsala screw: for intracapsular hip fracture; multiple, wide, threaded screws.

Venable screw: original vitallium screw.

Veseley-Street nail: for femoral shaft fractures; a splitting of a diamond nail both distally and proximally.

Virgin screw: for hip fractures; a compression screw using a proximal washer and spring.

von Bahr screw: for femoral neck fracture; a pin threaded at the tip for multiple screw fixation.

Watson Jones nail: for hip fractures; a triflanged nail with a small proximal pin through the nail and into lateral cortex.

Weiss spring: spring device used in some spinal fusions, particularly spondylolisthesis.

Williams nail: for hip fractures; a modified Küntscher cloverleaf "Y" nail using a locking nut to secure fixation.

Williams rod: for pediatric osteogenesis imperfecta deformity or congenital pseudarthrosis of tibia;

rod that is inserted through calcaneus into tibia after osteotomy.

Wilson plate: for spinal fusions.

Zickle nail: a curved 75- and 60-degree nail and screw device for femoral supracondylar fracture; or an intramedullary rod with transfixing nail for subtrochanteric fractures.

Zuelzer hook plate: commonly used in ankle fractures.

External Skeletal Fixation for Fractures

The use of external wires transfixed through bone to hold the position of a fracture is not new. Pins in plaster have been the usual method for holding bone fragments in proper position during the healing process. There has been increased use of multiple pins placed through one cortex or both cortices of bone and held by one external device. These external fixation devices are also known as **fixateurs** or **fixators.** This allows easy access to wounds, adjustment during the course of healing, and more functional use of limb involved. The devices used have increased in number and include the following.

Types by Configuration

articulating frame: designed to bridge across a joint and allow joint motion.

bilateral: fixation on both sides of bone, pins cross entire limb.

C-clamp: occasionally used for emergent treatment of pelvic fractures.

circular: circular plates that hold thin through-and-through wires under tension to hold fracture or osteotomy fragments.

hybrid: different techniques are combined such as the combination of a ring system with half pin fixation.

quadrilateral: fixation on both sides of bone, pins may or may not cross entire limb, quadrilateral configuration for stability.

semicircular: curved plates holding thin through-and-through wires under tension to hold fracture or osteotomy fragments.

triangular: fixation on both sides of bone, pins may or may not cross entire limb; triangular configuration for stability.

unilateral: fixation on one side of bone, pins do not cross entire limb.

Types by Design and Manufacture

Ace-Colles	Kronner-ring
Ace-Fischer	Monticelli-Spinelli
Calandruccio	Murray
DeBasitiani	Orthofix
Denham	Rezaian
Four-bar	Roger Anderson
Ganz	Slatis
Hex-Fix	Sukhtian-Hughes
Hoffman	Videl-Adrey
Hoffman-Vital	Volkov-Oganesyan
Hughes	Wagner
Ikuta	Wasserstein
Ilizarov	

Electric and Magnetic Stimulation of Fracture Healing

The use of direct electric currents and magnetic impulses in the treatment of fractures has been studied for the effect on fracture healing. In the past, the presence of nonunion (extended failure of fracture healing) has often required extensive surgical attention, including bone grafts. Electric and magnetic stimulation in treating fractures has been approved by the Food and Drug Administration for established nonunion of long bones.

capacitive coupling: application of high-frequency surface electrodes that create smaller currents that stimulate fracture healing.

direct electric stimulation: a procedure involving small voltage and amperage electric currents passed through electrodes placed immediately at the fracture site. The source of current is a battery placed external to the body or under the fat, similar to a cardiac pacemaker. For the external battery devices, the electrodes can be placed directly through the skin, eliminating the need for an incision. The limb involved is usually held in a cast.

magnetic stimulation: large magnetic coils applied externally and connected to a specific pulsating

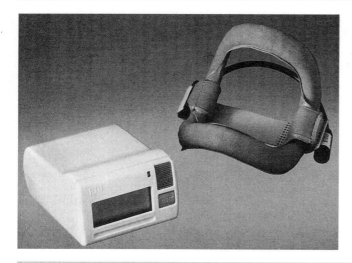

FIG 8-4 Saddle-shaped coil signal generation device. (Courtesy of EBI Medical Systems, Inc.)

current. The home treatment device, used to control the magnetic field, is a small box-like apparatus that is plugged into a standard 110-volt outlet; can be used up to 12 hours a day. As in electric stimulation, the affected limb is immobilized in a cast during the treatment period. Because pulsed electromagnetic fields are used, the abbreviation **PEMF** is often used (Fig. 8-4).

Internal Prostheses

Numerous devices composed mostly of alloys and plastic have been developed to aid in joint replacement efforts. Prosthetic replacements are now available for almost every joint in the body, and even a spinal segment can now be replaced. This field continues to rapidly expand, with a constant influx of new components and the outdating of others. Each is listed in the appropriate section by anatomy. Many of the prostheses listed may already be or soon will be obsolete. They are mentioned because they will still be found in some patients in the future and in their records. Chapter 13 discusses research efforts in internal prostheses.

The advent of a polymer called **methylmethacrylate** led to the development of new types of devices held firmly in place by polymers (glue). It is a cement-like substance that forms no chemical bonds but instead holds components to bones by space filling and locking effects. When applied, methylmethacrylate is soft and pliable, but it becomes very hard and firm within 15 minutes. Problems encountered with this method prompted further research and improvement in the development of joint resurfacing techniques.

The "cement" technique was originally a finger-packing process that was eventually called **first-generation technique.** The use of a "gun," a cement-holding device similar to a caulking gun, was used in the **second-generation technique.** The use of a vacuum to help remove bubbles from the cement, and thus strengthening the eventual cement construct, has been referred to as **third-generation cement technique.**

All internal prosthetic devices wear. The result is the production of microscopic particles that eventually cause a cellular response that leads to bone absorption and prosthetic loosening. The terminology for general material applications for all prosthetics is listed here.

adhesive wear: to the most common cause of polyethylene wear in hip replacement, microscopic size particle release into joint due to the tendency for adhesion between the opposing surfaces.

alumina: ceramic material used for total joints.

annealing: heating below the temperature of ultra high molecular weight polyethylene (UHMWPE).

beaded: tiny cobalt chrome beads bonded to surface of implants for bone ingrowth.

BFH: *b*ig *f*emoral *h*ead technology starting with 36-mm size and larger.

CAOS: computerized aided orthopaedic surgery. The design is to assist in accurate placement of prosthetic components.

cast components: larger grain size and softer.

ceramic-ceramic: bearing consisting of two like ceramics articulating with each other. Concern is bearing fracture.

crevice corrosion: breakdown of the metal that affects the grain structure, which ultimately leads to failure of the implant.

cross-linked UHMWPE: increased radiation to 10 megarads and elimination of free radicals causes cross linking of polyethylene for greater wear.

fibermetal: microtubular-like titanium coating of prostheses for bone ingrowth fixation.

forged components: smaller grain size and greater hardness.

fretting corrosion: corrosion occurring at the junction of two metal interlocking parts that have micromotion.

hemiarthroplasty: only one articular surface is replaced, leaving the native joint on the opposite side.

hybrid fixation: the use of cement fixation for one component of a total joint and bone ingrowth for the other component.

hypersensitivity reaction: allergic reaction related to metal ions that become attached to haptanes.

keel: portion of prosthesis, typically a tibial tray that has flanges that extend into the metaphysis.

metal-metal: bearing consisting of two metal surfaces articulating with each other. Concern is metal ion levels in blood.

micromotion: when applied to implants, motion of 28–50 μm, which allow for bone ingrowth.

minimally invasive surgery (MIS): procedures done through smaller incisions.

modular components (modularity): many prosthetic components, particularly the femoral components of hip replacements, have different sized interlocking parts to allow for different sizes and shapes of the femur.

oxidized zirconium: surface treatment that likely reduces surface wear of ceramic.

polymethylmethacrylate (PMMA): a relatively fast setting plastic that acts as grouting agent in the fixation of prosthetic components.

press fit: design to have a firm fixation based on firm abutment against three points of bone canal margins. Typically these have porous coats for bone ingrowth.

prosthesis of antibiotic-loaded acrylic cement (PROSTALAC): facsimile of a total hip prosthesis that has a very thin polyethylene acetabular cup that is loosely cemented.

remelting: heating above the melting temperature of ultra high molecular weight polyethylene (UHMWPE).

resurfacing arthroplasty: used mostly in hips, conserves the femoral head and neck by using a thin-walled acetabular component with typically metal on metal components.

salvage procedure: descriptive of revision procedures with innovative approaches to large bone defects or other anatomic loss.

stress shielding: although more commonly applied to prosthetic devices, this term is applied to the effect of any implant in which there is loss of bone integrity due to the biologic bone absorption secondary to the shield of stress by the implant.

stripe wear: caused by edge-loading of ceramic during stair climbing.

tantalum: a highly porous material with elastic modulus closer to bone allowing for initial stability.

taper: rounded top of the femoral stem component; designed as a slightly tapered cylinder that will accept a similarly "female"-shaped portion of the femoral head, which come in various sizes.

> *Eurotaper (12/14):* taper designed with a 12-mm tip and 14-mm base.

> *Morse taper:* specific type of taper used to accept femoral head component on the stem component.

third-generation ceramic: small grain size with increased density and each prosthesis proof tested to reduce likelihood of fracture.

third-body wear: wear due to particle of cement or metal between bearing surfaces.

total joint replacement: both articular surfaces are replaced with a prosthetic component.

two-body abrasive wear: hard surface on opposing soft surface wear.

zirconium: ceramic material used for total joints.

Arthro- (Joints)

Anatomy of Joints (Fig. 8-5)

bursa sac: helps tendons and muscles to glide easily over bones at the joint outside the synovial fluid.

capsule: the general fibrous and ligamentous tissues that act as encasements and enclose the immediate joint area.

cartilage: the strong smooth covering at the ends of the articular surface of bone. In highly mobile joints like the wrist, fingers, and elbows this cartilage is called *hyaline.* In less mobile segments, such as the intervertebral disk, *fibrocartilage* is present.

meniscus: in the knee, a crescent-shaped fibrocartilaginous disk between the two joint surfaces. There are other menisci and meniscal-like structures in the body. The medial and lateral menisci of the knee receive the most surgical attention.

subchondral bone: named for the bone immediately next to the joint cartilage. Also called **subchondral plate.**

synovium: inner lining of a joint cavity that is a one- or two-layer cell membrane (*synovial membrane*) on a bed of fat. The synovial membrane normally produces and absorbs a clear synovial fluid, which lubricates and feeds cartilage surfaces.

Types of Joints

Joints are the places of union between two or more bones. All joints are not alike in structure and fall into the following categories according to function.

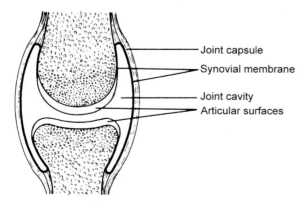

Joint capsule

Synovial membrane

Joint cavity

Articular surfaces

FIG 8-5 Typical structure of diarthrotic joint. (From Hilt NE, Cogburn SB: *Manual of orthopedics,* St Louis, 1980, CV Mosby.)

ball-and-socket j.: main points of articulation; femur to acetabulum of hip, humerus to glenoid of shoulder.

hinge j.: located in the elbows, fingers, and knees.

immovable j.: of orthopaedic concern, in the symphysis pubis and sacroiliac region.

synovial j.: two bones connected by fibrous tissue (capsules) with space between them and lined with synovial membrane.

weight-bearing j.: located in the lower spine, hips, knees, and ankles.

General Surgery of Joints

arthrectomy: excision of a joint.

arthrocentesis: needle puncture and aspiration of fluid from a joint.

arthroclisis: surgical breaking down of an ankylosis to secure free movement of a joint.

arthrodesis: a procedure to remove the cartilage of any joint to encourage bones of that joint to fuse, or grow together, where motion is not desired, for example, the spine. Also, an external fusion of a joint by means of a bone graft. The many types of arthrodeses are listed separately.

arthroereisis: a procedure to limit abnormal motion in a joint. Could be in any joint, but frequently referred to in the foot.

arthrogram: radiographic examination of the joint performed with radiopaque solution; commonly done on the shoulder, hip, and knee joints.

arthrokleisis: ankylosis of a joint by closure; production of such ankylosis.

arthrolysis: loosening adhesions in an ankylosed joint to restore mobility.

arthroplasty: reconstructive surgery of a joint or joints to restore motion because of ankylosis or trauma or to prevent excessive motion. This repair and reconstruction may use silicone, metallic, or other implants.

arthroscopy (arthroendoscopy) (Fig. 8-6): a surgical examination of the interior of a joint and evaluation of joint disease by the insertion of an optic device capable of providing an external view of the internal joint area. This technique represents a major advance in orthopaedic technology during the past two decades. The optical system is fiberoptic, giving the surgeon a high-resolution view of a

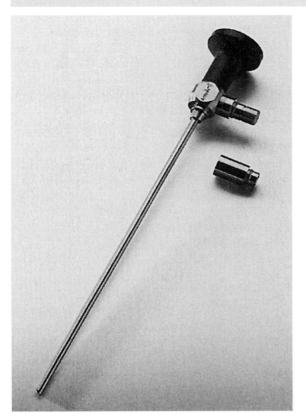

FIG 8-6 Arthroscope outside of sleeve that is used during surgery; close-up view of 30-degree angle for viewing difficult to see areas. (Wide-angle arthroscope, 4-mm diameter, 30-degree angle optic. Courtesy of Arthrex, Inc., Naples, FL.)

arthrotomy: surgical incision into a joint for exploration and removal of joint material; usually refers to knee exploration but can apply to any joint.

arthroxesis: scraping of diseased tissue from the articular surface of bone.

Arthrodeses

Three Basic Categories of Arthrodeses

compression: a general class of arthrodeses in which the pins on either side of the joint have some external compression device; the appliance is removed after fusion takes place.

extra-articular: fusion of the joint outside the joint capsule; rarely used.

intra-articular: fusion of a joint all within its capsule, with or without intra-articular bone grafts.

Specific Arthrodeses

Abbott-Fisher-Lucas: two-stage hip fusion that includes a delayed femoral osteotomy.

Baciu and Filibiu: intra-articular ankle fusion using dowel bone graft taken from the joint to include the medial and a portion of the lateral malleolus. The graft is rotated 90 degrees and reinserted.

Badgley: intra-articular and extra-articular hip fusion, using anterior iliac crest of bone.

Blair: a tibiotalar fusion, using an anterior sliding tibial graft.

Bosworth: a method of fusing the hip following tuberculosis infection.

Brett: extra-articular shoulder fusion, using tibial graft.

Brittain: four procedures have this name: (1) intra-articular knee fusion using anterior tibial grafts, (2) extra-articular hip fusion requiring a subtrochanteric osteotomy and tibial bone graft, (3) extra-articular graft to the medial side of the humerus of shoulder, and (4) intra-articular fusion of the elbow, using two crossed intraosseous grafts.

Campbell: extra-articular fusion of the ankle and subtalar joint.

Chandler: intra-articular and extra-articular hip fusion, using the deep portion of the greater trochanter.

Charnley: intra-articular type of ankle or knee fusion, using a temporary metallic external compression clamp.

Charnley and Henderson: intra-articular and extra-articular fusion of the shoulder, using the

joint, anywhere from a direct forward view to a view at 70 degrees to the end of the microscope, allowing the surgeon literally to see around corners. The arthroscopes vary in diameter from 2.7 to 5.0 mm. Miniature television cameras are attached directly to the arthroscope, allowing all operating room personnel to view the interior joint.

With the advancement of arthroscopic surgery, a wide variety of instruments has made it possible to remove synovium and plicas, repair peripheral tears, excise meniscal tissue, remove loose bodies, shave cartilage, and do many other procedures. The knee receives the most attention in arthroscopic procedures; however, the arthroscope is now used in ankle, shoulder, elbow, wrist, and other joint surgery.

glenoid and acromial surface abutting a split humeral head.

Chuinard and Petersen: of the ankle, using a wedge of iliac bone.

Compere and Thompson fusion: intra-articular hip fusion, using iliac crest and wing for bone graft.

Davis: intra-articular and extra-articular hip fusion, accomplished by using a live pedicle of iliac crest.

Ghormley: intra-articular and extra-articular hip fusion, using anterior iliac crest graft.

Gill: extra-articular and intra-articular fusion, using acromion bone graft from and to the shoulder.

Henderson: intra-articular and extra-articular hip fusion, using detached iliac cortical bone graft.

Hibbs: intra-articular and extra-articular hip fusion, using greater trochanter as a graft.

Horwitz and Adams: ankle fusion, using the distal fibula as a graft.

Key: knee fusion, using anterior inlay bone graft.

Kickaldy and Willis: intra-articular and extra-articular hip fusion, using iliac crest bone from the ischium to the inferior neck.

King procedure: intra-articular hip fusion, using iliac and tibial bone grafts.

Kuntscher modified: knee arthrodesis, using a bridging intramedullary rod.

Lucas and Murray: knee fusion, using patella for bone graft and held by an internal plate.

Marcus, Balourdas, Heiple: chevron-shaped tibiotalar fusion, using inlay graft taken from medial and lateral malleolus.

Müller: intra-articular shoulder fusion, using bent plates for fixation.

Potter: knee fusion, using a retrograde tibial rod and graft from the distal tibia.

Putti: (1) knee fusion, using anterior tibial graft; (2) extra-articular fusion, using the acromion of the scapula; (3) an intra-articular fusion of the shoulder.

Schneider: intra-articular hip fusion, using innominate osteotomy with greater trochanter for a bone graft.

sliding: anterior ankle fusion, using tibial bone.

Smith-Petersen: technique for fusion of the sacroiliac joint.

Stamm procedure: intra-articular hip fusion, using free iliac crest bone grafts.

Staples: intra-osseous and extra-osseous elbow fusion.

Steindler: intra-articular fusion of the shoulder or the elbow, using posterior bone graft.

Stewart and Harley procedure: for fusion of ankle, using lateral and medial malleoli as grafts.

Stone: intra-articular hip fusion, using a split acetabulum and bent plate from the ilium to the femoral neck.

Trumble: extra-articular hip fusion, using a tibial graft from the ischium to the femur.

Watson-Jones: intra-articular and extra-articular hip fusion, using a nail and iliac crest graft; also, a shoulder fusion, using a piece of acromion.

White: intra-articular hip arthrodesis, using posterolateral approach and iliac bone graft.

Wilson procedure: extra-articular fusion of the elbow.

Wolf blade plate: ankle arthrodesis performed with a specifically designed blade plate internal fixation device.

John C. Wilson: intra-articular and extra-articular hip fusion, using an iliac side graft.

Chondro- (Cartilage)

Cartilage (L. gristle) is a fine, glistening, resilient, *nonvascular fibrous connective* tissue that absorbs shock and facilitates the mechanics of joint motion. All mobile joint surfaces contain cartilage. *Perichondrium* is a connective tissue that covers cartilage in some places. Cartilage cells (*chondrocytes*) are widely separated and surrounded by matrix, also (*chondromucoid*) known as ground substance, composed of collagen and mucopolysaccharides. In the embryo, cartilage forms the temporary skeleton and is important to growth in providing the model in which most of the bones develop. Then, it is called ossifying or precursory cartilage.

Cartilage cannot be seen on radiographs; if open space is apparent between two bones on radiography, cartilage is present. However, if the radiograph shows two bones touching at a joint, such as the femur on the tibia, osteoarthritis and dissolution of the cartilage in that joint may have occurred.

Types of Cartilage

articular c.: thin layer of hyaline cartilage on articular surface of bones in synovial joints; **arthrodial c.**

calcified c.: in which granules of calcium phosphate and calcium carbonate are deposited in interstitial substance.

cellular c.: composed almost entirely of cells with little interstitial substances.

connecting c.: connects surfaces of an immovable joint; **interosseous c.**

diarthrodial c.: articular c.

elastic c.: yellow opaque flexible substance (more so than hyaline) in which cells are surrounded by a territorial capsular matrix, outside of which is an interterritorial matrix containing elastic fiber networks, collagen fibers, and ground substance; **reticular c., yellow c.**

fibrocartilage: contains Types I and II collagen fibers with a strongly basophilic ground substance in area of chondrocytes.

floating c.: detached piece of cartilage on medial or lateral condyle of femur or on patella.

hyaline c.: somewhat elastic, semitransparent cartilage, characterized by type II collagen and proteoglycan aggrecans. Seen in movable joint surfaces and the physis (growth plate).

Surgical Procedures on Cartilage

articular cartilage implant (ACI), articular cartilage transfer (ACT): cells harvested from a non-weight-bearing portion of the joint are suspended in cell culture for cell division. Weeks later, the expanded mass of cells are placed in the defect with a covering of neighboring periosteum.

chondrectomy: surgical removal of cartilage.

chondrodiastasis: for limb-length discrepancy; closed, gradual, and progressive distraction of the growth plate by using an external bone fixation device.

chondroplasty: plastic surgery on cartilage by repair of lacerated or displaced cartilage.

chondrosternoplasty: surgical correction of funnel chest.

chondrotomy: dissection or surgical division of cartilage.

  synchondrotomy: incision and division of an articulation that has no appreciable mobility and in which cartilage is the intervening connective tissue.

mosaicplasty: removal of plugs of cartilage and bone from a limited weight-bearing portion of the joint to be placed in the area of a defect.

shell osteochondral allograft: donor intact cartilage and subchondral bone is harvested from the same location as similar-sized donor and implanted in defect site. The term "shell" refers to the relatively thin 5-mm shell of bone that distinguishes this procedure from larger bony segments.

Capsulo- (Capsule)

A capsule is the circumferential sleeve surrounding a joint composed of a tough band of fibrous and ligamentous tissues. It may be referred to as a joint capsule or a capsular ligament.

Surgical Procedures on the Capsule

capsulectomy: excision of a joint capsule; most commonly done on the hip.

capsulodesis: imbrication of a capsule (see Chapter 10).

capsuloplasty: plastic surgery on a joint capsule.

capsulorrhaphy: suturing of a joint capsule. If used by itself, the term implies a procedure on the shoulder (glenohumeral joint) because this joint commonly has soft tissue reconstructions.

capsulotomy: incision into a joint capsule; **capsotomy.**

Bursae

A bursa (sac or sac-like cavity) is filled with viscid fluid and situated in places in tissue where friction would otherwise develop. Bursae act as cushions, relieving pressure between moving parts such as an **anserine bursa,** a goose-foot sac found between tendons of the sartorius, gracilis, and semitendinous muscles and the tibial collateral ligament. A bursal sac is easily recognized during surgery and is involved in only three procedures.

bursectomy: excision of a bursa.

bursocentesis: puncture and removal of fluid from a bursa.

bursotomy: incision into a bursa.

Other Specific Tissue(s)

The entire musculoskeletal system is made up of connective tissues, that is, cell elements that establish structure and shape. Bones and joints receive the most attention in orthopaedic surgery and therefore are listed separately.

All connective tissues have, to some degree, cohesion that is supplied by a protein structure called **collagen.** Collagen, in its most familiar form, is a household product, gelatin. However, when combined with other chemical and cell elements, it is the basic molecular matrix of bone, cartilage, tendons, and many other tissues. The connective tissue cells are the following.

adipose tissue: fatty tissue.
chondroblasts: cells that form cartilage.
chondroclasts: cells that remove cartilage.
chondrocytes: cartilage cells.
fibroblasts: cells that predominantly form collagen.
fibrocytes: cells seen in tendons, ligaments, and similar structures.
histiocytes: cells involved in removal of cellular or chemical debris; a type of phagocyte.
myoblasts: muscle-forming cells.
myocytes: muscle cells, voluntary (striated) and involuntary (nonstriated).

Myo- (Muscle) (Fig. 8-7)

Muscle is the contractile tissue essential for skeletal support and movement. The anatomic features of muscles with associated tissues and surgery are presented here.

Muscle fibers are composed of small bundles of cells combined to form distinct muscular units. Terms often related to muscle include actin, myosin, sarcomere, nerve spindle, motor unit, neuromuscular junction, and spindle cell.

The smooth coordinated way in which muscles work together in the execution of a movement is called **synergy** (syn- [together] plus ergon- [work]). In particular, the muscles that play the part of **synergists** during any particular movement are concerned with obviating any unwanted movement that might result from the action of the **prime movers** or **agonists**. Muscles that pull in the opposite direction are called **antagonists**. Synergist muscles are usually classified as **corrective** if they obviate such unwanted movements, and **fixative** if they fix the point proximal to that at which the movement is taking place. **Muscle insertion** is the attachment of a muscle or its tendon to the part of the skeleton that the muscle moves when it contracts. **Muscle origin** is a fixed attachment or anchor of muscle allowing a muscle to exert power when it contracts. The many muscle groups are named and illustrated in Figure 8-7.

Surgical Procedures on Muscles

myectomy: excision of a portion of muscle.
myoclasis: intentional crushing of muscle; rare.
myomectomy (myomatectomy): surgical removal of tumors with muscular tissue components (myoma).
myoneurectomy: surgical interruption of nerve fibers supplying specific muscles; used for patients with cerebral palsy.
myoplasty: plastic surgery on muscle in which portions of partly detached muscle are used for correction of defects or deformities.
myorrhaphy (myosuture): muscle repair by suture of divided muscle.
myotenontoplasty: surgical fixation of muscles and tendons.
myotenotomy: surgical division of a tendon from muscle.
myotomy: incision or dissection of muscle or muscular tissue.

Aponeuroses

Aponeurosis is the name given to the end of a muscle that becomes a tendon. This muscular component is a white, flattened, ribbon-like tendon expansion that connects muscle with the parts it moves.

Surgical Procedures on Aponeuroses

aponeurectomy: excision of the aponeurosis.
aponeurorrhaphy: repair and suture of muscle and tendon; **fasciorrhaphy.**
aponeurotomy: surgical incision into the aponeurosis.

Teno- (Tendons)

The extension of muscle into a firm, fibrous cord that attaches into a bone or other firm structure is a tendon. Some muscles have a tendon at both ends, some have direct attachment to bone at one end, and a few attach directly to bone at both ends and have no tendon.

A **common tendon** serves more than one muscle; such as a **conjoined tendon** that is found in the inguinal region. The tendons that receive the most attention are the following:

Achilles t.: the common tendon of the gastrocnemius and soleus muscle inserted into the medial posterior surface of the calcaneus; **calcaneal t.** or **tendocalcaneus, heel t.**

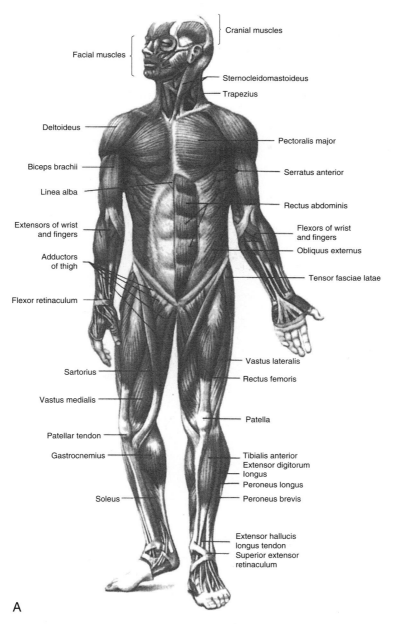

Cranial muscles

Facial muscles

Sternocleidomastoideus

Trapezius

Deltoideus

Pectoralis major

Biceps brachii

Serratus anterior

Linea alba

Rectus abdominis

Extensors of wrist
and fingers

Flexors of wrist
and fingers

Obliquus externus

Adductors
of thigh

Tensor fasciae latae

Flexor retinaculum

Vastus lateralis

Sartorius

Rectus femoris

Vastus medialis

Patella

Patellar tendon

Gastrocnemius

Tibialis anterior
Extensor digitorum
longus
Peroneus longus

Soleus

Peroneus brevis

Extensor hallucis
longus tendon
Superior extensor
retinaculum

A

FIG 8-7 Muscular system, **A,** Anterior view.

(*Continued*)

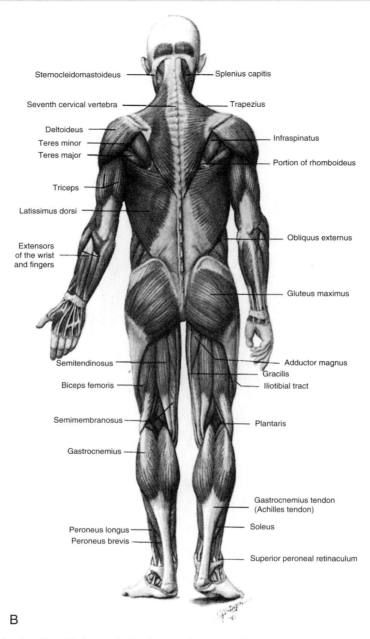

FIG 8-7 Cont'd. B, Posterior view. (From *Mosby's medical and nursing dictionary*, ed 2, St Louis, 1986, CV Mosby.)

hamstring t.: one of the tendons that bind the popliteal fossa laterally and medially. The inner hamstring includes tendons of the gracilis and sartorius muscles, and the outer hamstring is the tendon of the biceps flexor femoris muscle.

patellar t.: anterior or inferior ligamentum patellae.

Sharpey fibers: fibers of a tendon attached to bone that actually penetrate the periosteum and cortex of bone, and thus make a very strong attachment.

Surgical Procedures on Tendons

The nomenclature of surgical procedures on tendons has a certain amount of overlap, because several prefixes are used—teno-, tendo-, and tendino-. Therefore, the same surgical procedure may have several forms of spelling. The preferred term for a surgical procedure is listed first, with the related term appearing after the definition.

tendon release: surgical transection of a tendon, with or without repair.

tenectomy: excision of a lesion (ganglion or xanthoma) of a tendon or of a tendon sheath.

tenodesis: tendon fixation by suturing proximal end of a tendon to the bone or by reattachment of the tendon to another site.

tenolysis: surgically freeing a tendon from adhesions; **tendolysis.**

tenomyoplasty: procedure involving repair of tendon and muscle; **tenontomyoplasty.**

tenomyotomy: excision of a portion of tendon and muscle.

tenonectomy: excision of a portion of tendon with or without excision of a portion of tendon to shorten it.

tenontomyotomy: incision into the principal tendon of a muscle, with partial or complete excision of that muscle.

tenoplasty: surgical repair of a ruptured tendon; **tendoplasty, tendinoplasty, tenontoplasty.**

tenorrhaphy: union of a divided tendon by a suture; **tenosuture, tendinosuture.**

tenosuspension: surgical repair that fashions a soft tissue sling to hold the tendon in a specific place.

tenosynovectomy: resection or excision of excessive synovial lining within the tendon sheath.

tenotomy: incomplete or complete division of a tendon, as in clubfoot; **tendotomy.**

Desmo- (Ligaments)

Ligaments are bands of strong fibrous connective tissue that bind together the articular ends of bones and cartilage at the joints to facilitate or limit motion. Also, they give support and attachment to fascia, viscera, and muscles. An **accessory ligament** is one that supports another ligament on the lateral surface outside the joint capsule where excessive motion occurs. In the knee, elbow, and wrist, the **medial, lateral,** and **collateral ligaments** provide additional support. There are many others, but the knee receives the most attention. Because ligaments tie bones together, the prefix syn- (together) is used with desmo (ligament) for ligament surgery. **Syndesmosis** is the name for an articulation in which the bones are united by ligaments (e.g., the distal tibiofibular articulation).

Surgical Procedures on Ligaments

desmotomy: surgical division of a ligament or ligaments.

syndesmectomy: excision of a ligament or portion thereof.

syndesmopexy: surgical fixation of a dislocation by using the ligaments of a joint.

syndesmoplasty: ligaments sutured together.

syndesmorrhaphy: suture or repair of ligaments.

syndesmotomy: dissection or cutting of ligaments.

Fasciae

Fasciae (pronounced fash'-e-e) (fascia, sing.) are sheets of dense connective fibrous tissue that act as a restricting envelope for muscular components and bind groups of muscles, blood vessels, and nerves into bundles. Generally, the fascia does not play any role in the movement of joints and bones. The exception to this is the **fascia lata** of the outer thigh; this fascia has its own muscle (**tensor fascia lata**) that, when tightened, will pull through the fascia to points across the knee.

Surgical Procedures on Fasciae

fasciaplasty: plastic surgery of fascia; **fascioplasty.**

fasciectomy: excision of strips of fascia.

fasciodesis: suturing a fascia to another fascia or tendon.

fasciorrhaphy: suturing and repair of lacerated fascia; **aponeurorrhaphy.**

fasciotomy: surgical incision or transection of fascia, commonly done for forearm and leg injuries, in which the pressure in the compartment surrounded by the fascia has become very high.

Neuro- (Nerves)

Nerves are cord-like structures that convey impulses between a part of the central nervous system and some other region of the body. Structural components of the nerves include epineurium, perineurium, nerve sheath, axon, Schwann cell, and myelin. **Innervation** refers to the nerve supply to any tissue. Nerves are usually named for the anatomic area involved. Hilton law states that a nerve trunk that supplies any joint supplies the muscles moving that joint and the area over the skin over that joint.

Orthopaedic Surgical Procedures on Nerves

Mellesi cable graft: for neuroma excision and replacement with grafts of specific length of fascicular gap.

neurectomy: resection of a segment of a nerve.

neurolysis: destruction of a perineural adhesion by a longitudinal incision to release the nerve sheath.

neuroplasty: plastic repair of a nerve.

neurorrhaphy: suture of a severed nerve; repair.

neurotomy: division of a nerve or nerves.

neurotripsy: surgical crushing of a nerve.

rhizotomy (radicotomy, radiculectomy): procedure dividing the nerve roots close to their origin from the spinal cord; rhizo- refers to root of the spinal cord.

Vascular (Blood Vessels) System
(Fig. 8-8)

There are thousands of miles of blood vessels in the human body and approximately 2000 gallons of blood per day coursing through these vessels, likened to a road map with its major arteries, tributaries, and branches. The **arteries** are the major pipelines that distribute oxygenated blood from the heart to the various organs.

In each group, the main artery resembles a tree trunk that gives off numerous branches and these branch forming smaller vessels called **arterioles,** which branch again forming microscopic vessels called **capillaries.**

The **veins** are an extension of the capillaries in that capillaries unite into vessels of increasing size to form **venules** and eventually **veins.** Their function is to carry deoxygenated blood from the various organs back to the heart. Veins differ from arteries in that they have **valves** that create a unidirectional flow. Arteries and veins often have the same name for their location in the body, for example, femoral artery and femoral vein. The following terms relate to blood vessels.

adventitia: loose outer lining of a blood vessel; outermost wall of artery.

artery: blood vessel that carries oxygenated blood away from heart on its way to various organs and tissues in the body.

arterioles: smallest vessels considered arteries (0.2 mm diameter) made mostly of smooth muscle; blood flows through arterioles and moves to capillaries.

capillaries: tiny network of blood vessels supplying oxygen directly to cells of body. At this level, oxygen and other nutrients are delivered to cells, and carbon dioxide and waste materials are passed from the tissues back to the bloodstream.

cardiovascular: pertaining to blood vessels (arteries and veins) and the heart.

cerebrovascular: pertaining to blood vessel circulation of the brain and to the brain.

collateral circulation: named and unnamed secondary vessels supplying blood to an organ or extremity through indirect channels. These collateral vessels become particularly important when the main artery is damaged (occluded), for example, genicular arteries around the knee in support of an occluded popliteal artery.

diastole: filling or relaxation phase of the heart cycle.

intima: the innermost lining of the arterial wall.

lipid: one of many chemical compounds normally found in blood that are considered fats and have a relationship between the amount and kinds of lipids in the blood and hardening of the arteries.

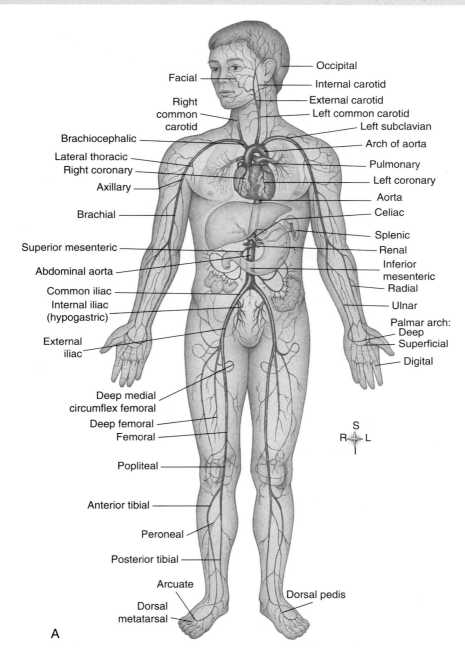

FIG 8-8 A, The arteries of the body distribute oxygenated blood from the heart to the body. The name of each artery corresponds to the organ or region served. The pulmonary arteries pumps deoxygenated blood to the lung.

(*Continued*)

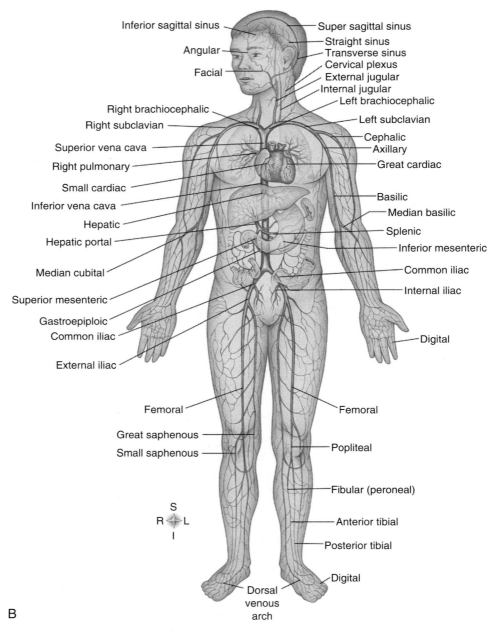

Inferior sagittal sinus

Angular

Facial

Right brachiocephalic
Right subclavian
Superior vena cava
Right pulmonary
Small cardiac
Inferior vena cava
Hepatic
Hepatic portal
Median cubital
Superior mesenteric
Gastroepiploic
Common iliac
External iliac

Femoral
Great saphenous
Small saphenous

Super sagittal sinus
Straight sinus
Transverse sinus
Cervical plexus
External jugular
Internal jugular
Left brachiocephalic
Left subclavian
Cephalic
Axillary
Great cardiac
Basilic
Median basilic
Splenic
Inferior mesenteric
Common iliac
Internal iliac

Digital

Femoral
Popliteal
Fibular (peroneal)
Anterior tibial
Posterior tibial
Digital

Dorsal venous arch

S
R L
I

B

FIG 8-8 Cont'd. B, The major veins are named to correspond to the regions of the body they drain: blood is returned by these veins to the heart. The oxygenated blood returns to the heart via the pulmonary vein. (From Thibodeau and Patton: *Anatomy and physiology,* ed 6, St Louis, 2006, Mosby.)

lumen: the space inside a blood vessel, duct, or hollow viscus.

patency: refers to an open blood vessel (artery or vein) in which blood is flowing.

systole: contraction phase of cardiac cycle.

vascular: pertaining to vessels. Can also refer to amount of blood supply to an organ, such as a very vascular tumor, that is, good blood supply.

vein: blood vessel that carries blood from the various organs in the body back to the heart. Veins usually have valves creating a unidirectional flow, whereas arteries do not. Small veins are then called **venules.**

vena cava: either of the two main veins that convey blood from other veins to the right atrium of the heart.

Vascular Surgical Procedures (Arteries/Veins)

Peripheral vascular surgery procedures center around the treatment of disorders of the blood vessels, that is, the arteries and veins (not including the heart), and may be performed in conjunction with orthopaedic procedures, such as the repair of a disrupted popliteal artery following knee dislocation. An understanding of peripheral vascular surgery is also necessary in diagnosing patients with vascular disease who come to the orthopaedic surgeon. For example, a patient may see an orthopaedic surgeon for a painful foot believing it to be a bony problem, only to find it is "rest pain" from occluded arteries in the thigh and calf. In this case, the patient is referred to the vascular surgeon for further evaluation and treatment. Because these two specialties overlap in diagnosis, treatment, and surgery, vascular procedures are included for reference.

Most peripheral vascular surgical procedures performed today are done to correct the problem of arteriosclerosis (hardening of the arteries). In this regard, the problems can usually be corrected by a bypass, by replacing the artery, or by cleaning it out (endarterectomy). The terms relating to blood vessel surgery follow.

aortofemoral bypass (AFB): surgical procedure whereby the narrowing or occlusion of the abdominal aorta and iliac arteries (from arteriosclerosis) is bypassed with a graft (usually Dacron) going from just below the renal arteries down to the femoral arteries in the groins. This is considered one of the bigger vascular procedures, requiring opening the abdomen (taking from 3 to 6 hours). Separate bypass grafts may be taken off the main aortofemoral graft to increase the blood supply to the kidneys, intestines, or pelvic viscera to include the male genitalia.

aortoiliac bypass: a bypass graft going from just below the renal artery down to the iliac arteries. This procedure is usually performed for abdominal aortic aneurysms (AAAs).

aneurysmorrhaphy: a repair of an aneurysm in which it is left in place, but disconnected from the circulation, and a graft is sewn in its place. Following this, the aneurysm wall can either be wrapped around the graft or left in place. (Totally removing the aneurysm is rarely done because it may jeopardize adjacent organs.)

arthrectomy catheter (Simpson): a vascular procedure for a localized endarterectomy in which a device is passed percutaneously or intraoperatively to an area of stenosis, using a small circular knife blade.

autogenous saphenous vein graft (ASVG): the greater saphenous vein of the lower extremity is removed and used to either bypass or replace a diseased segment of artery or vein elsewhere in the body. When the vein is removed and placed in a different location, care must be taken to ensure that the valves of the vein are either destroyed or that the vein is put in a reversed fashion so that the arterial blood will flow unimpeded.

axillofemoral bypass (AxFem): an extra-anatomic bypass whereby either Dacron or polytetrafluoroethylene (PTFE) graft is used to carry blood from the axillary artery (under the arm) down to one or both common femoral arteries. This procedure is usually performed in lieu of an aortofemoral bypass because the abdomen is inaccessible resulting from infection in the abdomen, for example, infected aortofemoral graft, severe cardiac disease, or severe pulmonary disease. The patency rate for these grafts is not nearly as good as that for a usual aortofemoral bypass graft.

balloon angioplasty: a procedure whereby a balloon catheter is passed up to an area of stenosis in an artery to widen vessel, a balloon is inflated, and the area of the stenosis (stricture) is dilated. This procedure is augmented by adding a stent or wire mesh inside the artery to support the dilated segment; **percutaneous transluminal angioplasty (PTA).**

carotid endarterectomy: an opening up and cleaning out of the common carotid and internal carotid artery in the neck. During this procedure, the diseased intima and portions of the media are removed to open and smooth out the channel of blood flow to the brain. The procedure removes the roughened irregular buildup of atherosclerosis and is done to prevent transient ischemic attacks (TIAs) and strokes.

carotid subclavian bypass: procedure involving either vein or prosthetic material whereby a bypass graft is placed between the carotid artery and subclavian artery. It is done to improve the blood flow in the subclavian artery to the arm and hand by bringing blood up the carotid artery and down into the subclavian, bypassing a "narrowing" at the origin of the subclavian artery. (See also **subclavian carotid bypass.**)

coronary artery bypass graft (CABG): procedure on the blood vessels of the heart whereby narrowed areas in the arteries leading to the heart muscle itself are bypassed with a vein graft going directly from the aorta to more distal portions of the coronary (heart) arteries. This procedure, performed by cardiac surgeons, is done while the patient is on a cardiac bypass machine.

distal bypass: procedure performed with either synthetic material or vein whereby blood is brought from either the common femoral or superficial femoral artery down to the small named blood vessels below the knee. The procedure is usually performed to prevent amputation of an extremity from severe ischemia. The patient frequently has severe pain and skin breakdown before the operation.

endarterectomy: an opening up and cleaning out of blood vessels diseased by hardening of the arteries, which begin in the intima and progress down through the media. In this procedure, the diseased intima, fatty deposits, and much of the media are removed; the roughened irregular surface of the blood vessel can produce a surface on which blood

clots will collect and break off, moving downstream, or a surface on which more clot can form and occlude (close off) the artery.

endovascular grafting: reconstruction of aneurysms and, in some cases, occlusive disease by passing balloon expandable synthetic grafts into the aneurysm and opening the graft. The graft is held in place with stents or other devices. Fluoroscopy and angiography ensures proper positioning. Limitations and complications (early and late) are the focus of current active development.

endovascular therapy: catheter-based endovascular approach to quickly dissolve clots and blockages. An ultrasound-enhanced drug delivery system is used composed of tiny transducers situated on hair-thin wires (catheters) that dissolve blood clots in the pelvis and limbs, and stroke causing blood clots in the brain. Now, clot-busting drugs are infused at the site of the clot in the pelvic arteries or limbs.

end-to-end anastomosis: a joining of two vascular structures-arteries, graft and artery, or vein and artery-to bypass an occluded or damaged segment; the end of one structure is sewn to the end of the other.

end-to-side anastomosis: a joining of the end of an artery or vein or prosthetic material to the side of another vein, artery, or prosthetic material to bypass an occluded or damaged segment.

extra-anatomic bypass: bypass graft in which prosthetic material or vein is used to route blood between the two arteries or two veins. The route of the graft is other than a usual anatomic position, such as axillofemoral or femoral-femoral bypass.

extracranial/intracranial bypass (ECIC): a procedure performed by neurosurgeons whereby severely narrowed or occluded blood vessels within the brain are bypassed. The usual procedure is to take the superficial temporal artery, which is a branch on the scalp, make a bone flap in the skull, and move the distal end of this artery down into the brain to supply blood flow directly into the brain.

femoral-femoral bypass (fem-fem bypass): a bypass procedure using a synthetic or vein graft material whereby one femoral artery is used to supply the blood to both lower extremities. This could be done to bypass an infection, or to provide blood flow from one undiseased iliac femoral system to another femoral system. It is considered an extra-anatomic bypass.

femoral popliteal bypass (FPB): bypass graft from the femoral artery to the popliteal artery. The distal end of the graft can go to a portion of the popliteal artery above the knee or the popliteal artery below the knee. May be performed with vein or prosthetic material. It is done to correct an occluded superficial femoral artery. Indications for this procedure are claudication, rest pain, or threatened limb loss.

vena cava filter: for venous thromboembolic disorders, an umbrella-shaped metallic device that is inserted into the inferior vena cava to prevent clot from breaking off from legs or pelvis and going into the lungs (pulmonary emboli), for example, **Greenfield filter.**

***in situ* bypass:** instead of removing the greater saphenous vein and reversing it, it is left in place and the valve destroyed through a variety of techniques. The proximal end is sutured into the inflow artery, and the distal end of the vein is sutured into the recipient artery. The side branches of the vein are ligated in distal artery of leg. This technique provides better patency than taking the vein out and reversing its course.

laparotomy: a procedure whereby the abdomen is opened for exploration or to conduct another surgical procedure.

limb salvage: a general category of procedures performed on a lower extremity to improve the blood supply and prevent amputation. Skin ulceration and gangrene are often present.

patch angioplasty: a local procedure whereby the artery is opened, the inside of the vessel is cleaned out and a patch of vein or prosthetic material is used to widen that area of the artery. This procedure is also done in the repair of traumatic injuries.

polytetrafluoroethylene (PTFE): a plastic graft that has gained popularity in bypassing and replacing occluded arteries throughout the body.

reversed vein bypass graft: a technique in which a vein, usually the greater saphenous, is removed and used as a bypass. The small end of vein is sutured to proximal artery (inflow) and distal (large) end of vein is sutured to outflow artery. The vein must be turned around in this fashion to obviate the function of valves.

subclavian carotid bypass: bypass procedure between the subclavian artery and carotid artery to correct a severe narrowing at the origin of the common carotid artery. This allows blood to flow up the subclavian artery, along the graft, into the carotid artery, and into the brain without interrupting blood flow to the arm or hand.

sympathectomy: division of sympathetic chain to allow some dilatation of small extremity blood vessels. Not considered adequate treatment of claudication but may be a useful adjunct in limited situations. Sometimes helpful in upper extremity vasospastic disorders (Raynaud's or reflex sympathetic dystrophy [RSD]).

thrombolytic therapy: a dissolution of thrombus in an artery or vein with urokinase or streptokinase. Has been most useful in recent thromboses, but some contraindications must be considered.

Specific Anatomy and Surgery by Location

The Shoulder

Shoulder separations and shoulder dislocations are very distinct injuries and involve two different joints. Palpating the collar bone (clavicle) and working the fingers laterally, a distinct bump is felt—the acromioclavicular (A/C) joint, which is the junction between the collar bone and shoulder blade (Fig. 8-9). The acromion is the part of the shoulder blade that connects with the collar bone. Injury of this joint is often called a shoulder separation. However, a person dislocating the shoulder has disrupted the ball-and-socket joint between the arm and the shoulder blade (glenohumeral joint). The orthopaedist may not be able to feel this joint dislocation under the numerous muscles, but its presence is apparent through pain and an inability to place the arm behind the back or raise it over the head.

Anatomy
Bones
clavicle (cleido-): collar bone.
   acromioclavicular joint: between clavicle and scapula.
   sternoclavicular joint: at the junction of the clavicle and breast bone.

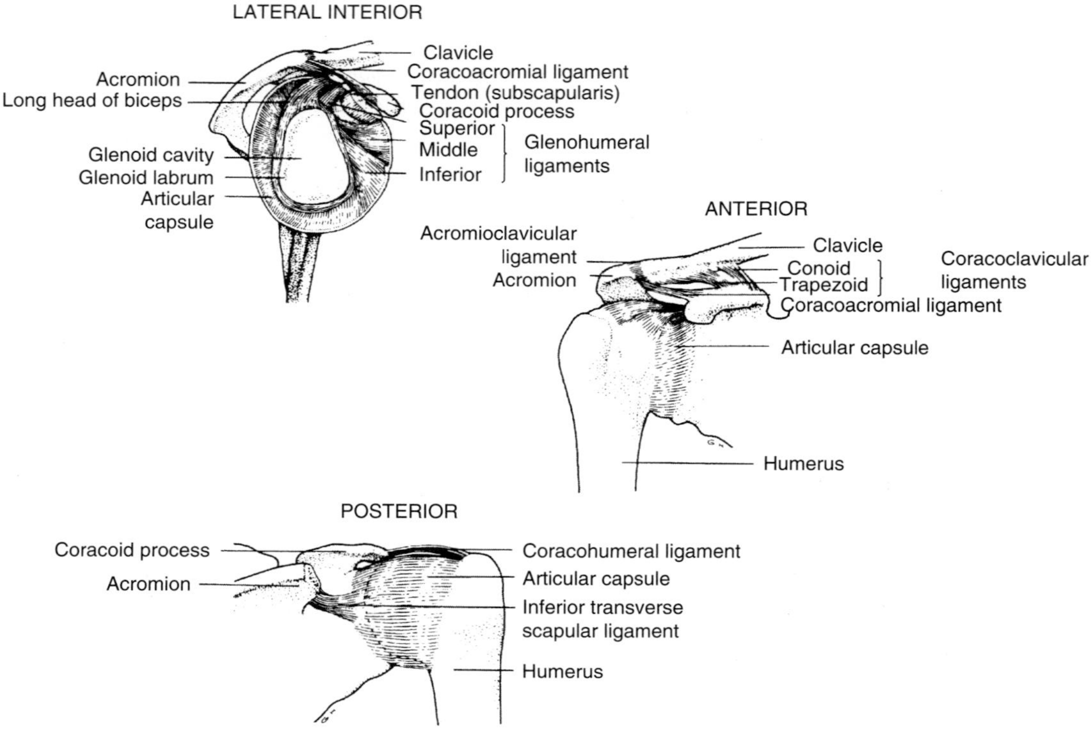

LATERAL INTERIOR

Acromion
Long head of biceps

Clavicle
Coracoacromial ligament
Tendon (subscapularis)
Coracoid process

Glenoid cavity
Glenoid labrum
Articular capsule

Superior ⎤
Middle ⎬ Glenohumeral
Inferior ⎦ ligaments

ANTERIOR

Acromioclavicular ligament
Acromion

Clavicle
Conoid ⎤ Coracoclavicular
Trapezoid ⎦ ligaments
Coracoacromial ligament

Articular capsule

Humerus

POSTERIOR

Coracoid process
Acromion

Coracohumeral ligament
Articular capsule
Inferior transverse scapular ligament
Humerus

FIG 8-9 Shoulder joints. (From Hilt NE, Cogburn SB: *Manual of Orthopaedics*, St Louis, 1980, CV Mosby.)

humerus: arm bone between the shoulder and elbow.

anatomic neck: point of attachment of shoulder capsule (humerus).

biceps groove: groove for the long head of the biceps muscle; **bicipital groove.**

greater and lesser tuberosity: points of attachment for the rotator cuff.

humeral head: half-circle-shaped portion of the humerus for the shoulder joint.

surgical neck: most common point of fracture of the humerus.

rhomboid fossa: an inconsistent feature on the medial side of the clavicle. It is the attachment of the costoclavicular or rhomboid ligament and has importance only because it may be mistaken for a tumor.

scapula: shoulder blade.

acromion process: outermost tip of the shoulder.

coracoid: knob of bone attached to the anterior scapula just medial to the shoulder.

glenoid fossa: saucer-shaped depression of the scapula that has direct contact with the humerus and glenohumeral joint.

glenoid labrum: ring of fibrocartilage of connective tissue attached to rim of margin of glenoidal cavity of shoulder blade to increase its depth.

spine: outcropping portion of the posterosuperior scapula.

spinoglenoid notch: small fingernail-sized V-shaped groove in the superior border of the scapula through which the suprascapular nerve courses.

Muscles Around the Shoulder

axilla: often the armpit, the axilla is bordered in the front by the pectoral muscle and in the back by the latissimus dorsi.

coracobrachialis: from the coracoid of the scapula to the inner distal humerus; pulls the arm across the midline.

deltoid: triangular muscle arising from the acromion that attaches to the lateral arm; elevates, flexes, and extends the arm.

infraspinatus: from the posterior upper scapula to the posterior superior humerus; externally rotates the arm.

latissimus dorsi: from the lower thoracic and lumbar spine to the anterior upper humerus; pulls the arm down and helps depress the humeral head.

levator scapula: from central midneck to the superior medial scapula; controls scapular elevation and rotation.

pectoralis major and minor: from the clavicle (major) and coracoid (minor) to the anterior chest wall; pulls the scapula forward.

rhomboideus major and minor: from the midline of the thoracic spine to the medial scapula; pulls the scapula back toward the midline.

rotator cuff: arrangement of four muscles from the scapula to the humerus, which, with the capsule and glenoid labrum (a cartilaginous margin of the joint), hold the shoulder together. The muscles of the rotator cuff are supraspinatus, infraspinatus, teres minor, and subscapularis.

serratus anterior: from the medial scapula to the chest anteriorly; holds the scapula into the body during shoulder motions.

shoulder girdle: a general term for the soft tissue around the glenohumeral joint.

sternocleidomastoid: from the base of the skull to the sternum and medial clavicle; turns head and flexes the neck.

subscapularis: from the anterior scapula to the lesser tuberosity; strong internal rotator of the shoulder.

supraspinatus: from the top of the scapular spine to the greater tuberosity of the humerus; abducts the arm and depresses the humeral head.

teres major and minor: from the lateral scapula to the humerus; pulls the arm in with the minor externally rotated as a part of the rotator cuff.

trapezius: kite-shaped muscle from the base of the neck to lower spine to scapular spine; controls scapular motion.

Ligaments around the Shoulder Region At the sternoclavicular joint, the **sternoclavicular l.**

At the acromioclavicular joint, the **acromioclavicular l.** and **coracoclavicular l.** (the **conoid** and **trapezoid l.**).

At the glenohumeral joint:

anteroinferior glenohumeral l.: lower of the three anterior glenohumeral l.

anteromedial glenohumeral l.: most substantial of the three anterior glenohumeral l.

anterosuperior glenohumeral l.: most superior of the three anterior glenohumeral l.

conjoined tendon: the common origin of two tendons from the coracoid process of the scapula leading to the arm and forearm. In surgery it is detached temporarily to gain access to the shoulder joint.

coracohumeral l.: starting at coracoid and crossing over humeral head.

glenoid labrum: meniscus-like rim of cartilage that deepens the glenohumeral joint.

rotator interval: area of thin tissue under coracohumeral l. and between the subscapularis and supraspinatus tendons.

transverse humeral l.: covering long head of biceps tendon over the bicipital groove.

Main Arteries, Veins, and Branches Around the Shoulder

axillary artery: a continuum of the subclavian artery in the axillary area that branches into highest thoracic, lateral thoracic, anterior humeral circumflex, posterior humeral circumflex, thoracoacromial, and subscapularis.

brachial artery: a continuum of the axillary artery and main artery of the arm. The branches are listed in the Arm and Forearm section.

cephalic vein: large vein between the deltoid and pectoralis muscles.

subclavian and axillary vein: the continuous vessel running alongside the subclavian and axillary arteries. The branches are not consistent and are rarely described in orthopaedic procedures.

subclavian artery: main artery from the chest leading down through the arm that branches into internal thoracic, vertebral, thyrocervical, transcervical, superior intercostal, and suprascapular.

Nerves

anterior thoracic n.: from the lateral cord, supplies the pectoral muscles.

axillary n.: arising from the posterior cord, supplies the upper arm, particularly the deltoid and teres minor.

brachial plexus: a large complex of nerves from the lower cervical and upper thoracic (C5 to T2) spinal segments. This nerve plexus includes:
Superior, medial, and inferior *trunk*
Anterior and posterior *division*
Medial, lateral, and posterior *cord*
Lower and upper subscapular nerve
Musculocutaneous nerve
Radial nerve
Ulnar nerve
Dorsal scapular nerve
Axillary nerve
Medial nerve
Scapular nerve
Long thoracic nerve

dorsal scapular n.: from the fifth nerve root, supplies the rhomboids.

long thoracic n. (nerve of Bell): from the fifth, sixth, and seventh cervical root, supplies the serratus anterior.

lower scapular n.: from the posterior cord, supplies the lower scapular and teres major muscles.

median n.: from the lateral and medial cord, supplies the finger and wrist flexors, except the fourth and fifth profundus and flexor carpi ulnaris, and the thumb intrinsics, except the adductor.

musculocutaneous n.: from the lateral cord, supplies the biceps coracobrachialis, brachialis, and lateral cutaneous nerve of the forearm.

radial n.: from the posterior cord, supplies the triceps, anconeus, supinator, and hand and wrist extensors.

suprascapular n.: from the superior trunk, supplies the supraspinatus and infraspinatus.

thoracodorsal n.: from the posterior cord, supplies the latissimus dorsi muscle.

ulnar n.: from the medial cord, supplies the fourth and fifth profundus and flexor carpi ulnaris along with the hand intrinsics including the thumb adductor, but not the other thumb intrinsics.

upper subscapular n.: from the posterior cord, supplies the subscapularis muscle.

Surgery of the Shoulder
Prosthetic Procedures
Bechtol p.: for replacement of the glenohumeral joint.

DANA (Designed After Natural Anatomy) total shoulder: a plastic component for glenoid associated with metallic-stemmed prosthesis for humerus.

Gristina and Webb p.: nonarticulated, semiconstrained shoulder prosthesis.

Michael Reese p.: replacement for shoulder joint involving an interlocking device.

Neer p.: shoulder replacement prosthesis.

reverse shoulder: for degenerative arthritis of the shoulder with cuff insufficiency, a "socket" is on the humeral side with a "ball" attachment to the glenoid.

Roper-Day p.: an unconstrained metal on plastic shoulder replacement.

Eponyms
The following list of eponyms for surgical procedures is arranged according to the area of injury or deformity. In most instances, the arthroplasties can be referred to as capsulorrhaphies of the shoulder.

Arthroplasties for Acromioclavicular Separations
Bosworth
Dewar and Barrington
Mumford-Gurd
Neviaser

Arthroplasties for Anterior Shoulder Dislocations

Bankart	Magnuson-Stack
Bristow	Nicola
Cubbins	Putti-Platt
de Toit and Roux	Speed
Eden-Hybbinette	Trillat

Arthroplasties for Posterior Shoulder Dislocations
McLaughlin
Scott
Wilson and McKeever

For High-Riding Scapulae (Sprengel Deformity)
Chang and Farahvar
Green
Inclan-Ober
Robinson
Schrock
Woodward

Arthrodeses for Shoulder Stabilization

Brittain	Steindler
Gill	Watson-Jones
Putti	

Muscle Transfers for Paralysis of Scapula

Chaves His-Haas

Chaves-Rapp	Whitman
DeWar and Harris	Saha
Dickson	Vastamäki
Henry	

Posterior Bone Block Elbow

Boyd

Putti

Putti-Scaglietti

Shoulder Procedures

acromionectomy: excision of all or part of the acromion, usually in cases of rotator cuff injuries.

acromioplasty: repair or partial removal of the acromion.

Armstrong p.: for rotator cuff impingement; resection of entire acromion.

Bankart p.: capsular repair in the glenoid for chronic anterior dislocation of the shoulder.

Bateman p.: for paralysis of the deltoid; a trapezius muscle transfer to the greater tuberosity.

Bosworth p.: screw fixation of the clavicle to the coracoid for acromioclavicular separations.

Boyd and Sisk p.: for stabilization of recurrent posterior shoulder dislocation; transfer of long head of biceps to posterior glenoid.

Braun p.: for partial ankylosis of the shoulder; open tenotomy of the subscapularis. Also, for painful shoulder in stroke patients; section of subscapularis and pectoralis major tendons.

brisement p.: a closed manipulation of a stiff shoulder.

Bristow p. (Bristow-Laterjet p.): coracoid process transfer for chronic anterior dislocation of the shoulder.

Brittain p.: extra-articular fusion of the shoulder.

Brooks and Saddon p.: for paralysis of biceps; transfer of pectoralis major tendon to biceps.

Bunnell p.: for paralysis of elbow flexion; transfer of triceps anterior to radial tuberosity. Also, for paralysis, biceps transfer of sternocleidomastoid to long head of biceps.

Burrows p.: for dislocation of sternoclavicular joint; use of subclavian muscle to hold reduction.

Chaves-Rapp p.: for long thoracic nerve palsy; transfer of the pectoralis major to inferior scapula.

clavicectomy: excision of all or part of the clavicle.

clavicotomy: surgical division of the collar bone.

Cofield p.: for rotator cuff tear; resection of distal clavicle, acromioplasty, and V-Y repair of rotator cuff or subscapularis substitution.

Copeland and Howard p.: for shoulder paralytic instability; fusion of scapula to ribs using tibial cortical grafts.

costectomy: excision of part or all of a rib for purposes of either a bone graft or approach to thorax.

costotransversectomy: excision of the transverse process of a vertebra and the neighboring rib for approach to the spine or cord.

Cubbins p.: passage of the coracohumeral ligament through the humeral head for an old anterior dislocation of the shoulder.

Das Gupta p.: technique of excision of scapula.

Debeyre p.: for repair of rotator cuff tear; superior approach to supraspinatus to advance tendon.

Dewar and Barrington p.: transfer of the coracoid tip to the clavicle for acromioclavicular separations.

du Toit and Roux p.: a stapling procedure of the anterior shoulder capsule for chronic anterior dislocation of the shoulder.

Eden-Hybbinette p.: a bone block to the anterior glenoid for chronic anterior dislocation of the shoulder.

Eden-Lange p.: for spinal accessory nerve palsy; transfer of levator scapulae, rhomboid major, and rhomboid minor.

Eyler p.: for paralysis of elbow flexor; transfer of flexor wad of five proximally on humerus facilitated with tendon fascia lata graft.

Fairbanks and Sever p.: for internal rotation and adduction contraction of shoulder; resection of tendinous portion of pectoralis major and minor, coracobrachialis, and short and long head of the biceps.

Gill p.: intra-articular and extra-articular fusion of the shoulder.

girdle resection: various resections of proximal humerus and/or scapula in an attempt to preserve the shoulder in ablative tumor surgery.

Green p.: soft tissue release and repair for high-riding scapulae.

Harmon p.: for partial paralysis of deltoid; transfer of posterior origin to anterior part.

His-Haas p.: for long thoracic nerve palsy; transfer of teres major from humerus to chest wall.

Hitchcock p.: tenodesis of long head of biceps into biceps groove.

Hovanian p.: for paralysis of biceps; transfer of latissimus dorsi to radial tuberosity. Also, for triceps weakness; transfer of latissimus dorsi to triceps muscle.

Inclan-Ober p.: soft tissue release and repair for high-riding scapulae.

Janecki and Nelson p.: for scapular malignancy; radical resection that includes a portion of the clavicle, proximal humerus, and entire scapula.

Jobe and Kvitne p.: for recurrent anterior dislocating shoulder; a criss-cross and overlapping imbrication of capsule to help recreate a labrum.

Kristiansen and Kofoed p.: for proximal humeral fractures; percutaneous pin is used to reduce fracture, and an external fixation is then applied.

L'Episcopo Zachary p.: for internal rotation and adduction contracture of the shoulder; resection of anterior capsule and tendon of pectoralis major with transfer of triceps and latissimus dorsi tendon.

Magnuson-Stack p.: stapling of the subscapularis for chronic anterior dislocation of the shoulder.

Marcove, Lewis, Horos p.: for scapular malignancy; radical resection that includes a portion of the clavicle, proximal humerus, and entire scapula.

McKeever p.: for open fixation of clavicle fracture, using a threaded wire.

McLaughlin p.: for rotator cuff injury of shoulder, a technique of repair; a transfer of the subscapularis into a hatchet head deformity of the humerus for old posterior dislocation of the shoulder.

McShane, Leinberry, and Fenlin p.: for rotator cuff impingement; excision of 50% of the inferior surface of the anterolateral acromion.

Moberg p.: for paralysis of triceps; posterior transfer of deltoid.

B. H. Moore p.: for muscle imbalance in shoulder caused by stroke; posterior transfer of part of deltoid muscle.

J. R. Moore p.: for posterior dislocation of humeral head in stroke; multiple anterior tendon and anterior capsule resection with bone graft to glenoid.

Mumford-Gurd p.: resection of the distal clavicle for a chronic acromioclavicular separation or arthritis.

Neer p.: for recurrent multidirectional anterior dislocating shoulder; capsular lateral advancement with superior placement of distal flap.

Neviaser p.: transfer of the coracoacromial ligament to the clavicle for acromioclavicular separation. Also a Knowles pin fixation of the clavicle, especially for nonunion of a fracture.

Nicola p.: transfer of the long head of the biceps tendon through humeral head for chronic anterior shoulder dislocation.

Ober and Barr p.: for weakness of triceps; transfer of brachioradialis.

O'Brien p.: for multidirectional anterior dislocating shoulder, superior and inferior placement of laterally based flaps in capsular repair.

Phelps: for tumor; technique of partial resection of the scapula.

Putti p.: fusion of the shoulder by two different methods.

Putti-Platt p.: subscapularis muscle and capsular repair for chronic anterior dislocation of the shoulder.

Rockwood p.: for chronic acromioclavicular separation; resection of distal clavicle and repair with acromioclavicular ligament, and 12-week fixation with a lag screw to coracoid.

Roger p.: for paralytic internal rotation deformity of the shoulder; a proximal derotation osteotomy of the humerus.

Rowe and Zarins p.: for chronic anterior shoulder dislocation; open reduction and fixation by a number of temporary means including sling.

Saha p.: for paralysis of deltoid; transfer of trapezius and distal acromion to humerus below greater tuberosity. Also, for paralysis of subscapularis; transfer of two superior digitations of serratus anterior or transfer of pectoralis minor. Also, for paralysis of supraspinatus; a transfer of levator scapulae or sternocleidomastoid. Also, for paralysis of infraspinatus or subscapularis; a transfer of latissimus dorsi or teres major.

scapulectomy: excision of all or part of the scapula.

Schrock p.: soft tissue release and repair for high-riding scapulae.

Scott p.: wedge bone block procedure for chronic posterior dislocation of the shoulder.

Speed p.: ligamentous repair for sternoclavicular joint separations. Also, for chronic dislocation elbow; reduction and stabilization, using a folded expansion of triceps muscle.

Spira p.: for paralysis biceps; transfer of pectoralis minor.

Steindler p.: intra-articular fusion of the shoulder.

Stewart p.: for acromioclavicular joint separation; resection of distal clavicle with repair of coracoacromial ligament.

Swafford and Lichtman p.: for suprascapular nerve entrapment; release of ligamentous tissue at the suprascapular notch.

Tikhoff-Linberg p.: for scapular malignancy; radical resection that includes a portion of the clavicle, proximal humerus, and entire scapula.

Trillat p.: for anterior shoulder dislocation; osteotomy of coracoid with attachment to glenoid to act as bone block.

Watson-Jones p.: shoulder fusion using a piece of acromion.

Weaver and Dunn p.: for acromioclavicular separation; transfer of coracoacromial ligament to distal clavicle.

Weber osteotomy: for recurrent shoulder dislocations associated with large posterior humeral head defects; internal rotation osteotomy of proximal humerus.

Whitman p.: for long thoracic nerve palsy; stabilization of scapula with fascial strips attached to spinous processes.

Wilson and McKeever p.: K-wire (Kirschner wire) fixation after open reduction of an old posterior shoulder dislocation.

Woodward p.: soft tissue release and repair for high-riding scapulae.

Zeir p.: for long thoracic nerve palsy; pectoralis minor transferred to scapula using a tensor fascia lata graft.

Arm, Elbow, and Forearm

Specifically, the arm is the portion of the upper limb between the shoulder and the elbow, and the forearm is between the elbow and the wrist. Most surgical procedures on the arm and forearm are of a general type, that is, nerve and vessel repairs and fracture fixations. Most forearm tendon transfers are considered in Chapter 10.

Anatomy
Bones

humerus: the humerus, the arm bone, extends from the shoulder to the elbow (Fig. 8-10).

capitellum: provides articulation with the radial head.

epitrochlea: medial epicondyle.

medial and lateral epicondyles: large prominences on either side of the elbow.

olecranon fossa: thin portion of the bone with an opening above the elbow joint.

spiral groove: groove in the bone for the radial nerve.

trochlea: provides articulation with the ulna.

radius (Fig. 8-11): The radius is the bone on the thumb side of the forearm.

biceps tuberosity: point of insertion of biceps tendon.

Lister tubercle: a prominence on the distal dorsum of the radius.

radial head: the articular portion of the radius to the elbow.

styloid process: the distalmost portion of radius.

ulna: The ulna is the bone of the forearm on the little finger side of the wrist, prominent at the elbow (Fig. 8-11).

coronoid process: anterior part of the ulna at the elbow joint at the brachialis insertion.

olecranon: prominent ulnar portion at the elbow.

styloid process: the most distal portion of the ulna, prominent on turning the wrist downward.

Muscles of the Arm

arcade of Struthers: a fibrous expansion of the medial distal triceps muscle; a potential area of entrapment for the ulnar nerve.

biceps m.: a two-belly muscle that flexes the elbow; extends from the scapula to the radius.

brachialis m.: flexes the elbow from the arm to the ulna.

coracobrachialis m.: pulls the arm in and up; extends from the scapula to the arm.

rotator cuff: see under Shoulder anatomy.

triceps m.: a three-belly muscle that extends the elbow; its origin is at the scapula, down the arm to the ulna.

Muscles of the Forearm

Many muscles of the forearm that affect hand function are discussed in Chapter 10. Others that relate to forearm function are the following.

anconeus: small muscle on the ulnar side of the elbow.

extensor wad of three: muscles that extend the wrist and flex the elbow.

brachioradialis muscle: located on the lateral side of the forearm; helps flex the elbow.

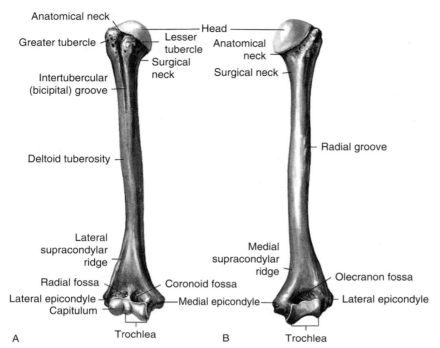

Anatomical neck
Greater tubercle
Lesser tubercle
Head
Surgical neck
Anatomical neck
Intertubercular (bicipital) groove
Surgical neck
Radial groove
Deltoid tuberosity
Lateral supracondylar ridge
Medial supracondylar ridge
Radial fossa
Coronoid fossa
Olecranon fossa
Lateral epicondyle
Capitulum
Medial epicondyle
Lateral epicondyle
Trochlea
Trochlea
A
B

FIG 8-10 Right humerus. **A,** Anterior view. **B,** Posterior view. (From Seeley RR, Stephens TD, Tate P: *Anatomy and Physiology,* St Louis, 1989, Times Mirror/Mosby College Publishing.)

extensor carpi radialis brevis: short muscle that extends the wrist.

extensor carpi radialis longus: long muscle that extends the wrist.

flexor wad of five: muscles that flex the wrist and fingers and pronate the forearm—flexor carpi ulnaris, palmaris longus, flexor digitorum superficialis, pronator teres, and flexor carpi radials; see Chapter 10.

pronator quadratus: flat muscle at the distal forearm that turns the palm down in pronation.

supinator muscle: located at the proximal forearm; brings the palm up in supination.

Blood Vessels (Fig. 8-12)

basilic vein: branches upward and laterally from ulnar side of forearm to front of elbow, winding around ulnar border of forearm to join the brachial vein, which becomes the axillary vein.

brachial artery: main artery of the arm that divides at the elbow into the radial and ulnar arteries.

brachial vein: branches off axillary.

cephalic vein: branches off from an axillary artery and vein on radial side; runs upward and medially to front of elbow and winds around and enters the axillary vein.

median cephalic vein: near elbow area (where blood is drawn).

median basilic vein: near elbow area.

profundus: deep anterior brachial artery of the arm.

radial artery: one that travels deep into the muscle on the thumb side of the forearm.

radial vein: branches off from cephalic vein.

ulnar artery: one that travels deep into the muscle on the little finger side of the anterior forearm.

Other Blood Vessels

Elbow

Ulnar collateral

Anterior and posterior ulnar recurrent

Anterior and posterior radial recurrent

Forearm

Anterior and posterior interosseous

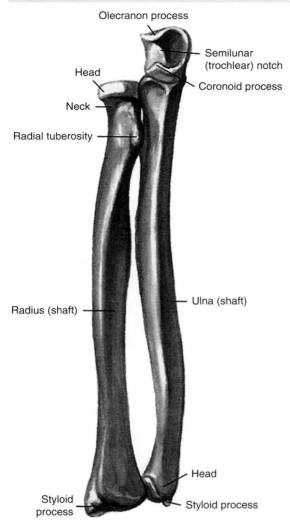

Olecranon process

Semilunar (trochlear) notch

Head

Coronoid process

Neck

Radial tuberosity

Radius (shaft)

Ulna (shaft)

Head

Styloid process

Styloid process

FIG 8-11 Ulna and radius of the right forearm. (From Seeley RR, Stephens TD, Tate P: *Anatomy and physiology*, St Louis, 1989, Times Mirror/Mosby College Publishing.)

Nerves

The nerves leading to the forearm and hand are all listed in the section on shoulder anatomy. Some specific branches to the arm and forearm are listed here.

anterior interosseous n.: branch of the median nerve; supplies the deep index finger and thumb flexor and pronator quadratus.

cutaneous n. of the arm (brachial cutaneous nerve): posterior, medial, and lateral.

cutaneous n. of the forearm (antebrachial cutaneous nerve): posterior, medial, and lateral.

posterior interosseous n.: branch of radial nerve that passes through supinator muscle and then supplies some of the deep muscles of the posterior forearm.

superficial radial n.: does not go through supinator; supplies no muscles but supplies sensation for the dorsal radial side of the hand and thumb.

Ligaments

arcade of Frosche: tunnel for posterior interosseus nerve that travels through the supinator.

cubital tunnel (arcade of Struthers): expansion of fibers from medial epicondyle to proximal dorsum of forearm; is a potential source of entrapment of ulnar nerve.

interosseous membrane: thick, fibrous tissue between most of the length of the radius and ulna.

laceratus fibrosus: expansion of fibers of the biceps tendon at the elbow; becomes an important structure in some injuries.

oblique ligament: a part of the radial collateral ligament of the elbow.

orbicular ligament: surrounding the radial head and holding it to the ulna at the elbow.

Osborne fascia: covering fascia over the ulna nerve between the medial humeral epicondyle and the olecranon.

ulnar and radial collateral ligament: on the medial and lateral side of the elbow.

Surgery of the Arm and Forearm
Prostheses

The classification of elbow prostheses is similar to that used for knee prostheses. They are generally categorized as constrained, semiconstrained, or unconstrained. Because there is such a wide list of manufacturers' names for these devices, they are not listed. These are typically specific to individual hospitals and the trade names can be found in the operating room supply section.

Eponymic

Amspacher and Messenbaugh p.: for malunion of humeral fracture; a distal rotation osteotomy.

Aronson and Prager: for supracondylar fracture in children; percutaneous pin fixation.

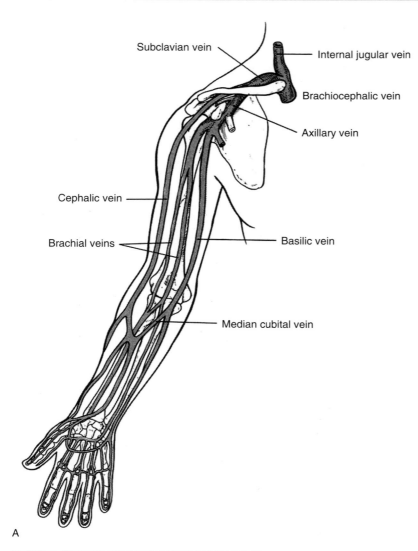

Subclavian vein

Internal jugular vein

Brachiocephalic vein

Axillary vein

Cephalic vein

Basilic vein

Brachial veins

Median cubital vein

A

FIG 8-12 Blood vessels of the upper limb. **A,** Veins of the upper limb—the subclavian vein and its tributaries. The major veins draining the superficial structures of the limb are the cephalic and basilic veins. The brachial veins drain the deep structures. Blood vessels of the upper limb.

(Continued)

arthrodeses of the elbow: two procedures are Staples and Steindler arthrodeses.

Baumgard and Schwartz p.: for lateral epicondylitis; percutaneous or small open incision release of origin of extensor carpi ulnaris and extensor carpi radialis brevis and longus.

Blount p.: for supination deformity of forearm; closed osteoclasis of both bones of forearm setting at 45 to 90 degrees of pronation.

Bosworth p.: resection of a portion of the radial head ligament and muscle attachment for tennis elbow.

Bowers "hemi" resection: for radioulnar joint arthritis; resection of distal radial side of ulna with interposition of fascia.

Boyd and Anderson p.: for biceps distal tendon rupture; a method of reattachment.

Boyd and McLeod p.: for tennis elbow; excision of a part of the orbicular ligament.

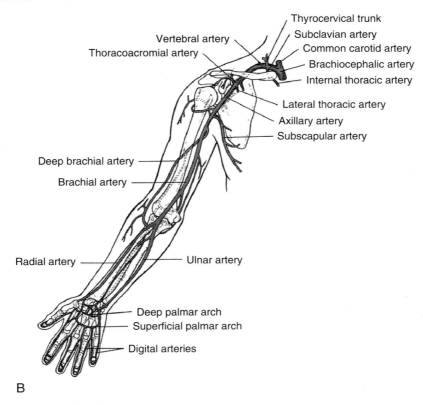

Thyrocervical trunk
Subclavian artery
Common carotid artery
Brachiocephalic artery
Internal thoracic artery

Vertebral artery
Thoracoacromial artery

Lateral thoracic artery
Axillary artery
Subscapular artery

Deep brachial artery

Brachial artery

Radial artery — Ulnar artery

Deep palmar arch
Superficial palmar arch

Digital arteries

B

FIG 8-12 Cont'd. B, Arteries of the upper limb—the brachiocephalic, subclavian, axillary, and brachial arteries and their branches. (From Seeley RR, Stephens TD, Tate P: *Anatomy and Physiology*, St Louis, 1989, Times Mirror/Mosby College Publishing.)

Brady and Jewett p.: for proximal cross-union of radius and ulna; resection of radial head and 4-week screw fixation to separate radius and ulna.

Campbell p.: for arthritic radial capitellar joint; resection of capitellum and radial head with imbrication of capsule over bone. Also for malunited Colles fracture; resection of distal ulnar side of ulna to use as graft correcting radial deformity.

Campbell and Akbarnia p.: for tumor of distal radius; resection of distal radius with replacement using tibial bone graft.

capitellocondylar p.: an unconstrained elbow prosthesis designed to allow greater supination and pronation.

De Rosa and Graziano p.: for varus deformity in elbow; closing step cut osteotomy of distal humerus.

Ellis p.: for reduction of intra-articular volarly displaced wrist fracture; a technique of screw plate fixation.

Feldon wafer resection: for radioulnar joint arthritis; resection of thin portion of bone and joint of distal ulna, preserving the styloid.

Fernandez p.: for dorsal and radial shortening of a radius fracture; dorsal wedge resection with radial replacement to correct both deformities.

Flynn p.: for nonunion or delayed union of minimally displaced lateral condylar fractures in children; open reduction, peg bone graft, and fixation.

Fowles p.: for chronic posterior dislocation of elbow; a posterolateral approach with detachment of all tight structures and possible V-Y plasty of triceps.

French p.: for malunion of ulna; distal ulnar osteotomy with screw and wire fixation.

Froimson and Oh (keyhole) p.: for chronic tendonitis of long head of biceps; a keyhole is fashioned in the bicipital groove and then used to insert a knotted portion of biceps tendon.

Gaille p.: for recurrent anterior dislocation shoulder; use of fascia lata graft to replace anterior capsule.

Gill p.: for nonunion of ulna; a massive sliding graft technique.

Hall and Pankovich p.: for mid-humeral fracture; use of multiple small Ender nails in antegrade or retrograde fashion.

Hassman, Brunn, and Neer p.: for recurrent elbow dislocation; plastic repair of lateral capsuloligamentous structures.

Hirayama p.: for chronic dislocation of the radial head with ulnar deformity in a child; osteotomy of the proximal ulna.

Hitchcock p.: for rupture of the long head of biceps; a method of reattachment.

Hovanian p.: for restoring elbow flexion; transfer of latissimus dorsi to olecranon.

Hohmann p.: for tennis elbow.

Kapel p.: triceps and biceps tendon formed into ligaments for a chronic dislocated elbow.

Liebolt p.: for subluxing distal radial/ulnar joint; using tendon graft.

MacAusland p.: arthroplasty of the elbow for a recurrent dislocation.

Manktelow; Ikuta p.: for loss of forearm flexor muscle mass; free neurovascular pedicle transfer of pectoralis major.

McKeever and Buck p.: for olecranon fracture with adequate remaining joint surface; excision of olecranon fragment and reattachment of triceps mechanism.

Milch p.: for radial shortening; an ulnar shortening by step cut resection of distal shaft of ulna. Also, for pronation deformity; an osteotomy of distal ulna with fixation in supinated position. Also humeral osteotomy for cubitus valgus deformity.

Milch shortening osteotomy: for radioulnar joint arthritis; resection of circular section of distal ulnar shaft with plate fixation and resultant shortening of ulna.

Mital p.: for spastic muscle contracture of elbow; Z-plasty of biceps tendon and release of brachialis sheath and joint capsule.

Mizuno, Hirohata, and Kashiwagi p.: for displaced distal humeral epiphysis; posterior open reduction and pin fixation.

Nirschl p.: for chronic lateral epicondylitis; excision of hypercapsular tendon segment of extensor carpi radialis brevis and decortication of anterolateral condyle.

Osborne and Cotterill p.: capsular reefing for a chronic dislocated elbow.

Outerbridge-Kashiwagi p.: for osteoarthritis of the elbow; debridement arthroplasty using posterior approach and fenestration of olecranon fossa.

Reichenheim-King p.: transplantation of the biceps tendon into the coronoid process for a chronic dislocated elbow.

Sauve-Kapandji p.: distal radioulnar joint arthritis; fusion of distal radius and ulna with creation of an ulnar pseudoarthrosis proximal to the fusion.

Sherk and Probst p.: for proximal humeral epiphyseal fracture; reduction and percutaneous pinning.

J.S. Speed p.: for old dislocation of radial head; fashioning of sling from a portion of triceps expansion.

Speed and Boyd p.: for irreducible Monteggia fracture; reconstruction of orbicular ligament and plating of ulnar fracture.

Spittler p.: for forearm amputations; a biceps muscle cineplasty.

Steindler flexorplasty: transfer of the flexor wad of five muscles in the elbow to a higher level for loss of voluntary elbow flexion; **Eyler flexorplasty** is a variation of this procedure.

Stewart p.: for radial navicular arthritis; excision of radial styloid.

Weber-Vasey p.: for comminuted olecranon fracture; combined use of bent pin and figure eight wire fixation.

Wilson p.: for extra-articular ankylosis of elbow in flexion; release of anterior structures with Z-plasty of biceps tendon.

Zancolli p.: for supination deformity of forearm; suturing of biceps tendon after lengthening.

(The anatomy and surgery of the hand and wrist are found in Chapter 10.)

Pelvis and Hips

The pelvis is a large basin-like structure that supports the lower abdominal viscera, contains the birth canal, and acts as a weight-bearing bridge between the spine and the lower extremities. It is often referred to as the **pelvic girdle.** It is composed of a bilateral set of three bones that are completely fused and are on either side of the sacrum. The largest and uppermost bone is the ilium, the lowermost and strongest is the ischium, and the anteriormost is the pubis. In the outer center of these fused bones is the hip socket, called the acetabulum, the "true" anatomic hip and socket for the ball-and-socket joint.

Most hip surgical procedures involve structures immediately neighboring the acetabulum. The anatomic structures involving the pelvis that are occasionally encountered in hip procedures are listed first, followed by anatomic structures directly related to hip procedures.

Anatomy of the Pelvis
Bones
ala of the ilium: the outer flair of the ilium; resembles a wing.

anterior inferior iliac spine: prominence in the deep ilium just above the hip is origin of rectus femoris.

arcuate ligament: arcuate, meaning arch-shaped. The arcuate line of the pelvis is the iliac continuation of the iliopectineal line; the arched inferior edge of the posterior layer of the rectus sheath.

calcar: a spur. **Calcar femorale** is a bundle of cancellous laminae of bone in the neck of the femur, serving to strengthen it.

greater sciatic notch: the large notch on the posterior surface of the ilium below the posteroinferior iliac spine where the sciatic nerve exits.

gluteal lines: refers to the three curved lines across the outer surface of the ilium, anteriorly, posteriorly, and inferiorly.

iliac crest: the outer uppermost margins of the ilium, two of the four iliac spines arise from the crest; the **anterior superior iliac spine** is the origin of the oblique abdominal muscles and sartorius; the **posterior superior iliac spine** is a part of the origin of the gluteus maximus.

iliopectineal line: a ridge inside the pelvis that denotes the entrance into the birth canal, with a concave inner surface called the **iliac fossa.**

ilium: wide plate-like bone that forms the top of the pelvis just below the waistline; generally referred to as "the hips."

inferior pubic ramus: lower portion of the pubic bone.

innominate bone: composed of three fused bony subunits, called the ilium, pubis, and ischium, that are attached to the sacrum and coccyx to form the pelvis.

ischial spine: prominence of bone of strong ligamentous attachment above the tuberosity; main significance is in obstetrics.

ischial tuberosity: the prominent, hard portion of bone at the base of the ischium, felt when sitting erect.

ischium: a U-shaped bone of the lower part of the pelvis, which forms a ring.

obturator foramen: refers to the large opening of the innominate bone almost entirely occluded by the obturator membrane. It is the two muscles that cover the large opening of the anterior pelvis; also pertains to the nerves and vessels penetrating this orifice. The cartilage ring turns to bone in childhood, and the ischium and pubis become a solid bony continuum, producing a hole or ring that is the largest foramen in the body.

pelvic girdle: a general term that denotes the entire bilateral bony pelvis; the ring that the pelvis makes with its articulation to the sacrum (sacroiliac joint) is called the **pelvic ring.**

posterior inferior iliac spine: prominence of posterior inferior ilium away from sacrum; attachment of ligaments.

pubis (pubic bone): the anterior increased shape of bone of the pelvis, which meets its counterpart from the other side at a point called the **symphysis pubis.**

sacroiliac: joint space between the sacrum and the two ilia; junction of the pelvis to the spine.

superior pubic ramus: top portion of the pubic bone.

symphysis pubis: the junction of the two pubic bones just above the genital area.

Muscles
Most of the pelvic muscles affect the hip or abdominal motion and are described in this section. However,

those muscles of the lower abdominal wall surrounding the bladder, uterus, and rectum are sometimes encountered in orthopaedic procedures; they are the levator ani, pubococcygeal, transverse urethral, and cremaster (in scrotum).

sphincter ani: muscle that controls defecation; loss of control of this muscle is a serious sign of herniated disk disease.

Ligaments

anterior sacroiliac l.: large ligament between the sacrum and the ilium.

Poupart inguinal l.: anterior ligament at the groin fold from the anterosuperior iliac spine to the pubic tubercle.

sacrospinous l.: from iliac spine to sacrum.

sacrotuberous l.: ligament from the sacrum to the ischial tuberosity; small sacrosciatic.

Blood Vessels

Most large blood vessels within the pelvis are not encountered in orthopaedic practice. The aorta divides into the common iliac arteries at about the level of the fourth lumbar vertebra. Branches within the pelvis include the hypogastric, superior and inferior gluteal, iliac (which becomes the femoral to the inguinal ligament), and pudendal.

Nerves

cluneal n.: inferolateral, inferomedial, and superior sensory nerves of the buttocks and thighs.

lumbar plexus: arises from the second through fourth lumbar vertebrae, with two major nerves.

  femoral nerve: arises from L2, L3, and L4 and supplies most of the knee extensors.

  obturator nerve: arises from L2, L3, and L4 and supplies many of the thigh adductors.

pudendal n.: arising from just below the sacral plexus, traveling along the ischium (Alcock canal), and supplying the lower pelvic muscles that do not affect hip motion but affect sexual function.

sciatic n.: the large nerve developed by the sacral plexus supplying the hip rotators, knee flexors, and entire leg and foot muscles and most of the sensation.

sciatic plexus: the major plexus of nerves arising in the pelvic area to include nerves from L4 and L5 and

nerves of the first three sacral levels. Major injuries or disorders of this plexus are rare, but it is important to understand that this plexus forms the sciatic nerve, which eventually becomes the tibial and common peroneal nerves. Most "sciatica" is actually a nerve root irritation in the spinal column.

Miscellaneous Terms

inguinal: refers to the area of the groin. The precise line is from the anterosuperior iliac spine to the pubis; this is the line of the natural fold of skin in the groin. Terms relating to the area include inguinal nerve, hypogastric nerve, ilioinguinal nerve, and inguinal canal.

peritoneum: inner membrane lining of the abdominal cavity.

Anatomy of the Hip

The average person refers to the prominent part of the pelvis that flares out just below the waistline (iliac crest) as the "hip." However, the hip portion of the pelvis is the lesser part of the entire pelvic mass; it is 5 inches below the iliac crest and is called the acetabulum, or "true" hip. The three bones of the pelvis merge to form the cup-shaped depression of the hip joint, which holds the femoral head in place. The proximal femur (thigh bone) and its components are described here as the major elements of the hip function and not as part of the lower extremities.

Bones

acetabulum: cup-shaped depression in the mid-outer pelvis known as the hip; this is the socket of the ball-and-socket joint of the hip.

acetabular notch: a cup-shaped defect in the lateral iliac wall above the acetabulum seen in infants who go on to progressive hip dysplasia.

  fovea centralis: central depression in the center of the acetabulum and origin of the ligamentum teres.

  posterior lip: posterior part of the acetabulum, which sometimes breaks off in a dislocation of the hip.

  superior dome: the weight-bearing portion of the acetabulum.

  triradiate cartilage: structure present only during growth; the meeting point of the ischium, ilium, and pubis.

digital fossa: a deep depression on the inner surface of the greater trochanter; the site of the insertion of the obturator externus and posterior aspect of the superior border of the greater trochanter.

femoral head: the ball and topmost part of the ball-and-socket joint of the hip; in a growing child may be referred to as the **capital epiphysis.**

femoral neck: the area below the femoral head where the bone narrows into a tube-like structure about 2 inches long.

femur: as related to the hip, is considered the upper, proximal 4-inch segment of bone.

greater and lesser trochanters: part of the femur just distal to the neck where the bone widens into two large prominences, the lower, smaller, and medial of which is the lesser trochanter; the greater trochanter is the larger, lateral prominence. In thin persons the greater trochanter can be felt at about the level of the palm of the hands when the arms are resting by the sides. It is often used as a landmark in physical and x-ray examinations.

intertrochanteric: refers to any region between the two trochanters; a large number of fractures of the hip occur in this region.

piriformis fossa: small, shallow depression located at the tip of the greater trochanter; site of insertion of the piriformis tendon.

subtrochanteric: refers to the widened part of the shaft just below the lesser trochanter.

Muscles

adductors: a group of five muscles that pulls the thigh inward (adduction); these include the adductor magnus, adductor longus, adductor brevis, pectineus, and gracilis muscles.

external and internal rotators: a group of muscles originating at the pelvis around the hip, helping to control internal and external rotation; these muscles are the internal and external obturator gemelli (superior and inferior gemellus), quadratus femoris, and piriformis.

gluteus maximus m.: the large buttock muscle that helps to extend the hip.

gluteus medius and minimus muscles: the deeper significant muscles that abduct the hip and prevent a waddling gait.

iliopsoas m.: a combination of the iliacus and psoas muscles arising from the anterior back and inserting into the lesser trochanter. These large hip flexors are often involved in hip reconstructive procedures.

rectus femoris m.: anterior thigh muscle of the quadriceps group; attaches across the hip joint.

sartorius m.: the muscle stretching from the anterolateral pelvis (anterosuperior iliac spine) to the medial tibia, crossing two joints; it enables the person to assume a cross-legged position.

tensor fascia lata m.: the most lateral hip abductor muscle.

Ligaments

Bigelow ligament (anterior iliofemoral ligament): major ligamentous expansion of the capsule covering the femoral neck.

labrum: fibrocartilaginous rim that surrounds the outer margin of the acetabulum, particularly prominent in the superoanterior portion.

ligamentum teres: the round ligament between the middle of the femoral head and the center of the acetabulum (fovea centralis).

Arteries

femoral a.: the major artery from the point of exit from the pelvis to the point of exit behind the knee. Near the hip, it gives off a branch called the **deep femoral (profundus) artery.** The lateral circumflex artery arises from the lateral deep profundus and supplies the lateral and anterior femoral neck. This is the major blood supplier to the femoral head in late childhood and adult life. A branch of the femoral artery is the **medial circumflex artery,** which arises from the deep femoral artery and supplies the posterior femoral head.

inferior gluteal a.: large artery from the internal iliac artery within the pelvis; supplies the gluteus medius and minimus.

obturator a.: a branch from within the pelvis that supplies some of the adductor muscles after exiting through the obturator foramen.

superior gluteal a.: a large artery from the internal iliac artery within the pelvis supplying the gluteus maximus and lesser muscles outside the pelvis.

Nerves

All three nerves supplying the thigh and leg also supply the hip. As a result many patients with hip problems complain of thigh, calf, and even foot pain. The large nerves passing near the hip are the following.

femoral n.: supplies sensation to the anterior thigh, medial leg, and the muscle for knee extension.

obturator n.: supplies sensation to the medial side of the thigh and the muscles for pulling the thigh inward (adducting).

sciatic n.: supplies sensation to the posterior thigh and hip extensors; the more distal branches (common peroneal and posterior tibial) are discussed under nerves of the lower limbs.

Surgery of the Pelvis and Hips

Most of the surgery performed on the hip is directed toward making the hip a mobile, painless, weight-bearing joint. Surgical procedures designed to remodel the hip or replace the parts involved are described in this section. Surgical procedures to fuse the hip or to change the direction of alignment of the femur or pelvis are defined in the following sections.

Hip Arthroplasty

A hip arthroplasty is a procedure designed to directly change the contour of or to replace the hip joint (acetabulum) and/or femoral head. This term is so general that it includes most procedures for developmental dysplasia of the hips (DDH) and all procedures that involve prosthetic replacement. For example, the term **total hip arthroplasty** is used often to denote the total joint replacement procedure. Nonprosthetic procedures are listed first.

shelf procedure: a bending of the outer acetabulum (hip joint) so it more completely covers the femoral head. This is commonly done for DDH in which the acetabulum is not well rounded and allows the femoral head to displace. It is necessary, in many instances, to reduce the hip and then perform a shelf procedure, using a bone graft to maintain a new position of the lateral acetabulum. Some types of operative shelf procedures are listed. This term specifically means the creation of a bony shelf at the edge of the acetabulum. However, femoral head coverage is sometimes accomplished by pelvic osteotomy with or without the addition of a bone graft to create a shelf.

Albee	Hay-Groves
Bosworth	Lance
Chiari	Lowman
Colonna	Pemberton
Eppright Wagner	Salter
Frank Dickson	Steel
Ghormley	Sutherland
Gill (Type I, II, III)	Weston
Hall Kalamchi	Wiberg

capsular arthroplasty: many procedures for a dislocation of the hip involve soft tissue manipulation only and include curetting of the acetabulum and muscle transfers but do not involve bony osteotomies such as are seen in the shelf procedures. One of these procedures is the **Colonna capsular arthroplasty.**

Joint Replacement Surgeries

Short straight stem femoral components designed to replace the femoral head are now obsolete. The original effort to replace the hip joint was centered around the femoral head component. One of the first femoral head components was made of acrylic attached to a metal stem (Judet). These became loose fairly rapidly. As bone remodeling and response to stress became better understood, the devices were no longer used. This led to the development of single femoral canal stem devices. Although the cartilage on the acetabular side would often disappear over time, many of these prostheses lasted for years. In addition, they were fairly easy to replace. These prostheses are still used in some cases for femoral head replacement in hip fractures. Because of loosening problems and loss of articular cartilage in the hip socket total joint replacement surgery was developed. The names of these devices can be found for historical reference in previous editions of this dictionary. The range of manufacturer's brand names for joint replacement devices is so large that incorporation here is not practical. Related terms specific for hip replacement surgery follow (Fig. 8-13).

bipolar hip replacement: large femoral head on a stem in which there is a "head within a head" using a high molecular weight polyethylene interface. No acetabular component. These can be used for primary femoral neck fractures and some salvage circumstances.

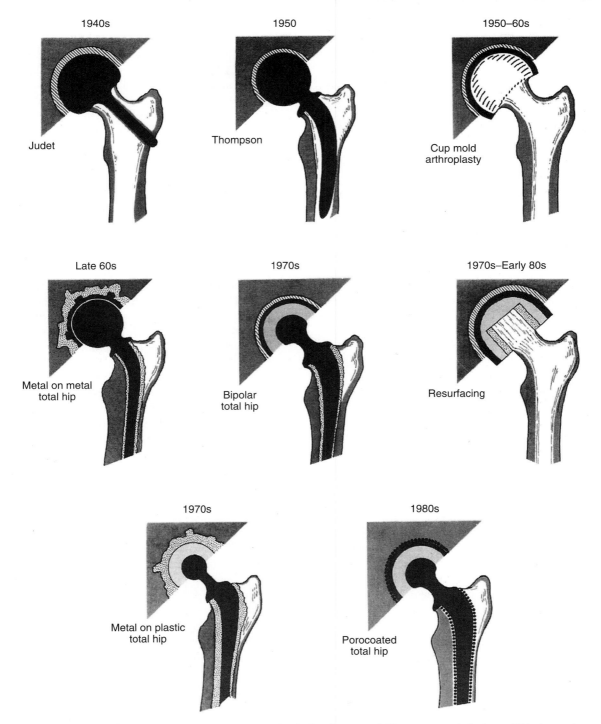

FIG 8-13 Development of the total hip prosthesis in the past four decades has shown remarkable improvement in fixation and biologic acceptance. Lined areas are cartilage, grossly stippled areas are cement (methylmethacrylate), finely stippled areas are plastic, and solid black areas are metal. More recent alternative bearing surfaces are porocoated with metal on metal, ceramic on plastic, and ceramic on ceramic. (Drawing by Frances Langley, USUHS.)

cage: typically used in hip socket replacement where large bony defects occur, this is a metal device, designed to hold multiple screws and other fixation components. The acetabular component is then cemented into the cage.

composite beam model: stem is held in place with collars and roughened surface finish, designed to load the proximal femur.

constrained liner: for prosthetic hip instability, locks femoral head inside of acetabular component.

cup arthroplasty: surgical remodeling of the femoral head and the acetabular socket with the insertion of a metal cup. This procedure is usually reserved for younger persons with severe deforming diseases of the hip after trauma; **mold arthroplasty.**

distal coated stem: term usually applied to porous coating where the coating is on the entire stem.

double bubble: term applied to acetabular hip components designed to accommodate bone defects.

dual geometry: radius of acetabular component is larger at the periphery than the dome and designed to maximize rim fit.

equatorial contact: seen in metal on metal articulations in which equal contact is made over entire femoral head.

femoral head prosthesis: insertion into the femoral shaft of a metallic or synthetic component that resembles the femoral head. In present use, it replaces the femoral head in an older person who has a normal acetabulum, but a recent fracture of the hip. This may be unipolar or bipolar.

first-generation cementing: the use of methylmethacrylate by finger-packing into the femoral canal though the exposed neck.

mat finish: roughened finish on stem.

mid-coated stem: term usually applied to porous coating in which the coating is only on the proximal and mid-part of the stem.

polar contact: seen in metal on metal articulations in which top portion of head has a higher amount of contact.

proximal coated stem: term usually applied to porous coating in which the coating is only on the proximal part of the stem.

resurfacing procedures: the purpose of research into resurfacing rather than replacement was to leave as much bone stock as possible. The effort that is required to remove a preexisting total hip prosthesis often destroys a fair amount of surrounding bone. The advantage of the resurfacing procedure was that it did not require removal of the femoral head and placement of a stem with methylmethacrylate down the femoral canal. However, the acetabular cap was held with methylmethacrylate and the portion placed over the reshaped femoral head was also held with methylmethacrylate. The problem with this procedure has been an eventual loss of the femoral component because of absorption of bone. If the method did fail, replacement with other total hip devices was easier, with more bone available for fixation. With metal on metal bearings this procedure is being done more frequently.

second-generation cementing: the use of methylmethacrylate by lavage of the canal, plugging canal, and retrograde filling of the canal.

surface finish: range of finish from smooth mirror-like finish to roughened (mat) finish.

taper slip design: stem subsides in cement mantle taking advantage of viscoelastic properties of cement.

third-generation cementing: the use of methylmethacrylate by lavage of the canal, plugging canal, and retrograde filling of the canal pressurization, vacuum mixing, and proximal and distal centralizers to center the prosthesis with the best possible cement mantle.

total hip arthroplasty (low friction arthroplasty): a joint replacement involving an internal prosthesis by removing the diseased joint and replacing the acetabular component with either metal or plastic materials and a metal prosthesis of the femoral segment. This type of procedure is usually reserved for older individuals who are suffering from osteoarthritis, avascular necrosis, or other degenerative diseases of the hip. Bearing surfaces include metal on plastic, ceramic on plastic, metal on metal, and ceramic on ceramic. Fixation can be by bone ingrowth or methylmethacrylate.

unipolar: large femoral head on a stem without acetabular component.

Closed Hip Reduction Procedures for Developmental Dysplasia of the Hip (DDH)

These are manipulations in an infant or child to reduce a dislocated hip. The method of reduction, followed by the casted position after reduction, varies.

Crego: use of skeletal traction until a closed manipulation with minimal force becomes possible.

Lange: positioning the hip in abduction, internal rotation, and extension after a closed reduction.

Lorenz: both a method of reduction and the frogleg position cast applied following the reduction.

Ridlon: method of reducing a congenitally dislocated hip and then using a Lorenz cast.

Wingfield frame: used in a gradual method of closed reduction.

Open Hip Reduction

An open hip reduction is a procedure that, when listed by itself, implies the need to reduce a hip under direct surgical vision but with minimal reconstruction of the capsule. Some open techniques include **Calandriello, Ferguson, Howorth, Scaglietti,** and **Somerville.**

Iliopsoas Transfers

This strong hip flexor is sometimes transferred to act as a hip abductor in conditions of muscle imbalance and hip dislocation. Two such procedures are the **Mustard** and the **Sharrard.**

Osteotomies

The osteotomies of the hip are listed here for reference, but some are defined more fully in this chapter under Osteotomy.

Amstutz and Wilson	MacEwen and Shands
Bernese	McCarroll
Blount	McMurray
Blundell Jones	Müller
Borden, Spencer, and Herndon	Osgood
Brackett	Pauwels
Chiari	Pauwels Y
derotation	Pemberton
dial	Platou
Dimon	Salter (innominate)
Gant	Sarmiento
Ganz	Schanz
Ghormley	Schede
Hass	Southwick
Irwin	Steel-triradiate
Langenskiöld	Sutherland-Greenfield
Lloyd-Roberts	Whitman
Lorenz	

Arthrodeses

The arthrodeses are listed for reference but some are defined more fully under General Surgery of Joints.

Abbott	Ghormley
Abbott-Fisher-Lucas	Henderson
Albee	Kickaldy and Willis
Badgley	Schneider
Blair	Stamm
Brittain	Trumble
Chandler	Watson-Jones
Davis	John C. Wilson
Gant	

Other Pelvic and Hip Procedures

acetabuloplasty: any surgical remodeling of the cup side of the hip joint.

Asnis p.: for mild chronic slipped capital femoral epiphysis; fixation with a cannulated screw.

Baxter and D'Astous p.: for hip contracture in myelomeningocele; resection of proximal femur and interposition of muscle mass.

Bleck p.: for excessive hip internal rotation when walking; a recession of the iliacus and psoas tendon to anterior capsule of hip.

Campbell p.: for abdominal and hip flexion contracture; excision of a part of the anterior ilium after a soft tissue release.

Canale p.: for mild chronic slipped capital femoral epiphysis; cannulated screw fixation.

Castle and Schneider p.: for spastic cerebral palsy hip dislocation; interposition of muscles over joint following resection of femur proximal to subtrochanteric line.

Chandler p.: for hip adduction gait; intrapelvic obturator neurectomy.

Couch, DeRosa, and Throop p.: for hip adduction gait; transfer of the adductor tendon to ischial tuberosity.

coxotomy: surgical opening of the hip joint.

Dimon and Hughston p.: for comminuted intertrochanteric hip fracture; a method of reduction with valgus placement and use of a high angle nail.

Dunn p.: for displaced slipped capital femoral epiphysis, removal of "hump" and fusion of epiphysis.

Fish p.: for chronic slipped capital femoral epiphysis; resection of dome-shaped wedge at femoral head.

Girdlestone resection: excision of the femoral head and neck for a fractured intertrochanteric hip joint and other diseases.

Graber-Duvernay p.: boring holes leading to the center of the femoral head for the purpose of promoting circulation.

hebosteotomy: incision into the pubis; hebotomy.

Heyman-Herndon p.: for displaced slipped capital femoral epiphysis, a shortening of the femoral neck with correction of deformity.

ischiectomy: surgical excision and removal of a part of the ischium.

ischiohebotomy: surgical division of the ischiopubic ramus and ascending ramus of the pubis.

ischiopubiotomy: incision into the ischial pubic junction.

Karakousis and Vezeridis p.: for malignancy of pelvis; resection of hemipelvis and head of femur, preserving neurovascular structures.

King and Richards p.: for posterior acetabular fracture; oblique screw fixation.

Kramer, Craig, and Noel p.: for chronic slipped capital femoral epiphysis; osteotomy and wedge resection at base of femoral neck.

Legg p.: for paralysis of gluteus maximus; posterior portion of tensor fascia lata muscle is transferred to a more posterior position.

Lyden p.: for mild chronic slipped capital femoral epiphysis; use of cannulated screw; **Lehman p.**

Lynne and Katcheria p.: for spastic cerebral palsy subluxation of hip; ipsilateral iliac crest used as a graft in pelvic osteotomy.

Martin p.: for chronic, severe slipped capital femoral epiphysis; a closed-wedge osteotomy at base of femoral head.

Malta and Saucedo p.: for sacral fracture; reduction and fixation with posterior screws placed lateral to medial.

McCarty p.: for chordoma of sacrum; resection of a portion of sacrum.

Menson and Scheck p.: for osteoarthritis of the hip; release of the pericapsular muscles. Also called **"hanging hip" procedure.**

Morrisay p.: for mild chronic slipped capital femoral epiphysis; percutaneous single screw fixation.

Ober-Barr p.: for paralysis of gluteus maximus; a fascia lata graft still attached to fascia lata and flap transferred to erector spinae m.

pubiotomy: surgical incision and division in the pubic bone.

Radley, Liebig, and Brown p.: for malignancy of ischium; resection of tuberosity and lower portion of pubis.

Root p.: for spastic cerebral palsy with tight hip adductors; transfer of adductors to ischial tuberosity.

Root and Siegel p.: for valgus and internal rotation deformity of hip; varus derotational osteotomy of proximal femur.

Sarmiento p.: for intertrochanteric fracture of the hip; use of osteotomy cut in the distal fragment to achieve valgus nail plate fixation.

Selig p.: for hip adducted gait; intrapelvic obturator neurectomy.

Soutter p.: for abdominal and hip flexion contracture; release of the soft tissues about the iliac crest.

Staheli p.: for developmental hip dysplasia; shelf procedure using iliac crest bone graft for buttress.

Stee p.: for spastic cerebral palsy internal rotation and flexion hip deformity; transfer of gluteus medius to vastus intermedius.

Stener and Gunterberg p.: for chordoma of sacrum; resecting portion of sacrum.

Sutherland p.: for internal rotation deformity of the hip; transfer of semitendinosus and semimembranosus to lateral posterior septa of thigh.

Taylor, Townsend, and Corlett p.: technique of vascularized free iliac crest graft.

Thomas, Thompson, and Straub p.: for gluteus medius paralysis; transfer of external abdominal oblique to the tensor fascia lata.

trochanteric slide: an osteotomy of the outer portion of the greater trochanter done from an anterior direction so that it and the attachment of the gluteus medius and vastus lateralis can be retracted posteriorly as a single flap and then replanted with wire fixation following a hip procedure.

trochanterplasty: surgical excision of a ridge of bone to form a new femoral neck.

Veleanu, Rosianu, and Lonescu p.: for hip adduction gait; combination of adductor tenotomy and obturator neurectomy.

Ward, Thompson, and Vandergriend p.: for vertical shear fracture of pelvis; posterior iliac to sacral screw fixation after reduction.

Webb p.: for separation of symphysis pubis; two-screw and plate fixation after reduction.

Weber, Brunner, and Freuler p.: for displaced hip fracture in children; cancellous screw fixation after initial fixation with Kirschner wires; **Boitzy p.**

The Lower Limbs

Anatomy

Bones

adductor tubercle (adductor tuberosity): the knobby prominence of the medial femoral condyle, which is easily felt by pressing on the medial side of the knee 5 cm above the joint.

anterior and posterior tibial spines: little prominences of bone inside the knee joint; attachment for the anterior and posterior cruciate ligaments.

anterior tibial tubercle: the large knob just below the anterior knee joint; the point of insertion for the quadriceps (knee extensors) muscles.

Chaput tubercle: the anterolateral tubercle of the distal tibia at the ankle joint for the strong attachment of the anterior tibiofibular ligament; **tubercle of Tillaux-Chaput.**

femoral condyles: the two prominences at the distal end of the femur, called the medial and lateral femoral condyles. The space between the condyles, called the **intercondylar notch,** contains the cruciate ligaments within the knee.

femur (Fig. 8-14): thigh bone; largest bone in the body.

fibula (Fig. 8-15): the smaller bone on the lateral side between the knee and ankle.

fibular facet (proximal tibiofibular facet): the flat portion of bone on the lateral side of the proximal tibia for articulation with the fibula.

fibular neck: narrow part of the fibula just below the proximal enlargement of the bone.

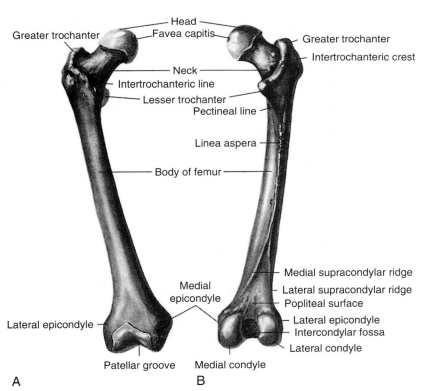

Greater trochanter
Head
Favea capitis
Greater trochanter
Intertrochanteric crest
Neck
Intertrochanteric line
Lesser trochanter
Pectineal line
Linea aspera
Body of femur
Medial supracondylar ridge
Lateral supracondylar ridge
Popliteal surface
Medial epicondyle
Lateral epicondyle
Intercondylar fossa
Lateral condyle
Lateral epicondyle
Patellar groove
Medial condyle
A
B

FIG 8-14 Right femur. **A,** Anterior view. **B,** Posterior view. (From Seeley RR, Stephens TD, Tate P: *Anatomy and Physiology*, St Louis, 1989, Times Mirror/Mosby College Publishing.)

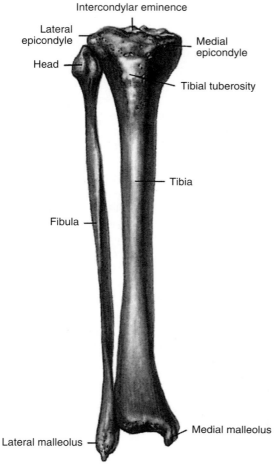

Intercondylar eminence
Lateral epicondyle
Head
Medial epicondyle
Tibial tuberosity
Tibia
Fibula
Medial malleolus
Lateral malleolus

FIG 8-15 Right tibia and fibula, anterior view. (From Seeley RR, Stephens TD, Tate P: *Anatomy and Physiology*, St Louis, 1989, Times Mirror/Mosby College Publishing.)

Gerdy tubercle: prominence of bone superior and lateral to the anterior tibial tuberosity; used as reference point in some knee surgery.

lateral malleolus: the distal end of the fibula, which is the outer prominence of the ankle.

linea aspera: a line of prominent bone on the lateral side of femur in the posterior proximal and middle femur for insertion of the gluteus maximus.

medial malleolus: the large prominence on the inner side of the ankle and part of the tibia.

patella (Fig. 8-16): the kneecap, a round to ovoid bone within the quadriceps (knee extensor) tendon. It has a posterior cartilaginous surface for articulation with the femoral condyles known as the **medial** and **lateral facets.**

posterior malleolus: a structure that cannot be seen or felt but is the posterior joint aspect of the tibia. It may fracture by itself or, more commonly, in association with other ankle fractures.

tibia (see Fig. 8-15): the large leg bone on the medial side between the knee and ankle.

tibial eminence: prominence of bone for attachment of anterior cruciate ligament on tibial plateau.

tibial plateau: the surface that articulates with the femur; may be subdivided into the medial and lateral plateaus.

trochlea: the groove that holds the patella in line on the distal femoral joint surface.

Muscles

adductor m.: the medial muscle of the thigh responsible for pulling the thigh toward the midline.

hamstring m.: three posterior thigh muscles, originating mostly at the pelvis and posterior femur, that help flex the knee. They are given this common name

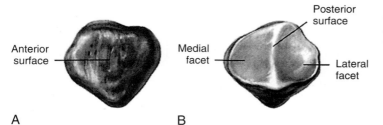

Anterior surface
Medial facet
Posterior surface
Lateral facet

A   B

FIG 8-16 Right patella. **A,** Anterior view. **B,** Posterior view. (From Seeley RR, Stephens TD, Tate P: *Anatomy and Physiology*, St Louis, 1989, Times Mirror/Mosby College Publishing.)

because when they reach the knee joint they are mostly tendinous. The three hamstring muscles are:

biceps femoris: outer hamstring.

gracilis: inner hamstring.

semimembranosus: inner hamstring.

semitendinosus: inner hamstring.

pes anserinus: the distal tendon portion of the gracilis, sartorius, and semitendinosus muscles, which at their attachment on the proximal medial tibial side are similar to a goose's foot in appearance.

popliteus m.: a muscle in the posterior superior tibia that has its tendon insertion into the posterior femur. It is important in lateral injuries of the knee in that the structure may be involved or encountered on arthrographic examination or as a part of surgical procedure.

quadriceps m.: the four divisions of muscles that are the bulk of the anterior thigh that become a tendon that surrounds the patella and ends on the tuberosity of the tibia. They function in extending the knee and, in the case of the rectus femoris, help to flex the hip. The quadriceps femoris group of muscles includes the **vastus lateralis, vastus medialis, vastus medialis obliquus (VMO), vastus intermedius,** and **rectus femoris (direct head** and **indirect head).**

Muscle Compartments

Muscles act in groups to bring about movements, primarily as agonists, antagonists, synergists, and prime movers. There are many muscle groups and compartments throughout the body. The most commonly referred to muscle groups are in the leg, because swelling within the compartments can lead to irreversible muscle change and loss of motor function. Therefore, the four compartments of the leg are defined here and the function and names given of the muscle groups of the lower extremity.

Achilles tendon: the tendinous heel cord that is the extension from the **triceps surae** group of muscles.

anterior c.: contains the muscles responsible for dorsiflexion of the ankle and the large and lesser toes; included are the **tibialis anterior, extensor hallucis longus, extensor digitorum longus,** and **peroneus tertius.**

deep c.: contains the flexors of the toes and ankle and are known as the **tibialis posterior, flexor digitorum longus,** and **flexor hallucis longus.**

gastrocsoleus muscle: refers to the combination of the two largest muscles contributing to the Achilles tendon.

lateral c.: contains the muscles that evert or plantar flex the ankle; they are the **peroneus longus** and the **peroneus brevis.**

posterior c.: contains the **triceps surae** muscles, which make up the bulk of the calf; included are the following:

> **gastrocnemius:** the most posterior muscle of the calf, leading to the Achilles tendon, that flexes both the ankle and knee.

> **plantaris:** the smaller ankle flexor that leads to the Achilles tendon over the medial side.

> **soleus:** the larger deep ankle flexor of the calf leading to the Achilles tendon.

Ligaments

The knee is an encapsulated joint that has several layers of fascial tissue. The deeper layer is referred to as the **joint capsule,** but numerous ligaments and tendons make up this capsule (Fig. 8-17).

anterior and posterior cruciate l.: the two deep ligaments within the knee that are crossed.

arcuate ligament: curved ligament in posterolateral corner of the knee.

fabello-fibular ligament: between fabella in lateral head of gastrocnemius and posterior fibular head.

infrapatellar l.: the infrapatellar tendon. Because this "tendon" bridges two bones and not a muscle to bone, it is more correctly referred to as the infrapatellar ligament. Its bursa is the infrapatellar bursa.

lateral collateral l.: strong fibrous ligament of the lateral knee joint with fibers from the femur to the tibia and fibula. This ligament is sometimes called the **tibial collateral,** but caution should be taken to distinguish this from the ankle ligaments.

ligaments of Henry and Wrisberg: small ligaments of attachment for the meniscus in the posterior knee.

ligamentum mucosa: not a true ligament but the thin, filmy membrane that sometimes divides the knee joint.

medial collateral l.: strong fibrous ligament on the medial side of the knee connecting the femur with the tibia. There is a **superficial** and a **deep ligament** in most knees. The posterior oblique ligament is

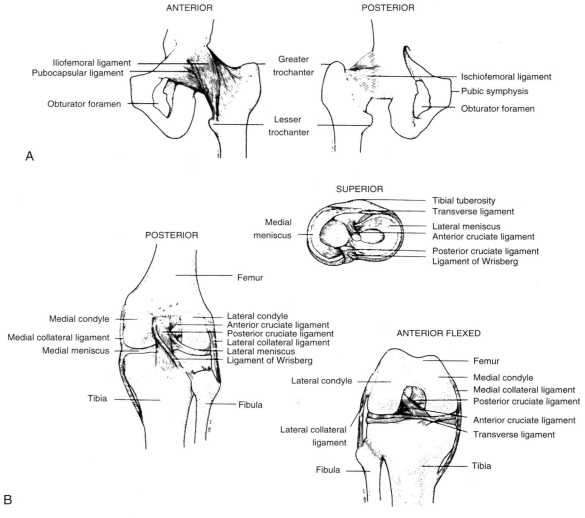

FIG 8-17 Major joints in terms of disease and surgical sites. **A,** Hip. **B,** Knee. (From Hilt NE, Cogburn SB: *Manual of Orthopedics,* St Louis, 1980, CV Mosby.)

composed of fibers that arise from the medial collateral ligament and attach more posteriorly in the joint.

menisco-femoral ligament: contribution of meniscal margin to medial collateral ligament leading to femur.

menisco-tibial ligament: contribution of meniscal margin to medial collateral ligament leading to femur.

proximal tibiofibular l.: ligament between the fibular neck and tibia.

tibiofibular l.: when used without distinction as to distal or proximal, refers to the ligaments just above the ankle; these ligaments are divided into the anterior, middle, and posterior tibiofibular ligaments.

Arteries and Veins (Fig. 8-18)

anterior tibial a.: main artery of the anterior leg supplying the extensors and peroneal muscles.

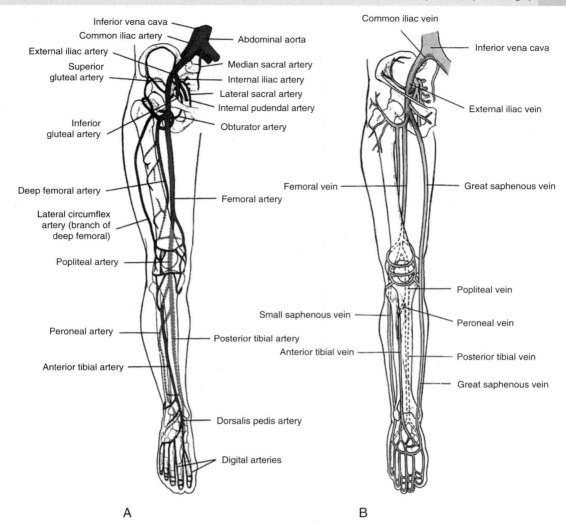

Inferior vena cava
Common iliac artery
External iliac artery
Superior gluteal artery
Inferior gluteal artery
Deep femoral artery
Lateral circumflex artery (branch of deep femoral)
Popliteal artery
Peroneal artery
Anterior tibial artery

Abdominal aorta
Median sacral artery
Internal iliac artery
Lateral sacral artery
Internal pudendal artery
Obturator artery
Femoral artery
Femoral vein
Posterior tibial artery
Small saphenous vein
Dorsalis pedis artery
Digital arteries

Common iliac vein
Inferior vena cava
External iliac vein
Great saphenous vein
Popliteal vein
Peroneal vein
Anterior tibial vein
Posterior tibial vein
Great saphenous vein

A

B

FIG 8-18 Blood vessels of the pelvis and lower limb. **A,** Arteries of the pelvis and lower limb—the internal and external iliac arteries and their branches. The internal iliac artery supplies the pelvis and hip, and the external iliac artery supplies the lower limb through the femoral artery. **B,** Veins of the pelvis and lower limb—the right common iliac vein and its tributaries. (From Seeley RR, Stephens TD, Tate P: *Anatomy and Physiology,* St Louis, 1989, Times Mirror/Mosby College Publishing.)

deep femoral a.: the largest branch of the femoral artery in the upper thigh that travels closely to the femur and gives off numerous circumferential branches around that bone; the branches are referred to as the **perforating arteries.**

femoral artery and vein: large artery and vein of the thigh that originate in the groin area; they penetrate posteriorly through fascia above the knee (Hunter canal) and become the popliteal artery and vein.

highest genicular a.: large branch from the femoral artery supplying the muscles and joints on the medial aspect of the knee. Branches above the knee may be referred to as medial and lateral superior genicular, medial and lateral inferior genicular, anterior and posterior tibial recurrent, and fibular arteries.

other arteries near the ankle: perforating, anterior and posterior medial malleolar, and anterior and posterior lateral malleolar arteries.

peroneal a.: travels along the posterior fibula supplying deep calf muscles and collateral circulation of the leg.

popliteal artery and vein: continuation of the femoral artery and vein as they emerge behind the knee, dividing distally to that joint and giving off the anterior tibial artery and posterior tibial artery.

posterior tibial a.: large artery of the posterior leg supplying most of the muscles of the calf and deep spaces; a major branch is the peroneal artery.

saphenous vein: large vein of the subcutaneous tissue in the medial thigh; continuous to the medial side of the ankle.

Other Structures

infrapatellar fat pad (retropatellar fat pad): a distinct mass of fat behind the patellar tendon extending into the anterior joint of the knee. Also called **Hoffa fat.**

medial and lateral menisci: referred to as the **semilunar cartilages,** which are fibrocartilaginous structures interfacing the medial and lateral rim of the femorotibial joint; serve to help distribute the weight load on the two cartilaginous surfaces by changing shape and position during motion.

interosseous membrane: a very strong fibrous membrane between the fibula and tibia, extending throughout most of the length of the bones.

plica: a fold, pleat, band, or shelf of synovial tissue; minor structures but may be large enough to produce symptoms and demand surgical attention. Specific locations include the transverse suprapatellar, medial suprapatellar, mediopatellar (also called medial patellar shelf), and infrapatellar plica (also called ligamentum mucosa, which does not produce symptoms).

prepatellar bursa: a bursa in the fat in front of the kneecap.

suprapatellar pouch: the extension of the anterior knee joint to about 12 cm above the joint line.

Nerves of the Lower Limbs

common peroneal n.: a brief segment of nerve that divides into the superficial and deep peroneal nerve just distal to the fibular head.

deep peroneal n.: nerve that supplies voluntary function of the toe and ankle extension; the sensory branch is between the first and second toes.

posterior tibial n.: nerve of the posterior leg that supplies the outer and deep calf muscles and eventually the muscles of the foot and sensation on the sole of the foot.

saphenous n.: nerve branch from the femoral nerve; supplies only sensation to the medial leg.

sciatic n.: nerve of the posterior thigh, supplying muscles of the posterior thigh and dividing into the common peroneal and posterior tibial nerves.

superficial peroneal n.: nerve that supplies the voluntary muscle function which turns the ankle out; also supplies sensation on the dorsum of the foot.

sural n.: large sensory nerve of the calf deriving branches from both the peroneal and posterior tibial nerves.

Surgery of the Lower Limbs
Eponymic and Named Procedures of the Femur and Tibia

Caldwell and Durham p.: for quadriceps rupture; a transfer of the biceps femoris tendon to quadriceps tendon.

D'Aubigne: for tumor of femoral condyle or tibial plateau; use of attached patella to act as graft for joint surface.

Enneking: for malignancy of distal femur or proximal tibia; resection of affected bone and use of graft taken from healthy bone and fixation with rod and patellar screws.

Gage p.: for spasticity of hamstring muscle; transfer of semitendinosus to rectus femoris.

Grant, Surrall, and Lehman p.: for spastic flexion contracture of knee; anterior closing wedge osteotomy of distal femur.

Lewis and Chekofsky p.: for malignant tumor of proximal femur; resection of proximal femur.

Moore p.: for malunion of distal femur in child; excision wedge of bone, using fragments as a graft after correcting deformity.

Sage p.: for hamstring spasticity with dislocating patella and internal rotation deformity of hip; lengthening of rectus femoris.

Sutherland p.: for hamstring spasticity with weak quadriceps muscle; transfer of semitendinosus and semimembranosus to patellar extensor mechanism.

Tachdjian p.: for hamstring spasticity in a child; lengthening of semitendinosus, semimembranosus, and biceps femoris.

Wagner p.: for correction of leg-length discrepancy (LLD); a method of shortening the femoral or tibial diaphysis, shortening the metaphysis of the femur or tibia, or lengthening the femur or tibia.

White p.: for leg-length discrepancy; a method of shortening the femur.

The Knee

Knee injuries account for a large percentage of the surgical procedures of the lower limbs because many muscles arising in the thigh and leg affect that joint. Often more than one procedure is indicated at the same time. Over the years, some of the combinations of procedures have acquired eponymic designations. To give a general purview of surgery of the knee, the single procedures and their modifications are listed first, and the combined procedures are listed last.

Knee Surgery for Internal Derangement

anatomic anterior cruciate ligament reconstruction (double bundle repair): uses a tendon or tendons to recreate the anterior to medial and posterior to lateral relationship that the normal anterior cruciate ligament has from proximal tibial to distal femur.

Andrews p.: for anterior cruciate laxity; extracapsular tenodesis by using iliotibial band.

Campbell p.: use of fascial strip from quadriceps tendon to replace anterior cruciate ligament.

Cho p.: for anterior cruciate deficiency; intra-articular use of semitendinosus tendon.

Clancy: for anterior cruciate-deficient knee; use of midpatellar tendon with attached patellar and tibial bone. Also, for posterior cruciate laxity; use of mid patellar tendon graft.

Drez p.: for anterior cruciate replacement; use of patellar tendon.

Ellison p.: extra-articular repair to replace anterior cruciate function; rerouting iliotibial band under the lateral collateral ligament.

Engebretsen p.: for anterior cruciate ligament deficiency; use of semitendinosus tendon with an ligamentous anterior dislocation (LAD) prosthetic graft as augmentation.

Ericksson p.: for anterior cruciate instability; midportion of patellar tendon and portion of bone redirected through tibia and into posterior lateral femoral condyle.

five-in-one repair: five procedures for severe ligamentous injuries to the knee; includes a medial meniscectomy, medial collateral ligament repair, vastus medialis advancement, semitendinosus advancement, and a pes anserinus transfer. Also called **Nicholas procedure.**

Fox-Blazina p.: extra-articular repair to replace anterior cruciate function by rerouting the iliotibial band under the lateral collateral ligament and placing it distal to original attachment.

Hey-Groves p.: a reconstruction of the anterior cruciate ligament using tensor fasciae latae graft.

Hughston and Degenhardt: for posterior cruciate-deficient knee; use of medial head of gastro-cnemius.

Hughston and Jacobson: for posterolateral instability; advancement of bony attachment of fibular collateral ligament and popliteus tendon to a superior and anterior direction.

Insall p.: for anterior cruciate laxity; use of iliotibial band and bone block as replacement.

Insall and Hood p.: for posterior cruciate ligament laxity; use of medial gastrocnemius and bone block as replacement.

Jones p.: repair of the anterior cruciate ligament using a portion of the patella and patellar ligament. A **Lam modification** of this procedure is also used.

LAD (ligamentous anterior dislocation) composite graft: a synthetic anterior cruciate replacement that was designed to be used with tissue graft.

Leeds-Keio: a prosthetic Dacron mesh that was designed to be a replacement for the anterior cruciate ligament.

ligamentous advancement: implies a soft tissue procedure only. The ligament is detached and then pulled up or down and reattached to bone. This is done for the medial and lateral collateral ligaments.

Lindeman p.: for anterior cruciate ligament rupture; gracilis tendon transfer as a replacement.

Loose p.: for anterior cruciate instability with pivot shift; portion of iliotibial band is redirected through lateral femoral condyle and around lateral joint.

MacIntosh p.: using infrapatellar and quadriceps tendon for transfer over posterior lateral femoral condyle for anterior cruciate ligament replacement. Also, iliotibial band used in reconstruction to provide anterior cruciate stability.

Marshall p.: for anterior cruciate ligament laxity; portion of patellar tendon and fascia is directed through notch and over lateral femoral condyle.

Mauck p.: detachment of a segment of the tibia containing the medial collateral ligament and replacement of that block of bone in a position that tightens the ligament.

meniscectomy: excision of the medial or lateral meniscus. There are other menisci in the body, but meniscectomies are usually done on the knee. A **partial meniscectomy** is the removal of the torn portion only or a definite attempt to leave meniscal margins of an even width.

Muller p.: for posterolateral instability; reinforcement with iliotibial band graft.

over-the-top p.: for anterior cruciate deficiency; any procedure that places the transferred ligament over the lateral femoral condyle rather than through the condyle.

Pagddu p.: for anterior cruciate-deficient knee; intraarticular use of gracilis and semitendinosus tendons.

Paulos p.: for anterior cruciate-deficient knee; use of medial patellar tendon and retinaculum through tibial grove.

reverse Mauck p.: detachment of a segment of the femur containing the medial collateral ligament and insertion of this block of bone into a position that tightens the ligament.

Slocum p.: a pes anserinus transfer (pes transfer). This is commonly done in association with other procedures and involves a change in the direction of pull of tendons inserting just below the medial knee joint; designed to help replace dynamic stability in ligamentous laxity.

triad knee repair (O'Donoghue p.): a repair involving the anterior cruciate ligament, medial collateral ligament, and a medial meniscectomy.

vastus medialis advancement: a procedure done rarely by itself but more commonly in association with procedures for ligamentous laxity of the knee and/or chronic subluxing patella. It is a tightening of the vastus medialis muscle.

Wirth Jager p.: for posterior cruciate ligament deficiency; use of proximally-based semitendinosus and gracilis tendon for replacement.

Yount p.: for severe contracture of posterior knee; division of iliotibial band and biceps tendon.

Zaricznyj p.: for anterior cruciate-deficient knee; use of double strand semitendinosus for replacement.

Zarins and Rowe: for anterior cruciate-deficient knee; simultaneous "over the top" of semitendinosus and iliotibial band with posteromedial and posterolateral capsular reefing.

Knee Surgery for Chronic Subluxation of the Patella

Campbell p.: fascial tissue transfer and vastus medialis reefing.

Elmslie-Trillat p.: medial displacement of anterior tibial tuberosity on a bone pedicle for subluxing patella.

Galeazzi p.: for chronic lateral subluxing patella; use of fold of medial strip of parapatellar capsule, strip is brought across inferior to superior patella and back again.

Hauser p.: inferomedial displacement of a block of bone with the infrapatellar tendon attached.

Hughston p.: lateral release with quadricepsplasty and patellar tendon transfer as needed.

Insall p.: lateral retinacular release and lateral advancement of vastus medialis.

Maddigan, Wissinger, and Donaldson p.: for chronic lateral subluxing patella; wide lateral advancement of vastus medialis.

Maquet p.: anterior tibial tuberosity displacement on bone pedicle for patella alta.

Roux-Goldthwait p.: medial displacement of the lateral portion of the infrapatellar tendon.

Sargent p.: lateral release and advancement of vastus medialis over patella with attachment to exposed, bleeding patellar surface.

Silfverskiöld p.: for knee flexion contracture (in cerebral palsy); transection of medial and lateral head of gastrocnemius muscle and motor branch to medial gastrocnemius.

Southwick slide p.: medial displacement of bony attachment of the patellar tendon, replacing the lateral defect with bone from the medial side.

Stanisavljevic p.: for congenital dislocating patella; massive patellar tendon and quadriceps refashioning.

West and Soto-Hall p.: patellectomy and medial advancement of the quadriceps mechanism for patellar osteoarthritis.

Patellar Surgery

Cave and Rowe p.: for osteoarthritis of the patella; partial patellectomy with fold of infrapatellar fat sewn onto the posterior patella.

Codivilla p.: for neglected quadriceps tendon rupture; direct repair and advancement of fold from superior quadriceps mechanism.

Houston and Akroyd p.: for sleeve fracture of patella; tension band wire fixation with two Kirschner wires.

Magnuson p.: for unstable fracture of the patella; arthroplasty of the knee (fascia) in an attempt to remodel, and use of encircling metal wire.

Martin p.: for patellar fracture; fixation with a wire loop.

McLaughlin p.: for quadriceps or patellar tendon rupture; a reinforcing encircling wire is attached to patella or tibia, respectively.

Miyakawa p.: patellectomy with fabrication of a fold taken from the thick tissue well superior to the patella and reinforcing the patellar area to provide better mechanical force.

patellar or femoral condylar shaving (skiving): direct removal of diseased cartilage from the patella and femoral cartilage, usually done in combination with treatment of other chronic knee injury problems.

patellectomy: removal of the kneecap.

patellectomy (partial): this procedure has two different meanings: (1) total removal of cartilage from the patella, and (2) removal of a portion of the bone following a fracture.

Scudari p.: for fresh quadriceps rupture; repair with reinforcing flap from superior quadriceps mechanism.

Quadricepsplasty

Any repair or reapproximation of the quadriceps mechanism is called a quadricepsplasty.

Judet quadricepsplasty: for knee fibrosis; parapatellar and intra-articular adhesion release with intraoperative manipulation.

Thompson quadricepsplasty: for knee fibrosis; isolation of vastus lateralis and medialis from rectos femoris and capsular incision.

Total Knee Arthroplasty

Total knee arthroplasty (TKA) is the replacement of both sides of the knee joint by metal or plastic components. See Internal Prostheses in this chapter for various types of prostheses.

Knee Prostheses (Fig. 8-19)

Knee prostheses are designed to replace portions or all of the knee joint. The original attempts involved solid metal to replace one side or the other of the joint. Metal with plastic interfacing, better joint mechanical design, and superior attention to detail in surgical applications have improved the relative success of knee joint replacements.

The listing of total knee devices is not practical because of the expansion of manufacturers and their variety of trade names. Previous editions of the dictionary list names of those devices that are possibly remaining in some joints or are still being used. Most hospital operating rooms have a limited list of devices and are a good resource for location of specific terminology. There are general terms that describe the basic types of knee replacement devices.

bicompartmental replacement: the medial and lateral side of the joint is replaced but there is no patellar-trochlear resurfacing. The breakdown of the patellar mechanism resulted in disuse of this design.

cruciate retaining: designs that retain the posterior cruciate ligament.

cruciate sacrificing (or substituting): designs that remove the posterior cruciate ligament and replace with a plastic post on the polyethylene component.

constrained: the prostheses are not necessarily totally constrained. Some are nonhinged and prevents posterior subluxation with a post and limits varus and valgus to less than 5 degrees. The term **fully constrained** implies no motion and actually denotes a block of anteroposterior shifting on lateral motion. Because there is restriction in at least one plane of

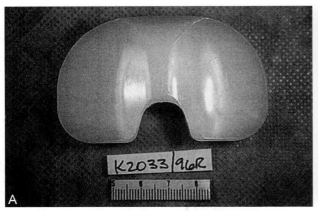
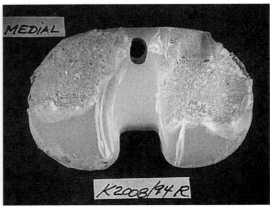

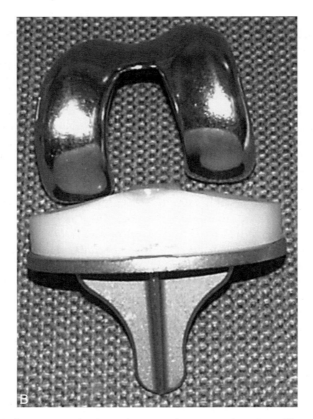

FIG 8-19 **A,** Total knee prosthesis showing accumulated wear that occurred over years of use. **B,** Total knee. (**A,** Courtesy of the Orthopaedic Research Laboratory, Good Samaritan Medical Center, West Palm Beach, FL.)

motion, there are forces that produce high stresses on the bone. These devices are more likely to become loose as the bone breaks down or the prosthesis itself fails. One design is a **hinged knee** design that locks components in place with a hinge and prevents any anterior posterior shift or varus/valgus motion.

high flex design: total knee replacements designed to allow up to 160 degrees of flexion.

meniscal bearing: plastic able to move anterior to posterior on a smooth groove on the tibial tray.

monoblock: one piece tibial component; metal-based plate is bonded to polyethylene liner.

patellar button: typically all plastic dome-shaped device to replace articular surface of the patella. Previously used devices were **fixed anatomic,** which was an anatomically shaped piece of plastic on metal backing. Another device was **rotating,** which is an anatomically shaped piece of plastic that is attached to a metal backing in such a way that the plastic can rotate during knee motion.

rotating platform: plastic fitted on a smooth tibial metal surface with central hole for the plastic insert, which allows rotation of the plastic on the tibial surface.

semiconstrained: the degree of constraint ranges from minimal to nearly full in any given plane. This is the design of many of the current pro-stheses.

tricompartmental: most knee replacements entail a design that replaces both tibial-femoral surfaces and the patella.

unconstrained: the most minimally constrained prosthetics with the maximal freedom of motion of the knee joint. These devices require good soft tissue stability.

unicompartmental: the unicompartmental design has evolved into a metal unicondylar component for the femur making contact with a plastic or plastic on metal tibial component. There are few patients for whom this limited procedure is appropriate.

Tendon Transfers

Surgical releases for muscle imbalance or knee contractures are referred to as tendon transfers.

Baker p.: patellar tendon advancement; semitendinosus transfer for knock-kneed gait caused by internal rotation deformity of the hip.

Bickel and Moe p.: translocation of the peroneus tendon.

Caldwell and Durham p.: for quadriceps paralysis; transfer of biceps femoris to quadriceps mechanism.

Chandler p.: patellar tendon advancement.

Ecker, Lotke, and Glazer p.: for neglected infrapatellar tendon rupture; transfer of gracilis and semitendinosus for reinforcement.

Eggers p.: transfer of the biceps femoris tendon associated with capsular releases and soleus neurectomy.

Galleazzi p.: for chronic subluxation of the patella; transfer of the semitendinosus.

Hughston p.: for chronic subluxation of the patella; patellar tendon transfer fixed by staple and redirection of vastus medialis.

Kelikian p.: for old patellar tendon rupture; transfer of the gracilis tendon.

Sutherland p.: for internal rotation deformity in hip affected by cerebral palsy; lateral transfer of medial hamstring.

Tachdjian p.: for hamstring tightness in cerebral palsy; plastic lengthening of hamstring sheaths and tendons.

Genu Recurvatum Procedures

Brett and Campbell: tibial osteotomies.

Heyman p.: reinforcement of posterior capsule using multiple tendon transfers; soft tissue release and transfers.

Perry p.: posterior capsular repair with multiple tendon transfers.

Knee Arthrodeses

Brittain
Charnley
Key
Lucas and Murray
Putti

The ankle arthrodeses are listed under foot and ankle procedures in Chapter 11.

Tibial Osteotomies

Campbell
Cotton
Coventry
Ferguson-Thompson-King
Brett
Pott
Lucas and Cottrell

Lower Limb (Below Knee) Surgery

Anderson p.: for unequal leg lengths; tibial lengthening using an external skeletal fixator.

Anderson and Hutchins p.: for unstable tibial fractures; a method of skeletal pins and casting for fixation.

beefburger p.: for failed total knee arthroplasty; debridement with interposition of acrylic cement between leveled edges of femur and tibia, followed by brace immobilization.

Bosworth p.: for anterior tibial epiphysitis; insertion of bone pegs into the tibial tubercle.

Brett p.: for malunited proximal tibial fractures with knee recurvatum; bone graft applied to opened anterior tibial plateau hinged posteriorly.

Brown p.: for congenital absence of tibia; transfer fibula to femoral intercondylar notch.

Carroll p.: bone graft replacement of the distal end of the fibula for tumors.

d'Aubigne p.: for tumors; a method of excision of femoral condyle or tibial plateau.

Fahey and O'Brien p.: for excision of tumor; technique of excision of a portion of the shaft of a bone.

Forbes p.: for nonunion tibial fracture; iliac bone graft to tibia.

Gilbert p.; Tamai p.: technique of obtaining vascular fibular graft by using lateral approach.

Gill p.: for long-bone nonunion; a half diameter slide graft of a 10- to 15-cm portion of bone.

Gruca p.: for congenital absence of the fibula; construction of an ankle mortise by splitting of the fibula.

Hsu and Hsu p.: for ankle flexion contracture in muscular dystrophy; percutaneous tendocalcaneus lengthening.

Irwin p.: for paralytic genu recurvatum; a closing wedge osteotomy of the proximal tibia.

Langenskiold p.: for partial absence of fibula; fusion of distal tibia and fibula.

Lee p.: for depressed tibial plateau fracture; anterosuperior iliac spine used to replace joint surface.

Malawer p.: for malignancy of proximal fibula; resection of proximal fibula.

Nicoll p.: for tibial or other long-bone nonunion; dual onlay bone graft with cancellous bone in the middle.

Russell p.: for central depression lateral plateau; proximal portion of fibular head is used to support depression of joint surface.

Taylor p.: technique of obtaining vascular pedicle fibular graft through posterior approach.

Van Ness p.: for proximal focal femoral deficiency; a derotation osteotomy of the tibia to fit the limb more readily with a prosthesis.

Wagner p.: for leg-length disparity; shortening of proximal tibia or distal femur.

Weber p.: for persisting acute valgus deformity tibial shaft fracture in children; open reduction and removal of tissue.

Weiland p.: technique of obtaining vascular fibular graft by using lateral approach.

Wilson and Jacobs p.: for comminuted tibial plateau fractures; replacement technique for the lateral side using iliac crest graft.

The ankle and foot procedures are covered in Chapter 11.

Skin Grafts

Skin grafts are of three major categories; split-thickness skin graft (STSG), full-thickness skin graft (FTSG), and pedicle and rotational flaps.

Split-Thickness Skin Graft

A split-thickness skin graft is 0.015 inch or 0.4 mm thick. Taking a graft this way leaves viable skin from the donor site and living cells in the graft. However, both donor site and the graft will appear different from normal surrounding skin. Names associated with skin grafts are **Blair-Brown, Douglas (mesh), Dragstedt,** and **Ollier-Thiersch.**

Full-Thickness Skin Graft

A full-thickness skin graft is a procedure that, throughout the entire surface of the graft, includes all the epidermis and, therefore, all the smooth skin coverage. This leaves behind a **donor site** that will need some form of closure or a split-thickness skin graft; for example, if a small necrosed area on a finger needs full skin coverage, a small ellipse of skin could be removed from the forearm; this is called a **pinch graft,** and the wound edges are closed.

Names associated with full-thickness skin grafts are **Braun, Davis, Esser (Stint), Krause-Wolfe, Reverdin,** and **Wolfe.**

Pedicle Grafts and Rotational Flaps

A pedicle graft is a layer of fat, dermis, and epidermis raised from a portion of the body having a sufficient blood supply to keep it alive. Pedicles are often used to cover large tissue defects, areas of exposed tendons, or areas where there will be considerable wear on the skin. The intended purpose of a pedicle is to eventually transfer this loose piece of skin and fat to cover another portion of the body. A flap is another name for pedicle, although the term connotes a local use in some cases; for example, a **rotational flap** is a rearrangement of the skin and fat in one area to cover a local defect. Pedicles may include muscle or bone.

A **delayed flap** is used for stimulation of the blood supply. An incision in the skin and fat with approximation of the wound margins into their original position is carried out. In a second or third procedure the flap is raised on a pedicle that is still attached, but now the distal part of that flap can be laid on another portion of the body. For example, a U-shaped incision is made in the leg and closed; 3 weeks later that skin is raised through the same incision and the flap that develops is laid on an open area of the opposite leg. This is called a **cross-leg pedicle graft.**

Other terms referring to pedicle grafts and flaps are bilobed, compound, compound lined, double pedicle, Verdan, jump, marsupial, tumbler, Tait, and island pedicle.

Surgical Blocks

The term **local anesthesia** is sometimes used to indicate a regional anesthesia. In precise parlance, **local anesthesia** indicates the injection of anesthetic agents at the site of the procedure. **Regional anesthesia** is infiltration of anatomic structure(s) proximal to the location of the procedure. Those used for orthopaedics are the following.

axillary b.: injection of anesthetic agent into the nerves immediately around axillary artery, approached from the axilla; used for elbow, forearm, and hand procedures.

epidural b.: infiltration of anesthetic agent into spinal canal but outside of the dura; can be used for so-called continuous drip anesthesia, in which a catheter is left in place during procedure so that if more anesthesia is required it can be administered without repositioning the patient.

intravenous b.: application of double tourniquet and the infiltration of anesthetic agents directly into vein to produce anesthesia in the limb below the tourniquet. Also called **Bier block.**

scalene b.: injection of anesthetic agent into brachial plexus at the point of scalene muscles; used for shoulder and other upper limb procedures.

spinal b.: infiltration of anesthetic agent into the spinal canal within the dura in the lumbar region. The proper positioning of patient during anesthetic infiltration is important in ensuring correct and sufficient anesthesia for procedures on the pelvis and lower limbs.

Surgical Approaches

A surgical approach implies the type of incision made by the surgeon to do a particular procedure. Many surgical approaches have been described by various surgeons whose names are applied to those approaches. However, those approaches are not all original and have been modified and improved over the years. Anatomically, the direction of the incision may be modified by another surgeon, whose name then becomes attached to that incision, although in fact it is designed for accessing the same area of the body. In many instances, an experienced surgeon may decide to plan an individualized approach in a given situation.

This prior consideration to surgical intervention may be described by the anatomic location and direction of the incision, for example, anterolateral or posterolateral approaches. More frequently, the anatomic terms are favored in describing where an incision is to be made, even though the eponyms are also used for a particular anatomic area described.

Approaches are listed by anatomic location, eponyms, and common uses for the incision. Those interested in the technique of an incision will use other references. At the end of this section is a list of common incision shapes.

Shoulder Approaches

anterior axillary a.: usually used for repair of anterior dislocations; **Roberts.**

anteromedial a.: used for repair of shoulder and acromioclavicular joint injuries; **Cubbins, Callahan and Scuderi, Roberts, Thompson and Henry, saber-cut.**

deltoid splitting a.: used to approach the rotator cuff and subacromial bursa.

posterior a.: used for repair of a posterior dislocation of the shoulder and lateral scapula. **Abbott and Lucas, Bennett, Harmon, Kocher, McWhorter, Rowe, Yee.**

transacromial a.: used to approach the rotator cuff and bursa; **Codman, Darrach-McLaughlin, saber-cut.**

Humerus Approaches

anterolateral a.: an approach to the bone and radial nerve; **Thompson** and **Henry.**

anteromedial a.: an approach to the median and ulnar nerves.

posterior a.: an approach used to visualize the humerus, triceps, and radial nerve; **Henry.**

Elbow Approaches

anterior and anteromedial a.: for exploration of the median nerve, brachial artery, and other soft tissues; often associated with fractures.

anterolateral a.: for exploration of the radial nerve; **Henry.**

medial a.: for exploration of the ulnar nerve and medial epicondyle; **Campbell, Molesworth,** and **Campbell.**

posterior: for fractures of the distal humerus; **Bryan** and **Morrey.**

posterolateral a.: for elbow dislocations, radial head and distal humeral fractures, and arthroplasties; **Kocher.**

Forearm Approaches

posterior a.: in the proximal forearm used for fixation of proximal ulnar fractures and an approach to radial fractures; **Thompson.**

posterolateral a.: approach used for radial head fractures, some ulnar fractures, and exploration of the deep radial nerve; **Boyd.**

anterior a.: used for visualization of most of the forearm muscles that flex the fingers and for internal fixation of fractures of the radius; **Henry.**

posterolateral (distal) a.: used for some distal forearm fractures, tendon transfers, and excision of the distal ulna; **Gordon.**

Pelvis Approaches

Avila a.: anterior approach along the iliac crest to reach the anterior sacroiliac crest.

Radley, Liebig, and Brown a.: to the ischium.

Hip Approaches

anterior approach: Smith-Peterson using interval between sartorius and rectus muscle in front of hip.

anterolateral a.: for open reduction and internal fixation of the femoral neck, prosthetic replacement, and some congenital dysplasia surgery; **Smith-Petersen, Van Gorder, Wilson, Watson Jones, Cave, Callahan, Fahey.**

Hardinge a.: splitting gluteus medius and respecting anterior portion of that muscle with part of vastus lateralis.

Heuter approach (direct lateral): anterior hip exposure technique for arthroplasty techniques.

lateral a.: for internal fixation of hip fractures and prosthetic replacement; **Callahan, Charnley-Müller, Fahey, Harris, Hay, McLaughlan, Murphy, Ollier, Watson-Jones.**

medial a.: for congenital dysplastic hip surgery and other iliopsoas tendon approaches; **Ludloff, Young.**

posterior a.: for prosthetic replacement and repair of some pelvic fractures; **Abbot, Gibson, Guleke-Stookey, Kocher, Langenbeck, McFarland** and **Osborne, Moore, Osborne.** The **Kocker-Langenbeck** approach is a more extensive approach for access to pelvic fractures.

Senegas (modified Ollier): for acetabular fractures; an extensive exposure of the involving detachment of the greater trochanter.

trochanteric slide: removal of trochanter and portion of lateral proximal femoral shaft for improved access in prosthetic revision surgery.

two-incision anterior approach: a combination approach in which the anterior approach is used for cup placement and percutaneous posterior approach for the stem.

Femur Approaches

anterolateral a.: used for rod or plate fixation fractures; **Thompson.**

lateral a.: used for fracture fixation; **Eycle-Shymer** and **Shoemaker.**

posterior a.: used for some muscle surgery and fixation of fractures; **Bosworth.**

posterolateral a.: used for muscle procedures, fracture fixation, and nerve explorations; **Eycle-Shymer** and **Shoemaker, Henry.**

Knee Approaches

All approaches to the knee are for ligamentous and bony reconstruction, meniscectomies, and vascular explorations. The posterior approaches are more specifically devoted to neurovascular surgery but may also be used in ligamentous and bony reconstructive procedures.

anterior a.: Coonse and Adams, Bosworth, Putti, Jones and Brackett, Insall.

anterolateral a.: Kocher, Henderson.

anteromedial a.: Abbott and Carpenter, Langenbeck.

lateral a.: Bruser lateral, Aufranc, Henry, Hoppenfield, deBoer, Pogruna and Brown.

medial a.: Aufranc, Cave, Henry, Bosworth.

Midvastus a.: vastus medialis muscle fibers are split in their midsubstance.

Parapatellar a.: typically medial for knee approach in knee replacement.

posterolateral a.: Henderson.

posterior a.: Abbott, Osgood, Bracket and Osgood, Putti and Abbott.

posteromedial a.: Banks and Laufman, Henderson.

quad snip a.: for difficult joint replacement knee approaches; cutting the quadriceps tendon proximal to the patella at a 45-degree angle.

quad sparing a.: avoidance of cutting the quadriceps in the approach.

transverse a.: Cave, Charnley, Cozen, Sir Henry Platt, McConnell.

trivector retaining a.: for extensive knee surgery such as a total joint replacement; an incision that is medial to the standard parapatellar incision cutting into a portion of the vastus medialis muscle.

Lower Limb Approaches

anterior a.: for internal fixation of fractures; this is an exploration of the anterior deep spaces.

posterior a.: approach to the superomedial region of the tibia and gastrocnemius muscle; **Banks** and **Laufman.**

posterolateral a.: for peroneal nerve and muscle surgery and for some bone grafts; **Harmon, Henry, Huntington.**

posteromedial a.: for neurovascular exploration and internal fixation of fractures; **Phemister.**

Surgical Incisions Described by Appearance

J shaped	curvilinear
L curved	double
S-flap	linear
T shaped	longitudinal
T-tube saber-cut	saber-cut
U shaped	split
Y incision	transverse
Z-plasty	

Replantation Microsurgery

Microsurgery, the use of a binocular microscope to assist in intricate surgery, is another challenge for the skilled orthopaedic surgeon and is adapted to a variety of orthopaedic conditions. Microtechniques are applied to nerve and vascular repair, replantation, and free tissue transfers, as well as knee and spine surgery.

The integration of this technique provides the surgeon with a three-dimensional telescopic view of the operating field at magnifications of structures 2½ to 25 times the size. Nylon sutures of high tensile strength, finer than human hair, are used to reattach small blood vessels and nerves. To keep vessels open and carefully avoid constriction are the goals of this procedure. Use of the technique requires extreme patience and perseverance on the part of the microsurgical team.

Replantation of traumatically severed extremities has become a common practice in orthopaedic surgery and in musculoskeletal trauma management. The reintegration of tissues by way of microsurgical techniques has successfully restored functional use and eliminated the need for amputation in many cases. Hand and knee surgery have benefited greatly from microsurgery.

Replantation is truly a team effort, involving many hours of work with no room for compromise. The surgeon must spend many hours practicing and developing the skill, applying extreme patience and good judgment during application. The team approach is used to allow replacements during the long procedures.

Although other tissues heal in a short time, the regeneration of nerves may take from 1 to 2 years. Other technologic developments, such as the **laser scalpel,** are also useful in surgical procedures.

Treatment of Tumors

The prognosis for musculoskeletal tumors has improved with the addition of various chemotherapies and other interventions. Some of these therapies are used in conjunction with amputation and wide excisions.

adjuvant therapy: a method of treatment (i.e., radiation or chemotherapy) combined with another treatment (surgery) to improve therapeutic success.

chemotherapy: the use of drugs to treat tumors.

intralesional resection: surgical removal of tumor from within the surrounding capsule.

marginal resection: surgical removal of tumor through the capsule.

radiation therapy: the use of ionizing radiation to treat tumors.

radical resection: removal of an entire anatomic compartment, which includes tumor, tumor capsule, and all muscle, bone, nerve, and artery found within that compartment.

wide resection: surgical removal of tumor capsule and surrounding margin of tissue.

Amputations

The least desirable procedure for any surgeon is an amputation of a part; however, sometimes it becomes necessary. An **amputation** is the removal of a part through bone, and a **disarticulation** is the removal of a part through a joint space. Both of these terms are interpreted by most as the same procedure, but there is a distinction.

Most amputations take place in the lower limbs and may be indicated by traumatic injury, burns, infection, loss of blood supply, or malignancy. Amputation may also be indicated when a nonfunctioning limb could be replaced by a functional prosthetic device or when a congenital defect could be improved cosmetically or functionally by the removal of a part.

The level of amputation is often based on preservation of as much of the residual limb as would heal well with the vascular and peripheral circulation intact. The most common levels fall into the following categories: above elbow (AE), above knee (AK), below elbow (BE), and below knee (BK).

In the present nomenclature, the description for limb absences can be reversed, that is, a leg, complete, is a complete leg amputation; if there is a partial amputation, it can be stated as to the level, for example, partial arm (upper one-third). Any amputation through an epiphysis or closer to a joint is considered a complete amputation; an amputation of the distal third to the distal growth plate (growth plate scar in an adult) is considered a complete leg amputation (Tables 8-2 and 8-3).

Following such a procedure the patient is often fitted right away with an artificial limb for the remaining residuum. The after treatment of the residual limb is most important in the adjustment and rehabilitation of the amputee, as are the psychologic aspects.

Before and after a prosthesis (artificial limb) is prescribed for an amputee, the physical medicine and rehabilitation team is an important link in teaching the patient prosthetic training. Prostheses have come a long way in appearance, fit, and functional use, and often it is not evident that a person is using a prosthesis. Chapter 7 discusses the many types of prostheses available. The following list of general terms applies to amputations.

TABLE 8-2 Amputation Levels, Upper Limbs

New Terms (with Abbreviations)	Current Terms	Eponyms
Shoulder (Sh), complete	Forequarter	Littlewood
Arm (Arm), complete	Shoulder disarticulation	Larrey, Dupuytren, Lisfranc
Arm (Arm), partial (upper ⅓)	Short (upper-third) AE	
Arm (Arm), partial (middle ⅓)	Medium (mid-third) AE	
Arm (Arm), partial (lower ⅓)	Long (lower-third) AE	
Forearm (Fo), complete	Elbow disarticulation	
Forearm (Fo), partial (upper ⅓)	Short (upper-third) BE	
Forearm (Fo), partial (middle ⅓)	Medium (mid-third) BE	
Forearm (Fo), partial (lower ⅓)	Long (lower-third) BE	
Carpal (Ca), complete	Wrist disarticulation	
Carpal (Ca), partial	WD, with some carpals still present	
Metacarpal (MC), complete		
Metacarpal (MC), partial	Partial hand amputations, usually without precise differentiation	
Phalangeal (Ph), complete		Kutler
Phalangeal (Ph), partial		

From Kay HW: A nomenclature for limb prosthetics, Orthot Prosthet J 28(4):37-47, 1974.
Note: An amputation at the metacarpophalangeal (MCP) joints of the ring and little fingers would be designated as Ph, 4,5, complete; an amputation of the same two fingers at the proximal interphalangeal (PIP) joints would be Ph, 4,5, partial. AE, above elbow; BE, below elbow; WD, wrist dislocation.

General Amputations

cineplastic (kineplastic) a.: amputation that includes a skin flap built into a muscle (the biceps being the most common); a portion of the prosthetic mechanism is activated by the muscle.

circular a.: one in which a perfect circular incision is made with single flaps.

closed a.: any amputation in which the wound is closed at the time of initial or secondary surgery.

disarticulation: any amputation in which the limb is severed through a joint.

guillotine (chop) a.: amputation making a straight cut through the limb.

Marquardt technique: to broaden bone support for below-knee stump, an iliac crest bone graft is inserted in the distal tibia.

open a.: any amputation in which the wound is left open for drainage, as opposed to a closed amputation.

skew flap a.: for below-knee amputation, creating better coverage of anteromedial tibia with a fish mouth in which the axis of amputation creates a posterolateral flap.

stump revision: any surgery designed to revise the shape or scar of a residual limb.

Syme a.: the term is used to describe a special method of incision and closure for amputations at other locations but most commonly the term is used for an amputation through the ankle where the heel pad is closed over the tibial and fibular stump to give a firm walking surface.

Associated Surgical Terms

ablate: to completely excise or amputate; the surgical removal of a part is referred to as **ablative surgery,**

TABLE 8-3 Amputation Levels, Lower Limbs

New Terms (with Abbreviations)	Current Terms	Eponyms
Pelvic (Pel), complete	Hemicorporectomy	
Hip (Hip), complete	Hemipelvectomy	King and Steelquist, Jaboulay, Gordon-Taylor, Sorondo-Ferré
Thigh (Th), complete	Hip disarticulation	Béclard, Boyd, Pack
Thigh (Th), partial (upper ⅓)	Short (upper-third) AK	Alouette
Thigh (Th), partial (middle ⅓)	Medium (mid-third) AK	
Thigh (Th), partial (lower ⅓)	Long (lower-third) AK	Kirk
Leg (Leg), complete	Knee disarticulation	Gritti-Stokes, Morestin, Callander, Pollock, Carden, Batch, Spittler and McFaddin
Leg (Leg), partial (upper ⅓)	Short (upper-third) BK	
Leg (Leg), partial (middle ⅓)	Medium (mid-third) BK	
Leg (Leg), partial (lower ⅓)	Long (lower-third) BK	Came
Tarsal (Ta), complete	Ankle disarticulation	Syme, Pirogoff, Guyon, Hancock, MacKenzie
Tarsal (Ta), partial		Chopart, Le Fort, Malgaigne, Vladimiroff-Mikulicz, Tripier
Metatarsal (MT), complete	Known collectively as partial foot amputations	Lisfranc, Hey
Metatarsal (MT), partial		
Phalangeal (Ph), complete		
Phalangeal (Ph), partial		

From Kay HW: A nomenclature for limb prosthetics, Orthot Prosthet J 28(4):37–47, 1974.
AK, above knee; BK, below knee.

for example, the excision of a large tumor mass and the surrounding soft tissue.

advancement: surgical or traumatic detachment of muscle, tendon, or ligament structure followed by reattachment at a more advanced point.

anastomosis: restoration of continuity of any vessel or organ; usually refers to the suturing of a tubular structure such as a blood vessel creating the passage between two distinct parts, such as end-to-end anastomosis.

anesthesia: loss of sensation with or without loss of consciousness as a direct result of the administration of a systemic drug agent. The term also describes the local or systemic loss of sensation caused by trauma or other injury.

antibiotic beads: methylmethacrylate impregnated with antibiotic and place on a suture for later removal in the treatment of deep wound infections.

approximate: to bring together or into apposition; this term is commonly used to refer to suturing of tissues or the repositioning of fractures.

aseptic: free from bacteria; aseptic technique is any technique designed to prevent contamination by bacteria.

aspiration: withdrawal of fluid from any open or closed space.

attenuate: to make thin, small, or fine; reduce in size.

autopsy: a postmortem and pathologic examination of the body by dissection; **necropsy.**

biopsy: the excision of a section of living tissue for microscopic examination and diagnosis. This may be performed on any tissue; for example, a bone marrow biopsy is performed by closed method (use of a needle or trocar); the terms **needle biopsy** and **closed biopsy** are often used. In the same sense, an **open biopsy** is one in which the tissue is examined before excision, and all or a sample of that tissue is sent for microscopic inspection. The purpose of a biopsy is to determine the etiology and test for systemic, neoplastic, or reactive conditions. A biopsy is not made on normal anatomic tissue or where there is trauma or inflammation.

brisement: the forcible breaking up of joint capsule, usually for conditions of partial fibrous ankylosis such as frozen shoulders (pronounced breez-maw).

broaching: the act of widening a bone medullary canal in such a fashion that it will accept the stem of a specific implant. The instrument used to do this is a **broach.**

callotasis: for limb-length disparity, a transverse section of the bone of the short limb is stabilized with an external skeletal fixator and then the limb is gradually lengthened over a period of weeks.

catheterization: insertion of a tube into a cavity or blood vessel for drainage.

cauterization: the use of an electric current to stop local bleeding. This term also denotes the use of caustic materials such as silver nitrate to reduce local tissue granulation, as seen in open wounds.

cautery: an instrument designed to stop bleeding by destroying tissue through heat, electricity, or corrosive chemicals.

chamfer: applied to the act of smoothing off soft edges or rounding the end of a bone by making small cuts.

costoplasty: correction of rib deformity by osteotomies of rib, often used for correction of scoliosis deformities.

curettage: procedure in which a sharp, scraping instrument is used to remove abnormal tissue, to obtain diagnostic specimens, or to obtain donor bone or marrow.

curette: sharp, scraping, spoon-shaped instrument used in curettage.

débridement: cleansing a wound of devitalized, contaminated, or foreign material.

decompression: surgical relief of pressure to any structure.

dehiscence: a separation or splitting of the edges of a surgical wound, in which the expectation was for the wound to remain closed.

delayed primary closure (secondary closure): the closure of an open wound by intention after the initial surgery or injury; this is often done when the risk of infection is very high.

diaplasis: obsolete term for the reduction of a fracture or dislocation by surgical means.

dismemberment: amputation of a limb.

dissection: separation of tissue for any reason. **Sharp dissection** is the use of a sharp instrument to facilitate dissection. **Blunt dissection** refers to the separation of tissues along natural lines of cleavage by the use of the fingers or other blunt instruments.

drainage: removal of fluid from a cavity. This term is often used to refer to material arising from open surgical wounds. **Dependent drainage** is an active effort to position a patient so that gravity will carry fluid away from the wound via catheterization.

ebonation: stripping of one tissue from another. In orthopaedics, this refers to a surgical or pathologic removal of hard, bony loose cartilage from the surface of bone.

electrocautery: surgical instrument used to control bleeding of a surgical wound. The use of this instrument is called **electrocauterization.**

enucleate: to remove whole and clean in its entirety an organ, tumor, or cyst by shelling out.

evacuate: to empty a cavity.

excise: to cut out.

exploration: the examination by direct surgical visualization; surgery done for the express purpose of examining tissue is called exploratory surgery.

extirpation: the removal in its entirety of diseased tissue, a structure, or mass; **excision.**

extraction: process of removal by pulling out.

extubation: the removal of a tube; used to refer to the tube inserted into the windpipe during anesthesia.

fixation: as applied to orthopaedics, implies the use of internal or external fixation, which is the use of metallic devices inserted into or through bone to hold a fracture in a set position and alignment while it heals.

fulguration: the use of high-frequency electrocautery to destroy tissue during surgical procedures.

fusion: the uniting of two bony segments, whether a fracture or a vertebral joint.

granulation: the proliferation of numerous small blood vessels at a wound site to give the general appearance of a raw, red tissue. This is a normal healing process in that this rich vascular bed can modulate into normal tissue or act as a base for skin grafts or primary closure. **Granuloma** is a pathologic reaction to a foreign body or organism and should not be confused with granulation.

imbrication: the overlapping of tissue structures in closure of a wound and in repair of defects to improve the tightness of a structure.

implant: any substance inserted into the tissue for an indefinite period; this includes all internal prostheses, internal fixation devices, and other materials not absorbed by the body.

incision and drainage (I&D): surgical incision into a cavity, usually for purpose of removing purulent (infected) material; most common example is the lancing of an abscess.

infiltration: usually refers to local injection of anesthetic solutions or fluids that then permeate soft tissue; may be a result of failure of intravenous fluids to go into the vein correctly.

infusion: introduction of any solution such as saline into a blood vessel or cavity.

injection: introduction of material, nutrients or medicine into tissues of the body by the use of a syringe and needle.

in situ: in orthopaedics, the fixation of a fracture in the position that it presents at the time of injury, usually a nondisplaced fracture; also used to describe a lesion that is highly localized.

in toto: in total; removal of an organ, cyst, or tumor in its entirety.

intubation: insertion of a tube into the trachea for entrance of air during surgical procedure; for example, endotracheal intubation.

in vitro: cells or tissue maintained in an artificial environment such that they can survive outside the living body usually for experimental purposes. (This term is sometimes italicized in the literature.)

in vivo: within the living organism, such as an experimental drug being used on an animal or human subject. (This term is sometimes italicized in the literature.)

irrigation: washing out of a wound or cavity with a solution. **Closed suction irrigation** is a specific system by which irrigating tubes are surgically implanted in a wound and used continuously after the time of surgery.

laser (*light amplification by stimulated emission of radiation*): a device used in surgical procedures consisting of a resonant optical cavity in which a substance is stimulated to emit light radiation and a mirror that reflects the rays back and forth so molecules will emit more radiation. Finely directed laser light sources can be used to cut tissue, coagulate vessels, or cause the adhesion of one tissue surface to another.

lavage: the copious washing out or irrigation of a wound or cavity.

ligamentotaxis: use of strength of ligaments to bring about reduction of fracture fragments by using external skeletal fixation.

ligation: tying off; used particularly in reference to the tying of blood vessels at a surgical wound.

ligatures: sutures used to tie off blood vessels.

manipulation: the planned and carefully managed manual movement of a joint or fracture to produce increased joint motion or better position and alignment of the fracture. This term is sometimes used to denote a precise sequence of movements of a joint to determine the presence of disease or to reduce a dislocation.

marsupialization: incision into a cystic lesion with incorporation of the walls of the cyst to the exterior edges of the skin to produce constant drainage.

matte finish: a fine-ground-glass-appearing finish, designed for better cement to metallic surface fixation of internal prosthetics.

morcellation: breaking up or subdividing tissue for easier removal; also, to leave in place but in a refashioned shape such as cortical or cancellous bone graft material.

palliative: surgical procedure or use of medications to treat the symptoms without curing the disease process; used relative to the treatment of terminal conditions seen in cancer.

paracentesis: needle puncture into a cavity to aspirate fluid; usually done in the abdominal and thoracic cavities.

parenteral: the introduction (injection) of substances into the body by way of intravenous, intramuscular, subcutaneous, or intramedullary route, other than through the alimentary canal.

per primam: the healing of a surgical or traumatic wound by first intention, after closure. This means that the closure of the wound is successful and that there is no reopening of the wound due to failure of healing.

-pexy (suffix): fixation by solid tissue attachment. In orthopaedics, the most common term using this root is **scapulopexy,** a procedure whereby the scapula is fixed directly to the ribs.

phantom pain: the sensation of pain following amputation that seems to be in the part that has been removed. Eventually, the patient is able to localize the pain to the stump and loses the sense of the presence of the amputated part.

plication: taking tucks in a structure to shorten it; folds. **Fundoplication** is a combination of shortening and being part of the anatomy.

polyacetyl rod: synthetic polyester rod used for fracture fixation. The rod is bioabsorbable.

portal: small stab incision used for introduction of arthroscope or instrument into a joint.

primary closure: the closure of the wound edges at the time of trauma or surgery.

prosthesis: this term has a very broad meaning and includes all artificial limbs as well as materials implanted in the body to replace the structure, function, or appearance of the missing structure.

reefing: a folding in or overlapping of soft tissue by surgical suture designed to make that structure tighter.

reflect: in the surgical sense, to fold back tissue such as a muscle belly to expose deeper structures.

regimen: a system of therapy regulated to achieve certain results (e.g., diet, exercise following surgery).

release: incision into any soft tissue to produce relaxation of that tissue, for example, tendon release.

resection: partial excision of soft tissue or segment of bone; also, the removal of a portion of diseased nerve tissue, called a nerve resection.

retraction: a pulling back of tissue, whether done mechanically at the time of surgery or by scar formation after surgery; for example, a scar that is indented inward toward the body is considered a retracted scar.

revision: any surgical reconstruction of soft or hard tissue. A revision may be done at the time of initial trauma if damaged tissue is removed and normal structures are repositioned to compensate for that destruction. The term is more commonly used to describe a later surgical effort to reposition various tissues.

rongeur: to cut into bone with a sharp biting instrument called a rongeur, usually to remove bone that is diseased or obstructing visualization of deeper structures.

saucerization: creation of a saucer-like depression in bone in an effort to remove diseased bone. This is most commonly done for bone infections, and the wound is usually left open for drainage; it is also a saucer-like collapse of a crushed vertebrae on the horizontal surface.

scaffold: a support, usually of an absorbable fiber, for the ingrowth of tissue.

secondary closure: closure of a wound that had been left open after previous trauma or surgery. This is also called **delayed primary closure** and is done often when there was initially a high risk of infection.

sepsis: the presence of bacterial infection in blood or tissue from any source. This term is often used to describe the systemic condition resulting from an infection, for example, septicemia.

septic: contaminated with bacteria. A septic wound, otherwise known as a **dirty wound,** is one in which there is an existing infection with purulent material.

-stasis (suffix): to control flow or progression (e.g., hemostasis).

stasis: condition arising from a static circumstance. For example, a stasis ulcer is one that is created in a patient kept in the same position for any length of time in which blood or fluids stagnate.

stent: a support, flexible or rigid, usually biodegradable, designed to relieve excessive strain during graft or other tissue repair and remodeling.

subcutaneous: the fatty and fibrous tissues beneath the thick layers of skin.

subcuticular: the thick layer of skin below the epidermal layers. A subcuticular suture is used to close the skin by a continuous suture that pulls the deep layer of skin together, with the suture exiting at each end of the wound only.

sulcus: any normal groove or depression in bone or soft tissue.

suspension: usually refers to a soft tissue procedure designed to help hold some anatomic structure in a more functional position; tenodesis.

suture: any thread-like, pliable material that is used to close soft tissue; catgut, nylon.

tamponade: method to control bleeding by direct pressure.

-tome (suffix): any instrument that cuts.

tourniquet: any instrument used to compress blood vessels to slow or stop circulation. If light pressure is applied by tourniquet, there will be congestion in the venous system. This is often used to help draw blood for laboratory testing. More secure tourniquet pressure, designed to stop all blood flow to a part, is used to prevent bleeding.

toxic: poisonous. This term is often used to describe the systemic condition of a patient with infection.

transect: to cut across the long axis of a tissue. For example, a tendon transection is often done to release the pull of that tendon at its point of insertion.

transfusion: term commonly used to describe the intravenous infusion of whole blood or blood components; however, any solution may be transfused.

transposition: the repositioning of an intact and attached tissue segment from one place to another. This term is often used in describing soft tissue and bone graft procedures.

-tripsy (suffix): surgical crushing, for example, an osteotripsy is a procedure done in the foot to relieve a corn or callus caused by prominence of bone under the skin.

vest-over-pants closure: closure of fascia, particularly near joints, in which one layer is closed on top of another to produce tightening or pull on the joint capsule.

viable: alive or capable of living; used to describe healthy tissue that appears to be intact.

The Spine

9

The spine consists of three basic elements: bones, joints, and neural tissue. Together these components allow the spinal column to perform a variety of functions in the human body. The weight of the body is transferred through the vertebrae and disks, motion occurs through the intervertebral joints and disks, and the brainstem, spinal cord, and spinal nerves that travel in and around these bones and joints are allowed to function in a protected environment.

The body has three main neural components: the central, peripheral, and autonomic nervous systems. The **central nervous system** consists of the brain, brainstem, and spinal cord. Protecting the spinal cord and spinal nerves are the meninges, composed of the dura mater, pia mater, and arachnoid. These protective layers help protect and isolate the central nervous system from the outside world. The brainstem and spinal cord travel within a tunnel-like structure called the spinal canal. The spinal cord gives rise to 31 pairs of spinal nerves or nerve roots that branch off along the length of the spinal cord and exit from the spinal canal through a tunnel called the foramen. After these nerve roots exit from the spine, they join other nerves to become **peripheral nerves.** Peripheral nerves contain the sensory fibers, voluntary muscle fibers, and fibers of the autonomic nervous system. The **autonomic nervous system** is composed of small nerve branches arising from the central nervous system and supplying **ganglia,** which are clusters of cells near but outside the bony limits of the vertebrae. The **sympathetic** and **parasympathetic nervous systems** are subdivisions of the autonomic nervous system, which is involved in the control of visceral organs and blood vessels. Most spinal nerves and peripheral nerves contain a mixture of sensory and motor fibers that supply specific muscles and provide sensation in particular locations in the body. By treating the anatomy of the spinal cord and its peripheral branches like a road map, a physician can often determine the cause of numbness, tingling, or weakness found on a sensory and motor examination.

The spine is made of bony segments known as **vertebrae.** These are separated by intervertebral disks and **facet joints** that permit motion. A complex arrangement of ligaments and muscles provide stability and motion of the spinal column. Neural elements exit and enter the spinal column through openings called **foramina.**

Each component of the spinal column depends on the others to function normally. If one part of the spine changes in character, such as in a fracture or a disk herniation, other structures can be affected, leading to arthritis, muscle fatigue, nerve or spinal cord damage, or irritation resulting in pain, numbness, weakness, or even paralysis in severe cases.

General Anatomy of the Spine

The 32 vertebrae composing the spinal segments are divided into five regions, with the segments numbered from top to bottom. They are the cervical, thoracic, lumbar, sacral, and coccygeal regions of the spine (Fig. 9-1).

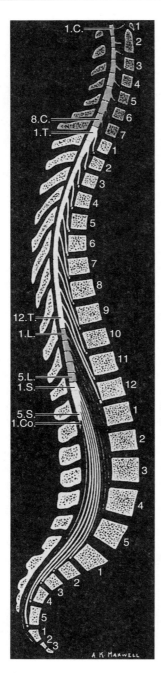

FIG 9-1 Diagram showing the relation of the segments of the spinal cord and nerves to the segments of the vertebral column. (From Hamilton WJ, editor: *Textbook of Human Anatomy*, ed 2, London, England, 1976, The Macmillan Press, Ltd.)

It is very important to understand the designation of vertebrae, intervertebral disks, and nerves when making reference in writing. The proper description is as follows.

Vertebrae	Disks	Roots
C-1, L-5	C-2–3, L-4–5	C-2, L-5
T-4, S-2	T-3-4, S-1-2	T-3, S-2

These specific designations may be abbreviated without first being written out in tables and clinical or technical data, but it should be clear as to what part of the spinal anatomy reference is being made.

cervical spine: seven spinal segments (C1–C7) and eight cervical nerve roots (C1–C8) between the base of the skull (occiput) and the thoracic spine. The cervical spine differs from the rest of the vertebrae in one major aspect: the numbered nerve roots exit the spinal canal above the correspondingly numbered vertebra's pedicle instead of below it.

thoracic (dorsal) spine: 12 spinal segments (T1–T12) incorporating the 12 ribs of the thorax. Other than a slight increase in size from top to bottom, they are fairly uniform in appearance.

lumbar spine: five mobile segments of the lower back (L-1 to L-5). These are the largest of the vertebral segments.

sacral spine (sacrum): five fused segments of the lower spine that connect to the pelvis and have four foramina on each side.

coccygeal spine (coccyx): remaining three or four, somewhat fixed, fused segments at the end of the spine (tailbone) that articulate with sacrum above.

Except for the coccyx, sacrum, and the first cervical spine, there are anatomic parts that are common to all 32 spinal segments. Moving from anterior to posterior (front to back), the main vertebral parts are the following.

facet joint (zygapophyseal joint): small articular cartilage-surfaced joints connecting the posterior elements of one spine to the posterior elements of the neighboring spine.

foramen: an opening allowing for the egress of spinal nerve roots from between two vertebrae.

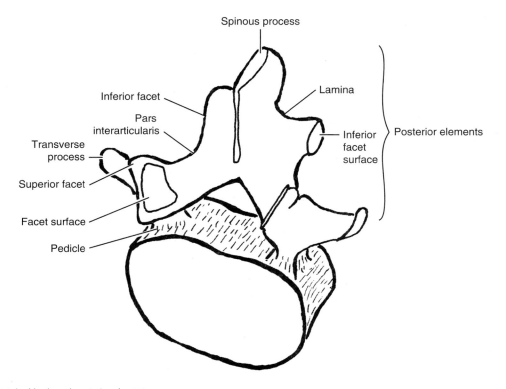

Spinous process

Inferior facet

Pars
interarticularis

Transverse
process

Superior facet

Facet surface

Pedicle

Lamina

Inferior
facet
surface

Posterior elements

FIG 9-2 Vertebral body and posterior elements.

intramedullary: refers to medullaris, marrow; (1) within the medulla oblongata of the brain, (2) within the spinal cord, and (3) within the marrow cavity of bone.

lamina: the posterior part of the spinal ring that covers the spinal cord or nerves.

pars interarticularis: the posterior continuation of the spinal arch from the pedicle; the superior and inferior facets are connected to each other by the pars interarticularis.

pedicle: the first portion of the posterior spine arising from the vertebral body.

spinous process: the most posterior extension of the spine arising from the laminae.

transverse process: bony process arising from midportion of the spinal ring just posterior to the pedicle and pars interarticularis.

vertebral body (Fig. 9-2): from a lateral view, it is the main rectangular portion; from an overhead view, oval.

Cervical Spine Anatomy

Bones and Landmarks

atlas: the first cervical vertebra (C1), lying directly under the skull, through which the head articulates with the neck. The main connection to the vertebra below is a pivot around the odontoid process that is an upward projection of the body of the second cervical vertebra. The atlas is held to the odontoid by a ligament complex attaching it to the odontoid anteriorly and facet joints posteriorly, allowing rotation, flexion, and extension between C1 and C2.

axis: the second cervical vertebra (C2), about which the first cervical vertebra rotates, allowing head movement. It bears the **odontoid process,** the projecting part of the second cervical vertebra, which allows the first cervical vertebra (atlas) to rotate.

carotid tubercle: prominence of the transverse process of C6 felt on the lateral side of neck.

cricoid ring: cartilage ring above the trachea and below the thyroid cartilage; the first cricoid ring is at the level of C6.

hyoid bone: small, vertically oriented bone lateral to trachea, located at the level of C3.

joints of Luschka (uncovertebral joints): unique to the cervical spine, these joint-like structures are formed by the apposition of posterolateral portions of adjacent vertebral bodies; forms the anterior portion of the canal where nerves pass through.

lateral mass: the lateral expansion of the spinal ring in the cervical spine, consisting of the facet joints and intervening bone as well as a tunnel through which the vertebral artery travels in the second through seventh cervical vertebra.

occiput: the base of the skull.

thyroid cartilage: widening expanses of cartilage above the trachea, the top marks the level of C4, the bottom C5.

Muscles

longissimus colli: long muscle immediately anterior to the cervical spine.

platysma: thin outermost muscle layer of the anterior neck.

posterior neck muscles: splenius, spinalis, and semispinalis.

scalenus: the deep lateral muscles of the anterior neck, including anterior scalene m. (scalenus anticus), middle scalene m. (scalenus medius), and posterior scalene m. (scalenus posticus).

sternocleidomastoid: large externally visible muscle of the anterior neck, enabling head to turn to either side.

strap muscles: a general term applied to the ribbon-like muscles in the anterior neck; they include omohyoid, sternohyoid, sternothyroid, and thyro-hyoid.

Arteries and Veins

carotid artery: main artery to the head that divides into external and internal carotid arteries.

jugular vein: large obvious vein in the neck.

other arteries and veins: transcervical, facial, superior thyroid, and inferior thyroid.

vertebral artery: large artery that travels in the lateral masses of the cervical spine and eventually supplies the lower brainstem.

Nerves

cervical plexus: plexus of nerves that supply the neck muscles with branches named by muscles supplied, a portion of which is called the ansa cervicalis.

occipital nerve: nerve from the back of the neck that supplies motor function and sensation to the forehead; two parts—greater and lesser.

other nerves (twelfth cranial): transcervical, supraclavicular, posterior rami, facial, greater auricular, and hypoglossal.

phrenic nerve: nerve arising from three cervical nerve roots (C3–C5); supplies the diaphragm.

spinal accessory nerve (eleventh cranial): the nerve from the brainstem that supplies the sternocleidomastoid muscles.

vagus nerve (tenth cranial): the long nerve in the anterior neck traveling with the carotid artery; responsible for many organ functions in the chest and abdomen.

Other Structures

esophagus: portion of the gut between the mouth and stomach in the anterior neck.

interspinous ligament: ligament between each of the spinal processes.

nuchal ligament: large posterior midline ligament in the neck from the base of the skull to the seventh cervical vertebra.

thyroid gland: near the "Adam's apple"; responsible for secretion of hormone that is involved in regulation of the rate of the metabolism.

trachea: the windpipe.

triangles: for surgical approaches and other considerations, the anterior half of the neck is divided into triangles—anterior, digastric, posterior, submental, and carotid.

Thoracic Spine Anatomy

costo-: combining form denoting relation to ribs.

costochondral junction: junction of the rib into cartilage in the anterior chest. NOTE: Most of the ribs have attachment to the cartilage rather than a direct junction with the breast bone.

costovertebral angle: juncture of tissue inferior and lateral to the twelfth rib and vertebral body.

costovertebral joint: junction of the rib with the thoracic spine.

diaphragm: the muscle between the abdomen and thorax; main muscle of normal breathing.

intercostals: the muscles between the ribs.

other thoracic spine and chest muscles: pectoralis, semispinalis, rotators, latissimus dorsi, and spinalis.

sternum: the breast bone; further divided into three segments.

    manubrium: upper portion, proximal end.

    sternum: main portion, medial portion.

    xiphoid: the dagger-like tip of the sternum, distal end.

thorax: the chest or rib cage; also refers to the space containing the lungs and heart. There are 12 vertebral segments and ribs; the lower two are called **floating ribs.**

Lumbar and Lower Spine Anatomy

Bones

lumbar spine: the five movable spinal segments of the lower back and largest of the spinal segments.

sacral spine (sacrum): the five segments fused together as a solid bone and below the last lumbar segment position.

coccyx: the three, and sometimes four, segments of bone just below the sacrum; referred to as the tailbone; the end of the spinal column.

sacroiliac joint: the junction between the sacrum and the ilium; resembles a large ear.

sacral ala: lateral portions of the sacral bone.

Disk and Spinal Canal

intervertebral (interspinal) disk: the structure that normally occupies the space between two moving vertebrae. It is more prominent in the cervical and lumbar spines. It is much like a radial tire. The centermost portion of the disk (**nucleus pulposus**) is normally composed of a gelatinous material that varies in consistency from a firm jelly material to a very thick and less pliable substance. This core is then surrounded by numerous layers of fibrous (fibrocartilaginous) material called the **annulus fibrosus.** That structure goes to the normal margins of the vertebral body, called the **anterior longitudinal ligament,** and to those on the spinal canal side posteriorly, the **posterior longitudinal ligament.**

ligamentum flavum: a band of yellow elastic tissue that runs between the laminae from the axis to the sacrum; it assists in maintaining or regaining erect position and serves to close in the spaces between the arches. It is important as a surgical structure in that a portion is usually removed during an exploration of the spinal canal.

spinal canal: the space between the vertebral body anteriorly and the lamina and spinal process posteriorly. The spinal cord extends to the level of the second lumbar segment in adults and the second sacral segment in infants. Below this level are numerous spinal nerves from the spinal cord. This lower portion resembles a horse's tail and is referred to as the **cauda equina** (horse's tail in Latin). The lower tip of the spinal cord is attached to the end of the spinal canal by a single filament called the **filum terminale.** The brain, spinal cord, and spinal nerves float in a water-like substance called the cerebral spinal fluid. This fluid is contained in a thin sac called the **meninges.** The thick, outer portion of that sac is called the **dura** or **dura mater.** The more flimsy inner coverings are the **arachnoid** (Latin for spider-like) and pia. The dura extends over the nerve roots out into the foramina. This sac-like covering is called the **nerve root sleeve.** The dura also extends within the spinal canal down to the level of the second sacral segment. Any space within the dura from the first cervical to the second sacral level is considered **intradural.**

spinal cord: the part of the central nervous system below the level of the brainstem and above the cauda equina in the regions of the cervical, thoracic, and upper lumbar spines. Usually, the orthopaedist does not deal with the spinal cord—that is for the neurosurgeon. Based on training, both the orthopaedist and neurosurgeon deal with spinal cord problems. Many of these conditions can result in peripheral neuromuscular disorders.

dorsal column: the main, normal sensory tract to the brain.

dorsal lateral column: the main tract of position and tone to the brain.

gray matter (anterior and posterior horns): the nerve cell bodies to muscle and sensory outflow and input, respectively.

long tracts: the nerve fibers that connect the spinal cord with the brain; main spinal nerve pathways.

pyramidal tract: carries the voluntary muscle messages from the brain.

spinal thalamic tract: the main tract of pain to the brain.

Muscles

abdominal muscles: important for support of the spine, these muscles are the rectus abdominis, external oblique, internal oblique, and transversus.

iliopsoas muscle: large muscle starting at L1 and becoming wider as it picks up segments from the lower lumbar spine; combines with the iliacus muscle before attaching to the lesser trochanter of the hip.

posterior spinal muscle segments: upper and lower posterior serratus m., spinalis m., semispinalis m., and rotators.

quadratus lumborum: a muscle lateral to the iliopsoas muscle of the spine running from the lower ribs to the ilium.

Artery

artery of Adamkiewicz: an important source of blood supply to the lower portion of the spine, usually occurring at the levels of T9 to T11; however, it is not the only blood supply to the cord at that level.

Diseases and Structural Anomalies

Back and Neck Diseases

The spine is a complex organ that is a series of joints with attending bone, nerve tissues, muscles, and ligaments. In addition, there are two elements not common to other joints, namely, intervertebral disks and the spinal cord and nerves in the bony spinal canal. The nerves may be affected by either bone or disk disease; therefore, this section is divided into discussions of diseases affecting bone, nerves, spinal cord, vertebral disks, and congenital disorders.

Diseases of the spine may be treated by other medical specialties, particularly neurosurgery in the case of spinal cord and nerve lesions and injuries. However, the orthopaedist treats many diseases and conditions of the spine such as scoliosis, spina bifida, and degenerative disk disease. Treatment may last for years in the correction of some deformities.

General Bone Diseases of the Spine

The Latin word *vertebra* and the combining form *spondylo-* both denote the bony spinal segments. In some word combinations, the root word is assigned only to a specific part of the vertebra, such as spondylolysis in which the defect is always at the pars interarticularis. However, spondylo- in general means vertebra.

Spondylo- Root Diseases

spondylalgia: pain in vertebra(e).

spondylarthritis: arthritis of the spine.

spondylarthrocace: tuberculosis of the spine; spondylocace.

spondylexarthrosis: dislocation of a vertebra.

spondylitis: inflammatory disease involving the spine with inflammation of vertebrae, including types such as ankylosing, rheumatoid, traumatic, spondylitis deformans, Kümmell, and Marie-Strümpell d.

spondylizema: depression or downward displacement of a vertebra, with destruction or softening of one below it.

spondylodynia: pain in vertebra(e).

spondyloepiphyseal dysplasia: disorder of growth affecting both the spine and the ends of long bones.

spondylolisthesis: anterior displacement of one vertebra on the adjacent lower vertebra. A general term with multiple distinctions:

anterior displacement: forward movement of the superior segment on the inferior one.

lumbar lordosis: angle made by lines drawn from the superior surface of the first and fifth lumbar vertebra.

lumbosacral joint angle: angle between the inferior surface of the fifth lumbar vertebra and the top of the sacrum.

rounding of the cranial border: relationship of the height to the width of the rounded portion of the superior sacrum.

sacral inclination: relationship of the sagittal plane of the sacrum to the vertical plane.

sacrohorizontal angle: angle between the top of the sacrum and the horizontal line.

sagittal rotation: denotes an abnormal angular relationship between the body of the fifth lumbar vertebra, and the sacrum; **sagittal roll, lumbosacral kyphosis, slip angle.**

wedging of olisthetic vertebra: measure obtained by dividing the height of the anterior border of the fifth vertebra by the height of its posterior border, multiplied by 100.

spondylolysis (Fig. 9-3): a fracture or defect in the pars interarticularis (a portion of bone between each of the joints of the spine), allowing one vertebral body to slide forward on the next. May be referred to as **pars interarticularis defect.**

A classification system for spondylolysis and spondylolisthesis has evolved:

dysplastic: congenital abnormalities of the arch of the sacrum or the arch of L5 that permit the slipping to occur.

isthmic: the lesion is in the pars interarticularis. Three types occur:

a. lytic, fatigue fracture of the pars interarticularis.

b. elongated but intact pars interarticularis.

c. acute fracture of the pars interarticularis.

degenerative: the lesion results from intersegmental instability of long duration.

traumatic: results from fracture in other areas of the bony hook than in pars interarticularis.

pathologic: generalized or localized bone disease is present.

spondylomalacia: softening of vertebrae; **Kümmell disease.**

spondylopathy: any vertebral disorder.

spondylopyosis: infection in vertebra(e).

spondyloschisis: congenital fissure (splitting) of vertebral arch.

spondylosis: bony replacement of ligaments around the disk spaces of the spine, associated with decreased mobility and eventual fusion; **marginal osteophyte.**

Rachio- Root Diseases

Rachio-, as relating to spine, is less frequently used than more specific combining forms.

rachialgia: pain in the vertebral column.

rachiocampsis: curvature of the spine.

rachiochysis: effusion of fluid within the vertebral canal.

rachiodynia: pain in the spinal column.

rachiokyphosis: humpbacked curvature of spine; kyphosis.

rachiomyelitis: inflammation of the spinal cord.

rachioparalysis: paralysis of the spinal muscles.

rachiopathy: any disease of the spine.

rachioplegia: spinal paralysis.

rachioscoliosis: lateral curvature of the spine.

rachisagra: pain or gout in the spine.

rachischisis: congenital fissure of the spinal cord.

Miscellaneous Spinal Disorders

alar dysgenesis: abnormality in development of the sacroiliac joint.

anisospondyly: different abnormal shapes of the vertebral bodies.

ankylosing spinal hyperostosis: arthritic disorder in which bridging osteophytes located anteriorly and posteriorly on the vertebral body bind two or more vertebrae together; **Forestier disease.**

anterior spurring: ligament turning to bone on anterior side of vertebral body.

Baastrup d. (kissing spine): false joint formed by wide posterior spinous processes of the lumbar spine. This may become a source of pain.

camptocormia: severe forward flexion of upper torso, usually an excessive psychologic reaction to back pain.

cervical rib: rib-like structure in the seventh cervical vertebra that may cause nerve root irritation.

coccyalgia: pain in the coccyx region; **coccygodynia, coccyodynia, coccydynia.**

crankshaft phenomenon: progressions of a spinal curve due to continued growth of the unfused anterior aspect of the spine following a posterior spine fusion for scoliosis in children. The deformity can be severe with increased lordosis and rotation despite little change in the curve as measured on an anterior-posterior (AP) radiograph.

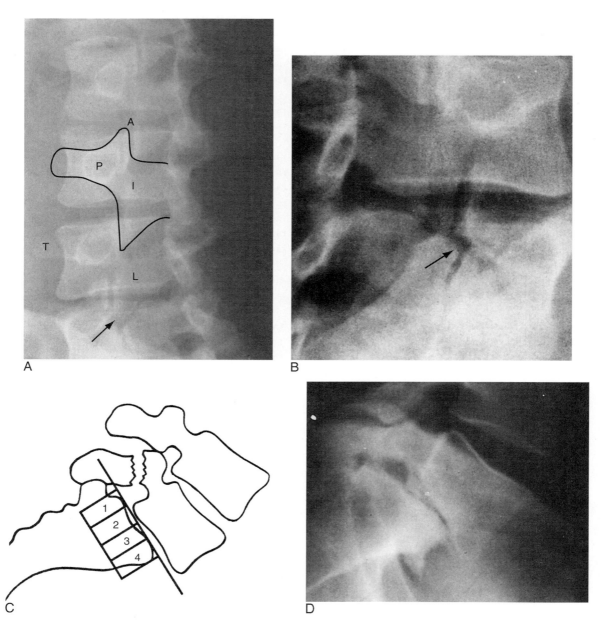

FIG 9-3 A, Oblique view: *A,* Articular facet joint; *I,* isthmus or pars interarticulars; *T,* transverse process; *L,* lamina; *P,* pedicle. The oblique view visualizes the so-called Scottie dog. Spondylolysis occurs through the isthmus (*arrow*). **B,** Bony defect (*arrow*) in the isthmus or neck of the Scottie dog present in spondylolysis (oblique view). **C,** Meyerding's classification of spondylolisthesis. The amount of slippage is graded 1–4. Grade 1 represents 25% forward displacement; grade 2, 25%–50%; grade 3, 50%–75%; and grade 4, greater than 75%. **D,** Spondylolisthesis of the lumbosacral junction. (From Mercier: *Practical Orthopaedics,* ed 5, St Louis, 2000, Mosby.)

dysraphism: dysraphism: any failure of closure of the primary neural tube. This general category would include the disorder **myelomeningocele.** This definition includes the conditions in which there is an abnormal midline structure in the neural axis. Hence, **diastematomyelia,** in which the midline structure has fused, but the term also implies a bony spike from the anterior-lying vertebral body.

facet tropism: asymmetrical orientation of the facets comparing right to left side.

Grisel syndrome: subluxation of the atlantoaxial joint from inflammatory ligamentous laxity due to infection. Can result in neurologic complications.

interspinous pseudarthrosis: formation of a false joint between two spinous processes.

limbus annulare: a mass of bone situated at the anterosuperior margin of a vertebra. Arises from failure of fusion of the primary and secondary ossification centers.

lumbago: archaic term meaning back pain.

lumbarization: partial or complete formation of a free-moving first sacral segment so that it looks like a lumbar vertebra.

marginal osteophytes: excess bone formation at the margin of the vertebral body; **spondylosis.**

olisthy: slipping of bone(s) from normal anatomic site; for example, a slipped disk.

paravertebral muscle spasm: spasm in the muscles on either side of the spinous processes (midline of the back); the term may be used to describe a physical finding or improperly used to define a disease process.

pseudoclaudication: increased pain and decreased strength in lower limbs associated with physical activity. Complaints are similar to those caused by an insufficient blood supply to the limb but are caused by diminished blood supply to the nerves in a narrowed spinal canal.

retrolisthesis: posterior displacement of the vertebra on the one below.

rudimentary ribs: nubbins of ribs seen below the level where the last rib normally occurs.

sacralgia: pain in the sacrum.

sacralization: fusion of L5 to the first segment of the sacrum, so that the sacrum consists of six segments; with this abnormality, it is called **Bertolotti syndrome.**

sacralized transverse process: one or both of the lumbar spinous transverse processes abnormally joining with the sacrum; **sacralization.**

sacrodynia: pain perceived to be in the area of the sacrum but may originate elsewhere; **referred pain.**

sacroiliitis: inflammation of the sacroiliac joint. A very painful, often one-sided sacral area pain that follows delivery, is not due to sepsis, and will subside gradually and completely; **acute postpartum sacroiliitis.**

sciatica: pain radiating down the sciatic nerve into the posterior thigh and leg; can be caused by irritation of a nerve anywhere from the back to the thigh.

scoliorachitis: disease of the spine caused by rickets; abnormal bone mineralization.

Spinal Deformities

Spinal deformity is the abnormal angulation of the spinal column when a person is viewed from the back or the side. It can occur from a variety of causes and at any age. An **inclinometer** is a device used to measure the amount of trunk rotation on examination.

Structural Anomalies

Scoliosis is a general term that applies to any side-to-side curve in the back, that is, a lateral and rotational deviation of the spine from the midline. Such a curve may be termed **fixed curve,** which means that any attempt to eliminate the curve by motion is not successful. Curves may be C-shaped or S-shaped (Fig. 9-4).

A **compensatory curve** has a flexible segment above or below the fixed curve; this compensation will place the spine (above or below) into a vertical position with the head at the midline. The rotation of the spinous process is away from the apex of the curve. **Levorotatory scoliosis** means that this rotation of the most dorsal element of the spine is to the left if one is looking at the patient from behind. **Dextrorotoscoliosis** is the opposite condition. The apex of a curve is called the *convex side,* for example, a right lumbar scoliosis is a lateral deviation of the spine in the lumbar region, with the apex of that curve to the right; the *concave side* of the curve is the opposite side.

Scoliosis may be associated with vertebral anomalies (missing parts of the vertebrae) and with forward bending (round back); the latter is called **kyphoscoliosis.** Scoliosis may occur at birth (*congenital*), occur

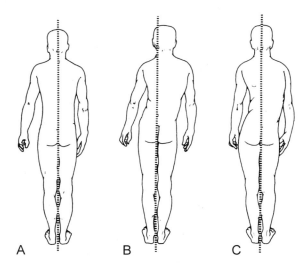

FIG 9-4 Scoliosis. **A,** Normal. **B,** Right convex curve, uncentered. **C,** Right convex curve, centered. (From the American Orthopaedic Association: *Manual of Orthopaedic Surgery,* ed 5, Chicago, 1979, The Association.)

from known causes or diseases (*acquired*), or occur from unknown causes (*idiopathic*). An example will best illustrate the terminology. In a right thoracic, left lumbar, **uncompensated rotatory scoliosis,** viewed from behind, the upper back curves to the right and the lower back to the left, there is rotation of the spine, which may or may not be in both curves (unless so stated), and the center of the head is not in the midline when the patient is standing.

Other Spinal Deformities and Conditions

adolescent scoliosis: lateral curvature of the spine occurring during adolescence.

adult scoliosis: scoliosis occurring after skeletal maturity.

chin-on-chest deformity: seen in ankylosing spondylitis, a marked kyphosis with fixed posturing of chin on chest.

compensatory curve: a curve located above or below a rigid structural curve to maintain normal overall body alignment.

congenital scoliosis: scoliosis due to bony abnormalities present at birth involving either failure of formation of a vertebra or separation of adjacent vertebrae.

double curve: two lateral curves in a single spine; **double major curve** is two lateral curves of equal magnitude, and **double thoracic curve** is two thoracic curves.

flattening of normal lumbar curve: condition in which the hollow of the back becomes shallow or even straight.

functional scoliosis: any scoliosis that is caused by leg length or other functional disorder and not by a primary curvature of the spine.

gibbus: most commonly used for spine deformity a hump or exaggerated convexity.

idiopathic scoliosis: structural lateral curvature of an unknown cause.

infantile scoliosis: lateral curvature of the spine that begins before age 3.

juvenile scoliosis: begins between the ages of 3 and 10 years of age.

kyphoscoliosis: lateral curvature of the spine associated with forward inclination of the spine.

kyphosis: round shoulder deformity, humpback, dorsal kyphotic curvature; may refer to any forward-bending area or deformity of the spine.

lordoscoliosis: lateral curvature of the spine associated with backward bending of the spine.

lumbar curve: curve with apex between the first and fourth lumbar vertebrae.

lumbar kyphosis: reverse of the normal curve of the low back.

lumbosacral curve: a lateral curve with its aspect at or below the fifth lumbar vertebra.

neuromuscular scoliosis: scoliosis caused by a muscle or central nervous system disorder.

reversal of cervical lordosis: change in the normal curvature of the cervical spine as seen on lateral radiograph. This is usually a straightening of the normal lordotic curve or an actual reversal and is most commonly caused by muscle spasm, indicating cervical disk abnormality.

structural curve: a fixed lateral curve of the spinal column.

thoracic curve: a spinal curvature with its apex between the second and eleventh thoracic vertebrae.

thoracolumbar curve: a spinal curve with its apex at the first lumbar or twelfth thoracic curve.

segmental instability: abnormal response to applied loads characterized by motion in the motor segment beyond normal constraints.

spinal stenosis: general term denoting narrowing of the spinal canal in the lumbar area leading to nerve root compromise; term often used for developmental abnormality that leaves a narrow, bony canal. There are four subgroups of this condition:

achondroplastic stenosis: increased vertebral thickness, marked concavity of the vertebral body, and short pedicles.

constitutional stenosis: normal-stature individuals with congenital variance in vertebral structure leading to a narrow canal.

degenerative stenosis: gradual hypertrophy of the vertebral body margin, facet joints, and ligamentum flavum leading to stenosis.

combined stenosis: for congenital or developmental reasons, the midsagittal diameter is decreased.

temporomandibular joint syndrome: complex of symptoms often seen in cervical sprain conditions. Symptoms include clicking in the jaw on opening and closing the mouth, soreness in the jaw, headaches, buzzing sounds, changes in hearing, stiffness in the neck and shoulders, dizziness, and swallowing disorders. It is believed that much of the reason for this symptom complex relates to change of the mandibular posture and the resultant change in cervical posture, or vice versa; **TMJ, craniomandibular cervical syndrome.**

thoracic outlet syndrome: mechanical problem related to the exit of arteries and nerves at the base of the neck leading down the arm, and can also involve the vein bringing blood back from the arm. Compression of these structures as they pass through a narrow foramen between the scalenus anterior muscle and first rib. Problem may be exacerbated by congenitally present additional cervical rib. An early sign is pain in the hand or shoulder. Arteries may be damaged in the process and cause an aneurysm in the area with possible breakoff of clot from the aneurysm.

traction spur: bony excrescence appearing on the anterolateral surface of the vertebral body near but not at the body margin that arises as a result of disk degeneration.

transitional vertebra: vertebra whose structure features some of the characteristics of the two adjacent vertebra. A common example is the fifth lumbar vertebra that has partial sacral components.

wedging: deformity of vertebral body, caused by trauma or gradual collapse, resulting in wedge-shaped vertebra; can also occur congenitally.

Eponymic Spinal Disorders

Marie-Strümpell d.: inflammation of the spine, occurring as a rheumatoid-type disease in children.

Pott d.: tuberculosis of the spine, usually in the lower thoracic segments.

Scheuermann d.: inflammation of the anterior cartilage of the bodies of the lower thoracic and upper lumbar segments, causing pain in some older, growing children. There is more than 5 degrees of wedging of at least three adjacent vertebrae as seen on radiographs.

Schmorl nodes: developmental change resulting in inferior or superior extension of the intervertebral disk into the vertebral bodies.

Nerve Root Diseases of the Spine

The nerve roots in the spinal canal lie in close contact with the vertebrae and emerge through openings called **foramina.** In the neck, nerve root irritation may be localized at the place where it exits through the foramen, whereas in the lumbar spine, nerve root irritation usually occurs one level above the point of nerve exit.

Vertebrae and nerve roots of the spine are the same in number, except for the cervical spine. There are seven cervical vertebrae and eight cervical nerve roots (Fig. 9-1). This occurs because the first cervical nerve exits between the skull and the first cervical vertebra. Therefore, between C-7 and T-1 the eighth cervical nerve makes its exit. After this level, all nerves exit in conformance with the vertebra above the point of exit. When the examiner speaks of the *nerve roots* of the spine, it is recorded singularly as C1 or C2, whereas if the examiner is speaking of the *intervertebral disk* between the vertebrae, it is recorded in combination as C1-2 or C2-3. The vertebrae are recorded individually as C1 or L4.

This section is concerned with the local spinal processes and the wide range of neurologic diseases seen by an orthopaedist and especially by a neurosurgeon.

cauda equina syndrome: sufficient pressure on the nerves in the low back to produce multiple nerve root irritation and commonly loss of bowel and bladder control.

compression of nerve root: mechanical process resulting from a tumor, fracture, or herniated disk; the resultant irritation is called **radiculitis** if there is actual inflammation around the nerve. Pain from this type of disorder is called **radicular pain.** A common lay term for pressure on the nerve is **pinched nerve,** as sometimes used by examiners. After surgery and a normal healing process, the patient may still have some irritation of the nerve, which is often referred to as **residual nerve root irritability. Sciatica** and **neuritis** may be used in describing these disorders, but the terms are not discrete in that the irritation of the nerve is not necessarily from within the spinal canal.

dermatome: refers to the distribution of sensory nerves near the skin that are responsible for pain, tingling, and other sensations (or lack of). The afferent nerve fibers (leading to the spinal cord) and cutaneous branches arise from a single posterior spinal nerve root and contain sensory fibers.

Loss of sensation in a **dermatomal** distribution may indicate damage to a nerve root that is caused by a disk prolapse.

> ***sclerotomal pain:*** more diffuse and ill-defined pain arising from voluntary muscles in spasm (**myotomic** distribution).
>
> ***referred pain:*** sclerotomic in distribution and felt distant from its origin (e.g., bursitis in the shoulder produces pain in the lateral arm, and sciatic-like leg pain can be referred from the low back area).

neurofibroma: fibrous tumor of a nerve, which may affect a nerve root and thus give the appearance of herniated disk disease.

radiculopathy: disease of the nerve roots in or near the spinal canal as a result of direct pressure from a disk or inflammation of the nerve roots due to disk or spinal joint disease.

root sleeve fibrosis: scar tissue surrounding a nerve in the spinal canal or neural foramen; **epineural fibrosis.** If it is within the nerve, it is called **intraneural fibrosis.**

sacral cyst: abnormality in the spinal fluid sac in the sacrum.

Disk Diseases

A disk is described as having a soft or fluid-like center called the **nucleus pulposus** and is surrounded by radial, circular, and longitudinal fibers that are firm, like gristle in meat. These intervertebral disks (IV disks) are situated between the vertebrae and act as shock absorbers. Any portion of the disk may herniate or extrude into the spinal canal, causing irritation and pressure on a nerve (Fig. 9-5).

cartilage space narrowing: narrowing of any cartilage space; also called disk space narrowing.

degenerative disk disease: gradual or rapid deterioration of the chemical composition and physical properties of the disk space. This may involve a simple increase in the rigidity of the nuclear material to be more involved with cellular removal of abnormal tissue and an inflammatory response. If the ligaments around the disk space ossify, they are often referred to as bony "spurs." Because the disk changes in its physical properties, some clinicians

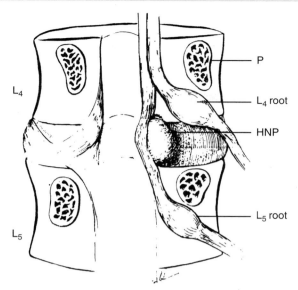

L₄

P

L₄ root

HNP

L₅ root

L₅

FIG 9-5 Diagram of herniated nucleus pulposus (*HNP*) as seen from back with spinous processes and laminae removed from pedicles (*P*). Note that disk protrusion between fourth and fifth lumbar vertebrae impinges on fifth lumbar nerve root. (From Brashear RH, Raney BR: *Shand's Handbook of Orthopaedic Surgery*, ed 9, St Louis, 1978, Mosby.)

will describe the condition as a disorganized disk; that is, the normal property of a soft center surrounded by more rigid, fibrous tissue is disrupted. The inflammation and muscle spasm that may result over a prolonged period are often referred to as a chronic cervical sprain, reflecting the abnormal stresses on the ligaments.

diskitis: inflammation or infection of the disk space.

diskogenic pain: back pain resulting from the disk itself. This pain is mechanical in nature and worse with sitting rather than standing. May be due to annular tears.

disk space infection: infection in the space normally occupied by an intervertebral disk.

herniated intervertebral disk (HID): outpouching of a disk.

herniated nucleus pulposus (HNP): fibrous extrusion of semifluid nucleus pulposus through a ruptured intervertebral disk; damage results from pressure on the spinal cord or nerve roots, causing pain and disability; **HID, ruptured disk, slipped disk.** There are four recognized degrees of disk displacement:

> ***intraspongy nuclear herniation:*** bulge of the disk within the annulus fibrosus.

> ***protrusion:*** displaced nuclear material causes a discrete bulge in the annulus, but no material escapes through the annular fibers.

> ***extrusion:*** displaced material reaches the spinal canal through disrupted fibers of the annulus, but remains connected to the central disk material.

> ***sequestration:*** displaced material escapes as free fragment(s), which may migrate elsewhere.

intervertebral disk narrowing: narrowing of the space between any two vertebral bodies.

Naffziger syndrome: intervertebral disk disease, cervical rib, or some other disorder causes the scalene muscles to go into spasm, resulting in pressure on the major nerve plexus of the arm, causing pain in the neck, shoulder, arm, and hand; **scalenus anticus syndrome.**

Diseases of the Spinal Cord

Because *myelo-* is the Greek root for marrow, and because it was originally thought that the spinal cord was a part of the bone marrow, many words seem to denote bone diseases but actually refer to an affliction of the spinal cord. For that reason, the term *myelitis* is not used alone in this discussion; for example, it may be used to denote a disease of the bone marrow (osteomyelitis) or a disease of the spinal cord (polio-myelitis). This section contains a mixture of terms, some of which may not necessarily relate to the spine. Disorders that are most commonly congenital problems are discussed in a following section.

Myelo- Root Diseases, Acquired

myelalgia: pain in the spinal cord.

myelanalosis: wasting of spinal marrow; **tabes dorsalis.**

myelapoplexy: hemorrhage within the spinal cord.

myelasthenia: loss of nerve strength caused by some disorder of the spinal cord.

myelatrophy: atrophy (wasting away) of spinal cord because of lack of nutrition, causing it to diminish in size.

myelauxe: abnormal increase in size of spinal cord.

myeleterosis: abnormal alteration of the spinal cord.

myeloencephalitis: inflammation of spinal cord and brain; **myelencephalitis.**

myelomalacia: softening of the spinal cord. A term that may be used to describe a whitish magnetic resonance imaging (MRI) finding on T2 images, which are related to ischemic changes in the cord.

myelomeningitis: inflammation of spinal cord and meninges (spinal membranes).

myeloneuritis: inflammation of spinal cord and peripheral nerves.

myeloparalysis: spinal paralysis.

myelopathy: functional disturbance and pathologic changes in the spinal cord. The myelopathies are defined as follows:

Nurick scale: classification scale for spinal cord compression due to spondylosis.

Grade 0: signs and symptoms of root involvement but without evidence of spinal cord disease.

Grade 1: signs of spinal cord disease but no difficulty in walking.

Grade 2: slight difficulty in walking but does not prevent full-time employment.

Grade 3: severe difficulty in walking that requires assistance and prevents full-time employment and avocation.

Grade 4: ability to walk only with assistance or with the aid of a frame.

Grade 5: chairbound or bedridden.

modified Frankel classification: scale for cord damage due to any cause.

Grade A: complete motor and sensory involvement.

Grade B: complete motor involvement, some sensory sparing including sacral sparing.

Grade C: functionally useless motor sparing.

Grade D: functional motor sparing.

Grade E: no neurologic involvement.

myelophthisis: wasting of the spinal cord; reduction of cell-forming function of bone marrow.

myeloplegia: spinal paralysis.

myeloradiculitis: inflammation of spinal cord and nerve roots.

myeloradiculopathy: disease of spinal cord and spinal nerve roots.

myelorrhagia: spinal hemorrhage.

myelosclerosis: hardening of the spinal cord.

myelosyphilis: syphilis of the spinal cord.

Other Spinal Diseases or Conditions, Acquired

central cord syndrome: most common of the incomplete traumatic cervical spinal cord syndromes characterized by motor impairment that is proportionately greater in the upper limbs than in the lower, with bladder dysfunction and a variable degree of sensory loss below the level of the cord lesion.

ependymoma: tumor of the spinal cord.

hematomyelia: effusion of blood (hemorrhage) into the substance of the spinal cord.

hematorrhachis: spinal apoplexy; hemorrhage into vertebral canal.

hyperlordosis: increase in the normal anterior concavity of the cervical or lumbar spine.

leptomeningitis: inflammation of the pia mater and arachnoid of the brain and spinal cord.

leptomeningopathy: disease of the arachnoid or pia mater of the brain and spinal cord.

lordosis: not a disease state, but the normal anterior concavity of the neck or low back.

meningioma: tumor arising from meninges, usually benign, does not recur if totally removed.

meningismus: apparent irritation of brain or spinal cord in which symptoms simulate meningitis but in which no actual inflammation of the membranes is present; **meningism.**

meningitis: inflammation of the meninges of the brain or spinal cord, caused by infectious agents such as bacteria, fungi, or viruses.

meningocele: local cystic protrusion of meninges through a cranial fissure; may be congenital or acquired.

meningoencephalomyelitis: inflammation of brain and spinal cord and their membranes.

meningomyelitis: inflammation of spinal cord, its enveloping arachnoid and pia mater, and sometimes the dura mater.

piriformis syndrome: a clinical diagnosis based on complaints of pain and abnormal sensations in the buttocks region with extension into the hips and posterior thigh as would be seen in sciatica. This is due to tightness of the piriformis muscle with pressure on the sciatic nerve.

syringomyelia: cavities filled with fluid in spinal cord, usually involving upper segments initially and involving the shoulder muscles.

Congenital Disorders of the Spine
Myelo- Root Diseases, Congenital

myelatelia: imperfect development of the spinal cord.

myelocele: herniation and protrusion of substance of spinal cord through defect in the bony spinal canal.

myelocystocele: cystic protrusion of substance of the spinal cord through a defect in the bony spinal canal.

myelocystomeningocele: cystic protrusion of substance of the spinal cord, with meninges, through a defect in the spinal canal.

myelodiastasis: archaic term for softening or other destruction of the spinal cord.

myelodysplasia: defective development of any part of spinal cord.

myelomeningocele: herniation of cord and meninges through a defect in the vertebral column.

Other Spinal Disorders, Congenital

diastematomyelia: congenital defect associated with spina bifida in which the spinal cord is split in half by bony spicules or fibrous bands, each half being surrounded by a dural sac.

failure of segmentation: failure of a portion or all of two or more adjoining vertebrae to separate into normal units.

hemivertebra: incomplete development of one side of a vertebral body, resulting in a wedge shape. If two hemivertebrae are near each other, they may be **balanced,** that is, the two wedges point in opposite directions, and a lesser curve or no curve results. **Unbalanced** means that there is no opposing wedge for one or more hemivertebrae, and the net result is an abnormal curve.

interspinous pseudarthrosis (Baastrup d.): formation of a false joint between two lumbar spinous processes due to the congenitally large size of those processes.

sacral agenesis: failure for normal development of the sacrum. The Renshaw classification is:

  Type I: partial or total unilateral agenesis.

  Type II: partial sacral agenesis with a partial but bilateral symmetric defect and a stable articulation between the ilia; first sacral vertebra is normal or hypoplastic.

  Type III: variable lumbar and total sacral agenesis; ilia articulate with the sides of the lowest vertebra present.

  Type IV: variable lumbar and total sacral agenesis; caudal end plate of the most distal vertebra rests above either fused ilia or an iliac amphiarthrosis.

segmental spinal dysgenesis: a rare set of distinct spinal anomalies including focal stenosis at the level of the dysgenesis with the spinal segments below that point being normal.

spina bifida: congenital defect common in the low back (lumbosacral region) of infants in which part of a vertebra does not fully develop (and in severe cases, nerve tissue) leaving a portion of spinal cord exposed. There are four forms of spina bifida:

  spina bifida occulta (SBO): congenital defect consisting of the absence of a vertebral arch of the spinal column; normally, there are no symptoms.

  myelocele (meningomyelocele): severe form.

meningocele: not as severe.

encephalocele: rare.

symmetric fusion: equal fusion throughout the vertebral body.

unsegmented bar: fusion on one side or the other of the vertebrae, which may involve the posterior elements or vertebral bodies; may occur at multiple levels and skip vertebral segments and may result in severe curves.

Eponymic Congenital Spinal Disorders

Arnold-Chiari syndrome: congenital combination of brain herniation and exposed spinal cord in the lower back. Two types are described:

Type I: cerebellum displaced caudally, brainstem normal, hydrocephalus occasionally present, onset of symptoms in adolescence.

Type II: commonly associated with myelomeningocele, caudal displacement of entire brainstem, cerebellar dysplasia, hydrocephalus in 90%, symptoms in infancy.

Jarcho-Levin syndrome: extensive defects of the spine with associated defects in the ribs leading to a small, stiff thorax and pulmonary compromise.

Surgery of the Spine

The two types of back surgery as applied to orthopaedics are the removal of disk fragments, bone, or ligaments causing pressure on neural elements from the spinal canal and fusion of two or more vertebral segments. The definitions of disk surgery are given to present some important distinctions between procedures of the cervical spine as compared with those of the lumbar spine and to clarify the misuse of terms related to spinal surgical procedures.

Before **invasive spine surgery** takes place, such as removal of a herniated disk, conservative measures are often initially taken in the form of medications, physical therapy, activity modifications, and often interventional blocks (i.e., epidural corticosteroid injections, root injections, facet blocks). Tests to determine the cause of the symptoms are usually performed prior to interventions. These can include plain radiographs (x-rays), myelography followed by computer axial tomography (CAT), magnetic resonance imaging (MRI), and occasionally discography.

For **myelography,** the patient is placed on a tilting table, and a needle is introduced into the subarachnoid space in the lower lumbar spine or upper cervical spine. Cerebrospinal fluid can be withdrawn for analysis and then one of several types of radiopaque contrast material injected. Currently, this material is water soluble. The contrast material infiltrates up and down the spinal canal to outline the nerve roots, nerve sleeves, dural sac, and, at higher levels, the spinal cord.

Multiple plain radiographs can be obtained at different angles and any given level to best outline the offending structure. A CAT scan is then taken to obtain better definition of the areas in question. MRI is often used as a substitute for myelography and CAT scanning because it does not require injection of contrast material into the spinal column. MRIs are performed and images reconstructed in axial or sagittal views. This exam can be performed in different modes or spins to give labels such as T1 and T2 images and can be done with contrast such as gadolinium to assess vascular tumors or scar tissue.

The following spinal surgical procedures are performed by orthopaedic surgeons.

chemonucleolysis: a little used, but once common procedure for lumbar disk herniation. Under direct radiographic control, a chemical that denatures the protein or protein sugar complex in the disk space is injected. The injected disk tends to dissolve itself, and the remaining cartilage cells repopulate the disk and produce ground substance similar in composition to normal nucleus pulposus, or continued degeneration and scar formation takes place. This procedure is designed to speed up the process of relief of compression of the nerve root without surgery. The procedure carries a risk similar to standard diskectomy via laminectomy.

decompression: in relation to the spine this procedure is carried out to relieve pressure on the spinal cord or nerve roots. The pressure may result from fracture fragments, disk fragments, tumors, or infections. The approach may be anterior, lateral, or posterior.

decompressive laminectomy: a decompression done by removing the lamina and spinous process.

discectomy: the removal of intervertebral disk material placing pressure on neural elements. If the annulus of the disk is torn, the disk is protruded. If the fragment of the disk material is torn through a hole in the ligament, it is called an extruded fragment or extruded disk. If the fragment has migrated completely through the ligament, it is termed a sequestered disk or free fragment. The term **herniated nucleus pulposus (HNP)** is a catchall phrase for all of these conditions. In the neck, a fresh (soft) disk excision is sometimes done through a posterior approach (laminotomy). However, many cervical disk problems are approached anteriorly and include a spinal fusion.

foraminotomy: a procedure carried out alone or in conjunction with disk surgery. The foramina (tunnels or openings for the individual nerves to pass from the spine) may become narrowed because of disk impingement, intervertebral collapse, and spondylolisthesis. This surgical widening of the foramen is an attempt to relieve pressure on the nerve roots from a variety of causes.

kyphoplasty: for osteoporotic collapse fractures of the spine, a minimally invasive procedure with vertebral reduction using an inflatable balloon tamp, and space is then injected with methylmethacrylate.

laminectomy: removal of the lamina, the bony element covering the posterior portion of the spinal canal. This procedure removes the lamina on both sides of and including the spinous process. It may be performed at more than one level to approach the spinal cord and nerves for conditions including tumors and herniated disks. The spinal canal is approached from both sides of the spinous process, and the term is often inappropriately used in reference to the following two lesser procedures.

hemilaminectomy: the excision of only one side of the lamina (right or left) relative to the spinous process.

laminotomy (Fig. 9-5): formation of a hole in the lamina without disrupting the continuity of the entire lamina to approach the intervertebral disk or neural structures. This is the most common approach to a herniated disk and is often mistakenly called a laminectomy when in fact it is a **partial laminotomy.**

laminoplasty: the lamina are hinged laterally, opened like a door, and secured in their new position with suture or bone to enlarge the spinal canal. Most often used in the cervical spine.

LISS: *less invasive spine surgery.* Surgery that is done through smaller incisions using special retractors or access systems. Also an acronym for a *less invasive stabilization system* where the screws are locked into the plate for long bone fracture fixation.

microsurgery: microdiscectomy using a microscope during the surgical procedure or to accomplish the procedure.

MISS: *minimally invasive spine surgery.* Often described as being done with minimal disruption to surrounding tissue yet still getting access to a surgical site. This type of surgery may be accomplished with special retractor systems, endoscopes, or done percutaneously.

vertebroplasty: for vertebral fracture and collapse in osteoporosis, in which methylmethacrylate is percutaneously injected through a pedicle directly in defect to stop the pain due to movement at the fracture site.

Spinal Fusions

A procedure in which two or more adjacent vertebrae are induced to grow together as a single, solid bone by destroying the intervening joints or disks and adding bone and/or bone substitutes that eventually heal into a solid bone bridge between the vertebrae. The fusion can be done anteriorly, posteriorly, or both. Spinal hardware or instrumentation is often used to stabilize the vertebrae, which helps with bone growth between them. The indications for fusion are spinal instability (due to disease or iatrogenic from extensive decompression), arthritis, deformity correction, and in some instances pain. The excision of an intervertebral disk does not necessarily lead to symptomatic chronic degenerative arthritis or instability and is not in itself an indication for spinal fusion. However, it is often the case that disk surgery and spinal fusions are done concurrently for a variety of reasons. Fusions are sometimes done to restore adequate stability when it has been disturbed by a fracture, tumor, infection, or surgery. The lumbosacral region is the most common area for spinal fusions.

anterior spinal fusion: approaching the spine from the front, the intervertebral disk and/or vertebral body is removed and bone graft is inserted. Some variations of this procedure include the **Smith-Robinson, Cloward,** and **dowel procedures.**

cervical spinal fusion: spinal fusion involving the seven cervical segments. This may include the base of the skull, the occiput, and the first thoracic spine. The fusion may be anterior or posterior, with or without bone graft, and with or without fixation.

Aebi, Etter, and Cosica: anterior approach to inferior C2 to fractured dens with screws.

Bohman: posterior triple spinous process wiring technique in the cervical spine to secure bone graft.

Brattstrom: use of acrylic cement for C1 to C2 fusion.

Brooks and Jenkins: loops of wire around lamina of C1 and C2 to hold bone graft between lamina.

Callahan: individual wire fixation of a strut bone graft to involved facets.

de Andrade and MacNab: anterior approach for cervical occipital fusion.

Gallie: wire around lamina of C1 and spinous process of C2.

Halifax: clamp across lamina of C1 and C2.

Mageri: wire looped around lamina of C1 and C2.

Magerl: transarticular facet screw fusion for posterior C1 on C2 with the use of bilateral screws directed from inferior posterior lateral mass to anterior superior C1.

McAffee: anterior retropharyngeal approach to upper cervical spine; often used for fusion, allowing excision of tumor.

Meyer: for C1 on C2 instability, posterior fusion using vertical strut grafts and wires.

Newman: C1 to C2 posterior fusion without fixation.

Overton: a dowel graft that is applied across facet joints.

Robinson and Riley: an extensive anterior approach for fusion of C1 to C3 or lower.

Roy-Camille: for stabilization between the skull and C2; posterior bone graft with wire and parallel vertical screw plate fixation from occiput to C3.

Simmons: use of keystone-shaped graft in anterior fusion.

Spetzler: approach to anterior C1 to C3 by using a transoral approach for fusion following excision of tumor.

Wertheim Bohlman: for occipital cervical fusion; use of iliac crest graft and wire fixation from occiput to C2.

Whitecloud and Larocca: anterior technique for cervical spine fusion using fibular graft.

Hibbs spinal f.: a lumbar spinal fusion that includes fusing the spinous process, lamina, and facet for stabilization.

posterior cervical spinal f.: spinal fusion done from the back, using the lamina, facets, and spinous processes of the neck.

Roger f.: posterior cervical fusion using iliac cortical and cancellous grafts.

Southwick: a posterior fusion with wire attaching bone graft to the facet joints.

posterior lumbar spinal f.: spinal fusion done from the back using the lamina, the facets, and spinous processes of the lower back.

Albee: fusion of the spine using grafts across the spinous processes in spondylolisthesis.

Bosworth: fusion using an H-shaped bone graft in spondylolisthesis.

Dwyer-Hartsill p.: for failed lumbar degenerative disk disease; pedicle screws wired to a rectangular frame along with posterolateral fusion.

Gill: removal of the posterior spinal arch in spondylolisthesis.

Gill, Manning, and White: a procedure sometimes combined with a posterolateral spinal fusion.

posterior spinal f.: a fusion of the cervical, thoracic, or lumbar regions primarily fusing the lamina and sometimes the facet joints, using iliac or other bone graft.

posterolateral f.: a fusion of both the lamina and transverse process, using the iliac bone for graft, usually in the lower lumbar and first sacral segments.

posterolateral interbody f. (PLIF): lumbar spine fusion that involves an interbony fusion accomplished through the posterior approach.

transforaminal lumbar interbody fusion (TLIF): lumbar spine fusion that involve anterior interbody fusion done through the transforaminal route.

Material Used for Bone Grafting in Spinal Fusion

In order for bone to grow between two vertebrae, one must provide material to do this. The material can be **osteoinductive,** which means it can induce bone to form, that is, like autograft, which contains precursor cells that form bone. The material can be **osteoconductive,** which means it works as a scaffolding for bone to grow through. Autograft or bone from the patient is both osteoinductive and conductive. There are several sources and types of graft that are important in spine surgery.

autograft: bone taken from the patient who is being operated on. The sites of graft harvest can be the bone from the local area, that is, bone removed during decompression, or from separate sites, which may include additional incisions such as from the iliac crest, fibula, tibia, or occasionally from a vertebral body.

> **structural vs. morselized graft:** the material can be structural or morselized. Structural graft is needed to hold up disk spaces or replace vertebrae that may be removed. Morselized graft is used in posterior or posterolateral fusions where structural support is not required. It can also be used to fill a structural device such as a cage. (See instrumentation.) The problems with autograft usually have to do with insufficient quantities for large surgeries, morbidity or problems at the site where it was harvested (i.e., fracture or infection), or pain at that site, which is most common.

allograft: human bone harvested from cadavers that can be processed into several types of usable forms. It can be made into morselized graft, putties, or granular material. It can also be made into spacers for the lumbar, thoracic, or cervical spine to fit into disk spaces or replace vertebral bodies. Most allograft used today is processed to prevent disease transmission. The lumbar replacements are often made of femoral rings and can be called femoral ring allograft (FRA). The cervical spacers are made of fibulas, ulnas, or from the radius cut into rings. Allograft is osteoconductive and osteoinductive by the presence of proteins, which can induce bone formation as the cells are dead. Not as effective as autograft but quantity is not limited by what you can harvest and there is no graft site pain or complications.

xenograft: graft material from other animals such as bovine (cow bone) used in the past. There are better products available that are used today.

Calcium phosphates are inert materials that are osteoconductive and can be used to expand the graft, that is, to make it more bulky when there is insufficient quantities, or on its own.

bone marrow aspirate: this is a syringe of blood withdrawn from the marrow areas such as the iliac crest and containing cells, which can form bone, that is, osteoinductive. This is often added to allograft.

bone morphogenic proteins (BMPs): osteoinductive proteins included in the superfamily of transforming growth factor-beta (TGF-β). Human BMP was discovered several decades ago by Marshall Urist at UCLA. Since then, human BMP extracted and purified from cadaver bones has been used to accomplish fusions. Human BMP is of limited quantities. Through the use of recombinant genetic technology, a set of proteins, designated rhBMP-1 through rhBMP-9, have been produced to obtain unlimited quantities. One of these recombinant proteins, rhBMP-2, was found to promote new bone and cartilage growth. They are osteoinductive and are often used with a osteoconductive collagen scaffold, which also binds the proteins.

> **rhBMP-2:** recombinant human bone morphogenic protein number 2, sold as INFUSE commercially, and is Food and Drug Administration (FDA) approved for anterior interbody fusions with a lumbar-tempered (LT) cage.
>
> rhBMP-7 sold as OP-1 is approved for use in posterior lumbar fusions.

> **platelet gels:** by centrifuging blood there is a buffy coat layer that is rich in platelets and platelet derived factors. This also has osteoinductive ability and is used to form bone often with local graft or allograft.

trabecular metal: this is an implant made of tantalum with a porous structure that allows bone to directly grow into it. Ideally in this case two vertebra could be fused together by simply attaching on both sides of this device obviating the need for graft material.

Spinal Instrumentation

Spinal instrumentation is comprised of metal, plastic, carbon fiber, or resorbable devices that are used to stabilize the spine, correct deformity, take the place of removed elements such as disks or vertebral bodies, and now attempt to replicate spinal function. The commonest types of instrumentation systems are listed and defined with respect to where they are used.

screws: usually used in conjunction with a plate or rod system to hold vertebrae stable. Screws are the anchoring devices into vertebrae and then they are connected to the rods or plates with connecting devices. Screws can be used on their own in the spine in several situations: as compression screws during the treatment of type 2 odontoid fractures, isthmic screws in hangman fractures, translaminar screws, or facet screws in lumbar fusions.

    anchoring screws: these screws are placed into the vertebral body, occiput, or pelvis and secured to a rod or plate system, which holds them and the vertebral bodies they attach to together.

    occipital screws: placed in the midline at the back of the skull during occipital cervical fusions.

    lateral mass screws: usually used from C2-C6 and connected to a rod or plate construct.

    cervical pedicle screws: are placed in C2 or C7 most commonly and connected to a rod screw construct.

    pedicle screws: for placement in thoracic and lumbar spines.

    sacral screws: can be pedicle screws often in S1 or S2 or alar screws, which angle out into the sacral ala.

    Iliac screws: often used to fix long spinal fusions with rods to the pelvis. In the Galveston technique, the rods themselves are bent and placed into the iliac wings to secure the system to the pelvis on each side.

Other anchoring devices include wires such as Luque wires, which are placed around the lamina and secured to long rods during scoliosis surgery by twisting the wires. This type of fixation is most commonly used for neuromuscular scoliosis.

plates and screws: used for anterior fusions to buttress interbody fusions or vertebral replacements. The plates are commonly locking plates, which means the screw can be fixed to the plate and make the construct rigid. Posterior fusions sometimes use a plate and screw device such as the Steffi plate in the lumbar spine or lateral mass plates in the cervical spine. For occipital cervical fusion, plate devices are still used in the occiput.

cages: spacers that provide structural support to nonstructural bone grafting material until it heals into solid bone. Cages can be described by:

- *what they replace:* removed disks, that is, intervertebral spacers or vertebral body replacements.
- *what they are made of:* metals, such as titanium, tantalum, or steel, and in the past, plastics such as polyetheretherketone (PEEK), carbon fiber, or even resorbable materials, which disappear once bone has grown through them.
- *how they are inserted:* anterior lumbar interbody fusion (ALIF) cages, posterior lumbar interbody fusion (PLIF) cages, transforaminal lumbar interbody fusion (TLIF) cages.
- *by their shape:* box cages, cylindrical cages.
- *by what they do:* that is, expandable cages.

Nonfusion Devices

There are new implants that are being designed to replace anatomic elements of the spine but trying to maintain the original function unlike fusion devices.

disk replacements: currently metal-backed devices that try to mimic the function of the intervertebral disk once it has been removed for pathology. Designed primarily for the lumbar and cervical spine. Their use has increased dramatically over the last 10 years. Currently the Charite disk, and Prodisc are the only FDA approved devices in the United States, but there are a multitude of companies and artificial disks that may be available in the future.

nucleus replacement: a technology not yet perfected but designed to replace the nucleus pulposus after herniation or degeneration; to reconstruct the spring-like component of the intervertebral disk, which is lost once the disk has been damaged.

Ligament replacement devices or nonrigid stabilization devices, which are often anchored by pedicle screws to the vertebral body.

Names of Instrumentation Systems

AO fixateur interne: a posteriorly placed spinal fixation device.

Banks-Dervin rod: for scoliosis fixation; a multiple level rod that is fixed with oblique spinous process to contralateral lamina screws.

Cotrel-Dubousset: posterior fixation device for spinal deformity, fracture, tumor, and degenerative conditions.

Dwyer: anteriorly placed screws and band device for correction of spinal deformities.

Edwards: a posterior rod and sleeve device used in stabilization of traumatic spinal conditions.

Harrington rod: an instrumentation and fusion using a straight, stiff rod for distraction or compression; associated with a posterior spinal fusion in the thoracic or thoracolumbar spine for scoliosis or trauma.

Isola: a posterior fixation device.

Jacobs locking hook: thick, threaded rods for fixation of various spinal deformities.

Kaneda: an anteriorly placed fixation device for spinal deformities.

Knodt distraction rod: for distraction stabilization of thoracic and lumbar spine.

Kostuick-Harrington: anteriorly placed device for spinal deformity correction.

Long Beach pedicle screw: posterolateral fusion screw and rod device.

Luque: a posterior method of fixation.

Luque ISF: for posterolateral fusion fixation; a pedicle screw and plate device.

Rogozinski: a combined anteroposterior device used in correction of spinal deformities.

Roy-Camille: posterior pedicle screw and plate device for spinal stabilization.

Steffee plate: for posterolateral fusion fixation; plate and screw device.

Texas Scottish Rite Hospital: instrumentation used anteriorly and posteriorly.

Vermont (Krag): posteriorly placed internal fixation device.

Wiltse plate: screw plate device for posterior spinal stabilization.

Wisconsin (Drummond) interspinous segmental spinal: series of wires, rods, and buttons for multi-segmental spine stabilization.

Zielke: a metho of fracture treatment with transpedicular fixation.

Miscellaneous Procedures on the Spine

Bradford: for kyphoscoliosis deformity; staged anterior and posterior approach for interbody fusion and correction of deformity.

Capner: draining of thoracic spinal abscess through an anterolateral approach.

coccygectomy: excision of the coccyx (tailbone).

coccygotomy: incision into the coccyx (tailbone).

commissural myelorrhaphy: a longitudinal division of the spinal cord to sever crossing fibers.

cordotomy: transverse incision into the spinal cord.

corpectomy: excision of vertebral body usually combined with interposition of prosthesis or bone graft.

Dunn: for myelomeningocele spinal deformity; use of *contouring L-rod* for posterior stabilization.

eggshell: excavation of vertebral body for correction of deformity that is combined with spinal fusion.

facetectomy: excision of an articular facet of a vertebra.

Getty: for decompression of lumbar spinal stenosis; excision of lamina and portion of facet.

Goldstein: for scoliosis deformity graft incorporating posterior elements, including facet joints and ribs.

Hodgson: anterior approach to C1 and C2 area for drainage of tuberculous abscess.

kyphectomy: for kyphotic deformity in myelodysplasia; excision of kyphotic portion of lumbar spine combined with spinal fixation.

Leeds: for scoliosis, segmental wiring of a contoured square-ended Harrington rod.

Localio: for sacral tumor; a method of partial excision of the sacrum.

Loughheed and White: for drainage of lower abdominal abscess; coccygectomy and drainage from space anterior to sacrum.

MacCarthy: for sacral tumor; a method of excision of the sacrum.

myelotomy: a procedure for severing tracts in the spinal cord.

rachicentesis: lumbar puncture for examination of the spinal fluid; rachiocentesis.

rachiotomy: incision into a vertebral canal for exploration.

rachitomy: surgical or anatomic opening of the vertebral canal.

radiculectomy: excision of a rootlet or resection of spinal nerve roots.

rhizotomy: division of the roots of the spinal nerves.

Risser: for scoliosis deformity; particular attention to fusion of facet joints and use of cast stabilization.

Roaf, Kirkaldy-Willis, and Cattero: drainage of thoracic spinal abscess through dorsolateral approach.

Schollner costoplasty: for rib deformity or scoliosis; multiple rib partial excisions.

Scott: use of cross-wire fixation transverse process to inferior pedicle in stabilization of spondylolysis fusion.

Seddon: drainage of thoracic spinal abscess through anterolateral approach with partial resection of rib.

Simmons: for cervical spinal kyphosis; a posterior osteotomy.

Smith Peterson p.: for correction of kyphotic deformity in ankylosing spondylitis; lumbar spine osteotomy.

Speed p. (Kellogg Speed): for spondylolisthesis spine fusion and anterior interbody fusion by using tibial cortical graft.

spondylosyndesis: surgical immobilization or ankylosis by fusion of the vertebral bodies with a short bone graft in cases of tuberculosis of the spine; **spondylodesis, Albee procedure.**

spondylotomy: incision into a vertebra or vertebral column; **rachiotomy.**

Tsuli: for severe cervical spondylosis; an expansive, multiple laminectomy.

Wiltse: a bilateral lateral spine fusion for spondylolisthesis.

Winter: for hemivertebra deformity; anterior and posterior approach with stabilization. Also a procedure for correction of congenital kyphosis, by using an anterior approach and strut bone grafts.

Spinal Approaches

anterior a.: when used to approach the cervical, cervicodorsal, dorsal, and lumbar spines, it is designed to provide sufficient surface for multiple segmental spinal fusions; **Hodgson, Roaf.**

anterior a.: for specific cervical spinal explorations and fusions; **Southwick** and **Robinson, Bailey** and **Badgley, Whitesides** and **Kelly, Henry** (to the vertebral artery).

anterolateral a.: an approach to the dorsal spine by rib resection to explore the spine anteriorly and in some cases to do spinal fusions and decompressions of the spinal cord.

dorsolateral a.: an approach to the dorsal spine by costotransversectomy, usually done for fractures and other affections of the spinal cord.

posterior a.: used for laminectomies and spinal fusions at any level; **Hibbs, Wagoner.**

The Hand and Wrist

10

Where is there available a precision instrument that can either gently pick up eggs or lift 200 lb; detect the weight of only four grains of sand, temperature differences of 1 degree, and the distance between two points less than 0.1 inch; be remote controlled, self-powered, and transportable to any part of the world? This priceless tool is available at no cost to almost all humankind—the hand.

A description of the intricate anatomic features of the hand and wrist is presented with illustrations. The sequence of definitions given here will help to define the basics of hand control, kinematics, and function. The chapter reflects changes in the anatomy format, with an explanation of zones, pulleys, and other miscellaneous names specific to the hand.

There are many abbreviations used in hand anatomy because of the lengthy Latin names, for example, flexor pollicis longus (FPL) tendon or metacarpophalangeal (MCP) joint. Usually the Latin name is spelled out initially and abbreviated subsequently. Appendix A (Orthopaedic Abbreviations) lists the many hand abbreviations used to simplify the terminology.

Anatomy of the Hand and Wrist

Bones (Fig. 10-1)
accessory bone: an extra bone that may develop in the carpus of the wrist as seen on radiographs; an anomaly.

carpal bones: the eight bones of the anatomic wrist, arranged in a proximal and distal row, and held firmly together by ligaments. The proximal row from lateral to medial (radial to ulnar) includes the **scaphoid (navicular), lunate (semilunar), triquetrum (triangular),** and **pisiform.** The distal row leading from the thumb side is composed of the **trapezium (greater multangular), trapezoid (lesser multangular), capitate,** and **hamate.**

carpus: the wrist; term applied to the structures of the wrist including the carpal bones.

DRUJ (distal radial ulnar joint): acronym commonly used to describe that joint (pronounced "drudge").

fossae (fossa, sing.): the scaphoid and lunate fossae are normal recesses in the articular surface of the distal radius that allow articulation of the scaphoid and lunate, respectively.

metacarpals: the five long bones of the hand in the palm area. The bases of the metacarpal bones articulate proximally with the distal row of carpal bones.

phalanges: the bones of the thumb and fingers. Each phalanx has a body, proximal base, and distal head. There are two phalanges in the thumb (proximal and distal) and three phalanges in each of the four digits (proximal, medial, and distal).

sesamoids: small bones on the medial and lateral side of the base of the proximal phalanx of the thumb (metacarpophalangeal [MCP] joint). The sesamoids articulate with the head of the metacarpal bone to

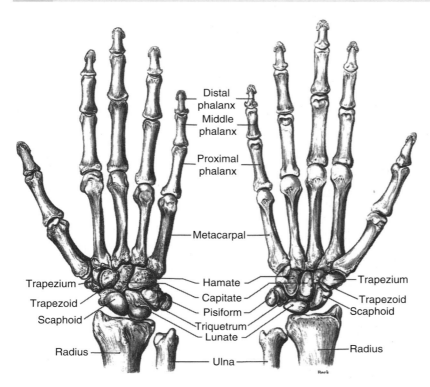

FIG 10-1 Bones of the right hand and wrist, dorsal surface. (From Anthony C, Kolthoff N: *Textbook of Anatomy and Physiology*, ed 9, St Louis, 1975, Mosby.)

Distal phalanx
Middle phalanx
Proximal phalanx
Metacarpal
Trapezium
Trapezoid
Scaphoid
Radius
Hamate
Capitate
Pisiform
Triquetrum
Lunate
Ulna
Trapezium
Trapezoid
Scaphoid
Radius

which muscles are attached. A sesamoid bone may also be found on the lateral side of the MCP joint of the index finger and medial side of the MCP joint of the little finger.

sigmoid notch: the articular surface on the distal radius that accepts the ulna in the distal radioulnar joint.

styloids: bony protuberances off the radius and ulna that act as attachment sites for the radial and ulnar collateral ligaments, respectively. The ulna styloid is also an attachment for the triangular fibrocartilage complex.

tubercles: bony prominences that provide ligamentous attachment. In the hand, these include the **scaphoid, trapezium, Lister tubercle,** and the **hook of the hamate.**

tuft: the terminal bony expansion of the distal phalanx.

Joints

The joints of the hand are remarkable for the variability of motion that supports the fingers and thumbs in many tasks (e.g., the carpometacarpal [CMC] joint of

the thumb can move in all planes). The joints of the phalanges are the proximal, medial, and distal joints and are referred to as follows:

Carpometacarpal (CMC)
Distal interphalangeal (DIP)
Metacarpophalangeal (MCP)
Midcarpal (MC)
Proximal interphalangeal (PIP)
Radiocarpal (RC)

volar plate: a thickening of the joint capsule of the volar aspect of the MP and IP joints that prevent hyperextension of these joints. Proximally, these begin with the "check-rein" ligaments.

Muscles

There are large muscles in the forearm that insert into the bones of the hand by means of their tendons (Figs. 10-2 and 10-3). These **extrinsic muscles** cause the hand and

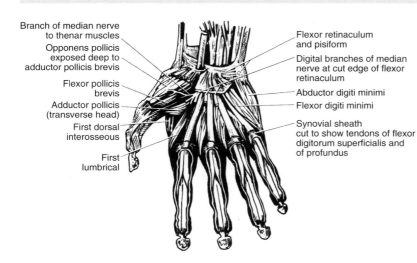

Branch of median nerve
to thenar muscles

Opponens pollicis
exposed deep to
adductor pollicis brevis

Flexor pollicis
brevis

Adductor pollicis
(transverse head)

First dorsal
interosseous

First
lumbrical

Flexor retinaculum
and pisiform

Digital branches of median
nerve at cut edge of flexor
retinaculum

Abductor digiti minimi

Flexor digiti minimi

Synovial sheath
cut to show tendons of flexor
digitorum superficialis and
of profundus

FIG 10-2 Muscles of the anterior aspect of the human hand; the palmar aponeurosis has been removed. (From DiDio LJA: *Synopsis of Anatomy*, St Louis, 1970, Mosby.)

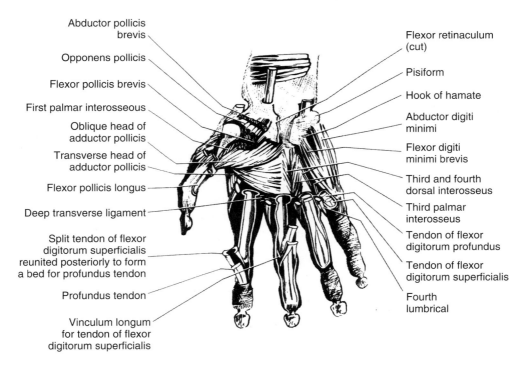

Abductor pollicis
brevis

Opponens pollicis

Flexor pollicis brevis

First palmar interosseous

Oblique head of
adductor pollicis

Transverse head of
adductor pollicis

Flexor pollicis longus

Deep transverse ligament

Split tendon of flexor
digitorum superficialis
reunited posteriorly to form
a bed for profundus tendon

Profundus tendon

Vinculum longum
for tendon of flexor
digitorum superficialis

Flexor retinaculum
(cut)

Pisiform

Hook of hamate

Abductor digiti
minimi

Flexor digiti
minimi brevis

Third and fourth
dorsal interosseus

Third palmar
interosseus

Tendon of flexor
digitorum profundus

Tendon of flexor
digitorum superficialis

Fourth
lumbrical

FIG 10-3 Muscles of the anterior aspect of the human hand. (From DiDio LJA: *Synopsis of Anatomy*, St Louis, 1970, Mosby.)

fingers to flex and extend (close and open). The **intrinsic muscles** are small and originate within the hand. These control positioning and to a large extent functional coordination of the fingers. In normal hand function, all these groups work together in intricate unison.

Extrinsic Muscle Function

wrist flexors: flexor carpi ulnaris (FCU), palmaris longus (PL), flexor carpi radialis (FCR); insert on the metacarpals, carpal bones, and ligaments. They cause strong wrist flexion.

wrist extensors: extensor carpi radialis longus (ECRL), extensor carpi radialis brevis (ECRB), extensor carpi ulnaris (ECU); insert on the metacarpals.

finger flexors: flexor digitorum profundus (FDP), flexor digitorum sublimis or superficialis (FDS), flexor pollicis longus (FPL) (thumb); insert on either the distal or the middle phalanges of the digits and cause powerful finger or thumb flexion.

finger extensors: extensor digiti quinti proprius (EDQP), extensor digitorum communis (EDC), extensor indicis proprius (EIP); insert on the bones and extensor hoods of the fingers and cause extension of the digits.

thumb extensors: extensor pollicis longus (EPL) and brevis (EPB).

thumb abductors: abductor pollicis longus (APL) and brevis (APB).

thumb adductors: extensor pollicis longus (EPL) and adductor pollicis (add poll).

Intrinsic Muscle Function

hypothenar muscles: opponens digiti quinti (or **minimi**) (**ODQ/ODM**), **flexor digiti quinti brevis (FDQB), abductor digiti quinti** (or **minimi**) (**ADQ/ADM**); a less important group of intrinsic muscles that arise from the carpal bones and insert on the little finger, metacarpal, and proximal phalanx.

intrinsic muscles: lumbricals, dorsal interossei, volar interossei; arise from the metacarpals or from the flexor tendons and insert into the finger dorsal (extensor) mechanism and base of the proximal finger bone. They are responsible for spreading and bringing together the fingers and for firm coordination of motion at each finger joint.

thenar muscles: opponens pollicis (OP), abductor pollicis brevis (APB), flexor pollicis brevis (FPB) deep and superficial head, the deep head sometimes called first palmar interosseous (intrinsic muscles of the thumb); arise from the carpal bones and ligaments at the base of the palm and insert on the proximal phalanx or on the thumb metacarpal. They function to bring the thumb out and away from the palm and to oppose it to the other fingers. One intrinsic muscle arises from the metacarpals and crosses deep in the palm to the thumb. This adductor pollicis muscle pulls the thumb forcefully back in toward the palm (adduction).

Associated Forearm Muscles and Tendons

other muscles in the forearm: brachioradialis, pronator teres (PT), supinator, anconeus, and pronator quadratus (PQ); these do not extend to the hand but affect the position of the hand by actions such as rotation of the forearm (pronation and supination).

aponeurosis: term usually used to denote the whitish or silvery thick membranes that separate muscles, but in the hand is a description of the entire extensor apparatus of the digits distal to the metacarpophalangeal joint to its insertion on the proximal end of the distal phalanx.

extensor carpi radialis intermedius: an anatomic variant (a third radial wrist extensor) that can be used to restore thumb function in paralytic disorders when present.

extensor digitorum brevis manus muscle: an anatomic variant of the extensor indicis proprius muscle originating from the dorsal lip of the distal radius inserting on the extensor indicis proprius.

flexor wad of five: five muscles with a common origin in the medial elbow: pronator teres (PT), flexor digitorum profundus (FDP) and sublimis (FDS), palmaris longus (PL), and flexor carpi radialis (FCR).

flexor tendons of the wrist: flexor carpi radialis (FCR) is the radial wrist flexor that travels in its own tunnel and inserts at the base of the second metacarpal. The **flexor carpi ulnaris (FCU)** (the ulnar wrist flexor) is the more important and powerful. It has a primary insertion on the pisiform but will send fibers distally to intermesh with the hypothenar muscle fascia. These tendons, with a synovial lining, glide back and forth through the tunnel as the fingers and wrist are moved.

radial sagittal bands: transverse tendinous structures on the radial side of the central extensor tendon slip in the region of the metacarpophalangeal joint to prevent ulnar subluxation of the extensor digitorum communis with flexion of the metacarpophalangeal joint.

retinacular ligament: fibrous bands that cover tendon tunnels such as extensor retinaculum and flexor pulleys.

Zones

A surgical zone system has been established for the fingers, hand, wrist, and forearm. The anatomic zones are important in determining technical considerations for each zone, surgical approaches, and corrections for different disorders. The clinical importance of anatomic zones is that, if an area is left unrepaired, specific deficits will occur in the extensor or flexor tendon zones.

zone I: from flexor digitorum profundus (FDP) insertion to flexor digitorum sublimis (FDS) insertion, anatomic structures found distal to the insertion of the sublimis tendon into the middle phalanx.

zone II: called **"no man's land,"** the anatomic structures found in the region just proximal to the A1 pulley up to zone I.

Camper chiasm: a bifurcation of the flexor digitorum sublimis (FDS) in zone II that allows passage of the flexor digitorum profundus (FDP) through it. This occurs just proximal to the insertion of the flexor digitorum sublimis (FDS) in the middle phalanx; **chiasma tendinum.**

zone III: anatomic structures at the origin of the lumbricals in the region of the arterial arch, from the carpal tunnel to zone II.

zone IV: the carpal tunnel.

zone V: anatomic area of the wrist proximal to the carpal tunnel.

Pulleys

Pulleys are thickened portions of flexor tendon sheaths that hold tendons in place. They are labeled as annular or cruciate, depending on the orientation of the fibers

of the pulley. The most proximal pulley is located on the distal metacarpal and is labeled annular 1 (A1) and then annular 2 through 4. The cruciate pulleys are similarly labeled C1 through C3 (Fig. 10-4).

A1	zone II	C1	zone II
A2	zone II	C2	zone I
A3	zone II	C3	zone I
A4	zone I	AO	zone IV (palmar fascia)

Ligaments and Fascia

There are numerous ligaments named for the bones to which the ligaments are attached.

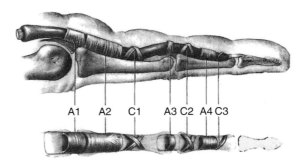

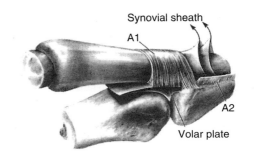

FIG 10-4 This anatomic diagram of various parts of flexor sheath is helpful in understanding gliding of tendon. Maintenance of second annulus (A2) and fourth annulus (A4) is essential to retain appropriate angle of approach and prevent "bowstringing" of flexor tendons or tendon graft. (From Doyle JR, Blythe W: In American Academy of Orthopaedic Surgeons: *Symposium on Tendon Surgery in the Hand,* St Louis, 1975, Mosby.)

deep transverse metacarpal l.: specific distal ligaments between the second, third, fourth, and fifth metacarpophalangeal (MCP) volar plates.

juncturae tendinum: tendinous interconnection between extrinsic extensors over the dorsum of the hand. These allow synchronized digital extension; **connexus intertendineus.**

transverse carpal l.: the strong ligamentous band that lies across the arch of the carpal bones forming the roof of the carpal tunnel. It covers the median nerve and binds down the nine long flexor tendons of the thumb and fingers.

triangular l.: interconnecting fibers that join the two lateral bands dorsally and hold them in place. They are located over the proximal end of the middle phalanx just distal to the insertion of the central slip of the extensor tendon; **triangular fibrocartilage complex.**

vincula longa and breva: vascular and fibrous connections from the floor of the flexor tunnel to each of the two flexor tendons. The vincula breva lie close to the tendon insertions.

volar carpal l.: the ligament that spans and covers the median nerve and canal of Guyon and runs from the transverse carpal ligament radially to the hypothenar fascia ulnarly. This ligament binds down the nine long flexor tendons of the thumb and fingers.

Extrinsic Wrist Ligaments

dorsal radiocarpal l.: (radiolunatotriquetrum).

volar l.: deep radioscaphocapite, long radioscapholunate, short radioscapholunate, and radiolunate and ulnar lunate.

Intrinsic Wrist Ligaments

arcuate (deltoid) l.: a major stabilizer of the midcarpal joint; ulnar arm (triquetrocapitate l.), radial arm (distal to scaphocapitate l.).

deep transverse intermetacarpal l.: fibrous interconnections between metacarpal heads II through V.

intermediate l.: lunatotriquetrum, scapholunate, and scaphotrapezium.

long l.: volar intercarpal ("U," deltoid arcuate).

short l.: interosseous.

space of Poirer: a weak area of the midcarpal joint, that is, the arcuate ligament volar and distal to the lunate because the capitolunate l. is either absent or attenuated.

superficial transverse intermetacarpal l.: the expansion of the palmar fascia in the region of the distal metacarpals; **natatory l.**

Collateral Ligaments

The collateral ligaments of the elbow and wrist are supportive ligaments providing stability on the medial and lateral side of the wrist joint.

radial collateral l.: scaphocapitate l. (radial arm).

ulnar collateral l.: triquetrocapitate l. (ulnar arm).

Digital Collateral Ligaments

accessory l.: originates volar and deep to the main collateral ligaments and runs to the volar plate.

beak ligaments: volar ulnar ligaments that stabilize the carpometacarpal joint of the thumb; originates on the volar aspect of the triscaphe joint and inserts on the volar ulnar surface of the proximal thumb metacarpal.

dorsal extensor compartments: the six fascial compartments on the dorsum of the distal radius for the wrist extensors numbering from radial to ulnar; these are defined by extensor retinacular tunnels over the wrist.

I: abductor pollicis longus (APL) and extensor pollicis brevis (EPB).

II: extensor carpi radialis longus (ECRL) and brevis (ECRB).

III: extensor pollicis longus (EPL).

IV: extensor indicis proprius (EIP) and extensor digitorum communis (EDC) II-V.

V: extensor digiti minimi (EDM) or quinti (EDQ).

VI: extensor carpi ulnaris (ECU).

main l.: runs from the center of rotation of the metacarpal or phalangeal head to the proximal metaphyseal flair of the phalanx adjoining.

Palm
Palmar Fascial Compartments

flexor and extensor retinacula: special thickening of deep fascia where muscles of forearm become tendons and pass into the hand into a broad band of superficial fascia over the dorsum of the wrist; help to restrain the extensor tendons and prevent tendons from bowstringing away from wrist.

digital retinaculum: the covering fascia of the finger flexors.

hypothenar eminence: prominence caused by intrinsic muscle mass on little finger side of the palm.

hypothenar space: deep space overlying the fifth metacarpal that may or may not be connected to the thenar space proximally.

Kanavel spaces: two fascial spaces of the palm, one thenar and one midpalmar, lying deep to the long flexor tendons and separated by a septum.

Landsmeer l.: fibrous tissue bands on the lateral side of the fingers that help to synchronize the motion of the two distal joints; **oblique retinacular ligaments.**

midpalmar space: a deep potential pace that runs from the third to fifth ray.

natatory l.: another name for the superficial transverse intermetacarpal l.

palmar fascia: complex interwoven fascia in the palm of the hand that is a part of the expansion of the palmaris longus (PL) and protects the delicate structures in the hand.

palmar skin crease: the creases in the palm caused by natural folds in the skin. These are labeled as distal palmar crease (DPC), midpalmar crease (MPC), and thenar palmar crease (TPC), the "life line." The digital skin creases are labeled proximal, middle, and distal.

septa: two fibrous septa pass deeply from sides of palmar aponeurosis and separate muscles of the thenar and hypothenar deep spaces from midpalmar space.

thenar eminence: the prominence caused by intrinsic muscle mass on the thumb side of the palm.

thenar space: the potential space on the thumb side of the hand deep to the tendons and nerves.

web l.: expansion of the palmar fascia between the base of the fingers.

Bursa

All bursa are lined with synovial sheaths (tenosynovium). Following are the important ones in the hand.

intermediate bursa: occasionally seen anatomically as the bursa containing the index finger flexor tendon sheath.

radial bursa: sac containing the flexor pollicis longus (FPL) tendon sheath in the palm and thumb.

ulnar bursa: sac in the palm containing tendon sheaths of the index, long, ring, and little fingers and extending to the end of the little finger.

Miscellaneous

anatomic snuff box: the area of the lateral wrist formed between the extensor pollicis longus (EPL) tendon medially, and abductor pollicis longus (APL) and extensor pollicis brevis (EPB) tendons laterally. With the thumb abducted and extended, a triangular depression is made on the dorsum of the wrist at the radial border.

arcade of Frohse: tunnel through supinator muscle for the deep radial nerve; anatomic series of arches.

carpal tunnel: space in the wrist created by the volar carpal ligament. This space contains the flexor tendons of the fingers and thumb, as well as the median nerve.

Guyon canal: space between the hamate and pisiform bones at the wrist for the ulnar artery and nerve, covered by the ulnar side of the volar carpal ligament. Floor is the pisohamate ligament.

hook of hamate: bony prominence (tubercle) that provides ligamentous attachment.

ligamentum subcruentum: the loose richly vascularized connective tissue that sits near the ulnar styloid in between the limbs of the distal radial ulnar joint ligament.

Lister tubercle: bony prominence on the distal dorsal radius for ligamentous attachment.

radial lunate angle: an angle created by the line perpendicular to the line connecting the distal tips of the lunate on the lateral x-ray with the long axis of the radius. This is used to estimate *d*orsal *i*ntercalated *s*egment *i*nstability (DISI) and *v*olar *i*ntercalated *s*egment *i*nstability (VISI) deformities in wrist injuries.

slider crank mechanism: an engineering model of scaphoid motion in carpal kinematics.

The Fingers

central slip (tendon): the portion of the extensor tendon that inserts into the middle phalanx.

cutaneous l.: ligaments that restrain the skin during finger motion and include the following:

Cleland l.: fibrous tissue bands on the lateral side of the fingers that stabilize the skin during finger movement, dorsal to Grayson l.

Grayson l.: fibrous tissue bands of the finger extending from the volar distal interphalangeal (DIP) and proximal interphalangeal (PIP) joints to the lateral skin.

distal pulp: the mass of tissue of the volar distal finger. It is the soft cushion of the palmar surface of the distal phalanx.

dorsal expansion: the fibers spreading laterally at the base of the dorsal hood.

extensor hood: the fan-like expansion of the extensor communis tendon over the dorsum and sides of the *meta*carpo*p*halangeal (MCP) joints. This complex structure brings together intrinsic and extrinsic tendons to control interphalangeal (IP) joint extension and metaphalangeal (MP) joint flexion or extension.

interdigital commissure: floor of the webspace between two digits, which follow a very specific anatomic pattern and must be carefully reconstructed in syndactyly surgery.

knuckle pad: the thick skin over the dorsum of the distal interphalangeal (DIP) and proximal interphalangeal (PIP) joints of the finger.

lateral bands: the portions of the intrinsic muscle tendons that run laterally across the proximal phalanx to the dorsum of the distal interphalangeal (DIP) and proximal interphalangeal (PIP) joints.

septa: fibrous tissue structures in fat pad of the fingertips.

skin creases: indentations in the skin at the point of natural motion points of the finger. The digital skin creases are labeled proximal, medial, and distal.

webspace: the skin web area between the base of the fingers.

The Nail

cuticle: the skin edge immediately covering the base of the fingernail.

eponychium: thin skin covering (epidermis) at the base of the nails on the dorsal surface; **cuticle.**

germinal matrix: the cells that generate the tissues that eventually form the nail from the base of the nail; primitive stage of development.

hyponychium: the thickened epidermis immediately under the distal portion of the nail; **subungual tissue.**

lunula: the white crescentic (half-moon shaped) area at the base of the nail.

nail matrix: the proximal portion of the nail bed from which growth mainly proceeds; also, the tissue on which the deep aspect of the nail rests; **matrix unguis, nail bed.**

nail plate: the hard plate of the distal end of the dorsum of the fingers and thumbs. This rigid outer covering extends approximately 8 mm under the nail fold (perionychium) and arises from the nail bed (matrix unguis).

paronychium: a fold of skin (nail folds) that surrounds the nail at the base; the epidermis bordering the nail; **perionychium.**

subungual space: the potential space between the nail and nail bed; common site for a hematoma.

unguis: the horny cutaneous plate on the dorsal surface of the distal end of a finger; the **nail.**

Nerves and Arteries

antebrachial cutaneous nerve: medial/lateral and sensory to the thumb.

axolemma: a column of neuronal cytoplasm enclosed by cell membrane including cell body, dendrites, and the axon.

common digital arteries and nerves (Fig. 10-5): the main branch of the various nerves or arteries in the palm; these then divide into the proper digital arteries and nerves.

dorsal digital artery and nerve: common and proper, the branches of artery and nerve in the dorsum of the finger.

intercompartmental supraretinacular arteries: these are series of arteries that branch off of the radial artery and supply the dorsal aspect of the distal radius and are described by the relationship to the extensor compartment of the wrist and the extensor retinaculum. These are generally fairly superficial in nature, and are used in the formation of vascularized pedicle-based bone grafts.

intercostal nerves: an array of nerves that run between the ribs and are occasionally used in brachial plexus reconstruction.

ANTERIOR (PALMAR) VIEW

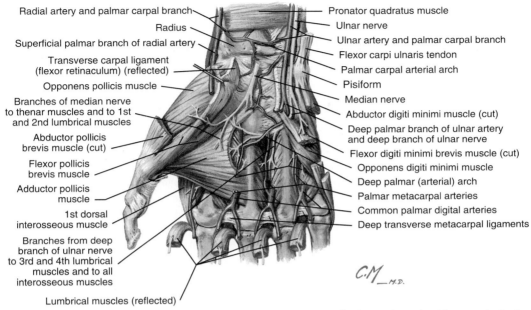

Radial artery and palmar carpal branch
Radius
Superficial palmar branch of radial artery
Transverse carpal ligament
(flexor retinaculum) (reflected)
Opponens pollicis muscle
Branches of median nerve
to thenar muscles and to 1st
and 2nd lumbrical muscles
Abductor pollicis
brevis muscle (cut)
Flexor pollicis
brevis muscle
Adductor pollicis
muscle
1st dorsal
interosseous muscle
Branches from deep
branch of ulnar nerve
to 3rd and 4th lumbrical
muscles and to all
interosseous muscles
Lumbrical muscles (reflected)

Pronator quadratus muscle
Ulnar nerve
Ulnar artery and palmar carpal branch
Flexor carpi ulnaris tendon
Palmar carpal arterial arch
Pisiform
Median nerve
Abductor digiti minimi muscle (cut)
Deep palmar branch of ulnar artery
and deep branch of ulnar nerve
Flexor digiti minimi brevis muscle (cut)
Opponens digiti minimi muscle
Deep palmar (arterial) arch
Palmar metacarpal arteries
Common palmar digital arteries
Deep transverse metacarpal ligaments

C.M ___M.D.

FIG 10-5 Major arterial and nerve supply to the hand. Note the median nerve crossing under the carpal tunnel and the separate structure of the Guyon canal. (Reprinted from Netter Anatomy Illustration Collection, © Elsevier, Inc.)

interscalene triangle: an anatomic space defined anteriorly by the anterior scalene, posteriorly by the middle scalene, and inferiorly by the first rib. This space facilitates the exit of the subclavian vein and brachial plexus in thoracic outlet syndrome.

lateral cutaneous nerve (of forearm): sometimes provides sensation to the lateral side of the thumb metacarpal area.

Martin-Gruber connection: a connection between the median and ulnar nerve in the forearm in which fibers that normally travel with the ulnar nerve from the brachial plexus distally, travel with median nerve until the midforearm and only enter the median nerve at that connection; **Martin-Gruber anastomosis.**

median nerve: the nerve that conducts sensations from the hand to the central nervous system and crosses under the small volar carpal ligament. Supplies some of the small muscles of the thumb including the opponens, the superficial head of the flexor pollicis brevis

(FPB), and the abductor pollicis brevis (APB) but not the adductor and the deep head of the flexor pollicis brevis (FPB); provides sensation for most of the palm and volar thumb, long and index fingers, and thumb side of the ring finger. The motor branch controls muscles surrounding the thumb.

Meissner's corpuscles: pressure receptors at nerve endings in the skin.

proper volar digital nerve and artery: the nerves and arteries after they have divided in the palm and travel along the two volar sides of the finger.

radial artery: major artery on the thumb side of the palm and wrist.

radial nerve, superficial branch: this nerve supplies sensation only; sensory distribution is over the dorsum of the thumb, index finger, long finger, and radial side of the ring finger.

Riche-Cannieu connection: the deep motor branch of the ulnar nerve may send a branch to join the motor branch of the median nerve. The relevance is that in injuries to the median nerve at the wrist, one may still retain motor function at the wrist.

superficial and deep palmar arterial arch: the superficial and deep connecting arcades of the radial and ulnar artery in the palm.

ulnar artery: artery on the little finger side of the palm and wrist.

ulnar nerve: the nerve crossing the wrist through the Guyon canal and supplying the adductor pollicis, deep head of the flexor pollicis brevis, and all small muscles of the hand, except the thumb and first two lumbricals. The sensation supplied is to the little finger and the little finger side of the ring finger.

Vater-Pacini corpuscle: pain pinpoint receptor.

vinculae: blood vessel bridges to the flexor tendons having a **vinculum brevum** and **vinculum longum.**

Diseases and Structural Anomalies

Most of the diseases that affect the bones and joints of the hand are described in Chapter 2. The specific terminology for deformities caused by rheumatoid arthritis, nerve injuries, and congenital defects related to the hand is listed here. The terminology for diseases of the hand comprises many words not specific to other parts of the anatomy and is divided as follows.

Arthritic Deformities

arthritis (degenerative): commonly seen in the following joints: distal interphalangeal (DIP) (Heberden nodes), proximal interphalangeal (PIP; Bouchard nodes), metacarpophalangeal (MCP; posttraumatic or infection), carpometacarpal (CMC) digits (associated with CMC bossing), trapeziometacarpal (thumb), intercarpal (triscaphe, radiolunate, triquetrohamate, lunatotriquetral), radioscaphoid (seen in postscaphoid nonunions or with scapholunate advanced collapse [SLAC] wrist).

scapholunate advanced collapse (SLAC): after untreated scaphoid nonunion or untreated scapholunate dissociation, there is rotatory subluxation of the scaphoid. Typically will have radioscaphoid arthritis, sparing the radiolunate joint with proximal migration of the capitate.

arthritis (inflammatory): rheumatoid hand deformities that include the following: flexor or extensor tenosynovitis, tendon ruptures, caput ulnar syndrome (Vaughn-Jackson syndrome), intercarpal collapse or volar carpal subluxation, metaphalangeal volar collapse with ulnar deviation, thumb digits, boutonnière deformity, swan-neck deformity, carpal tunnel syndrome, and intrinsic contractures.

arthritis mutilans: a form of rheumatoid arthritis manifesting extreme loss of bone stock; medullary, cancellous bones and markedly same with cortices.

attenuation (attrition) of tendons: erosion and eventual rupture of tendons by diseased synovium or bony spurs.

crystalline arthropathy (gout): with chronic hyperuricemia, there is recurrent joint inflammation, typically with fever and leukocytosis that affects fingers, wrists, and elbows; medical and surgical treatment indicated.

pseudogout: the deposition of calcium pyrophosphate crystals with episodic inflammation of wrist and metaphalangeal (MP) joints; chondrocalcinosis.

Grind test: a diagnostic test to clinically determine the presence of basal joint arthritis of the thumb by exerting axial pressure on the thumb metacarpal to the trapezium.

progressive systemic sclerosis (PSS): typically scleroderma, Raynaud's subcutaneous calcinosis, resorption of the distal tufts. Diffuse hand involvement with skin thickening and fibrosis.

psoriatic arthritis (PA): typically of the distal interphalangeal (DIP), but any joint can be affected. Joint pain and stiffness can have similar clinical picture to rheumatoid arthritis.

pyogenic arthritis: bacterial infection of a joint.

systemic lupus erythematosus (SLE): deformity similar to rheumatoid arthritis with pain and swelling in the midproximal interphalangeal (PIP) joints and the wrists. Usually systemic, there is relative sparing of articular cartilage until late.

Arthritic Deformities (Specific)

boutonnière deformity: a fixed deformity of the finger consisting of flexion of the proximal interphalangeal joint and extension of the distal interphalangeal joint. A result of rheumatoid destruction of the extensor tendon mechanism at the proximal interphalangeal joint and also secondary to trauma without arthritis. Can be moderate to severe and indicates that a separate classification system exists.

diabetic cheioarthropathy: hand arthritis associated with diabetes; characterized by flexion contracture of the metacarpophalangeal and proximal interphalangeal joints of the fingers, with thickening, induration, and a waxy appearance of the skin.

mallet finger: drop of the distal phalanx due to traumatic or arthritic avulsion to the extensor tendon over the distal interphalangeal (DIP) joint, drop finger.

opera-glass hand: a rare, very advanced stage of arthritis in which the joints are destroyed and the bones become thin, fragile, and shortened.

radial drift: the position toward which the metacarpals tend to drift in rheumatoid arthritis—the alignment of the hand deviates toward the thumb; may apply to the thumb but usually specified.

swan-neck deformity: a static or dynamic position of the finger that exhibits distal interphalangeal (DIP) flexion and proximal interphalangeal (PIP) hyperextension. Seen in posttraumatic or rheumatoid patients. Anatomically, there is failure of the distal extensor mechanism, tightness of the central slip, and proximal interphalangeal (PIP) volar plate laxity. In rheumatoid arthritis, the classification system is as follows:

  Type I: PIP joint flexible in all positions of MP joint.
  Type II: PIP joint is limited in certain positions.
  Type III: PIP joint is limited in all positions.
  Type IV: stiff PIP with gross articular destruction.

tophus: accumulation of any crystalline material in the soft tissue; seen commonly in gout.

trapeziometacarpal arthritis: an arthritis at the base of the thumb; often occurs in the absence of systemic disease or previous trauma. Most common in women.

ulnar drift: the position of the fingers in rheumatoid arthritis; the fingers point away from the thumb and are often associated with radial drift at the wrist.

Neuropathies

allodynia: a perception of nonpainful stimulus as painful. This is a symptom of complex regional pain syndrome.

Bouvier's maneuver: application of dorsal pressure over the proximal phalanx to passively flex the metacarpophalangeal joint resulting to straightening of the distal joint and temporary correction of a claw deformity in ulnar nerve palsy.

complex regional pain syndrome (formerly reflex sympathetic dystrophy): syndrome of abnormally intense, inappropriately prolonged pain, not a reflection of actual or impending tissue damage commonly seen after trauma, in a variety of neurogenic and vascular sequelae.

compressive neuropathy: loss of motor or sensory nerve function, acute or chronic, due to extrinsic compression. Entrapment can occur within tight fibroosseous tunnels or as a result of tumor, hemorrhage, or metabolic changes, causing swelling of soft tissues around the nerve.

dysesthesia: an unpleasant spontaneous sensation occurring in patients with chronic regional pain syndrome.

Halstead maneuver: a compression test of the thoracic outlet by moving the shoulders downward and backward with the chest protruding to draw the clavicle closer to the first rib, thus narrowing the thoracic outlet.

Horner's syndrome: strongly correlated with avulsion of the C8 and T1 nerve root in brachial plexus injury. This includes ptosis, meiosis, and anhydrosis.

hyperesthesia: increased sensitivity to a stimulus that would normally not be painful; seen commonly in chronic regional pain syndrome.

hyperpathia: a state of exaggerated and very painful response to stimulation seen in complex regional pain syndrome.

Jeanne's sign: hyperextension of the metacarpophalangeal joint of the thumb doing key pinch or gross grip due to paralysis of the adductor pollicis muscle, which acts as a first metacarpal adductor seen commonly in ulnar nerve palsy.

Klumpke's palsy: a paralysis due to isolated injury to the C8 and T1 nerve roots either in birth plexus injuries or traumatic injuries later in life.

phantom limb pain: a sensation after amputation of a limb. The patient may still have sensation that the amputated part is still present. This may be painful and may be due to representation of the limb in the terminal neuromatous stumps in the amputated part.

Pitres Testut sign: an inability to actively move the long finger in radial and ulnar deviation with palm placed flat on the table. Demonstrating paralysis of the second and third dorsal interosseous muscles in ulnar nerve palsy.

Pollock's sign: loss of extrinsic power with inability to flex the distal joint of the ring and little fingers due to the weakness of the flexor digitorum profundus through the fourth and fifth fingers in ulnar nerve palsy.

post-tourniquet syndrome: characterized by edema, stiffness, pallor and weakness without paralysis, and subjective numbness without objective anesthesia due to prolonged use of tourniquet in upper extremity surgery.

reflex sympathetic dystrophy (RSD): usually post-traumatic (major or minor) pain dysfunction syndrome. Thought to be due to abnormal modulation of afferent pain signals with possible short-circuiting of somatic and autonomic nerve fibers. Attendant autonomic nervous system hyperactivity will produce abnormal peripheral small vessel response to cold and heat stimulus. Symptoms include hyperpathia (increased pain at rest), allodynia (painful response to a nonpainful stimulus), erythema (brawny edema), joint stiffness, and loss of skin elasticity. Osteoporosis and complete loss of dexterity result. Bone scan and tomography are diagnostic, and treatment includes physical therapy, oral medications, and a sympathetic ganglion blockade; also called **autonomic dystrophy, shoulder-hand syndrome, Sudeck atrophy, causalgia,** and **sympathetic maintained pain syndrome (SMPS).**

Roo's classification: classification of thoracic outlet syndrome depending on the segment of the brachial plexus involved, either upper, lower, or combined compressions.

Roo's test: a clinical test to diagnose thoracic outlet syndrome where the patient abducts both arms 90 degrees and flexes with 90 degrees of elbow flexion, repeatedly opening and closing the hands to elicit numbness, tingling, or weakness in both hands.

Semmes-Weinstein monofilament tests: an array of monofilaments placed perpendicular to wooden or plastic rods that are held against the skin in progressive thickness and progressive skin resistance used to test innervation and density at the fingertips in nerve injury areas.

Spurling test: a clinical test for cervical nerve root compression by compressing the nerve root at the foraminal exit in the cervical spine. Compression is applied to the patient's head. A positive test represents a spray of numbness and pain shooting down the ipsilateral arm.

Sunderland classification (grades of nerve injury):

I neuropraxia: local conduction block, nerve in continuity, no wallerian degeneration, all have elements intact. No Tinel's sign.

II axonotmesis: axonal damage; wallerian degeneration distally; endoneurium, perineurium, and epineurium intact; nerve sprouting; progress excellent.

III axonotmesis: axon and endothelium are disrupted, perineurium intact. Nerve mismatching with regeneration. Recovery is dependent on degree of neural matching, unpredictable; advancing Tinel's sign and wallerian degeneration distally.

IV axonotmesis: axon, endoneurium, and perineurium violated. Nerve is grossly in continuity held by epineurium, advancing Tinel's sign, regenerative units trapped in scar; requires surgical intervention and traction (3-month wait before traction).

V neurotmesis: complete nerve transection requiring surgical intervention by repair graft or conduit.

VI neuroma in continuity: nerve grossly in continuity, but injured area is encased in nerve scar with varying degrees of nerve injury in each fascicle. The challenge is to identify the fascicles with a higher grade of injury and to repair these.

traction injury: refers to injury to nerve tissue from an overpull that exceeds 10% of resting length resulting in neuronal dysfunction, which is commonly seen in brachial plexus injuries. This injury may also pull the nerve root out of the cervical spine resulting in pseudoceles.

Median Neuropathy

anterior interosseous nerve syndrome: anterior elbow and forearm pain and motor weakness of the flexor digitorum profundus (FDP) II, flexor pollicis longus (FPL), and pronator quadratus (PQ). Electromyography may be helpful. Conservative therapy may be tried for several months, and, failing that, surgical decompression of the nerve is indicated.

carpal tunnel syndrome (CTS): a median nerve compression at the wrist caused by chronic synovitis surrounding the flexor tendons with repetitive finger motion or squeezing. Maximum pressure elevation occurs 3 to 4 cm distal to the volar wrist crease. Thenar motor loss may be included if untreated. Patient describes numbness, tingling, and dysesthesia in the hand at the median nerve distribution. Conservative therapy is indicated in chronic cases, and, failing that, surgical decompression of the carpal tunnel is necessary. Electromyograms (EMGs) and nerve conduction studies are usually diagnostic.

pronator syndrome: entrapment of the median nerve in the elbow causes anterior elbow and forearm pain, with numbness, tingling, and paresthesias in the median nerve distribution. Electrodiagnostics are occasionally helpful. Conventional therapy is tried for several months, and, failing that, decompression of the median nerve is indicated.

Radial Neuropathy

posterior intraosseous nerve syndrome: compression of the motor branch of the radial nerve near the **arcade of Froshe** that causes weakness of the finger and wrist extensors. Electrodiagnosis and conservative

treatment are not helpful. Surgical release of the radial nerve may improve function, but tendon transfers may be necessary.

radial sensory nerve entrapment (Wartenberg syndrome): the radial sensory nerve can become entrapped in the distal third of the forearm as it emerges between the brachioradialis and the extensor carpi radialis longus (ECRL). Patient experiences numbness and dysesthesia in the dorsoradial hand and wrist, provoked by hyperpronation of the forearm. Sensory nerve conduction studies are helpful, and surgical release is curative in most cases; **brachialgia statica paresthetica.**

radial tunnel syndrome: usually misdiagnosed as **resistant tennis elbow,** it is posterolateral elbow pain accentuated on resisted supination of the forearm or extension of the middle finger. Electromyography and nerve conduction studies are helpful. Treatment includes rest, splinting, and avoiding stressful activities.

wrist drop: a radial nerve palsy with loss of muscle control for wrist extension. This can be due to a variety of central and peripheral nerve conditions but is most commonly associated with radial nerve palsy; **posterior intraosseous nerve syndrome.**

Ulnar Neuropathy

cubital tunnel syndrome: entrapment of the ulnar nerve at the elbow due to fibrous tissue in the fibroosseous arcade and the two heads of the flexor carpi ulnaris (FCU) as a result of prolonged elbow flexion. Early on, symptoms are sensory and involve the fourth and fifth digits; later, intrinsic motor weakness predominates. Surgical compression and/or ulnar nerve transposition is necessary.

Charcot-Marie-Tooth disease: in the hand, spontaneous deterioration of the neuromuscular complex will affect the ulnar nerve and cause severe intrinsic wasting with a characteristic clawhand deformity; **intrinsic minus deformity.**

double (multiple) crush syndrome: compression of a peripheral nerve (i.e., median or ulnar nerve) in two or more locations. There is cervical root compression at C-6 or C-7 and carpal tunnel syndrome. Three types exist: multiple anatomic regions along a peripheral nerve, multiple anatomic structure access to peripheral nerve with anatomic region superimposed on a neuropathy, or a combination of the above. These complex conditions require a multifactorial approach. Prognosis is guarded.

focal dystonia: a condition whereby muscles become imbalanced when some muscles are used more than others. This is due to repetitive motions of the hand, such as seen in musicians (pianists or string or brass instrumentalists). The brain does not send proper signals to the affected muscles, resulting in spasms and seizures of the hand. Sometimes the arm is affected. Treatment is in the form of electrical stimulation, ultrasound, exercise, or surgery.

intrinsic minus hand: in low ulnar nerve palsy, will cause intrinsic palsy with a characteristic metacarpophalangeal (MCP) hyperextension and proximal interphalangeal (PIP) and distal interphalangeal (DIP) sensory deformity. Results from any interruption of intrinsic function; intrinsic minus deformity, intrinsic plus deformity; **clawhand deformity.**

intrinsic plus hand: loss of extrinsic muscle function or intrinsic contracture will cause metaphalangeal flexion and interphalangeal extension.

monkey paw: an adduction and extension of the thumb in which it cannot be opposed. It is unable to touch the tips of the fingers due to weakness of the opposing muscles of the thumb, as in a lesion of the median nerve.

peripheral neuropathy: intrinsic axonal or myelin pathologic condition usually due to an underlying metabolic malfunction or toxic state (i.e., diabetes, renal failure, alcoholic neuropathy).

Saturday night palsy: localized pressure palsy (e.g., in an alcoholic who falls asleep on a rested arm on a hard object); a first-degree neuropraxia occurs, which is worsened by an underlying alcoholic neuropathy.

tardy ulnar palsy: delayed chronic ulnar neuropathy secondary to chronic stretching of the nerve in the cubital tunnel due to cubitus valgus deformity at the elbow.

thoracic outlet syndrome: a constellation of signs and symptoms with multifactorial etiology. Common complaints include aching pain and heaviness in the neck, shoulder, and upper arm with numbness and tingling mainly to the fourth and fifth fingers. Symptoms worsen with arm elevation to include chest pain, tightness, and headaches. Thoracic outlet syndrome is believed due to compression of the brachial plexus over the cervical rib and between the scalenus anterior and scalenus medius muscles; in early adult life with shoulder sagging, brachial plexus traction can result. Initial treatment must include physiotherapy. Surgery may be indicated if symptoms persist for more than 1 year. Related conditions are *brachial plexus compression, scalenus anterior syndrome*, and *hyperabductor syndrome.*

ulnar tunnel syndrome: entrapment of the ulnar nerve at the wrist (Guyon canal). Could be acute or caused by repetitive trauma. Electrodiagnostics studies are helpful. Surgical release may be necessary.

vibration white finger syndrome: digital arterial or nerve injury in the hand from using tools with at least 2000 to 3000 cpm; characterized by Raynaud's phenomenon: cold intolerance, numbness, tingling, and weakness with loss of dexterity.

Congenital Anomalies
Classification of Upper Limb Anomalies
The International Federation of Societies for Surgery of the Hand (IFSSH) has adopted a classification system for upper limb anomalies that affect hand function. An example is given for each group.

I. Failure of formation of parts.
Transverse congenital amputations, constriction band syndrome (amniotic Streeter bands).
Longitudinal (radial, ulnar) hemimelias, phocomelias, hypoplastic digits.
II. Failure of differentiation of parts (incomplete morphogenesis).
Shoulder: Sprengel deformity.
Arm and forearm synostosis: humeroradial, humeroulnar, radioulnar.
Hand synostosis: syndactyly, camptodactyly, congenital trigger digit, clinodactyly.
III. Duplication.
Polydactyly triphalangism, central polydactyly (polysyndactyly, mirror hand).

IV. Overgrowth (gigantism).

Macrodactyly, lipofibromas, hamartoma of nerve, limb hypertrophy, hemihypertrophy.

V. Undergrowth.

Brachydactyly.

VI. Constriction ring syndrome (amniotic Streeter bands).

VII. Generalized skeletal anomalies.

Dwarfism, arthrogryposis, chromosomal anomalies (i.e., Madelung deformity); **Klippel-Feil syndrome.**

Agenesis

acheiria: absence of the hand.

acquired thumb flexion contracture: in children, a thumb flexion contracture that usually develops *after* birth, and, if present for more than a year, can be relieved by release of the A1 pulley at the volar base of the thumb. The thumb rarely catches or snaps. Hence, the term **congenital trigger thumb** is not appropriate for this condition.

acrosyndactyly: terminal interconnection of the syndactylyzed digits. These may or may not be connected proximally. The connection may be simple (skin) or complex (bone or other associated structures). These are commonly seen in Apert syndrome.

adactyly: absence of the digits.

amelia: total absence of the upper limb (congenital amputation).

amniotic bands: congenital circumferential crease rings that may be present at a fingertip or at upper arm level, or anywhere in between. This can be isolated or in conjunction with associated anomalies such as club-foot or cleft palate. Neurovascular embarrassment depends on the depth of the crease and may be complete if the crease goes down to the bone. Four types are evident: (1) simple constriction rings; (2) rings associated with distal lymphedema or deformity; (3) rings associated with soft tissue fusion of distal parts; and (4) intrauterine amputations. If there is any question of neurovascular compromise, Z-plasty releases are initiated in at least two stages; **constriction bands, Streeter bands, Streeter dysplasia.**

Apert syndrome: hand anomalies that include delta phalanx, metacarpal synostosis, complex syndactyly, and other anomalies including skull and facial. Digits are usually short, deformed, stiff, and at the tips "spoon hand."

aphalangia: absence of phalanges.

arachnodactyly: long spider-like fingers seen commonly in Marfan's syndrome.

arthrofibrosis: joint capsular thickening and scarring with resistant stiffness seen in either posttraumatic situations, chronic spasticity, or an arthrogryposis.

arthrogryposis (arthrogryposis multiplex congenita): joint contractures present at birth; cause is not yet known. Muscle weakness with immobility leads to contractures. Absent skin lines give it a waxy appearance. There are three groups:

single localized deformity **(in upper extremity):** forearm pronation contracture, palm clutched thumb, selected loss of wrist and finger extensors, and intrinsic muscle contracture.

whole upper extremity involvement: no shoulder girdle musculature; thin, tubular arms and forearms; straight, stiff elbows; flexion and ulnar deviation of the wrist; and stiff fingers and adducted thumbs.

global rigidity with associated deformities: polydactyly or windblown deformity (intrinsic plus hand).

Bayne's classification: a range of radial longitudinal congenital deficiencies describing the spectrum of deficits on the radial side of the forearm from hypoplastic thumb to complete absence of all radial structures including the radial bone.

Beal's syndrome: a system to categorize the different types of camptodactyly and congenital contractures in fingers.

Bell's classification: spectrum of inherited anomalies that include brachydactyly as the dominant feature.

bifid thumb: a generic term for thumb duplication or preaxial polydactyly. Wassel classification is the most commonly used.

I: bifid distal phalanx (IP joint common).

II: duplicate distal phalanx (first proximal phalanx).

III: bifid proximal phalanx (MP joint common).

IV: duplicate proximal phalanx (first metacarpal most common).

V: bifid metacarpal (CMC joint common).

VI: duplicate metacarpal.

VII: triphalangeal thumb.

brachydactyly ("short fingers"): digital hypoplasia may result from an arrest of development and it may affect any or all component tissues in a digit. It can be isolated or in conjunction with other congenital anomalies.

camptodactyly ("bent finger"): congenital nontraumatic flexion contracture in the sagittal plane of the proximal interphalangeal joint of the little finger, usually accompanied by metacarpophalangeal joint hyperextension. This is usually associated with other anomalies; causes are multifactorial, treatment is difficult, and outcome is uncertain.

carpal coalition: a congenital fusion or synostosis between two carpal bones, most commonly lunate and triquetrum or capitohamate. These are usually asymptomatic.

clasped thumb: refers to a spectrum of congenital thumb abnormalities resulting from deficiency of the thumb extensor mechanism. Overactivity of thumb extrinsic and intrinsic flexors.

cleft hand: a central ray deficiency (ectrodactyly, oligodactyly) secondary to failure of formation of parts. High association with extraskeletal (i.e., cardiac) defects that may be metacarpal and carpal anomalies or deficiencies. These present deep clefts that may extend down to the carpus. Despite the cosmetic appearance, function may be surprisingly good; **lobster-claw hand** (archaic).

clinodactyly ("bent finger"): radial or ulnar deviation of the digit tip in coronal plane. Usually this is expressed as radial deviation of the little finger at the distal interphalangeal joint and is associated with other anomalies.

congenital trigger thumb: a congenital locking or clicking of the thumb with flexion posture of the interphalangeal joint. Nodular formation on the flexor pollicis longus tendon or tendon sheath thickening is common. Tendon sheath release is curative.

congenital ulnar drift: ulnar deviation of the digits at the metacarpophalangeal (MCP) joint with proximal interphalangeal (PIP) joint flexion deformity. Thumb webbing is also present. General muscular hypoplasia in the arm is present. Associated with craniofacial deformities and a markedly narrowed mouth; also called **windblown hand, whistling face syndrome, Freeman-Sheldon syndrome.**

delta phalanx: a triangular-shaped bone interposed in the digit between two normal phalanges. A C-shaped physis is common and will cause a sharp angular digital deformity.

Ellis-Van Crevel syndrome: a form of ulnar polydactyly that is postaxial (multiple digits coming out of the ulnar aspect of the hand).

Fanconi anemia: pancytopenia, hematophoretic anomalies associated with radial hemimelia (autosomal recessive).

flipper hand (phocomelia): congenital absence of the arms; the hands appear to arise directly from the shoulder.

floating thumb (pouce floutant): an unstable hypoplastic thumb that may be connected to the hand by skin and a simple neurovascular pedicle. These digits are generally useless and are best removed.

Freeman-Sheldon syndrome: a condition affecting the hands and feet with a characteristic appearance of arthrogryposis as a dominant feature.

hemimelia: absence of the forearm and hand.

heart-hand syndrome (Holt-Oram syndrome): cardiac septal defects, autosomal dominant and seen with radial ray deficiency.

hereditary multiple exostosis: autosomal dominant inheritable disease characterized by multiple osteochondromas growing from the physis of long bone, pelvis, rib, scapula, and vertebra. This commonly appears in forearm bones and short tubular bones of the hand.

hyperphalangism: an extra (fourth) phalanx interposed between the phalanges of a finger. There are no extra digits. The digits are usually short.

hypoplastic thumb: an incompletely developed thumb that can range from a short thumb to complete absence. This is usually seen in conjunction with many associated abnormalities. There are five types: short thumb, adducted thumb, abducted thumb, floating thumb, and absent thumb.

Kirner deformity: parrot-beak convexity of the nail bed due to volar bending of the distal phalanx. This may not be obvious until age 12.

macrodactyly: a disproportionately large digit apparent at birth or early childhood. In a "true" case, all structural components may be enlarged including vessels and nerves. Commonly, there is a marked increase in subcutaneous fiber or fatty tissue.

Madelung deformity: congenital growth plate disorder of the volar ulnar physis of the distal radius. This will cause a severe volar and ulnar bowing of the radius, initially normal at birth, and the deformity becomes evident by 8 to 12 years of age.

Marfan's syndrome: a disease of connective tissue that causes arachnodactyly (long, pencil-like fingers) without flexion contractures. Patients with this condition also have loose ligaments in their finger joints.

mirror hand (ulnar dimelia): the forearm contains two ulnas and has no radius. Typically, the patient presents with eight digits. This is a rare spontaneous genetic mutation that, when present, can be passed down in an autosomal dominant fashion.

monodactyly: a single-digit hand that may also be seen as part of a spectrum of cleft hand disease.

Poland syndrome: thumb ray or finger deformity associated with absence of pectoral muscle head.

polydactyly: extra digits that may be complete or partially formed. These can be postaxial (ulnar side of the hand) or preaxial (on the thumb).

polysyndactyly (central polydactyly): polydactyly of the index and ring fingers, usually associated with complex syndactyly. These are usually bilateral.

radial clubbed hand: total or partial absence of radial structures of the hand and forearm (preaxial). There are four types: (1) short distal radius; (2) hypoplastic radius; (3) partial absence of the radius; (4) total absence of the radius. These may be accompanied by thumb, index, or long finger anomalies. Muscle or neurovascular anomalies can be isolated as part of a syndrome complex (i.e., vertebral defects, imperforate anus, tracheoesophageal fistula, and radial and renal dysplasia [VATER], Holt-Oram syndrome). Hand is radially deviated; **talipomanus.**

radial deficiency: a series of congenital malformation affecting the radial aspect of the hand, wrist, and forearm with varying degrees of hypoplasia of the bones, joints, muscles and tendons, ligaments, nerves, and blood vessel. This may be associated with other systemic conditions.

radio-ulnar synostosis: a congenital or posttraumatic fusion of the radius and ulna seen generally near the proximal radial ulnar joint of the elbow, but it can occur distally as well.

supernumerary digits: extra nubbins of fingers and thumb with no function.

symbrachydactyly: literally shortened, stiff digits. Seen commonly in the spectrum of cleft hand disease.

symphalangism: hereditary dysplasia and ankylosis of digital joints, most notably the proximal interphalangeal (PIP) joint. There may be partial or total bone bridging.

syndactyly: a congenital joining of two or more digits; the connection may be complete or incomplete, simple or complex. Simple-shared element of skin and subcutaneous tissue. Complex shared element of skin, subcutaneous tissue, tendon, bone, and neurovascular structures.

synostosis: fusion between two adjacent parallel bones (i.e., metacarpals or radius and ulna). Term may also be used for humeral-radial fusion.

synpolydactyly: a congenital anomaly resulting in the formation of extra phalanges or digits within an conjoined digital nerve with syndactyly of skin and bony structures.

TAR syndrome: *t*hrombocytopenia, *a*bsent *r*adius; complete absence of the radius may be present (autosomal recessive).

trident hand: typical hand appearance of an achondroplastic dwarf where there is a persistent space between the ring and long fingers.

triphalangeal thumb: interposition of an extra phalanx between two normal phalanges of the thumb; can at times be functionally normal or cause marked deformity or malfunction. The extra phalanx can be normal or be a delta phalanx. Often seen with congenital heart disease.

triplicate thumb: a variant form of preaxial polydactyly involving three thumbs; all are markedly diminished in size and may lack one or more tissue elements.

ulnar (postaxial) deficiency: usually isolated with severe limitation of elbow function; hypoplasia of ulna, partial aplasia of the ulna (absence of distal or middle third of the ulna), total aplasia of the ulna; **radiohumeral synostosis.**

ulnar variance: relative position of the distal ulnar joint referred to the level of the ulnar side of the distal radial joint, as determined on an anteroposterior radiograph that is obtained with neutral pronation and supination. A longer ulna is called a **positive variance,** and a shorter ulna is called a **negative variance,** measured in millimeters.

VATER syndrome: *v*ertebral anomalies, *a*nal atresia, *t*racheo*e*sophageal fistula, *r*enal and vascular anomalies, accompanied by a radial clubhand.

whistling face syndrome: an autosomal dominant condition affecting the hands and feet with a characteristic facial appearance in the form of arthrogryposis, which is a congenital and pathologic stiffness of the arms or legs down to the hands or feet in characteristic postures.

Muscle and Tendon Disorders

trigger finger (acquired): entrapment of finger flexor tendons usually under the proximal A1 pulleys; usually due to a disproportion between the flexor tendon and the flexor tendon sheath. Usually, the cause is obscure, with thickening of the pulley tissues and/or nodular formation about the tendon. This can be secondary (i.e., due to diabetes, rheumatoid arthritis, or gout). Conservative measures and steroid injections may help, but surgery is usually curative.

boutonnière deformity (posttraumatic): usually due to a central slip rupture of the middle phalanx with an injury to the triangular ligaments. Volar subluxation of the lateral bands below the flexion axis of the proximal interphalangeal (PIP) joint will cause a fixed flexion attitude of the PIP joint.

carpal pedal spasm: an intrinsic plus position with wrist flexion usually seen in hypercalcemia.

de Quervain's disease: stenosing tenosynovitis of the first dorsal extensor compartment, usually involving the extensor pollicis brevis (EPB) and abductor pollicis longus (APL).

intersection syndrome: pain and swelling over the place where the muscles of the first dorsal extensor compartment cross over the muscles of the second compartment. This is believed to be a tenosynovitis of the second dorsal compartment.

Landsmeer test: a test that elicits a tight oblique retinacular ligament of Landsmeer as seen in boutonnière's deformity where passively extending the proximal interphalangeal joint sends the interphalangeal joint into a tight fixed extension posture. Also, the particular anatomy of Landsmeer's ligament is volar to the proximal interphalangeal joint and dorsal to the distal interphalangeal joint.

lumbrical plus finger deformity: a condition in which there is overactivity of the lumbricals creating a paradoxical extension of the proximal and distal interphalangeal joints with attempted flexion of the fingers.

peritendonitis stenosans/digitus saltans: an archaic term used to describe conditions of stenosing tenosynovitis such as those found in de Quervain's disease, flexor carpi radialis tendonitis, and trigger digits.

quadregia: in a setting in which the profundus tendon to a digit is contracted or repaired too tightly, there will be a limitation of proximal excursion of the remaining flexor digitorum profundus (FDP), causing a weak grip (as all the FDP tendons usually share a common muscle belly).

tendovaginitis: form of tendon entrapment seen in trigger digits and de Quervain's tenosynovitis by tight retinaculum or tenosynovitis obliterating the space between the tendons and the overlying retinaculum.

tetraplegia: neurologic injury secondary to cervical spine trauma. Altered functional capacity of the hand, depending on the level of injury. This will also dictate operative and nonoperative intervention. A system has been devised:

Tetraplegia International Classification

Functional Group	Root Level Intact
Brachioradialis	C-5, C-6
Extensor carpi radialis longus	C-7 (possibly C-8)
Extensor carpi radialis brevis	C-7, C-8
Pronator teres	C-7, C-8
Flexor carpi radialis	C-8
Extensor digitorum communis	C-8
Extensor pollicis longus	T-1
Partial digital flexion	T-1
Lacks intrinsics only	T-1
Miscellaneous (i.e., Brown-Séquard syndrome or syringomyelia)	

Volkmann contracture: contracture affecting the volar forearm musculature as a result of scarring after an ischemic insult. This is the usual sequela of an untreated volar muscle compartment syndrome (seen in muscle crush injuries or forearm fracture). Circulation is usually impaired in the center of the forearm. The flexor digitorum profundus (FDP) and flexo pollicis longus (FPL) muscles are most severely affected. There is a mild, moderate, classic, or severe type.

"no man's land": usually refers to an injury to the digital flexor tendons at zone II (under the A1 and A2 pulleys). Until recently, injury to this area was fraught with technical difficulty and poor results.

Vaughn–Jackson syndrome: rupture of ring and little finger extensors due to synovitis at the distal radial ulnar joint.

washer woman's sprain: an archaic description of de Quervain's tenosynovitis, tendonopathies of the tendons of the first dorsal extensor compartment.

Vascular Disorders

acrocyanosis: seen in Raynaud's phenomenon. With exposure to cold, the fingers become deep blue and cold. This is usually due to peripheral vasospasm.

Buerger disease (thromboangiitis obliterans): an inflammatory thrombosis seen in smokers, usually in men. Digital arteries are affected. The disease is progressive, leading to digital loss and possibly loss of the whole hand.

hypothenar hammer syndrome: an ulnar artery aneurysm or thrombosis due to repetitive striking of the hypothenar eminence and the hook of hamate region against a hard blunt object; typically, localized pain, digital pallor, and cold sensibility are common symptoms.

Kienböck disease: a posttraumatic, vascularly mediated avascular necrosis of the lunate with subsequent collapse, dislocation, and arthrosis. Magnetic resonance imaging (MRI) and bone scan have fine-tuned the classification; **isolated dislocation.**

Lichtman classification for Keinböck disease is as follows:

Stage I: normal radiographic findings, positive bone scan, questionable linear fractures.

Stage II: lunate sclerosis without collapse. MRI subclassification:

IIA: T2 focal signal intensity increase.

IIB: T2 focal signal intensity loss.

IIC: T2 generalized signal intensity increase.

IID: T2 generalized signal intensity loss.

Stage III: lunate sclerosis, fragmentation, and collapse.

Stage IV: stage III plus degenerative changes of the carpus.

Traumatic Disorders

annulus fracture: fractures of the hook of the hamate usually caused by compression force as a direct blow.

Barton's fracture: a intra-articular fracture involving either the dorsal or the volar lip of the distal radius resulting in either dorsal or volar subluxation of the lunate.

chauffeur's fracture: displaced fracture of the radial styloid accompanied by ulnar translocation of the carpus.

dye punch fracture: a type of intra-articular distal radius fracture involving the compression of the lunate facet of the distal radius.

factitious edema: history of minor trauma followed by persistent dorsal forearm pain, swelling, and tenderness due to repeated self-inflicted trauma; **secretan edema.**

fragment specific fixation: a method of repairing the distal radius using a small plate to fix small fractures to the main body of the bone.

gamekeeper's thumb: an abduction laxity of the thumb at the metacarpophalangeal joint due to acute or chronic disruption of the ulnar collateral ligament of the finger joint.

Herbert's classification of scaphoid fractures: a four-part classification describing scaphoid fractures, which includes stable acute fractures, unstable acute fractures, delayed union, and established nonunion.

Holstein-Lewis fracture: a fracture of the distal humerus in which the radial nerve is in particular jeopardy. The proximal spike of the spiral fracture breaks through the lateral cortex of the humerus near where the radial nerve is most grossly opposed to the bone.

Hotchkiss fracture: a classification system describing fractures of the radial head and neck in trauma situation.

interdigital contracture: results from extensive scarring about the hand resulting in cicatrix forming in between the digits preventing digital abduction; seen commonly in severe burns of the hand.

Jahss maneuver: a method of closed reduction of metacarpal neck fractures flexing the metacarpophalangeal (MCP) joint and the proximal interphalangeal (PIP) joint and pushing upward on the flexed PIP joint while applying a cast, flexing the MCP joint into maximal flexion. The PIP joint is usually then brought out into extension.

lunotriquetral dissociation: a condition whereby a lunate becomes volar-flexed in sagittal plane due to a dissociation between it and the adjacent triquetrum.

malrotation: a condition whereby there is a mismatch between the proximal and distal ends of a fracture of a tubular bone in which the distal end of the fracture rotates relative to the proximal end on its long axis. This can cause finger overlap.

Melone's classification: a four-part classification of distal radius fractures that identifies specific intra-articular fragments of the distal radius and rank them in order of severity based on displacement.

negative pressure therapy: a technique that uses a suction apparatus on a mangling high-energy wound. This technique removes exudates, decreases edema, closes the dead space, and promotes wound healing commonly seen in the treatment of wartime injuries.

Palmer classification: for *triangular fibrocartilage complex* (TFCC) injury.

Class 1: traumatic.

Type A: central perforation.

Type B: medial avulsion (ulnar attachment), with or without distal ulnar fracture.

Type C: distal avulsion (carpal attachment).

Type D: lateral avulsion (radial attachment), with or without sigmoid-notch fracture.

Class 2: degenerative (ulnocarpal impaction syndrome).

Stage A: TFCC wear.

Stage B: TFCC wear with lunate and or ulnar chondromalacia.

Stage C: TFCC perforation with lunate and or ulnar chondromalacia.

Stage D: TFCC perforation with lunate and/or ulnar chondromalacia and lunotriquetral-ligament perforation.

Stage E: TFCC perforation with lunate and or ulnar chondromalacia and lunotriquetral-ligament perforation, and ulnar carpal arthritis.

peritendinous fibrosis: scarring around a tendon.

pseudoclawing: an intrinsic minus position with metacarpophalangeal hyperextension and proximal interphalangeal joint flexion due to flexion malunion of metacarpal neck fractures.

radial styloidectomy: the excision of the radial styloid done usually in conjunction with scaphoid excision and four-poster fusions in the reconstruction of SLAC wrist.

Rolando fractures: comminuted intra-articular fractures of the base of the thumb metacarpal.

scaphoid ring sign: a scapholunate dissociation in which the scaphoid collapses into flexion and has a foreshortened view on the anterior-posterior (AP) x-ray. The distal end of the scaphoid appears to have radial band with a ring superimposed on it.

scaphoid shift test: a test that determines the integrity of the scapholunate ligament by mobilization from pressure supply to the palmar tuberosity of the scaphoid while the wrist is moved from ulnar to radial deviation. A positive test is seen in a patient with scapholunate dissociation. The scaphoid no longer can strain proximally and subluxes out of the scaphoid fossa of the distal radius. When the pressure is released, the scaphoid goes back into position and a typical snapping occurs.

scapholunate ballottement test: with the lunate stabilized with the thumb and index finger and the scaphoid held over the other hand, a dorsal volar alternating pressure between the scaphoid and the lunate elicits pain and crepitance as well as instability of the joint in scapholunate dissociation.

sheer testing for lunotriquetral dissociation: a ballottement test for lunotriquetral dissociation secondary to interosseous injury. The lunate and triquetrum are held stably by the thumb and index fingers of both hands shifted dorsally and volarly relative to one another. A positive test elicits crepitance, pain, and increased movement between the lunate and triquetrum.

skier's thumb: an acute rupture of the ulnar collateral ligament of the metacarpophalangeal joint of the thumb seen commonly in skiers, but generally seen in fall on outstretched hands, hyperabducting the thumb at the MP joint.

Stener lesion: in a complete tear of the ulnar collateral ligament of the metacarpophalangeal (MCP) joint of the thumb, the ligament may avulse distally and roll up proximally, causing an interposition of the adductor aponeurosis. Nonoperative treatment will usually result in a chronically unstable thumb.

turret exostosis: a painful mass on the dorsal aspect of the middle phalanx seen on lateral x-ray as an exostosis **(bone spur)**. This is believed to be traumatic in origin.

ulnar impaction syndrome: excessive pressure from the ulnar aspect of the carpus, notably the lunate onto the distal end of the ulna in those situations in which the distal radius has been shortened leaving an ulnar positive variance.

Specific Dislocations

Wrist Dislocations and Instability

In a distal radius dislocation, the radius is dislocated in reference to the ulna. However, the standard terminology describes the position of the ulna in relationship to the radius.

carpal instability dissociative (CID; Linsheid): a carpal collapse pattern due to a ligamentous disruption in the proximal carpal row (i.e., scapholunate lunotriquetral pattern).

carpal instability nondissociative (CIND): a carpal collapse pattern due to disruption of ligaments connecting the proximal and midcarpal row or due to other extrinsic factors (i.e., radial malunion; Dobyns).

Desault d.: involves the radiocarpal joint with dorsal displacement of carpus and ulnar styloid process.

dorsal intercalated segment instability (DISI): a zigzag collapse pattern seen best on the lateral views of the wrist. The lunate appears to send its distal face dorsally. This can occur as a result of displaced scaphoid fractures, scapholunate instability, a nondissociated carpal instability. Commonly, the lunate follows the triquetrum volarly without the scaphoid to contract its movement. The capitolunate angle is greater than 20 degrees and the scapholunate angle is greater than 70 degrees when the wrist is held in neutral posture.

lumbrical plus finger: posttraumatic contracture of the lumbrical will cause a paradoxical extension of the PIP and DIP joints each time an attempt is made to flex the digits.

lunate d.: volar semilunar dislocation in the wrist; a type of dislocation often not recognized.

perilunate d.: involves all carpals, which are shifted posteriorly, leaving the lunate in proper position; may be associated with a scaphoid fracture, in which case it is termed a **transscaphoid perilunate d.** Rarely do other carpi dislocate singularly or in association with fractures about the wrist. Wrist instabilities may be associated with fractures but specifically relate to ligamentous instabilities of the carpal bones. A devastating injury in which all the connecting ligaments between the lunate and its surrounding carpal bones are severed. Commonly, the capitate sits dorsal to the lunate. The lunate may dislocate volarly as part of the spectrum.

transscaphoid perilunate dislocation: similar to the perilunate dislocation except that the stress lines extend through the body of the scaphoid itself rather than the scapholunate ligament. The radial styloid may be fractured as well.

volar flexed intercalated segment instability (VISI): a zigzag collapse pattern with the lunate distal face turned volarly. This is seen best on lateral x-rays of the wrist. These can follow triquetral lunate instability or nondissociated instability patterns. An average reduced scapholunate angle of over 35 degrees.

Hand Dislocations

Dislocation can occur at all the small joints of the hand. Dislocations at the carpometacarpal (CMC) and metacarpophalangeal (MCP) joints generally occur in a dorsal direction. Dislocations at the MCP joints can sometimes be reduced without surgery. Dislocations in the hand are often associated with intraarticular fractures. Fracture-dislocations often require surgical reduction and fixation to realign joint surfaces.

Bennett d.: lateral or dorsal displacement of the first CMC joint.

boutonnière deformity: flexion contracture of the proximal interphalangeal (PIP) joint that may progress to subluxation. Associated with hyperextension contracture of the distal interphalangeal (DIP) joint. Deformity begins with rupture of the extensor tendon insertion of the PIP joint and later becomes a fixed deformity.

carpal instability: partial or complete dislocations between individual wrist bones, causing a click-clunk with wrist movement. Most often occurs at the scapholunate joint but can occur at the triquetrolunate, midcarpal, and even the radiocarpal joint.

gamekeeper's thumb: a hyperabduction injury with partial subluxation and instability of the thumb MCP joint due to traumatic rupture of the ulnar collateral ligament. Commonly due to a ski-pole strap injury; **skier's thumb.**

Nail and Skin Disorders

acanthosis nigricans: dull, gray, friable nails with leukonychia; can be an external marker of an internal malignancy.

acquired digital fibrokeratoma: benign tumors of fibrous tissue usually found on the hands and feet. These are flesh-colored with thorn-like projections with a raised erythematous skin rash at the base. These are otherwise known as acrofibrokeratomas.

acrolentiginous melanoma: an unusual variant of melanomas found on palmar surface of the hand and nail apparatus.

beak deformity (hook nail): with amputation of the tip of the distal phalanx, the nail may grow over the edge of the finger. It is unsightly and occasionally painful.

Bowen's disease: the eponym given to intra-epidermal squamous cell carcinoma known as squamous cell carcinoma *in situ.*

chromonychia: color changes in the nail unit.

clubbing: an increase in the unguophalangeal angle of greater than 180 degrees with fibrovascular hyperplasia of the nail unit.

digital fibrokeratoma: a benign tumor of fibrous tissue origin occurring on the tips of the fingers.

Dupuytren's contracture (palmar fibromatosis): inflammatory process of the palmar fascia, occasionally extending into the fingers, in which severe contractures and nodular proliferation (skin dimples) may result. There are three phases: proliferative (nodular), involutional, and resolved. In the resolved state, the remaining constricting tissue is referred to as bands.

epidermoid cyst: benign cyst composed of epidermal fragments that have been pushed to the deeper layers by minor trauma.

keratosis: premalignant lesions seen in sun-exposed fair skinned individuals causing skin atrophy and telangiectasias. If allowed to progress, it may become squamous cell carcinoma.

leukonychia: whitening of the nail plate.

macronychia: an unusually large or wide nail.

micronychia: small, short, or narrow nail.

nail horn: formation of a nail horn can be a complication of distal tip amputations in which a fragment of nail tissue grows a thin projection at the tip of the finger, which can be quite painful and requires complete excision of the nail-forming tissue.

onychalgia: nail unit pain.

onychia: inflammation of the nail plate.

onychogryphosis: nail plate hypertrophy that is horn-like resulting from trauma; **onychogryposis.**

onycholysis: distal separation of the nail plate from the underlying nail bed.

onychomadesis: proximal separation of the nail plate from the nail matrix.

onychomycosis: fungal infection of the nail unit.

onychophagia: nail biting.

onychoptosis: loss of the nail plate.

onychorrhexis: spontaneous longitudinal splitting of the nail plate.

pincer or trumpet nail deformity: a pathologic curling of the nail plate and nail bed with ingrowing of the nail plate into the nail folds and progressive pinching off of the soft tissue of the distal fingertips, which results in pain and deformity.

pitted nail: surface pits of nails less than 1 mm in diameter.

pterygium: scarring of the eponychial fold and the nail fold to the nail bed in nail trauma leading to functional and esthetic deformities such as absence of nail growth or splitting of the nail. This has also been associated with nail bed ischemia and collagen vascular disease.

racket nail: thumbnail shorter than it is wide. Usually, the distal ends of the fingers are also short.

reedy nail: fingernail marked by longitudinal furrows.

sclerodactyly: a scleroderma in which the fingers become thin and shiny with sclerotic skin at the tip, which is due to subcutaneous and intracutaneous calcinosis and diffused fibrosis of the collagen.

scleroderma: an autoimmune disease that causes the skin of the hands to become thin, tense, and shiny; interphalangeal joint stiffness, distal ischemic ulceration, and autoamputation are common.

spoon nail: a central depression of the nail with raised sides.

subungual exostosis: a bone spur emanating from the distal phalanx dorsally under the nail bed, causing pressure pain, necrosis, and possible infection of the nail bed.

subungual hematoma: usually posttraumatic with nail bed laceration under an intact nail. A collection of blood under the nail plate, under pressure, can destroy the nail bed unless decompressed by a hole drilled into the nail plate (i.e., a hot paper clip tip).

turtle-back nail: a distorted fingernail, being more convex than normal.

unguis incarnatus: ingrown nail.

watch crystal nail: a nail as broad as it is long and convex lengthwise and crosswise; seen in pulmonary osteoarthropathy.

Other Specific Terms

aponeurotic fibroma: fibrous lesions of the hands commonly seen in childhood and adolescence. They are benign but can be locally aggressive.

Bouchard node: thick nodular swelling due to bone spurs in the proximal interphalangeal joints, not necessarily associated with systemic arthritis.

carpal bossing: prominence seen particularly at the dorsal index carpometacarpal (CMC) joint; may be painful but usually causes no symptoms.

flexor origin syndrome (reverse tennis elbow): tendonitis of pronator teres and wrist and finger flexor muscle origin on medial epicondyle of elbow.

ganglion: a clear, viscid, fluid-filled sac found near the wrist joints or fingers, arising from capsuloligamentous structures; rarely associated with other diseases; most commonly found on dorsum of wrist.

glomus tumor: small vascular lesion that is usually very painful and associated with hypersensitivity to pressure or temperature; usually in fingertip.

hamartoma: unusual tumors of the peripheral nerves most commonly involving the median nerve of the hand. It starts as a slowly progressive swelling in the distal forearm of the palm; common symptoms of nerve compression may be present.

hand-foot syndrome: swelling in hands and feet as seen in sickle cell disease.

Heberden node: a thick nodular swelling due to bone spurs in the distal interphalangeal joints; not necessarily associated with systemic arthritis.

inclusion cyst: a noninfectious process following healing of laceration or puncture wound; germinal matrix of dermal growth, causing mass comprised of desquamated dermal cells.

Luck's classification of Dupuytren's disease into three phases: proliferative phase, involutional phase, and residual phase, based on the histologic behavior of Dupuytren's fibroblast.

mucous cyst: a misnomer; this is a ganglion of the distal interphalangeal joint, which makes a cyst under the skin in the eponychial area.

nodular fasciitis: an uncommon reactive lesion that may simulate a sarcoma usually seen on the volar surface of the forearm, usually a rapidly growing small nodule. This has been confused with fibrosarcoma or myxoid liposarcoma leading to overtreatment.

overlap syndrome: seen in scleroderma patients with associated findings characteristics of lupus, dermatomyositis, or rheumatoid arthritis.

Preiser disease: spontaneous loss of blood supply and collapse of scaphoid, usually seen in young adults.

Raynaud's disease: a condition characteristic of color changes in the tip of the fingers either blanching or cyanosis in both hands and may not be involved with vasospastic disease and not lead to ulceration of the fingertips.

Raynaud's phenomenon: a clinical sign describing intermittent color changes that occur after exposure to cold or stress. A condition characteristic of color changes in the tip of the fingers either blanching or cyanosis in both hands and may not be involved with vasospastic disease and not lead to ulceration of the fingertips.

stenosing tenosynovitis: a bulbous swelling of the tendon, causing the tendon to catch as it passes through the pulley (the thick fibrous tunnel that holds the tendon in place); sometimes caused by rheumatoid arthritis; **trigger fingers, snapping tendons.**

Infections

The hand has many structures that are vulnerable to infections. When edema and swelling place pressure on muscles, tendons, blood vessels, and nerves, function is disrupted and compartmental ischemia could result. Adhesions or fibrosis following infection may reduce hand function temporarily or permanently. Terms related to infections are the following.

barber's intradigital pilonidal sinus: a foreign body granuloma usually due to a reaction to hair implanted in the intradigital skin of the hand, first described in barbers.

collar-button abscess: a digital webspace infection usually in the subdermal fatty layers. Drainage is usually required; **shirt-stud abscess.**

dactylitis: nonsuppurative insidious chronic infections of the hands and fingers commonly seen in syphilis and tuberculosis.

deep space infection (palmar space infection): refers to infection of the thenar or midpalmar spaces.

ecthyma contagiosum: a chronic infection causing large tumor-like lesions in immunodeficient host; believed to be contracted from exposure to sheep and goats.

epidermoid cyst: benign cyst composed of epidermal fragments that have been pushed to the deeper layers by minor trauma.

eponychia: a nail-fold infection involving the entire eponychial fold and lateral nail fold. These are relatively rare.

fasciitis: a rapidly advancing necrotizing infection affecting the skin and subcutaneous tissue sparing the underlying muscle associated with high morbidity and mortality, seen commonly in group A *streptococcus* infections.

felon: a subcutaneous abscess involving the tissue of the distal fingertip. These may be under great pressure and require drainage, usually through a midlateral approach.

Hansen disease (leprosy): commonly involves the hands; caused by *Mycobacterium leprae*. Peripheral neuropathy predominates with intrinsic atrophy and clawing. Later, soft tissue necrosis can result in actual loss of digits.

herpetic whitlow: a fascicular outbreak with an erythematous rim seen usually in fingertips of health care workers. These are commonly misdiagnosed and mistakenly drained. Supportive treatment is the mainstay. These are usually self-limited.

hockey-stick incisions: incisions placed at the lateral and distal aspects of the finger to facilitate drainage of felons (abscesses) of the fingertips.

horseshoe abscess: in those hands in which thenar and hypothenar spaces are interconnected, an abscess may spread to both sides of the hand in the shape of a horseshoe. Palmar space infection usually results from a penetrating wound. The deep spaces of the hand may fill with purulent material. Drainage is the key.

interdigital granuloma: small pyogenic granulomas found in the hand of cow milkers due to penetration of bovine hairs into the skin of the hand causing a foreign body reaction.

interdigital pilonidal sinus: see **barber's interdigital pilonidal sinus.**

Kanavel's sign: for pyogenic flexor tenosynovitis; there is a flexed position of the finger, symmetrical enlargement of the finger, excessive tenderness over the course of the tendon sheath, and extreme pain on passive extension of the digit.

Meleney infection: life- or limb-threatening infection with anaerobic bacteria or microaerophilic streptococcus. Amputation is usually required to save the patient's life; **gas gangrene.**

paronychia: infection in the soft tissue folds around the nail that usually results from injection of *Staphylococcus aureus* by a sliver of nail tissue, a manicure instrument, or a tooth. Drainage is mandatory.

pyogenic flexor tenosynovitis: a closed space infection of the flexor tendon sheath of the fingers and thumb generally caused by *Staphylococcus aureus, Streptococcus,* or *Pasteurella* presented with Kanavel's signs, which are semiflexed position of the fingers, symmetrical enlargement of the whole digit, excessive tenderness limited to the flexor tendon sheath, and excruciating pain on passively extending the finger.

pyogenic granuloma: an exophytic friable growth over the surface of the skin. These are usually caused by *Staphylococcus aureus* and will require complete excision to effect a cure.

shooter's abscess: infections caused by parenteral drug abuse involving accessible sites on the hand and forearm. These appear as raised ulcers with cellulitis.

subungual abscess: a collection of pus under the nail plate or over the nail bed.

tenosynovitis: inflammation of the tendon sheath. Causes are multifactorial and include overuse, rheumatoid arthritis, infection, and nonspecific onset.

verruca vulgaris: a viral wart involving the nail or skin tissue. A carbon dioxide laser is usually curative.

Surgery of the Hand and Wrist

Surgical procedures of the hand and wrist are more commonly described anatomically than by eponyms. All terms, including eponyms, are listed according to the goals of the surgical procedure.

Arthrodeses of the Fingers

chevron a.: a rigid stable construction for interphalangeal (IP) joint fusion; a precise, chevron-shaped fitting of the bone cuts of the joint to be fused with resection of the joint surface.

interphalangeal a.: cup and cone technique useful for metacarpophalangeal (MCP) or interphalangeal (IP) fusion, allows for fine adjustment of angles and rotatory alignment after joint surfaces have been prepared.

Moberg dowel graft: for an interphalangeal (IP) arthrodesis in which there has been bone loss or nonunion. A finger joint fusion using a small squared bone peg.

Potenza a.: a finger joint fusion using bone peg taken from the adjacent phalanx or metacarpal.

trapeziometacarpal fusion: for advanced trapeziometacarpal disease in the thumb in young, active patients.

Arthrodeses of the Wrist

Haddad-Riordan technique: a wrist arthrodesis using a radial approach and an iliac crest strut graft.

intercarpal a.: for wrist instability or collapse patterns, Kienböck disease, rheumatoid arthritis, localized degenerative changes in the carpus. These include triscaphe (scaphotrapeziotrapezoid), scaphocapitate, capitolunate, scapholunate, lunatotriquetral capitohamate (four-poster fusion). Moberg dowel grafts are useful in securing these fusions.

radiocarpal a.: commonly a total wrist fusion with or without autogenous graft. Useful for (1) a heavy laborer with posttraumatic arthritis, (2) failed radiocarpal arthroplasty, (3) rheumatoid arthritis, (4) tetraplegia with deformity of the wrist, and (5) tendon transfer surgery to stabilize the wrist.

radioulnar fusion: for the creation of a one-bone forearm for advanced disease of the distal radioulnar joint.

SLAC procedure (scapho*lunate* advanced collapse): for the common combination of radioscaphoid and midcarpal arthritis often seen in chronic nonunions of the scaphoid; a midcarpal arthrodesis with excision of scaphoid.

total wrist a.: fusion of the distal radius and proximal and distal carpal rows. Useful salvage procedure for severe carpal arthritis.

triscaphe a.: of the scaphotrapeziotrapezoid (SST) articulation. Useful in localized arthritis and for rotatory subluxation of the scaphoid.

Arthrodeses of the Wrist (Eponyms)

Abbott a.: using only cortical bone grafts; Abbott-Saunders-Bost a.

Brockman-Nissen a.: intra-articular wrist fusion.

Carroll a.: rabbit ear–shaped bone graft fusion.

Feldon 2-pin wrist arthrodesis: a technique for fusing the wrist in rheumatoid patients using two thin Steinman pins inserted through the second and third webspaces between the metacarpal bones across the carpus and the intermedullary canal of the radius.

Gill-Stein a.: extra-articular fusion using the dorsal distal radius as the graft; **radiocarpal a.**

Haddad-Riordan a.: intra-articular fusion using iliac crest bone graft.

Liebolt a.: fusion using chips of bone graft.

Nalebuff a.: fusion that includes use of a Steinmann pin.

Seddon a.: intra-articular fusion involving resection of the distal ulna.

Smith-Petersen a.: fusion that includes resection of the distal ulna.

Wickstrom a.: fusion of the wrist using bone graft inserted into both the radius and carpus.

Arthroplasties

An arthroplasty is the reconstruction of joints to restore motion and stability. It involves the metacarpophalangeal (MCP), carpometacarpal (CMC), and proximal interphalangeal (PIP) joints of the fingers and wrist, often with implants. The hand specialist frequently treats joint destruction commonly found in rheumatoid arthritis.

An implant arthroplasty involves a prosthetic replacement of joints by metallic or silicone-rubber parts, usually for arthritic conditions or traumatic ankylosis. Swanson silicone-rubber arthroplasty is a popular choice. Other prosthetic devices for the hand and wrist are the AMC total wrist (**Volz, Steffe, Swanson**).

anchovy procedure (Carroll): rolled palmaris longus (PL) graft placed into the space that remains after trapezium excision for pantrapezial arthritis.

Blatt capsulodesis: dynamic rotatory subluxation of the scaphoid. A proximally-based flap of dorsal wrist capsule is attached to the distal pole of the scaphoid; this will prevent downward movement of the distal pole during radial deviation of the wrist; **dorsal capsulodesis.**

capsulectomy: proximal interphalangeal (PIP) joint flexion contractures unresponsive to conservative treatment; proximal release of the joint capsule (volar plate) will improve movement.

Carroll (Froimson) a.: an interposition rolled tendon (palmaris longus [PL]) used as a spacer when the trapezium is removed for pantrapezial arthritis.

Darrach resection: resection of the distal 1 to 1.5 cm of distal ulna at the wrist. Once considered as the standard procedure for the treatment of a myriad of distal radioulnar joint problems; now useful primarily in the elderly and for severe rheumatoid arthritis. (**Albright and Chase.**)

dorsal capsulectomy: the removal of the dorsal joint capsule; for example, in the treatment of distal radial ulnar joint fracture.

Eaton volar plate a: a chronic subluxation of the proximal interphalangeal (PIP) joint after a displaced large volar lip fracture of the proximal end of the middle phalanx, greater than 50% of the articular surface. If left untreated, a chronic subluxation results. The volar plate is then advanced into the fracture site and tightened to prevent subluxation.

flexible hinge implant: a design for silastic implant arthroplasty developed by Swanson used in MP and PIP arthroplasties.

Fowler metacarpophalangeal (MCP) a.: for arthritis of the MCP joint. The metacarpal is cut in the form of a chevron at the base of the proximal phalanx and then cut into a V shape, with an interposition of extensor tendon fusion.

hemiresection interposition arthroplasty (Bowers): for distal radioulnar joint arthritis, resection of the articular surface of the distal ulna and interposition of a rolled tendon graft.

matched ulnar resection: popularized by Watson; resection of the articular surface of the distal ulna to match the shape of the radial styloid notch. This is useful for the treatment of distal radioulnar joint instability and arthritis.

Neibauer prosthesis: silicone hinge joints with built-in ties; useful in metacarpophalangeal (MCP) joint arthroplasty.

perichondral autografts: use of osteocartilaginous grafts (from ribs) to resurface the injured articular surface of a small joint in the hand.

proximal row carpectomy: a salvage procedure whereby the scaphoid, lunate, and triquetrum are excised. This is useful in treating advanced arthritis involving the radiocarpal joint if wrist motion is still desired by the patient.

radial styloidectomy: excision of the tip of the radial styloid; useful in isolated radioscaphoid arthritis or as part of the SLAC wrist reconstruction.

Stefee thumb a.: a cemented metal polyethylene prosthesis useful in thumb metacarpophalangeal (MCP) arthroplasty.

Suave Kapanje (Lauenstein procedure): fusion of the articular surface of the distal radioulnar joint with proximal resection of a distal ulnar segment of approximately 1.5 cm to facilitate motion.

suspensionplasty (LRTI-Burton): for advanced trapeziometacarpal arthritis, removal of the trapezium, and placement of half of the flexor carpi radialis (FCR) as an anchor to the metacarpal and as a spacer. An improvement on the classic "anchovy" procedure.

Swanson a.: complete array of silicone implants for all digital articula, joints, carpal bones, total wrist arthroplasty, distal ulna, and proximal radius. This is most useful in rheumatoid arthritis for the reconstruction of metacarpophalangeal (MCP) joints. Its use in the carpus had to be discontinued because of concerns regarding silicone synovitis.

Swanson prosthesis (silicone): most useful for metacarpophalangeal (MCP) and proximal interphalangeal (PIP) arthroplasty in rheumatoid arthritis. In selected situations, a total wrist arthroplasty is useful (i.e., in bilateral involvement). Carpal silicone arthroplasty is now falling out of favor because of silicone synovitis.

trapezial hemiarthroplasty: resection of the distal half of the trapezium, sparing the scaphotrapezial joint; useful for trapeziometacarpal arthritis.

Tupper a.: in metacarpophalangeal (MCP) joint arthritis, the volar plate may be used as an interpositional material after excision arthroplasty.

Vainio metaphalangeal (MP): MCP joint resectional arthroplasty with interposition of the extensor tendon and collateral ligaments.

Voltz a.: a metal-polyethylene cemented total wrist arthroplasty useful in selected cases of end-stage degenerative or rheumatoid arthritis.

Zancholli capsuloplasty: a volar plate advancement of the metacarpophalangeal (MCP) joint of the thumb to treat congenital hyperextension.

Zancholli-Lasso procedure: transfer of the flexor digitorum sublimis tendon (FDS) to the lateral band or the A2 pulley to prevent MP hyperextension and clawing; found in low ulnar nerve palsy.

Zancholli static-lock procedure: a volar plate advancement (plication) for the treatment of MP hyperextension; seen in claw deformities in low ulnar nerve palsy.

Neurologic Procedures

cable nerve grafts: a method of uniting strands of nerve graft and interposing them into a gap to repair a polyfascicular nerve discontinuity (of historic interest).

epineural repair: repair of lacerated nerve segments by repairing the epineurium. This is useful in digital nerves or in oligofascicular proximal nerves.

epineurotomy: the opening of the epineurium during a neurolysis procedure. This can be useful in certain cases of chronic nerve compression.

funiculectomy: for chronic end neuromas; peeling back the epineurium and resecting nerve fascicles, with reclosure and ligation of the epineurium. May aid in the treatment of end neuromas.

group fascicular repair: a perineural repair; useful in treating laceration of mixed motor and sensory nerves. Presumably, exact anatomic reapproximation will facilitate maximal functional return.

hemi-pulp flap: neurosensory free flaps from the great or second toe indicated for large single pulp defect. This is indicated when sensory function is essential for proper hand function and protection. This is best indicated for thumb reconstruction.

hetero-digital flaps: a cross-finger flap of dorsal skin to cover a significant palmar surface defect in an adjacent defect. Digital island transfer of pedicle flaps that are lifted with its neurovascular bundle and transferred to a defect on an adjacent digit.

internal neurolysis: presumably, internal dissection of intraneural scarring will facilitate return of nerve function. Originally thought to be useful in the treatment of carpal tunnel syndrome but now found to be harmful in many cases. This technique, however, is useful in the removal of intraneural neurilemmoma.

medial epicondylectomy: one method to decompress the ulnar nerve in the cubital tunnel by removing its bony floor, the medial epicondyle of the distal humerus.

Moberg procedure (key pinch): for tetraplegia; to restore the ability of key pinch in group II or III level tetraplegia. This includes carpometacarpal (CMC) thumb arthrodesis, extensor pollicis longus (EPL) tenodesis, and flexor pollicis longus (FPL) tenodesis or transfer.

neurectomy: the resection of a portion of nerve of an end neuroma (and presumed buried in bone or muscle).

neurotization: in patients with a profound brachial plexus injury with a flare anesthetic arm, the use of a live intercostal nerve grafted to a distal neural segment of the brachial plexus has restored some upper extremity function in select patients.

Trauma Procedures

Bentzon procedure: attempt to convert a painful scaphoid nonunion to a painless pseudarthrosis by soft tissue (capsular flap) interposition; of historic interest.

Bevin Aurglass technique: a digital web-deepening procedure for the correction of burn syndactyly.

distal finger amputation revision: procedure performed following traumatic amputation involving the distal phalanx (fingertip) by the following techniques:

finger flaps: to preserve sensation.

    Atosoy: volar single V-Y advancement.

    cross-finger flap: a section of skin with its blood supply intact from a neighboring finger used to cover open area.

    Kutler: lateral double V-Y advancement.

    thenar flap: one raised from the thumb side of the base of the palm.

    Wolfe graft: free skin (pinch) graft; a section of full-thickness skin placed on the open area.

Fisk-Fernandez volar wedge: anterior cortical cancellous bone graft for the correction of scaphoid nonunion or malunion.

Gibraiel flap: a form of rotational skin flap using moving skin from the lateral aspect of the digit to the flexor surface with little or no movement of the pivot point.

Herbert screw osteosynthesis: the use of a dumbbell-shaped bone screw with variable pitch to affect rigid compressive internal fixation of a scaphoid fracture or nonunion. This can be used with or without bone graft.

Kapandji fixation: for distal radius fracture; use of two K-wires inserted at 90 degrees at fracture site lateral and posterior and then angled 45 degrees anteriorly.

metacarpal lengthening (Matev): useful for irretrievable thumb amputation at the metacarpophalangeal (MCP) joint level; metacarpal osteotomy, application of a distraction device, slow distraction, and later bone grafting will partially restore length of the thumb ray. Secondary first web deepening may be required.

Russe bone graft: for scaphoid nonunion fracture; cortical cancellous graft placed by a volar approach through a longitudinal trough in the volar surface of the scaphoid that will enhance bony union.

Microvascular Procedures

anastomosis: term used for the direct repair of nerves and blood vessels.

back wall first technique: a microsurgical procedure in which the vessel wall away from the surgeon is sutured first, most useful in vessels approximately equal size when one or both of the presenting ends cannot be rotated within a double clamp.

Chinese flap (radial forearm flap): a radial forearm rotation flap based on the radial artery to repair radial and hand defects.

cross-arm flaps: random flaps using tissue from random pedicle flap using tissue from the patient's upper arm to cover a large defect on the patient's contralateral hand.

denervation: the accidental or intentional removal of sensory or motor nerve input to a distal site in the hand or arm.

dorsalis pedis flap: a microvascular free flap using the dorsalis pedis artery of the foot as the donor artery used to cover small defects in the upper extremity.

fibrin clot glue: a method of augmenting nerve apposition by using fibrin clot glue to "cement" the suture line.

flipping technique: used in microsurgery repairing a small vessel that is freely mobile. One can flip the vessel and over end to repair the back wall. Used in vein grafting and free-tissue transfer technique.

four-flap Z-plasty: a double Z plasty used commonly in the reconstruction of the first webspace.

free flaps: a method of free tissue transfer using skin, muscle, or bone or all of the above. Tissue is transferred using its vascular pedicle and microsurgical anastomotic technique.

interposition graft: generally used for either nerve or vascular (vein) grafts to bridge a gap for direct microanastomosis of nerves and vessels.

laser Doppler fluximetry: this evaluates cutaneous microvascular perfusion. This evaluates the motion of the red blood cells in the area directly beneath the probe.

lateral arm flap: a free flap based on the posterior radial collateral artery; useful for covering large, full-thickness defects in the dorsum of the hand.

no reflow phenomenon: a microvascular anastomosis with arterial anastomosis. Disruption of the neurovascular tree may result in no venous return into the field.

sympathectomy: a method to improve peripheral-blood flow by ablating the central or peripheral sympathetic innervation to arteries in treatment of chronic regional pain syndrome by surgery.

toe-thumb transfer: complete transfer of a toe with its full complement of neurovascular, tendinous, and bone structures to the hand to add to a digit or thumb on a posttraumatic or congenitally deficient hand.

wraparound procedure: the medial aspect of the great toe with its neurovascular bundles is removed from the toe and wrapped around a free bone graft at the tip of an amputation stump. This is then reattached using microvascular techniques. The donor site is secondarily grafted to close its defect.

Congenital Deformity Repairs

Barsky macrodactyly reduction: (1) filleting out of the distal phalanx, then placing all distal structures on to the end of the middle phalanx (this will shorten the macrodactylous digit); (2) hemiresection of the middle phalanx and primary distal interphalangeal (DIP) joint fusion.

Bilhaut-Cloquet procedure: for Wassel II thumb duplication (bifid thumb). The narrow half of each thumb tip is united with the other, discarding the central units and allowing the thumb to become one phalanx.

Bonola technique: a dorsally based closing wedge osteotomy of the distal phalanx to correct a Kirner deformity.

Bracket resection: epiphyseal resection of the apex of a delta phalanx accompanied by fat grafting.

Carstan reverse wedge osteotomy: for the treatment of a delta phalanx; a central wedge is reversed and turned 180 degrees to straighten a digit.

callotasis: technique of one-stage bone lengthening by placement of an external fixator on both sides of osteotomy and stretching the bone out to lengthen short digits.

Cronin's technique: a technique for separating syndactylyzed digit using a combination of palmar and dorsal triangular flaps.

distraction lengthening: see **callotasis.**

Krukenberg procedure: in the congenital absence of a hand, the radius and ulna are surgically separated and covered with soft tissue so that the two bones will act as a claw.

physiolysis: the selective obliteration of the growth plate and area of uneven bone growth such as seen in Madelung's deformity. This is frequently accompanied by fat grafting to inhibit further bone growth.

radialization/centralization: an attempt to rebalance the hand and wrist on to the distal forearm in radial clubbed hand.

Skin, Nails, and Fascia Procedures

advancement flaps (Kleinert-Atosoy): called V-Y flaps; flaps cut either from the volar pad or from the radial and ulnar pad of the distal fingertip for the reconstruction of fingertip injuries with skin and subcutaneous loss.

axial cutaneous flaps (scapular flap): free or island flap on a subscapular artery pedicle for medium-sized defect coverage in the hand.

axial flag flaps: a rotational skin flap based on a dorsal digital artery used for digital skin and subcutaneous defects.

axial pattern skin flap: a long skin flap possible because of an underlying vascular supply running along its long axis underneath.

cocked-half flap (Gillies): reconstruction of a thumb amputation at the metacarpophalangeal (MCP) joint level with a local skin graft, iliac crest graft, and skin graft.

composite nail bed flap: a full-thickness nail bed graft from a toe to cover a defect in a finger nail bed.

cross-finger flap: the dorsal skin of one digit is flapped over itself to create coverage for a volar skin defect of an adjacent digit.

cryotherapy: a method of using extreme cold to freeze skin lesions such as actinic keratosis.

escharotomy: in the management of deep thermal burns, burned and contracted skin is incised to decompress deeper tissues and prevent further necrosis.

fasciectomy: generic term used to describe excision of the palmar fascia, usually when involved in Dupuytren's disease.

fasciotomy: (1) opening of muscle compartments and decompressing intrinsic muscle spaces in compartment syndrome; spaces to be decompressed are interosseus muscles (through dorsal incisions or volar thenar and hypothenar compartments); (2) incision into a Dupuytren's central cord to release contracture; this is useful in elderly and debilitated patients, but contracture recurrence is common.

flag flap: a rotational pedicle flap harvested on the dorsum of the finger and used to cover defects on adjacent fingers or over the metacarpophalangeal joint. The same can be performed as a volar flap as well.

Macindo procedure: a form of palmar fasciectomy for Dupuytren's contracture when the palmar skin is left open to granulate.

marsupialization: a technique used to expose the germinal matrix of a nail in patients with chronic paronychia in which a crescent of the eponychial fold is removed to uncover chronic fungal infection.

Moberg flap: useful in thumb tip reconstruction; the volar half of the thumb soft tissue is elevated with its neurovascular structures, and by flexing the interphalangeal (IP) joint of the thumb, the flap is then stretched over the thumb tip.

neurovascular island transfer: a method of transferring sensibility to an important part of the hand such as the thumb tip from a less important part of the hand, whereby a portion of skin is left connected to its neurovascular structures and passed subcutaneously to a different part of the hand.

onychectomy: removal of a fingernail.

onychotomy: the method of cutting into a nail, usually to remove a mass under the nail.

pedicle flap: a procedure that permits an island of skin and subcutaneous tissue to be transferred from one place to another on its own vascular supply, using multiple operative stages.

pedicle grafts: a term used for pedicle flaps but also includes *pedicle bone grafts*. *Island pedicle grafts* and *neurovascular pedicle grafts* are pedicle, skin, or subcutaneous tissue containing blood and nerve supply, thus providing sensation for the skin graft.

thenar flap (Smith-Albin): for fingertip coverage, an H flap is raised on the thenar eminence and the digit tip is flexed down to it. By 10 to 14 days, the flap provides a good skin and soft tissue coverage to the distal digit tip. However, digital stiffness is common.

Muscle and Tendon Surgery of the Hand

There are two types of tendon procedures: (1) restoration of tendon function by direct repair of a tendon, its advancement, or its transfer and (2) freeing of tendon from scar tissue, restrictive bands, or abnormal lining tissues. Because of these basic categories, tendon grafts and advancement procedures are listed here contextually and not in alphabetic order.

Aichef technique: a method of central SLIP reconstruction in Boutonnière deformity by designing a tendon flap using the central half of the lateral bands and bringing them toward the midline to recreate a central SLIP in which the central SLIP has been irreparably damaged due to trauma.

Bateman's procedure: indicated in axillary and suprascapular nerve palsy, which involves an acromial fragment to the humerus to facilitate shoulder abduction.

Brent-Moberg tenodesis: thumb flexor tenodesis to restore key pinch in quadriplegics. A technique using flexor or extensor tendon graft to restore and treat functions in ulnar nerve palsy.

Burkhalter transfer: threading digital flexors through the proximal phalanx to facilitate metacarpophalangeal flexion in low ulnar nerve palsy with claw deformities.

deltoid flap: a muscular-free flap using the deltoid to cover small to moderate deficits in the upper extremity.

Hammond's procedure: multiple muscle transfers for reconstruction of the paralyzed shoulder in brachial plexus injuries. Transfer of the posterior third of the deltoid to the lateral aspect of the clavicle and from the tendinous origins of the long head of the triceps and the short head of the biceps to the lateral aspect of the acromion to aid in shoulder abduction. Transfer of the latissimus dorsi to teres major tendons.

House reconstruction: complete array of reconstructions to facilitate hand function in patients with varying degrees of quadriplegia (tetraplegia) depending on the level of the lesion in the cervical spine.

Hui-Linscheid procedure: a tenodesis procedure designed to reconstruct the volar ulnar carpal ligament using a strip of flexor carpi ulnaris tendon particularly useful in primary ulnar-carpal instability or secondary distal radial ulnar joint instability.

Lasso procedure: flexor digitorum superficialis in a tenodesis mode to flex the metacarpophalangeal joint used commonly in tetraplegia and patients with hyperextension deformities of the metacarpophalangeal joint and with hyperextension of the proximal interphalangeal joint.

Lennox Fritschi technique: a palmaris longus motored four-tail transfer used in ulnar palsy to correct claw deformities to promote metacarpophalangeal flexion and proximal interphalangeal extension.

Littler-Eaton ligament reconstruction: method of stabilizing the base of the thumb metacarpal in stage I basal joint arthritis.

Littler's boutonnière reconstruction: includes dorsal transposition of the lateral bands and repair of the central SLIP to the base of the middle phalanx.

Mennen's opponensplasty: the extensor pollicis longus is passed through the interosseous membrane to the volar aspect of the forearm and backed out along the thenar eminence to the dorsal surface of the metacarpophalangeal joint, thus creating opponens function.

Parke's tenodesis: static tenodesis using wrist extensors as "grafts" to treat claw deformities to promote MP flexion.

Ranney's technique: an extensor digiti minimi transfer to the neck of the fifth metacarpal to restore the transverse metacarpal arch in ulnar nerve palsy.

Riordan's technique: a flexor carpi radialis transfer using a free graft passing from the flexor to the extensor side of the forearm, radial lateral bands of the fingers involved in claw deformity in low ulnar nerve palsy.

tendolysis: often called tenolysis; a tendon release. It describes two different types of procedures: (1) one in which the tendon is freed from scar tissue or entrapment so that it may move properly and (2) tenosynovectomy, whereby all or part of the sheath of a functioning tendon is excised.

tendon advancement: done when the damage segment of a tendon is so near its insertion that a direct tendon-to-bone rather than tendon-to-tendon repair is necessary. One such technique is the **Wagner** advancement of the profundus tendon.

tenosynovectomy: a procedure whereby the tenosynovium surrounding the tendon sheaths are removed such as in rheumatoid arthritis to prevent tendon rupture or to treat tendon entrapment.

tenodesis: the fixation of a tendon onto two bony locations to keep a joint from flexing or extending beyond a selected range. This procedure lends itself to prevention of hyperextension of the metacarpophalangeal joints in ulnar claw deformity. Two commonly done are the Fowler and Riordan procedures.

tenorrhaphy: the repair of a lacerated tendon, either immediate or delayed.

tenotomy: a procedure in which a tendon, either flexor or extensor, is sectioned purposely to correct a deformity to bring back the position or function of the hand or wrist.

Tendon Repair Techniques

Numerous techniques and types of sutures are used in repairing tendons. A tendon repair is any reapproximation of a partially or completely severed tendon. The specific technique is directed at gaining maximal strength with minimal scarring.

Becker: multiple cross-stitching technique for approximation of fresh tendon edges.

Bunnell opponensplasty: the use of the flexor digitorum sublimis IV as a donor motor for thumb opposition using the pulley in the region of the flexor carpi ulnaris and the pisiform.

Kleinert: modification of Bunnell technique, burying suture knot at tendon edge.

modified Kessler suture: a direct end-to-end grafting suture for flexor tendon lacerations, especially in zone II. These are usually augmented with epitendinous sutures.

Pulver-Taft weave: the strongest method of reattaching two tendons where space is not at a premium. It involves weaving tendon ends in and out of each other.

Tsuge: multiple cross-stitching technique for tendon reapproximation.

Verdan: multiple cross-stitching technique for tendon reapproximation.

Other specific techniques include **Tajima, Halsted, Salvage,** and **Silfverskiöld procedures.**

Tendon Grafts and Transfers

A tendon transfer is the relocation of a tendon from one place to another. The tendon retains attachment to its muscle. By contrast, free tendon graft requires complete excision of a tendon and its repositioning in a new location. Tendon transfers may be static or dynamic.

central slip repair/reconstruction: procedure designed to repair the common extensor insertion into the proximal dorsal end of the middle phalanx, thus restoring active proximal interphalangeal (PIP) extension.

Clark pectoralis major transfer: transfer of the sternocostal portion of the pectoralis major muscle for the restoration of elbow flexion in brachial plexus injury.

crossed intrinsic transfer: in rheumatoid arthritis, with ulnar deviation of the digits at the metaphalangeal joint, a conjoined ulnar intrinsic tendon is released from one digit and placed into the radial conjoined intrinsic tendon of the adjacent digit on its ulnar side.

Green transfer: flexor carpi ulnaris (FCU) to extensor carpi radialis brevis (ECRB) transfer to correct a wrist flexion deformity in cerebral palsy. Overcorrection is common.

Jones transfer: in radial nerve palsy, tendon transfer designed to restore thumb, digital, and wrist extension.

flexor pronator slide: release of the flexor pronator muscle group origin allowing the muscle to slide distally. This helps correct wrist and digital flexion deformity and forearm pronation deformity in cerebral palsy.

flexor tenolysis: method used to free flexor tendon from its surrounding scars approximately 4 months after flexor tendon repair with secondary tendon adherence.

Fowler tenodesis: static tendon grafts originating in the extensor retinaculum, passing volarly to the deep transverse metacarpal ligament, and inserting it into the radial lateral bands. A procedure to prevent hyperextension of the metacarpophalangeal (MCP) joint as seen in the claw deformity of low ulnar nerve palsy.

tenovaginotomy: procedure designed to release stenosing tenosynovitis by incising a retinaculum or flexor pulley.

static tendon transfer: transfer of a free tendon graft that is attached to two or more bony locations such that the active movement of one joint will cause the passive movement of some other joint. For example, a tendon appropriately inserted proximal to the wrist and in the fingers will cause flexion of the fingers if the wrist is extended.

dynamic tendon transfer: one that brings about motion by direct action of muscle contraction.

Tendon transfers are commonly required to replace or assist voluntary muscle function that is lost because of nerve injury, nerve disease, or direct and indirect sequelae of trauma to the muscle. Substantial numbers of transfers are used in central nervous system paralyses such as those caused by strokes and polio. Transfers are listed by categories that define function.

Camitz procedure: the palmaris longus, with its distal attachment tubularized, is passed under the thenar eminence and attached to the radial aspect of the base of the proximal phalanx of the thumb to act as an opponensplasty. This is useful in chronic carpal tunnel syndrome.

finger extension: Boyes procedure.

finger flexion: for flexion of the metacarpophalangeal joint (intrinsic transfer); Boyes, Fowler, Bunnell, Stiles-Bunnell, Riordan, and Pulver-Taft procedures, and Brand I and Brand II procedures.

Huber transfer: a procedure designed to restore thumb opposition based on a transfer into the thenar eminence of the abductor digiti minimi, that is, a neurovascular pedicle.

opponensplasty: the use of any of the intrinsic or extrinsic muscle tendon units to restore thumb opposition (i.e., in median nerve palsy); Brand, Burkhalter, Groves, Goldner, Riordan, Phalen-Miller, Littler, Huber, and Fowler procedures.

Steindler flexorplasty: in brachial plexus injury causing paralysis of elbow flexion (biceps and brachialis) with sparing of distal forearm musculature, the flexor pronator mass with the medial epicondyle of the distal humerus is transferred anteriorly and proximally on the humerus to effect elbow flexion.

thumb abduction: pulling thumb away from the side of the hand; Boyes procedure.

thumb adduction: pulling the thumb to side of index finger; Boyes, Bunnell, Edgarton-Grand, and Royle-Thompson procedures.

wrist extension: Boyes procedure, using pronator teres to the extensor carpi radialis brevis muscle.

Tenosynovectomy

Tenosynovectomy refers to the excision of thickened tendon sheath and other tissue surrounding a tendon, commonly seen in infection, chemical irritation, and rheumatoid arthritis (synovectomy). It also refers to the following two procedures in hand surgery.

abductor pollicis longus release: a release of the fibrous canal surrounding the abductor pollicis longus at the wrist for symptoms of de Quervain's syndrome (pain on abduction of the thumb). Also called **de Quervain's release.**

trigger finger release: a release of fibrous covering of tendon (pulley) at the base of the finger to prevent a tendon with nodular changes from snapping with motion of the finger. Also called **snapping tendon release.**

Other Tendon Procedures

boutonnière reconstruction: a classic extensor tendon reconstruction for boutonnière deformity, designed to restore active extension of the proximal interphalangeal (PIP) joint and to prevent its flexion posturing. This procedure is fraught with difficulty, and prognosis is guarded; Littler, Matev, Fowler procedures.

Hunter rod (active tendon implant): a silicone rubber tendon replacement that can function as a permanent tendon. This implant has a proximal loop that can be sewn into forearm motor muscles.

Kortzeborn procedure: a lengthening of the extensor tendons of the thumb and formation of a fascial attachment of the thumb to the ulnar side of the hand to relieve "ape hand" deformity.

passive tendon implant: a silicone-rubber tendon spacer or rod that is used to form a new synovium-filled channel. It is removed during a second-stage procedure, and a tendon graft that is threaded through. Useful as a two-stage procedure when the tendon bed is extremely scarred and a direct tendon graft is impossible.

swan-neck revision: surgery designed to eliminate a swan-neck deformity in the fingers by revision of tendons; Swanson revision, Littler modified tendon revision.

Other Hand and Wrist Procedures

capsular release (capsulectomy): an incision of a joint capsule done to regain lost motion caused by contractures.

capsulodesis: in hand surgery, the capsule, which may include the dorsal or volar plate, may be tightened to help hold an affected joint in a position that can no longer be held voluntarily. This is done often for nerve injuries and is commonly called the **Zancolli** procedure (for clawhand deformity); **volar capsular reefing, Blatt dorsal capsulodesis.**

carbon (pyrocarbon) implant: a new form of resurfacing arthroplasty for the metacarpophalangeal and proximal interphalangeal joints used commonly in osteoarthritis.

carpal tunnel release: a division of the strong ligamentous band (transverse carpal ligament) that covers the median nerve and flexor tendons of the finger and thumb. This is usually done to relieve pressure on the median nerve that may result from arthritis, trauma, or unknown causes. A *tenosynovectomy,* if necessary, may be done through the same incision.

carpectomy: the removal of the proximal row of carpal bones, usually indicated in some forms of arthritis or severe spastic contractures.

dermodesis: the removal of a segment of skin and then closure of the skin margins to shorten skin and restrict motion of a joint. It is frequently done in conjunction with a *Zancolli* capsulodesis for ulnar clawhand.

Dupuytren's contracture release: named after a French surgeon, this surgical procedure is the excision of the contracted fibrotic bands of the palmar fascia. However, the skin is often adherent and recurrent deformity is a problem. Specific techniques for resection of these bands are:

    Luck procedure: percutaneous transection of fibrotic bands without removal of tissue.

    McCash procedure: transverse skin incision with transection of bands and then passive stretch dressing applied, leaving the wounds open.

fishmouth incision: a wraparound incision over the distal end of the finger to facilitate drainage.

Foucher technique: a procedure for internal fixation of metacarpal neck fractures using multiple prebent Kirschner wires in a "wire-stacking technique."

ganglionectomy: the excision of a ganglion, which usually occurs on the dorsum of the wrist or the base of the fingers.

Hammond's procedure: multiple muscle transfers for reconstruction of the paralyzed shoulder in brachial plexus injuries. Transfer of the posterior third of the deltoid to the lateral aspect of the clavicle and from the tendinous origins of the long head of the triceps and the short head of the biceps to the lateral aspect of the acromion to aid in shoulder abduction. Transfer of the latissimus dorsi to teres major tendons.

infiltration technique: a method of axillary block for regional anesthesia in upper extremity surgery. The anesthetic is injected around the axillary artery inside the sheath of the neurovascular bundle spreading local anesthetic around the brachial plexus.

interscalene block: a brachial plexus block using a needle in the interscalene space to numb the brachial plexus to effect regional anesthetic commonly used in shoulder surgery.

island flaps: either pedicle or free flaps of small amounts of tissue either skin, bone, muscle, or a combination of both for the reconstruction of small area defects.

joint leveling procedures with ulnar lengthening and radial shortening: used to restore the anatomic relationship between the distal radius and distal ulna (generally, the ulnar variance seen on the contralateral "normal side").

kite flap: an island pedicle of flap proximally based on the first dorsal metacarpal artery designed on the radial side of the distal portion of the second metacarpal and metacarpophalangeal joint used to reconstruct defects on the dorsum of the hand usually on the radial side.

K-wire fixation: in a Kirschner wire (K-wire) fixation, small threaded or nonthreaded wires are used to transfix fractures or to produce traction with the use of an external appliance.

latissimus dorsi flap: a form of myocutaneous pedicle or free flap in which blood supply derives from the thoracodorsal artery and is used to cover large soft tissue defects.

mallet finger revision: designed to regain active extension of the distal interphalangeal joints of the finger.

    Fowler release: technique used at the proximal interphalangeal joint for a mallet finger.

palmar advancement flaps: known as *the Moberg's flap.* A proximally based flap used to cover distal soft tissue defects; most commonly used in the thumbs.

palmar fasciectomy, fasciotomy: the release, with or without resection of tissues, of shortened, thickened, and contracted fasciae in the palm or finger in flexion deformities resulting from Dupuytren's contracture.

phalangectomy: the excision of a part or all of a phalanx because of trauma or arthritis. Rarely performed in the hand, more commonly done in the foot.

pollicization: any operation replacing a congenitally or traumatically missing thumb by reconstruction of the index, long, ring, or little finger such that it acts or functions as a thumb; **Buck-Gramko, Riordan, Littler, Gillies,** and **Verdan procedures.**

random pattern flaps: skin flaps that are generally quadrilateral in shape and are raised by incising three of the four sides and it depends on the minute vessels of the subdermal and subcutaneous plexus.

RASL procedure: the reduction association of the scapholunate joint. This consists of an open reduction of the scapholunate articulation, repair of the ligamentous remnants, and protection of the repair by internally blocking the scapholunate joint with a transverse Herbert's screw for a year to provide intercarpal fibrosis.

ray amputation: a procedure to remove a metacarpal and all phalangeal segments of a finger distal to that metacarpal.

regional flaps: those derived from tissues not immediately adjacent to the primary defect but in its vicinity. They can be random or axial pattern flaps depending on their blood supply.

replantation: a microsurgical procedure that requires the reattachment of nerves, veins, and arteries to attempt restoration of function to a freshly severed part such as a finger.

revision polydactyly: polydactyly usually affects the thumb and little finger. Revision requires reattachment of specific tendons or ligaments; **Marks and Bayne.**

saphenous flap: a myocutaneous flap based on the saphenous artery and nerve. This is used to cover small- to medium-sized defects.

synovectomy: removal of synovium in joints. The procedure is done frequently for rheumatoid arthritis.

tendino-cutaneous flaps: vascularized tendon graft that can be transferred with a dorsalis pedis or radial forearm flap. This is indicated for one-stage reconstruction of degloving injury to the dorsum of the hand with loss of skin and extensor tendons for example.

Tikhor-Linberg procedure: an alternative to the arm amputation of well-localized tumors around the shoulder, which represents a resection of the shoulder girdle with preservation of the arm.

transposition flaps: skin flaps used to cover small deficits. These may be axial pattern or random pattern.

trapeziectomy: removal of the trapezium bone in the treatment of basal joint arthritis, which may be done alone or in concert with an interposition arthroplasty.

ulnar forearm flap: a fascial cutaneous flap that is based on the ulnar artery and is harvested from the ulnar aspect of the forearm used to cover deficits of the ulnar side of the hand or used as a free flap for distal defect.

wafer procedure: for ulnar plus wrist; resection of the distal 2 to 3 mm of the ulnar head, leaving the styloid intact.

Approaches
Wrist

dorsal a.: on the back side of the wrist, this approach is used for tendon transfers, fusions, and ganglionectomies.

Henry approach: for volar forearm.

volar a.: approach from the palmar aspect of the wrist, used for carpal tunnel releases, tendon explorations, and some bony procedures.

medial a.: an approach to the ulnar side of the wrist used for some tendon transfers and for the Darrach procedure; **Smith-Petersen.**

lateral a.: used on the radial side of the wrist for tendon transfers, radial styloidectomy, and visualization of the navicular bone.

Hand

Surgical approaches are too numerous and complicated to describe here. Refer to Edmonson AS, Crenshaw AH, editors: *Campbell's Operative Orthopedics,* ed 9, vol 10, St Louis, 1996, Mosby.

The Foot and Ankle

The human foot is a marvelous anatomic structure that provides a stable base to support large amounts of weight and shift in any direction while structural support is still maintained. The bones of the foot are so arranged as to allow balance of full body weight and the ability to walk on varying types of terrain. The average person will walk an estimated 20,000 to 46,000 miles in a lifetime and, for that reason, will seek at some time the expertise of a foot and ankle specialist in orthopaedic surgery or a podiatrist for foot-related problems.

The **orthopaedic surgeon** treats many major problems related to the feet—repair of congenital deformities (clubfeet), tendon lengthenings, fusions, and other complicated surgical procedures necessary for foot and ankle correction. Problems of the feet are so numerous that treatment and care has become a subspecialty of orthopaedics. The American Orthopaedic Foot and Ankle Society (AOFAS) and the American Academy of Orthopaedic Surgeons (AAOS) have been directly responsible for establishing a subspecialty devoted to injuries, diseases, and surgery of the foot and ankle. This subspecialization is now a part of many residency training programs.

The **podiatrist,** a doctor of podiatric medicine, is a specialist who may be board certified in foot and ankle surgery or primary care podiatric medicine. His or her practice is devoted to the diagnosis and treatment of diseases and disorders in the human foot, offering instructions to patients in proper shoe fit and foot care. This may involve conservative management, surgery,

biomechanics (prosthetic/orthotic corrections), or treatment of patients with systemic diseases (diabetes) that affect the foot.

The **pedorthist,** a board-certified specialist in special footwear modifications and orthoses, provides services such as footwear modifications and filling prescriptions for special lines of shoes, customized inserts, and numerous foot support orthotics in the treatment of a variety of conditions.

In larger institutions, the orthopaedist may work in association with a *podiatrist* and *pedorthist* in the care of patients with ankle- and foot-related problems. The current trend is toward a team approach with advantages being that all aspects of patient care can be addressed in one setting. This team includes the orthopaedist, podiatrist, pedorthist, orthotist, and physical therapist. These specialists work independently but may also make up the orthopaedic foot and ankle service team. For that reason, we have included many terms specific to podiatry along with the generally interchangeable terms of anatomy, diseases, and surgery of the foot and ankle.

Anatomy

The human foot is composed of 26 bones plus a varying number of ossicles or sesamoid bones and is divided into three functional units: the hindfoot (talus and calcaneus), midfoot (cuneiforms, cuboid, and navicular), and forefoot (metatarsals and phalanges).

The joints between the calcaneus, talus, navicular, and cuboid bones permit most of the motion in turning the foot inward (inversion) or outward (eversion).

The bones of the midfoot and hindfoot are part of the longitudinal arch that allows for smooth distribution of weight and compensates for uneven terrain throughout the supporting structure. As weight is systematically shifted from the heel to the ball of the foot, forces increase to as much as two to four times the body weight. The tarsals, metatarsals, and ligaments form an arch that is flexible when the heel strikes the ground and is rigid as body weight is shifted forward for push-off aided by the dynamic balance of coordinated muscular counter forces.

With weight-bearing on a normal foot, force is transmitted across the heel, the lateral border of the foot, and the ball of the foot. The great toe joint supports most of the body's weight in the thrust of push-off, and the heel absorbs the impact of heel strike. They all work together in supporting various gait patterns and weights and adjusting to different terrain, making the foot fascinating to study. Figures 11-1 to 11-4 will assist in understanding these structures. Injuries around the ankle joint receive the most attention and are discussed in Chapter 1.

Bones of the Ankle and Foot

accessory navicular (os tibiale externum): an "extra" bone or ossicle on the medial side of the navicula, present in up to 14% of the population, actually a tertiary center of ossification. It can be a source of pain between the small ossicle and main navicular bone.

calcaneus: the heel bone; largest of the bones of the foot, articulates with the talus and cuboid. The combining form is *calcaneo,* for example, calcaneotalar ligament, calcaneofibular, or fibulocalcaneal ligament.

cuboid: cube-shaped bone on the lateral side of the foot, just anterior to the calcaneus and articulating with the base of the fourth and fifth metatarsals.

cuneiforms: three wedge-shaped bones lying just proximal to the first three metatarsals and distal to the navicular bone. They form the transverse arch. These are called the first, second, and third cuneiforms or the medial, middle, and lateral cuneiforms.

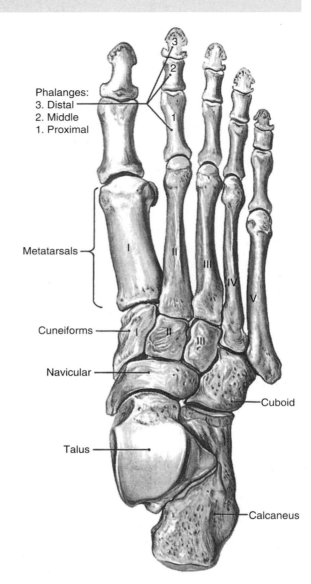

FIG 11-1 Bones of right foot viewed from above. Tarsal bones consist of cuneiforms, navicular, talus, cuboid, and calcaneus. (From Anthony C, Kolthoff N: *Textbook of Anatomy and Physiology,* ed 9, St Louis, 1975, Mosby.)

distal interphalangeal joint: the joint between the middle phalanx and distal phalanx of one of the lesser toes; **distal interphalangeal (DIP) joint.**

forefoot: portion of foot containing metatarsals, phalanges, and sesamoids.

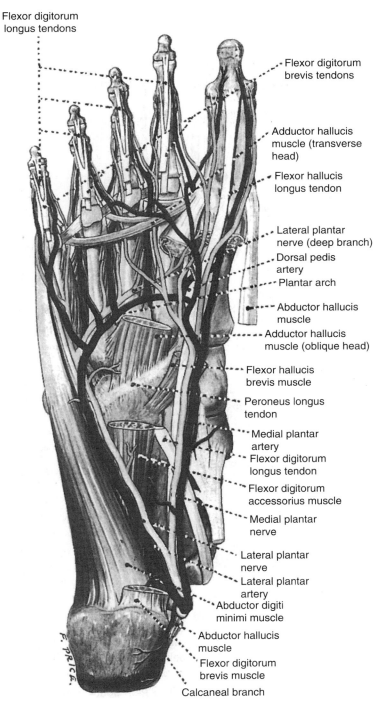

Flexor digitorum
longus tendons

Flexor digitorum
brevis tendons

Adductor hallucis
muscle (transverse
head)

Flexor hallucis
longus tendon

Lateral plantar
nerve (deep branch)

Dorsal pedis
artery

Plantar arch

Abductor hallucis
muscle

Adductor hallucis
muscle (oblique head)

Flexor hallucis
brevis muscle

Peroneus longus
tendon

Medial plantar
artery

Flexor digitorum
longus tendon

Flexor digitorum
accessorius muscle

Medial plantar
nerve

Lateral plantar
nerve

Lateral plantar
artery

Abductor digiti
minimi muscle

Abductor hallucis
muscle

Flexor digitorum
brevis muscle

Calcaneal branch

F. PRICE.

FIG 11-2 The arteries and nerves of the plantar surface of the foot. (Figure taken from *Textbook of Human Anatomy* copyright United Kingdom, 1976, W.J. Hamilton. Reproduced by permission of Macmillan Publishers, Ltd.)

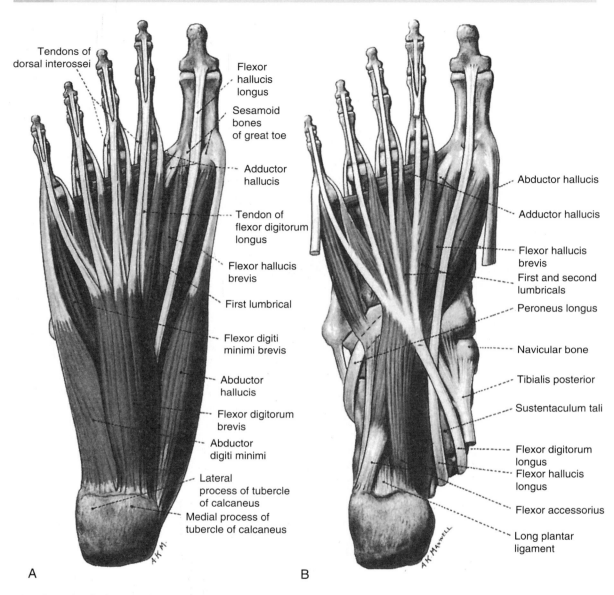

FIG 11-3 Muscles of sole. **A,** First layer. **B,** Second layer.

hallux (pl. halluces): the great toe.

hindfoot: calcaneal (heel bone) and talar (ankle bone) portion of the foot; **rear foot.**

interphalangeal joint: the joint between the proximal phalanx and distal phalanx of the great toe; **IP joint.**

malleolus: the prominence of bone on either side of the ankle. The medial and lateral malleoli come from the tibia and fibula, respectively. The posterior malleolus is deep to the Achilles tendon and is a part of the tibia.

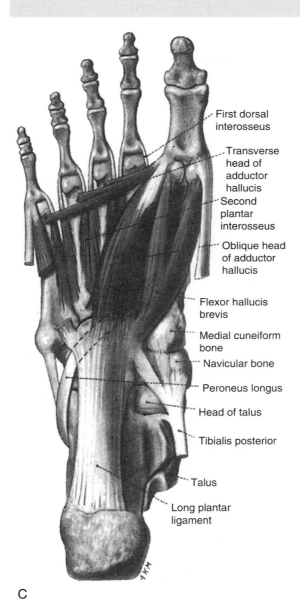

First dorsal interosseus

Transverse head of adductor hallucis

Second plantar interosseus

Oblique head of adductor hallucis

Flexor hallucis brevis

Medial cuneiform bone

Navicular bone

Peroneus longus

Head of talus

Tibialis posterior

Talus

Long plantar ligament

C

FIG 11-3 C, Third and fourth layers. (Figure taken from *Textbook of Human Anatomy* copyright United Kingdom, 1976, W.J. Hamilton. Reproduced by permission of Macmillan Publishers, Ltd.)

metatarsals: the five long bones of the foot between the tarsals and the phalanges.

midfoot: portion of foot containing the navicula, three cuneiforms, and cuboid.

midtarsal joint: comprises the talonavicular and calcaneocuboid articulations and permits adduction-abduction and inversion-eversion motions of the forefoot; **transverse tarsal joint, Chopart's joint.**

navicular: tarsal bone on medial side of foot that articulates proximally with head of talus and distally with three cuneiforms. Formerly called the **scaphoid.**

os: bone; also used in conjunction with a whole bone such as the calcis (calcaneus). However, os usually refers to small ossicles (small bones) or anatomic variants:

> **os intercuneiforme:** between the medial and intermediate cuneiform.

> **os intermetatarseum:** between the proximal fourth and fifth metatarsal.

> **os peroneum:** in the peroneal tendon at the proximal cuboid.

> **os sustentaculum:** the medial junction between the talus and calcaneus.

> **os talocalcaneus:** the large accessory bone bridging the lateral talus and calcaneus.

> **ossa tarsi:** the seven proximal bones of the foot connecting the tibia and fibula to the five metatarsals. The combining form *tarso* is used often, for example, tarsometatarsal joints and ligaments; **tarsus, bony tarsus, tarsus osseous.**

> **os tibiale externum:** medial navicular of foot; **accessory navicular.**

> **os trigonum:** posterior to talus; can be easily confused with a fracture of the posterior lateral tubercle of the talus; **Bardeleben bone.**

> **os vesalianum:** directly proximal to the fifth metatarsal.

phalanx: the toe; more specifically, the two distal bones of the great toe and three distal bones of the four small toes. It is not uncommon for the fourth or fifth toe to have the middle and distal phalanges fused and to have two phalanges only.

proximal interphalangeal joint: the joint between the proximal and middle phalanx of one of the lesser toes; **proximal interphalangeal (PIP) joint.**

sesamoid: two seed-shaped bones in the flexor hallucis brevis tendon located beneath the first metatarsal head, helping to plantar flex the great toe and protect the flexor hallucis tendon, which is situated between them.

subtalar joint: the main shock absorber for the foot; this joint comprises the talocalcaneal articulation and permits triplane movement of the hindfoot.

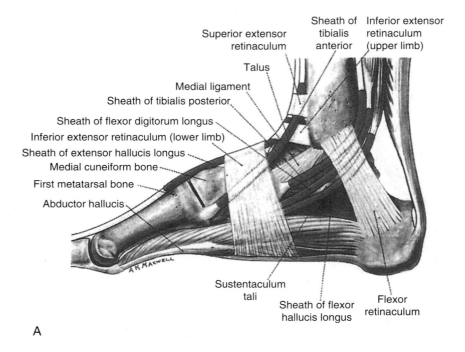

A

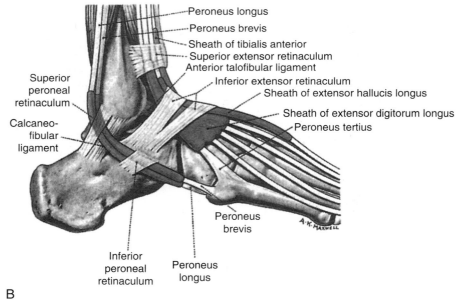

B

FIG 11-4 A, Retinacular and synovial sheaths of ankle region, medial view. **B,** Retinacular and synovial sheaths of ankle region, lateral view. (Figure taken from *Textbook of Human Anatomy* copyright United Kingdom, 1976, W.J. Hamilton. Reproduced by permission of Macmillan Publishers, Ltd.)

sustentaculum tali: a bony projection off the medial calcaneus that supports the talus.

talocalcaneal bar: a tarsal coalition that denotes a bony or fibrocartilaginous bridge between the talus and the calcaneus.

talus: large bone beneath tibia that helps make up one third of the ankle joint, permitting the foot to go up or down. The talocalcaneal (subtalar joint) below the ankle joint allows the heel to turn in and out. The talonavicular ligaments originate from the talus; **astragalus.** The spring ligament (the inferior calcaneonavicular ligament) extends from the sustentaculum of the calcaneus to the navicular and supports the head of the talus.

tarsal coalition: an abnormal bony, fibrocartilaginous, or fibrous bridge between the tarsal bones. It is present at birth, but does not manifest itself until after bony maturity.

tarsometatarsal joint: this joint comprises the tarsal and metatarsal articulations and is often referred to as **Lisfranc's joint.**

Muscles and Tendons

abductor hallucis: short muscle on medial side that pulls the great toe away from other toes and supports medial longitudinal arch.

Achilles tendon (heel cord): the long tendon of the calf composed of the gastrocnemius, soleus, and plantaris muscles and inserting into the calcaneus; **tendocalcaneus.**

adductor hallucis: short muscle that attaches to base of great toe, pulls it toward the second toe, and prevents splaying of metatarsal bones.

anterior tibial tendon (tibialis anterior): long tendon of anterior leg inserting into the medial cuneiform and first metatarsal; helps to dorsiflex the foot.

extensor digitorum longus and brevis: long tendon from limb and short tendon from foot that pull the lesser toes up in dorsiflexion (extension) and stabilize the lesser metatarsophalangeal joints. There is no brevis tendon to the fifth toe.

extensor hallucis longus and brevis: long tendon from limb and short tendon from foot that pull the great toe up in dorsiflexion (extension) and stabilize the first metatarsophalangeal joint.

flexor digitorum longus and brevis: long tendinous insertion from the tibia and short muscle from the foot that insert into the distal and middle phalanges and plantar flex the toes and metatarsal phalangeal (MTP) joints.

flexor hallucis longus and brevis: long tendons from fibula and short muscle (flexor digitorum longus) from foot to great toe that act as flexor of great toe in walking; support medial longitudinal arch of foot and are important in equilibrium.

interosseous muscles: the group of small muscles between the metatarsals that attach into the extensor hoods of the toes and extend the interphalangeal joints and flex the MTP joints.

intrinsic and extrinsic muscles: similar to the hand, the intrinsic muscles arise from the bones of the foot and the extrinsic muscles from the bones of the leg. The intrinsic muscles are:
- abductor hallucis
- abductor digiti minimi
- adductor hallucis
- dorsal and plantar interosseous
- extensor digitorum brevis
- extensor hallucis brevis
- flexor digitorum brevis
- flexor digiti minimi
- flexor hallucis brevis
- lumbricals
- quadratus plantae

peroneal muscles (peroneus longus and brevis): the tendons arising from these lateral compartment muscles travel posterior to the lateral malleolus and insert into the dorsolateral and plantar aspects of the foot. After crossing the plantar aspect of the foot, the longus inserts into the base of the first metatarsal, and the brevis inserts into the base of the fifth metatarsal. They plantar flex and evert the foot. The **peroneus tertius** is an anterior compartment muscle, which travels anterior to the lateral malleolus and inserts into the fifth metatarsal shaft. It dorsiflexes and everts the foot.

posterior tibial tendon (tibialis posterior): long tendon from posterior leg passing along medial side of the ankle, inserting diffusely into the navicular, medial cuneiform, and plantar aspect of the midfoot.

quadratus plantae: muscle of the plantar arch associated with the flexor digitorum longus.

Ligaments

Ligaments are named for specific bony attachments including the following:

collateral l.: of the phalangeal and metatarsophalangeal joints.
deep transverse metatarsal l.
dorsal and plantar cuneocuboid l.
dorsal and plantar cuneonavicular l.
dorsal and plantar intercuneiform l.
dorsal and plantar metatarsal l.
dorsal and plantar tarsometatarsal l.
talocalcaneal l.
talonavicular l.

bifurcated ligament: in the foot, this ligament arises from the upper anterior calcaneus and attaches to both the cuboid and navicula.
deltoid ligament: triangular ligament on the medial side of the ankle, running from the tibia to talus and calcaneus.
lateral collateral ligaments: three ligaments that give stability to the lateral aspect of the ankle joint; **anterior talofibular ligament, calcaneofibular ligament,** and the **posterior talofibular ligament.**
Lisfranc l.: a ligament passing between the medial cuneiform bone and second metatarsal bone.
long plantar l.: bridges the more proximal plantar aspect of the calcaneus to the cuboid, covering peroneal tendons.
short plantar l.: shorter of two plantar ligaments bridging the calcaneus and cuboid.
spring l.: very strong and key ligament of the arch; **plantar calcaneonavicular ligament.**

The Nail

eponychium (cuticle): the epidermal layer covering the nail root.
hyponychium: the thickened epidermis underneath the free distal edge of the nail plate.
lunula: half-moon-shaped (lighter) area at the proximal base of the nail next to the root.

nail matrix: the proximal portion of nail bed from which growth chiefly proceeds; also, the tissue on which the deep aspect of the nail rests; **matrix unguis, nail bed.**
nail plate (*unguis*): hard portion of epidermis on dorsal side of hallux and phalanges from which the nails grow.

Miscellaneous Foot Terms

ankle mortise: a rectangular cavity formed by the tibia and fibula; a joint space to receive the talus.
fat pad: thick fibrous collection of fat on the plantar surface of the foot.
Feiss line: the line that travels from the medial malleolus to plantar aspect of the first metatarsophalangeal joint.
Haglund's process: enlargement of the posterosuperior tuberosity of the calcaneus; usually congenital.
interdigital space: the area between the adjacent metatarsals and phalanges.
Meyer line: in a normal foot, a line that passes through the big toe to midpoint of heel.
plantar fascia: dense fascia of the plantar aspect of foot arising from calcaneus and inserting into base of proximal phalanges; **plantar aponeurosis.**
ray: complex of the metatarsals and phalanges that, on anteroposterior radiographs, appear as five rays.
sinus tarsi: small channel between the midanterior lateral calcaneus and talus; **tarsal sinus.**
tarsal tunnel: a fibro-osseous tunnel along the medial aspect of the tarsal bones that contains the flexor tendons and the branches of the posterior tibial arteries and nerves.
web space: web of skin between and at the base of each toe.

Arteries, Veins, Nerves

calcaneal branch of the posterior tibial a. and n.: supplies the heel (os calcis, calcaneus).
digital artery and nerves: terminal arteries and nerves that travel together on the sides of the toes in the interdigital spaces.
dorsalis pedis a.: branch from the anterior tibial artery, going into the dorsum of the foot.
malleolar a.: anterior, medial, and lateral branches supply the medial and lateral malleolus.

plantar a. (deep branch): supplies the plantar surface of the foot on medial and lateral side.

plantar arch: medial plantar artery that transverses the foot to anastomose with lateral plantar artery.

plantar nerve: terminal portion of posterior tibial nerve that divides into medial and lateral plantar nerves, giving off sensory branches to plantar side of foot and motor branches to intrinsic muscles of foot.

posterior tibial artery, nerve, and vein: travel through a fascial tunnel on the inner ankle (tarsal tunnel) and branch to supply the plantar aspect of the foot and toes.

Diseases and Conditions of the Foot and Ankle

The pathologic and neuromusculoskeletal changes that take place in the foot can be the result of multiple entities. For example, excessive weight, overuse, improper shoe fit, and similar causes can place stress and strain on the feet. Simple effects on the foot can relate to dermal abrasions, blisters, ulcers, fissures, bunions, corns, calluses, fungi, and other infections. The more severe problems involve peripheral vascular (ischemia) diseases, metabolic disorders (diabetes, gout), musculoskeletal changes (bunion and hammer toe deformities), and trauma (fractures, dislocations). All of these may cause or contribute to disability and inability to function. Diseases and conditions of the foot are listed alphabetically for reference. Other diseases are listed in Chapter 2.

Achilles tendonitis: dysfunction of the Achilles tendon due to inflammation of the surrounding tissue (peritendinitis) or degeneration of the tendon tissue itself (tendinosis). Retrocalcaneal bursitis refers to inflammation of the bursal sac between the calcaneus and Achilles tendon.

ainhum: a rare condition of unknown etiology, seen primarily in blacks where there is a constricting ring around a digit causing a very slow spontaneous lysis or autoamputation, usually of the fourth or fifth toe, but sometimes other toes; **dactylolysis spontanea.**

anonychia: absence of toenail(s).

athlete's foot (tinea pedis): fungal infection of skin on the plantar surface of the feet and between the toes and nails caused by one of the dermatophyte species (*Trichophyton* or *Epidermophyton*); disease consists of scaling, fissures, maceration, and eroded areas between the toes; **dermatomycosis pedis.**

Baxter's nerve: the first branch off the lateral plantar nerve, which is often entrapped deep to the plantar fascia and is implicated in heel pain syndrome.

blue foot syndrome: bluish discoloration of the feet most commonly caused by vascular disturbances.

bunion: joint deformity and enlargement of bone at the base of the MTP joint of the big toe with malposition of the first metatarsal, and overgrowth of bone at the first metatarsal head. This deformity, called **hallux valgus,** may or may not affect the position of the great toe. If the great toe is affected, then one of the following designations would be given: **hallux abductus** with bunion, **hallux adductus** with bunion, and **hallux abductovalgus** with bunion.

bunion (dorsal): overgrowth of bone (exostosis) on the dorsal surface of the first metatarsal head or a dorsal malposition of the first metatarsal.

bunionette: similar to the bunion deformity but affecting the fifth metatarsal, causing the metatarsal head to be prominent laterally; often referred to as a **tailor's bunion.**

bursitis: inflammation of a fluid-filled sac that is normally present around a bony prominence to cushion it.

calcaneal spur syndrome: a spur-shaped bony growth at the origin of the flexor digitorum brevis, quadratus plantae, and abductor hallucis on the inferior calcaneus, which arises as a response to tension and which can cause tenderness and pain and is exacerbated with weight-bearing.

callosity: hard, thickened skin on the bottom of the foot like a clavus; **tyloma, keratoma, callus** (pl. calluses).

Charcot foot: an acquired foot deformity secondary to multiple neuropathic fractures most often seen in diabetic patients; **Charcot arthropathy, neuropathic foot.**

clavus: any corn or hyperkeratotic tissue involving a toe; a reaction of skin to intermittent chronic pressure, producing extra layers of hard skin; caused by restrictive footwear or by abnormal position or motion of the toes.

clavus (soft): soft skin thickening between the toes, usually between the fourth and fifth toes; **heloma molle, soft corn, clavus mollis.**

clawtoes: fixed hyperextension of the metatarsophalangeal joints associated with flexion of the proximal and distal interphalangeal joints, producing a claw-like appearance; **claw toe deformity.**

clubfoot: congenital foot deformity resulting in the appearance of a golf club. The components include forefoot adduction with medial displacement of the talus, ankle equinus, and heel varus. The result is that the foot turns in with the sole of the foot and the heel pulled medially.

coalition: a bridge between two bones; may be fibrous (syndesmosis), cartilage (synchondrosis), or bone (synostosis), for example, a calcaneonavicular bar that is a bridge between the calcaneus and navicular bones; **tarsal bars.**

congenital bars: bridging of bone from one tarsal bone to another, with the most common being calcaneonavicular and talocalcaneal bars.

congenital rocker-bottom flatfoot: condition present at birth; abnormal equinus position of talus with valgus position of the heel, resulting in a foot that looks like a rocker and has a prominence below the medial ankle; **congenital vertical talus, congenital convex pes valgus.**

curly toe: a bilateral congenital deformity where one or more toes, usually the fourth toe, is supinated, medially deviated, and in plantar flexion.

dactylitis: infarcts in the small bones of the foot caused by sickle cell disease.

dorsiflexed metatarsal: a metatarsal that is deformed/malpositioned so that its head is higher than the adjacent metatarsal heads, resulting in increased plantar pressure over the adjacent metatarsal heads with limitation of motion of the involved metatarsophalangeal joint.

drop foot: paralysis or weakness of the dorsiflexor muscles of the anterior compartment of the leg innervated by the peroneal nerves, causing the foot and toes to drag when walking; **foot drop, peroneal nerve palsy.**

Dupuytren's fibromatosis: plantar fibromas of the plantar fascia of the foot; present as solitary or multiple nodules occurring most often along the medial border of the plantar fascia.

Egyptian foot: a foot with a long first ray.

equinus: abnormal position of plantar flexion and used in combining form with other words to denote the anatomic location; ankle equinus, forefoot equinus, metatarsus equinus.

exostosis: in children, a bony growth protruding from the surface of bone formed by endochondral ossification. It ceases to grow when growth plate closes; **osteochondroma, osteocartilaginous exostosis.**

flail foot: a foot with poor neuromuscular function and control.

flatfoot: a foot with a depressed longitudinal arch. This term covers a wide range of conditions. In most cases, a flatfoot is due to imbalances of the muscles and ligaments that control the arch and is referred to as a **flexible flatfoot.** If musculoskeletal changes occur during adult life or if there is an injury, the term **acquired flatfoot** might be used. Many individuals with flatfeet go through life with no functional interferences.

foot cramps: an involuntary action involving a muscle-tendon reflex contraction, stretching the tendon, which sends nerve messages to spinal cord, which in turn stimulates the muscle even more, producing a painful cramp. This can be related to abnormal levels of minerals (calcium, potassium, and magnesium), a decrease in blood supply to the muscle, a pinched nerve, holding the foot in pronation for a length of time, or a problem with the muscle itself.

forefoot equinus: describes a high-arched foot characterized by excessive plantar flexion of forefoot in relation to hindfoot.

forefoot valgus: describes pronated position of forefoot with respect to the hindfoot.

forefoot varus: describes supinated position of forefoot with respect to hindfoot.

ganglion: a benign soft tissue cystic mass filled with clear fluid, usually coming from a joint or a tendon sheath, usually in the midfoot or hindfoot.

gastrocnemius equinus: a tightness or contracture of the gastrocnemius muscle that restricts ankle dorsiflexion when the knee is fully extended; **Silverskold test.**

gout: a metabolic disorder deposits of uric acid crystals form in the joints, the kidneys, and the great toe, causing pain and inflammation. Aspiration of joint fluid can help differentiate gout from an inflammatory condition due to bacteria.

Greek foot: a foot with a short first ray.

Haglund's deformity: prominent posterosuperior aspect of the calcaneus; **retrocalcaneal exostosis** or a "pump bump."

Haglund's syndrome: pain on the superior and lateral side of the heel usually associated with a callus of the skin, bony prominence **(Haglund's deformity),** and retrocalcaneal bursitis. A variety of conditions and shoe types can contribute to this condition; **retrocalcaneal exostosis.**

hallux abductus: great toe pointing toward second toe (transverse plane deformity).

hallux adductus: great toe pointing toward midline of body (transverse plane deformity).

hallux elevatus: fixed dorsiflexed position of entire first ray.

hallux extensus: fixed dorsiflexed position of the great toe.

hallux flexus: fixed flexion position of great toe at the metatarsophalangeal joint.

hallux malleus: hammer toe deformity of the great toe; fixed flexion position of great toe at the interphalangeal joint.

hallux rigidus: painful, stiff metatarsophalangeal joint with limitation of motion and pain on dorsiflexion; caused by arthritic changes.

hallux valgus: great toe pointing toward second toe, often rotated in frontal plane so that the nail plate is facing away from second toe.

hallux valgus interphalangeus: a hallux valgus deformity caused by deformity of the proximal or distal phalanx.

hallux varus: great toe pointing toward midline of body, often rotated in frontal plane so that the nail plate is facing second toe.

hammer toes: descriptive of a variety of deformities of the second to fifth toes with increased flexion of the interphalangeal joints, causing prominence of the bones over the dorsal aspect of the interphalangeal joints. The term is more properly reserved for a toe with a fixed flexion deformity of the PIP only.

hard corn: a particularly hard, thickened area of skin over the dorsum of the toe; **heloma durum, clavus durum, hard clavus.**

heel pain syndrome: a common orthopaedic problem of the foot characterized by plantar fascial inflammation, entrapment neuropathy, heel spur, stress fracture of the calcaneus, or a painful heel pad caused by excessive loading on heel strike; **heel spur syndrome, plantar fasciitis, calcodynia.**

heel spur: osteophyte that protrudes from the plantar or posterior aspect of the calcaneus causing pain; **calcaneal spur.**

hindfoot equinus: characterized by plantar flexion of the calcaneus with a decrease of calcaneal inclination angle (low-arched, flatfoot, rocker-bottom foot).

ingrown nail: condition of the nail growing into the skin distally; **unguis incarnatus, onychocryptosis.**

intractable plantar keratosis: well-defined callous tissue with a central core located beneath a metatarsal head and usually the result of abnormal plantar pressure over a bony prominence; **IPK.**

lobster foot: congenital cleft secondary to the lack of the central three rays and middle and lateral cuneiforms producing a lobster claw appearance.

macrodactyly: enlargement of a toe or toes.

Madura foot: a severe deep fungal infection of the foot.

mallet toes: fixed flexion of the distal interphalangeal joint of the second to fifth toes, such that the toenails are pointing into the ground when walking.

malum deformans: a deep foot ulcer commonly associated with diabetes mellitus or other neuropathic conditions.

metatarsal cuneiform exostosis: an overgrowth of bone usually involving the dorsal surface of the first metatarsal base and first cuneiform.

metatarsalgia: pain in the plantar aspect of the metatarsal head area caused by a variety of disorders.

metatarsus abductus: turning out of the forefoot (metatarsals); **m. valgus.**

metatarsus adductocavus: forefoot turned inward in association with a high arch, usually seen in clubfoot deformity that includes heel varus (talipes equinovarus).

metatarsus adductus: turning in of the forefoot (metatarsals); **m. varus.**

metatarsus atavicus: abnormal shortness of the first metatarsal bone.

metatarsus equinus: see **equinus**.

metatarsus latus: broad foot due to spreading of the metatarsals; widened forefoot, splay foot.

metatarsus primus varus: refers to medial deviation of the first metatarsal with splaying between first and second metatarsals; can be the cause of a bunion deformity.

Morton foot: short first metatarsal and long second metatarsal that causes changes in the weight-bearing pattern of the foot.

Morton neuroma: a pseudoneuroma arising from the lateral branch of the medial plantar nerve with thickening of the digital nerves between the metatarsal heads. Usually found between the second and third interspaces; **interdigital neuroma.**

Morton syndrome: short, hypermobile first ray with insufficiency.

neuropathic fracture: fracture or fractures secondary to loss of protective sensation; **Charcot fracture.**

non-plantigrade foot: foot alignment with a portion of the weight-bearing sole not in alignment with the floor.

onychauxis: overgrowth and thickening of a nail plate with fragmentation and discoloration of the nail, most frequently the great toenail; **onychogryphosis.**

onychocryptosis: condition of nail growing into the skin distally; **ingrown nail, unguis incarnatus.**

onychomycosis: fungal infection of the nail plate.

osteochondrosis: disruption of the blood supply to a growth center of a bone. These have been given eponyms after the persons who first reported them:

Köhler's disease: osteochondrosis of the navicular bone.

Freiberg's infraction: osteochondrosis of the metatarsal head.

Sever's disease: osteochondrosis of the calcaneus apophysis.

overlapping toe: a toe that overlaps an adjacent toe; commonly affecting the second toe, which overlaps the great toe.

pachyonychia: extreme thickening of the toenails; usually congenital, the nails are more solid and regular than in onychogryphosis.

paronychia: an inflammation of the soft tissues around the nail plate, secondary to infection or trauma.

peroneal spastic flatfoot: overall descriptive term applies to many flatfeet, including congenital tarsal coalitions, in which the peroneals spasm secondary to pain from the underlying disorder, pulling the foot into pronation.

Persian slipper foot: the clinical appearance of the paralytic form of vertical talus in which the lateral column of the foot has an abducted plantar contour and the medial longitudinal column is elongated and convex. The lateral toes are elevated and clawed, which is the basis for the term.

pes: generally speaking, the term *pes* (foot) is used as a prefix to denote an acquired affection of the foot, for example, pes planus, better known as *flatfoot*. The terms *pes* and *talipes* are generally interchangeable.

pes cavus: high arches in midfoot, which may produce pain along the medial longitudinal arch (instep) after prolonged walking or standing.

pes planus: lowering of the longitudinal arch; flatfoot. There are two basic categories:

flexible pes planus: flatfoot with general laxity in which the foot appears normal when not bearing weight but flattens with weight-bearing.

rigid pes planus: nonflexible flatfoot that is present whether bearing weight or not.

pigeon toe: term that is often applied to any intoeing gait.

plantar fasciitis: inflammation of the plantar fascia.

plantar flexed metatarsal: a metatarsal that is malpositioned so that its head is lower than the adjacent metatarsal heads, resulting in abnormal pressure, which may produce a plantar callus.

plantar wart: an epidermal growth affecting the plantar surface of the foot caused by a papillomavirus; **verruca vulgaris.**

plantigrade foot: foot alignment with the weight-bearing sole in alignment with the floor.

podagra: although it literally means pain in the foot, this term is usually used for a painful attack of gout in the great toe.

polydactyly: congenital deformity, extra digits of the toes.

polysyndactyly: condition in which more than two toes are joined together.

posterior tibial tendon insufficiency: condition associated with acquired flatfoot deformity with loss of the longitudinal arch with peritalar subluxation of the navicular with abduction of the forefoot and heel valgus.

prehallux: accessory navicular (**os tibiale externum**).

pronation: a combination of motions including abduction and eversion of the foot that produces a *relaxing* of the arch for heel strike. This motion is normal during gait; however, excessive pronation can lead to pathologic changes of the foot (flexible flatfoot).

pump bumps: a thickening of skin forming a callus in the back of the heel above the calcaneus as a result of tight-fitting shoes and a **Haglund's deformity.**

rheumatoid nodule: potentially large painful synovial cysts, which can form on the weight-bearing surface of the foot.

rocker-bottom foot: deformity of the foot such that the arch is disrupted and resembles a chair rocker bottom. This may be a complication of clubfoot treatment, a neuropathic fracture deformity, or myelomeningocele.

skew foot: a complex deformity involving adduction and supination of the forefoot (metatarsus adductovarus) and hindfoot valgus. The condition is difficult to treat by nonsurgical methods; **z-foot.**

splay foot: abnormally wide forefoot caused by abnormally wide intermetatarsal angles.

squatter's talus: a dorsal articular facet on the talar neck found in cultures that are accustomed to squatting.

stiff ray: immobility of all joints of any toe or toes.

subungual exostosis: a benign osteocartilaginous bone spur that grows off a distal phalanx under the nail bed.

supination: a combination of motions including adduction and inversion of the foot that produces a stiffening of the arch for push-off. This motion is normal during gait; however, excessive supination can lead to pathologic changes of the foot (stiff cavus foot).

syndactyly: congenital anomaly of the foot (or hand) marked by a complete webbing between the toes; may involve two or more toes; may contain bone or merely soft tissue.

tailor's bunion: a pronounced prominence on lateral side of fifth metatarsal head. The term is derived from the historical cross-legged sitting behavior of tailors.

talipes: generally speaking, the term *talipes,* meaning ankle and foot, is used as a prefix to denote an affection of the foot, for example, talipes equinovarus (clubfoot).

> *talipes calcaneocavus:* high-arched foot with fixed dorsiflexion; **pes c.**
>
> *talipes calcaneus:* abnormally dorsiflexed hindfoot, with increased dorsiflexion of the calcaneus; **cavus foot, pes c.**
>
> *talipes calcaneovalgus:* abnormally dorsiflexed hindfoot with turning out of the heel; **pes c.**
>
> *talipes calcaneovarus:* abnormally dorsiflexed hindfoot with turning in of the heel; **pes c.**
>
> *talipes cavovalgus:* high arch and turning out of the heel; **pes c.**
>
> *talipes cavovarus:* high arch associated with turning in of the foot; **pes c.**
>
> *talipes equinovalgus:* plantar flexion and turning out of the calcaneus; **pes e.**
>
> *talipes equinovarus:* turning of the heel inward with increased plantar flexion. More precisely, a clubfoot, often having the components of talipes equinovarus with metatarsus adductus. This condition can result from a disease causing paralysis or from unknown causes; **clubfoot, pes e.**
>
> *talipes planovalgus:* depression of the longitudinal arch associated with heel valgus; **pes planovalgus.**
>
> *talipes planus:* depression of the longitudinal arch; no specified heel valgus is implied by this term; **pes planus, flatfoot.** A *flexible pes planus* is flatfoot with general laxity but no other specific disease process.

ulcer: a break down in the skin secondary to neuropathic or ischemic conditions; **neuropathic u., ischemic u.**

vertical talus: a spectrum of conditions in which the talus is oriented in a plantar flexed and medially directed position resulting in a flatfoot with heel valgus and a rocker-bottom or convex sole. In the more severe congenital form, congenital rigid flatfoot, it is usually associated with a neurologic disorder such as arthrogryposis or myelomeningocele; **congenital convex pes valgus.**

Surgery

Descriptions of Procedures

Akin p.: for hallux valgus or deformed great toe; an osteotomy of the proximal phalanx of the great toe.

Anderson p.: for lateral ankle instability, use of plantaris tendon for lateral ligament reconstruction.

Anderson and Fowler p.: for pes planus; an opening wedge osteotomy of the distal lateral calcaneus with tibial bone graft, closing wedge osteotomy of the medial cuneiform, and capsulotomy of the talonavicular joint.

arthroplasty: for hallux valgus or rigidus; can be hemiarthroplasty with resurfacing of the metatarsal head or base of the proximal phalanx or bipolar or total joint replacement.

arthroereisis: a general term for surgery of a joint. In the foot, it is a joint stabilization by implant (e.g., stabilization of subtalar joint in a pes planus deformity with expectation of removing the implant when the foot position has stabilized).

Austin p.: for hallux valgus; an osteotomy in the form of a chevron or "V" cut made in the distal aspect of the first metatarsal; **chevron procedure.**

avulsion of nail plate: a nonpermanent removal of the nail plate, either partial or complete, without disrupting the matrix cells that produce the nail plate.

Baker p.: for Achilles tendon tightness; relaxation of proximal tendon with a rectangular sliding slot incision.

Baker and Hill p.: for dynamic foot varus deformity due to cerebral palsy; transposition of posterior tibial tendon anterior to medial malleolus.

Banks p.: for nonunion medial malleolus; resection of nonunion, addition of locally obtained tibial cancellous bone, and screw fixation.

Barr p.: for paralytic clubfoot; transfer of the posterior tibial tendon to the third cuneiform or metatarsal.

Barr-Record p.: for clubfeet; subcutaneous plantar fasciotomy and tendon Achilles lengthening (TAL) done as separate procedures, with tibiotalar fusion.

Bartlett p.: for ingrown toenail; excision of wedge of skin with no excision of nail.

Batchelor-Brown p.: for flatfeet; fusion of the subtalar joint with a fibular bone graft.

Berman and Gartland p.: for metatarsus adductus; dome-shaped osteotomy of all five proximal metatarsals.

Bircher, Weber p.: for malunion ankle fracture with diastasis; osteotomy and corrective fibular lengthening with screw and plate fixation.

Bose p.: for ingrown toenail; excision of wedge of skin without excision of nail.

Bosworth p.: for repair of old rupture of Achilles tendon; fashioning direct tendon graft from median raphe (central portion of tendon).

Boyd amputation: an amputation at the ankle with tibial calcaneal fusion.

Brahms p.: for mallet toe; transfer of flexor digitorum profundus to dorsum of proximal phalanx.

Bridle p.: for foot paralysis; posterior tibialis tendon transfer through interosseous membrane to dorsum of foot, and dual anastomosis to anterior tibialis and anteriorly transposed peroneus longus.

Brockman p.: for clubfoot; a soft tissue release of the medial capsule of the foot as well as a release of the posterior tibial tendon.

Broström p.: for chronic lateral ankle instability; method of anatomic repair of lateral collateral ligaments; **Gould modification:** incorporates the extensor retinaculum with the repair.

Bugg-Boyd p.: for repair of old Achilles tendon rupture; use of fascia lata graft.

bunionectomy: for hallux valgus; a general class of many different operations that are designed to correct bunion deformity.

Campbell p.: for drop foot or talipes equinus of certain origins; creates a posterior bone block to prevent plantar flexion.

cheilectomy: for hallux rigidus; removal of an exostosis usually on the dorsal surface of the distal first metatarsal.

chevron osteotomy: for hallux valgus; an osteotomy in the form of a chevron or "V" cut made in the distal first metatarsal; **Austin.**

Chopart amputation: of the forefoot through the talonavicular and calcaneocuboid joint.

Chrisman-Snook p.: repair of lateral collateral ligament of ankle using peroneus brevis tendon. Also called modified **Elmslie procedure.**

Cincinnati incision: an incision to correct clubfoot.

Clayton p.: for deformity of toes in rheumatoid arthritis; resection of proximal phalanx and entire metatarsal heads of all toes.

closing abductory wedge osteotomy (CAWO): for hallux valgus; proximal metatarsal osteotomy with closure of wedge to bring first metatarsal closer to second metatarsal.

Cole p.: for cavus foot deformity; an anterior tarsal wedge osteotomy with fusion.

Coleman p.: for talipes valgus; soft tissue and tendon release associated with a subtalar fusion.

condylectomy: for painful callus; removal of a condyle from a metatarsal or phalanx.

cone arthrodesis: for fusion of the first metatarsophalangeal joint; the metatarsal head is shaped into a cone, and a cone wedge is cut into the proximal phalanx at a proper angle to accept the metatarsal head for fusion; **Wilson p., Johnson and Barington p.**

cotting: for ingrown nail; excision of a nail.

Cracchiolo p.: for deformity of toes in rheumatoid arthritis; silastic implant arthroplasty for MP joints of all toes.

crescentic osteotomy: for hallux valgus; a dome-shaped or crescentic osteotomy at the base of the first metatarsal to reduce the metatarsus primus varus.

cylindrical osteotomy: to shorten long bones; removal of a cylinder of bone.

Dias and Giegerich p.: for triplane fracture of ankle; open reduction with screw fixation when required.

Dickson-Diveley p.: for clawing of big toe; the interphalangeal joint is fused, and the extensor hallucis longus is transferred to the long flexor.

digital prosthesis: excision of interphalangeal joint with insertion of prosthetic device in that space.

Dillwyn-Evans p.: for severe resistant clubfoot deformity; Achilles and posterior tibial tendon Z-plasty, talonavicular joint capsulectomy, resection, and fusion calcaneocuboid joint.

DIP fusion: for mallet toes; removal of the distal interphalangeal joint and then fusion.

dorsal-V osteotomy: for plantar callosity; an osteotomy at the neck of a lesser metatarsal to allow the metatarsal to assume a slightly higher position.

dorsal wedge osteotomy: for plantar callosity; an osteotomy at the base of a metatarsal to allow the metatarsal to move to a higher position.

Drennan p.: for ankle flexion weakness; posterior transfer of anterior tibial tendon.

Dunn-Brittain p.: for paralytic clubfeet; a method of triple arthrodesis excising most of the head of the talus.

Dunn-Brittain triple arthrodesis: removal of entire navicular bone.

Durham p.: for flatfoot; closing wedge osteotomy/ fusion of cuneiform-navicular joint.

DuVries arthroplasty: for fixed hammer toes and mallet toes; resection of the head of the proximal phalanx (hammer toe) or middle phalanx (mallet toe).

DuVries plantar condylectomy: for plantar callosities; resection of plantar condyles from the lesser metatarsals.

DuVries p.: (1) for chronic instability of deltoid ligament of ankle; cross-shaped imbrication of deltoid ligament; (2) for hallux valgus; a modified McBride bunion procedure with vertical medial capsular imbrication and suturing of lateral capsule to second metatarsal head.

Dwyer p.: lateral closing wedge osteotomy of the calcaneus; associated with soft tissue release for clubfeet and other disorders.

Ellis Jones p.: for subluxing peroneal tendon; reconstruction of retinaculum using portion of Achilles tendon.

Elmslie p.: for lateral ankle instability; peroneal tendon used in ligament reconstruction.

Elmslie-Cholmely p.: double wedge osteotomy for certain high-arched feet.

Essex-Lopresti p.: for fractured calcaneus; use of a Steinmann pin or other metal pin to help achieve and hold fracture reduction.

Evans p.: for lateral collateral ligament instability of ankle; use of peroneus brevis tendon.

Evans p.: for severe flatfoot deformity; distal lateral opening wedge osteotomy of the calcaneus.

exostectomy: removal of any excess prominences of bone.

Farmer p.: for hallux varus; soft tissue repair with the use of a skin flap.

Fowler p.: for metatarsus varus with severe cavus deformity; plantar fascia and muscle release associated with an opening wedge osteotomy of the first cuneiform. Also, for deformity of toes in rheumatoid arthritis; resection of proximal phalanx and varying portions of metatarsal heads of all toes. Also, for ingrown toenail; excision of entire nail.

Freid-Green p.: for paralysis of posterior tibial muscle; transfer of the peroneus longus, flexor digitorum longus, flexor hallucis longus, or extensor hallucis longus to posterior tibial tendon.

Frost p.: for ingrown nail; a skin flap is made over the lateral nail bed, with removal of the nail and bed followed by closure of flap.

Fulford p.: for spastic valgus deformity of foot; peroneus brevis elongation.

Gallie p.: for malunion calcaneus; subtalar arthrodesis using a tibial bone graft.

Garceau p.: for clubfeet; anterior tibial tendon transfer.

Garceau-Brahms p.: for paralytic clubfeet; transection of the motor branches of the plantar nerve.

Gelman p.: for clubfeet; identical to the McCauley procedure, except that the inferior calcaneonavicular ligament is not incised.

Giannestras p.: for plantar callosity; proximal shortening of metatarsal.

Gill p.: for drop foot; wedge of bone taken from the superoposterior calcaneus with insertion of that block into the posterior tibiotalar joint.

Girdlestone p.: for flexible hammer toe deformities; transfer of the long flexors of the involved toe(s) to the extensor hood mechanism (top of toe).

Gould p.: for pes cavus due to tight plantar fascia; a double plantar fasciotomy through a lateral heel approach proximally and a distal medial approach.

Grice p.: for congenital talipes valgus; a soft tissue medial and lateral foot release procedure.

Grice-Green p.: for talipes valgus; tibial bone graft to subtalar joint. Also, for paralysis of gastroc-soleus; transfer of peroneus longus, peroneus brevis, and posterior tibial tendon.

Hark p.: for congenital talipes valgus; multiple extensor and flexor Z-tendon lengthenings with bony repositioning.

Harris-Beath p.: for flatfeet; talonavicular and subtalar arthrodesis.

Hauser p.: (1) for hallux valgus; excision of the medial exostosis and transfer of the adductor tendon from the proximal phalanx to the distal metatarsal; (2) for tight heel cord; division of proximal posterior and distal medial two-thirds of the Achilles tendon; (3) for Achilles tendon tightness; partial incision at two levels with passive stretching and casting.

Heifetz p.: for ingrown nail; excision of affected ingrown side of nail and nail bed.

hemiphalangectomy: for shortening or straightening of a toe; resection of a portion of the phalanx.

Herndon-Heyman p.: for congenital talipes valgus; medial and lateral foot release with tendon lengthening.

Heyman p.: for clubfeet; soft tissue release for clubfoot, including deltoid ligament.

Hibbs p.: for clawtoes and cavus feet; plantar fascia release with transfer of the extensor digitorum longus to the third cuneiform.

Hiroshima p.: for spastic equinus and equinovarus deformity; anterior transfer of long toe flexors.

Hoffer p.: for spastic inversion of foot; transfer of anterior tibial tendon to cuboid.

Hoffman-Clayton p.: resection of metatarsal head; resection of metatarsal heads and bases of proximal phalanges for cock-up deformities of toes as seen in rheumatoid arthritis.

Hoke p.: (1) triple arthrodesis done with reshaping of the head of the talus; (2) for flatfeet; navicular bone and two medial cuneiforms are fused.

Hoke-Kite p.: for calcaneocavovarus deformity; excision and fusion with some shortening of talonavicular joint and a posteriorly closing wedge fusion of the talocalcaneal joint.

Hueter-Mayo p.: for simple bunion deformity; resection of prominent portion of first metatarsal.

Ingram p.: for congenital talipes valgus; Z-plasty lengthening of peroneus brevis tendon, medial release, reduction of navicular bone, and anterior tibial tendon transfer.

intermediate phalangectomy: for hammer toe deformity; excision of the middle phalanx.

Jahss p.: for cavus foot with clawtoes; excision of metatarsotarsal joint with dorsal wedge closed to reduce cavus and with adequate bone excision to relax plantar fascia.

Jansey p.: for ingrown toenail; excision of wedge of skin without excision of nail.

Japas p.: for high-arched feet; a combination of plantar fascia release and dorsal wedge osteotomy of the tarsal bones.

Johnson and Spiegl p.: for hallux varus; fusion of interphalangeal joint great toe and transfer of extensor hallucis longus to lateral proximal phalanx.

Jones p.: for cock-up deformity of great toe and other problems; transfer of the extensor hallucis longus to the distal first metatarsal; currently done with a distal interphalangeal joint fusion.

Jones p.: an ankle repair of the fibular collateral ligament using the peroneus brevis muscle.

Joplin p.: for splay foot deformity; transfer of fifth toe flexor to first metatarsal.

Juvara p.: for hallux valgus; an oblique osteotomy at the proximal portion of the metatarsal to correct an abnormal transverse and/or sagittal plane deformity.

Karlsson p.: for lateral ankle ligament instability; reconstruction using original ligament; **Brostrum procedure.**

Kashiwagi p.: for malunion calcaneus fracture; lateral subtalar and calcaneocuboid joint fusion.

Kates-Kessel-Kay p.: for deformity of toes in rheumatoid arthritis; resection of metatarsal head only.

Kaufer p.: for spastic inversion of foot; transfer of posterior tibial tendon to peroneus brevis.

Keller p.: for hallux rigidus or hallux valgus; resection of the proximal phalanx of the great toe.

Kendrick p.: for metatarsus adductus; soft tissue release for all tarsal metatarsal joints.

Kessel-Bonney p. (Moberg p.): for lack of great toe extension; a closing wedged osteotomy of proximal phalanx.

Kidner p.: for an accessory navicular bone; removal of the accessory navicular bone with or without transfer of the posterior tibial tendon under the navicular bone.

Kiehn-Earle-DesPrez p.: for plantar ulcer; closure of ulcer and transfer of extensor digitorum longus to distal metatarsal shaft.

Lambrinudi p.: a triple arthrodesis done by resection of the head and inferior portion of the talus.

Lange p.: for metatarsus varus; simple oblique osteotomy of the second, third, and fourth metatarsals; lateral closing wedge osteotomy of the first metatarsal at the base.

Lapidus p.: for hallux valgus; arthrodesis of the first metatarsocuneiform joint and a distal soft tissue procedure.

Larmon p.: for rheumatoid foot deformity; arthroplasty by resection of medial metatarsal head and proximal phalanx of great toe and resection of plantar part of metatarsal head of lesser toes.

Liebolt p.: for paralytic equinus foot; a two-stage procedure involving a Hoke triple arthrodesis followed by an ankle fusion.

Lindholm p.: for repair of ruptured Achilles tendon; fashioning of fascial flaps from superior tendon.

Lipscomb p.: for deformity of toes in rheumatoid arthritis; resection of proximal phalanx and plantar metatarsal head of all toes.

Lisfranc amputation: amputation through the tarsometatarsal joint.

Lloyd-Roberts p.: for clubfoot deformity in early childhood; soft tissue release.

Lowman p.: for flatfeet; transfer of the anterior tibialis with navicular cuneiform fusion.

Ludloff p.: for hallux valgus; an oblique osteotomy of the first metatarsal from proximal dorsal to distal plantar.

Lynn p.: for repair of Achilles tendon rupture; use of fanned out portion of plantaris tendon to cover direct repair.

Ma-Griffith p.: for Achilles tendon rupture; percutaneous technique of suture repair.

Majestro-Ruda-Frost p.: for spastic posterior tibial tendon; intramuscular lengthening.

malleolar osteotomy: a procedure or approach that provides access to the lateral side of the ankle joint in fracture reductions or in excising abnormal bone or cartilage.

Mammon p.: first metatarsal osteotomy and bone graft for a dorsal bunion.

Mann p.: for hallux valgus; a modified McBride bunion procedure with a vertical medial capsular imbrication and suturing of lateral capsule to second metatarsal head; **DuVries p.**

matricectomy: for toenail deformity or chronic disease; excision of all or a part of the nail plate (matrix) to eliminate growth of the nail.

Mau p.: for hallux valgus; an oblique osteotomy of the first metatarsal from proximal plantar to distal dorsal.

Mayer p.: for deformity caused by poliomyelitis; transfer of peroneal tendon.

Mayo p.: (1) for bunion exostosis of first metatarsal head without significant angular deformity; excision exostosis; (2) for first MTP joint arthritis; oblique excision of the first metatarsal head.

McBride p.: for hallux valgus; excision of the medial exostosis, medial capsular reefing, fibular sesamoidectomy, and transfer of the adductor hallucis tendon into the distal first metatarsal.

McCauley p.: very extensive medial release of multiple joint capsules, tendon sheaths, and abductor hallucis and, if needed, posterior capsulotomy later.

McElvenny p.: (1) excision of a plantar nerve neuroma; (2) for hallux varus; lateral capsular reefing procedure associated with use of the extensor hallucis brevis tendon for repair.

McKeever p.: for hallux valgus or rigidus; fusion of the first metatarsophalangeal joint; **arthrodesis.**

McReynolds p.: for fractured calcaneus; open reduction and fixation with staples using a medial approach.

Meisenbach p.: for callosity on plantar aspect of foot; dorsal displacement of metatarsal head(s).

metatarsal head resection with prosthesis: removal of the metatarsal head to create an artificial joint with a silastic implant.

metaphyseal osteotomy: through the neck of the metatarsal head.

Miller p.: for severe flatfoot deformity; navicularcuneiform metatarsal fusion for hallux varus with repositioning of stump of adductor hallucis and transfer of abductor hallucis to lateral proximal phalanx.

Mitchell p.: for hallux valgus; a distal metatarsal osteotomy with a step cut and shifting of metatarsal head laterally with excision of exostosis and medial capsular reefing.

Naughton-Dunn p.: for severe foot deformity; a triple arthrodesis with wedge resection.

neurectomy: excision of a neuroma anywhere in the body; in the foot, excision of an interdigital neuroma between the second and third or third and fourth toes.

Ober p.: for paralytic clubfeet; a method of transfer of the posterior tibial tendon to the third cuneiform or metatarsal.

onychotomy: incision into the nail bed.

opening abductory wedge osteotomy (OAWO): for hallux valgus; osteotomy of the first metatarsal base with use of bone graft to open the wedge and bring the first metatarsal closer to the second.

opening wedge osteotomy: for hallux valgus; in orthopaedics, a variety of procedures with or without tendon transfers, with proximal cut in the metatarsal and reduction of the deformity.

Osmone-Clarke p.: for talipes valgus; soft tissue release of the medial and lateral foot with peroneus brevis tendon transfer.

osteotripsy: for callosities; may be any percutaneous reduction of a bony prominence.

panmetatarsal head resection: usually for severe arthritic deformity; resection of all of the metatarsal heads.

pantalar fusion: for instability of the hindfoot; fusion of the tibiotalar, subtalar, calcaneocuboid, and talonavicular joints.

partial ostectomy: to relieve pressure on the skin; removal of bony prominence.

Peabody p.: (1) for metatarsus varus; resection of the proximal portion of the second, third, and fourth metatarsals, with osteotomy of the fifth and capsular release of the first metatarsals; (2) for paralysis of gastroc-soleus complex; transfer of anterior tibial tendon to the calcaneus.

Perry p.: for talipes equinovarus; split transfer of anterior tibialis to proximal third metatarsal, and flexor hallucis longus to dorsum of fourth metatarsal.

phenolization: for nail deformity in which a permanent elimination of a part or all of nail plate is desired. Phenol is applied to the nail matrix after the nail plate is removed to destroy any further nail growth.

Pierrot-Murphy p.: for dorsiflexion of the ankle weakness; transfer of Achilles tendon anteriorly on calcaneus.

PIP fusion: operation commonly done for clawtoes or hammer toes; removal of the proximal interphalangeal joint and then fusion.

Pridie-Koutsogiannis p.: for flexible flatfoot with excessive heel valgus; medial displacing osteotomy of calcaneus.

Putti-Mayer p.: for treatment of polio foot deformity; transfer of posterior tibial tendon.

Quenu p. (Fowler p., Zadik p.): for ingrown toenail; excision of nail bed germinal matrix through skin flap incision, leaving distal nail intact.

Reverdin-Green p.: for hallux valgus; a closing wedge osteotomy of the first metatarsal head.

Richardson p.: for malunited calcaneal fracture; posterior subtalar fusion using iliac bone graft as necessary.

Rose p.: for ingrown nail; removal of the ellipse of soft tissue to ingrown portion of nail.

Ruiz-Mora p.: proximal phalangectomy of the fifth toe for cock-up (or curly toe) deformity.

Samilson p.: for calcaneocavus foot; a crescentic osteotomy of the calcaneus.

scarf p. : for hallux valgus; a midshaft osteotomy with a scarf overlapping cut to correct metatarsus primus varus.

shock wave therapy: the use of either low-energy or high-energy extracorporeal shock waves to treat chronic inflammatory conditions of the foot and ankle, that is, plantar fasciitis.

SERI p.: for hallux valgus; a distal metatarsal neck osteotomy through a minimal incision, stabilized with a longitudinal K-wire. Stands for *s*imple, *e*ffective, *r*apid, and *i*nexpensive. Popular in Italy.

Siffert-Foster-Nachamie p.: for paralytic clubfeet; triple arthrodesis.

Silver p.: excision of medial first metatarsal exostosis with lateral capsular release and medial capsular imbrication.

Staples-Black-Broström p.: for acute, severe ankle sprain; method of repair of lateral collateral ligaments.

Steindler matricectomy: for nail deformity; removal of a part of the nail matrix to eliminate one border of the nail plate.

Steindler p.: plantar release of the proximal muscles and fascia of the foot for high-arched feet.

step down osteotomy: for abnormally long lesser metatarsal; an osteotomy to shorten the bone.

Stone p.: for hallux rigidus; resection of the dorsal first metatarsal exostosis.

Strayer p.: for tight heel cord; gastrocnemius lengthening leaving soleus intact.

subtalar arthrodesis: for arthritis and other conditions of the talocalcaneal joint; fusion of the talus to the calcaneus.

subtalar arthroereisis: for severe flatfoot with calcaneal valgus; insertion of an inert spacer into the subtalar joint.

Suppan p.: for nail deformity; this is a name applied to a variety of procedures to eliminate all or a part of the nail matrix.

Syme's amputation: an ankle disarticulation with preservation of the heel pad for weight-bearing.

syndactylization: a soft tissue procedure in which two adjacent toes are intentionally joined together. Syndactyly is the condition of an abnormal fusion of two or more digits.

TAL (tendon Achilles lengthening): a variety of procedures used to lengthen a tight or spastic Achilles tendon.

talectomy: excision of the talus for severe soft tissue contractures.

Thomas p.: for malunion calcaneus; subtalar arthrodesis using an iliac crest graft.

Tohen p.: for spastic equinovarus deformity of foot; transfer of conjoined extensor hallucis longus and anterior tibial tendon to second or fifth metatarsal.

transmetatarsal amputation: an amputation through the midportion of the metatarsals.

triple arthrodesis: for flail hindfoot and other deformities caused by arthritis. Procedure involves fusion of the calcaneus to the cuboid, navicula to the talus, and talus to the calcaneus.

Turco p.: for clubfeet; soft tissue release of the posteromedial capsule as well as Achilles tendon lengthening.

Valpius-Compere p.: for Achilles tendon tightness; proximal inverted V-shaped lengthening.

V-Y plasty: for clawtoes; transection of skin in V-shaped incision with closure in the shape of a Y.

Warner-Farber p.: for trimalleolar fractures with large posterior fragment; detachment of the fibula from tibia to get screw fixation of posterior fragment.

Watson-Cheyne p.: for ingrown toenail; excision of vertical wedge avoiding bone; **Burghard p., O'Donoghue p., Mongensen p.**

Watson-Jones p.: for lateral ankle instability; use of peroneus brevis tendon in reconstruction of lateral ligament.

Weil p.: for a dislocated/subluxed lesser MTP joint or for a plantar callosity or metatarsalgia secondary to a long metatarsal; a distal oblique metatarsal shortening osteotomy.

Westin p.: for paralytic talipes calcaneus; a tenodesis of the Achilles tendon to the fibula.

White slide p.: for Achilles tendon tightening in spastic hemiplegia; anterior fibers of the Achilles tendon are cut distally, and medial fibers are cut proximally. The foot is then dorsiflexed, producing the slide.

Whitman talectomy p.: talectomy for calcaneovalgus foot.

Whitman-Thompson p.: for talipes calcaneus or talipes calcaneovalgus; complete excision of the talus.

Wilson p.: for hallux valgus; an oblique osteotomy of the first metatarsal neck area.

Wilson and Jacob p.: for tibial plateau fracture; use of patella and its cartilage surface for joint replacement graft.

Winograd p.: for an ingrown nail; excision of an ingrown portion of toenail, with curettement of the nail bed.

Wolf p.: for plantar callosity; proximal shortening of the metatarsal.

Wu p.: (1) for hallux valgus; an oblique osteotomy of the metatarsal neck with lateral and plantar displacement stabilized with a Herbert screw; (2) for hallux rigidus; a first MTP joint fusion with three Herbert screws for fixation.

Young p.: anterior tibialis transfer for flatfoot.

Z-plasty: for tight heel cord; complete Z-shaped cut requiring suturing of Achilles tendon.

Zadik p.: for ingrown nail; excision of the entire nail.

Ankle Prostheses

The forces acting on the ankle are biplanar, yet by design, the prosthetics are monoplanar. With the highly active forces that exist across the ankle joint, there are fewer occasions for replacement of that joint. Prosthetic fixation is not as secure for these lower limb joint replacements, with loosening a continuing problem. A historical list of prostheses is in previous editions.

Ankle and Foot Approaches

anterior a.: for tendon repairs, transfers, and some ankle fusions; **Kochler, Ollier.**

lateral and posterolateral a.: for repair of fractures, ligamentous injuries, and some tendon transfers; **Kocher, Gatellier and Chastang.**

medial and posteromedial a.: for ankle fractures, tendon transfers, and correction of clubfeet; **Broomhead, Colonna and Ralston, Koenig and Schaefer, Garceau.**

Physical Medicine and Rehabilitation: Physical Therapy and Occupational Therapy

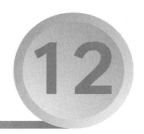

Physical Therapy

Physical medicine and rehabilitation (PM&R) is a medical specialty that is based on the fundamentals of neuromuscular physiology, exercise physiology, and functional anatomy.

The **physiatrist** is the physician specialist in PM&R certified by the American Board of Physical Medicine and Rehabilitation after completing a residency and other requirements. In some distinct centers for rehabilitation, a physiatrist is the medical director of the unit. However, some units are organized on a programmatic basis and have a group of other medical specialists overseeing individual programs; for example, a rheumatologist with the arthritis program, a neurologist with the neuromuscular disease program, and an orthopaedist with the musculoskeletal program.

The **physical therapist** is a health care professional who has completed an entry-level education program accredited by the Commission on Accreditation in Physical Therapy Education. Board-certified physical therapy specialties are in the following areas: cardiopulmonary, neurologic, clinical electrophysiologic, orthopaedic, pediatric, geriatric, and sports physical therapy.

In a hospital setting, the rehabilitation team may include the occupational therapist, speech therapist, rehabilitation nurse, social worker, and psychologist. Additional members might include a vocational counselor, special educator, prosthetist/orthotist, and numerous medical specialists depending on patient needs. The physical therapist assistant is a skilled technical health worker who, under the supervision of a physical therapist, assists in the patient's treatment program.

The goal of the rehabilitation team is to enhance each patient's physical capabilities by using the team members' individual professional skills, expertise, and knowledge to evaluate, plan, and implement treatment interventions tailored to the needs of the patient. In this patient-centered approach, the patient and/or family participates in setting realistic goals to be achieved during the rehabilitation process.

In association with orthopaedic surgery, the rehabilitation team works closely with and is considered an integral part of the orthopaedic rehabilitation program. The physical therapist consults with the orthopaedist and other primary care physicians in the evaluation and treatment of patients and establishes the treatment plan.

Services are provided for preoperative and postoperative care of the surgical patient after restorative surgery, trauma, or correction of congenital anomalies. In addition, treatments include the prevention of pulmonary complications after surgery. Strengthening and range of motion exercises are designed for patients with ligamentous tears and fractures. Amputees fitted with prostheses are instructed in their use and maintenance. The patient with a spinal cord injury is taught **activities of daily living (ADL)**, gait with braces, the use of assistive devices, and exercises to improve function. Large rehabilitation centers are designed to most effectively address these patients' needs.

Physical therapist services provide identification, prevention, remediation, and rehabilitation of patients with acute or prolonged physical dysfunction. Such intervention encompasses examination and analysis, therapeutic application of physical and chemical agents, exercises, and education to promote functional independence.

Physical therapy treatments may include the evaluation and treatment of abnormal gait patterns resulting from pathologic conditions, such as muscle weakness, paralysis, or biomechanical defects. Patients may also be referred for rehabilitative services for treatment of neuromuscular diseases (e.g., arthritis, stroke, or spinal cord injuries), temporomandibular joint (TMJ) syndrome, and chronic pain. The goal is to decrease pain, increase function, and prevent deformity.

Physical Therapy Services

Physical therapists practice in a variety of settings: acute care hospitals, rehabilitation centers, skilled nursing facilities, convalescent homes, home health, schools, industry, sports clinics, pediatric facilities, and private practice.

The following is a quick reference to typical services (although not inclusive) that are routinely provided by the physical therapist.

Evaluation (General)	
strength	coordination
functional ability	sensation
range of motion	ambulatory status
cognitive level	

Evaluation (Specific)	
manual muscle testing	posture
cardiopulmonary function	muscle tone
electroneurophysiologic	wound
neurodevelopmental	neonatal
isokinetic	thermography
gait	functional capacity evaluation

Treatment Techniques
Therapeutic Exercise
passive
active-assistive
active
resistive (isometric, isotonic, concentric, eccentric, isokinetic)
work hardening
Specific Techniques
proprioceptive neuromuscular facilitation (PNF)
Bobath (neurodevelopmental)
Rood
Brunstrom
Muscle Re-education
brushing
icing
tapping
quick stretch
neurodevelopmental training
Mobility
bed (bedbound patient)
transfer techniques
wheelchair mobility and safety
ambulation—parallel bars, walker, crutches, cane, prosthetic, orthotic
Hydrotherapy
cold/ice
heat (moist)
whirlpool (for increasing circulation, decreasing pain, debriding open wounds)
therapy pool (for gravity-free exercise and ambulation)
paraffin
Physical Modalities
electrical stimulation
functional electrical stimulation (FES)

diathermy

transcutaneous electrical nerve stimulation (TENS)

ultrasound

infrared

ultraviolet

Mobilization

soft tissue

joint

Cardiac Care

cardiac rehabilitation

cardiac stress testing

Pulmonary

bronchial drainage

breathing exercises

Pediatric

neurodevelopmental

scoliosis care (education and exercise, preoperative and postoperative care)

musculoskeletal

Intermittent Compression

edema control

Traction

cervical

pelvic

extremity

Patient Education (an essential element of most treatment plans)

Consultation Services

Consultative services are available for patients with special or extraordinary needs that require the recommendations of a multidisciplinary group.

Physical Therapy Modalities

cervical traction: a means of separating the cervical vertebrae 1 to 2 mm to help relieve painful neck conditions or cervical radiculopathies; may be intermittent or continuous.

contrast baths: alternately exposing affected limb to warm and cool water for specified periods. This is a means of reducing swelling, diminishing pain, and improving joint range of motion.

diathermy: electromagnetic waves with a specific wavelength (shortwave diathermy, microwave diathermy) used as a means of producing heat deep inside tissues; no longer in use.

electrical stimulation:

alternating current: sinusoidal or faradic; stimulates normally innervated muscles to relieve pain and relax muscle spasm.

galvanic: direct current used to stimulate denervated muscles and for ion transfer (iontophoresis).

high-voltage pulsed galvanic: to relieve pain and relax muscle spasm. Stimulates normally innervated muscles.

iontophoresis: the use of direct current (DC) to drive water-soluble ions through the skin. Dexamethasone and Xylocaine (lidocaine) are commonly used to treat acute and subacute localized inflammation and pain.

MENS (microamperage electrical nerve stimulation): microamperage current that is below patient's threshold; to relieve pain.

TENS (transcutaneous electrical nerve stimulation): self-contained, modulated galvanic current (low voltage) that seems to block painful afferent nerve impulses. Helps to control pain so patient may exercise.

fluidotherapy: the use of forced warm air through a container holding fine cellulose particles to provide dry heat and exercise to upper and lower extremities. Both the temperature and the particle agitation can be controlled for edema and desensitization of hypersensitive area.

hot packs: silicone gel, clay, or other material in bags that can be heated to provide superficial heat for tissues.

Hubbard tank: a large full-body water tank used to assist in range of motion and endurance exercise.

hydrostatic bed: essentially a waterbed that supports the patient for specific therapies.

hydrotherapy treatments: as commonly used today, immersion of affected limbs (sometimes including the trunk) in a tank of water at a specified temperature. The water may be moving (whirlpool), which is one means of debriding tissue. There are also tanks in which patients may sit (Lo-Boy) and in which they may be almost totally immersed (Hubbard tank). In a pool, the buoyancy of water can assist patients with partially paralyzed legs to walk. Some therapists refer to the **Archimedes principle** because the buoyancy in the water supports the weight, eliminates shock, and decreases the concern for need of balance.

interferential current: application of two medium-frequency alternating currents that interfere with each other. Used for pain control and muscle stimulation.

intermittent compression: a boot or sleeve that encloses the leg or arm and is alternately pressurized with air and then deflated. The inflate/deflate action provides a pumping effect that reduces disabling edema. It is often prescribed for breast cancer patients after a mastectomy and for lymphedema that may result.

paraffin bath: a combination of wax and mineral oil at 126°F used as a means of heating the hands or feet.

pelvic traction: for low back pain; application of pelvic belt with caudad pull, which may be continuous or use greater force intermittently.

phonophoresis: the use of ultrasound to drive molecules of medications through the skin to the underlying tissues.

RICE: an acronym for the initial treatment of an injury; *r*est, *i*ce, *c*ompression, and *e*levation.

ultrasound: ultrahigh-frequency sound waves that mechanically vibrate soft tissue. Secondary deep heat may develop according to method of application.

whirlpool: a form of hydrotherapy using fast moving water that is usually heated.

Physical Therapy Procedures

acupressure: sustained deep pressure over muscular trigger points.

aerobic exercises: exercises in which oxygen is inhaled at a rate sufficient for a continuous process of energy production for muscle contraction; the goal is to increase endurance required for long-distance running or after cardiac complications.

agility training: to improve balance and coordination; trains in the ability to make rapid changes in movement and direction.

anaerobic exercises: exercises in which the expenditure of energy is at a faster rate than that for which the muscles can function without a period of recovery before there is further exertion.

aquatic exercise: exercise performed in a pool or large hydrotherapy tank that uses the buoyancy of water.

closed chain exercise (closed kinetic chain): exercise that occurs when the distal segment of an extremity is fixed, such as performing a squat, in which the foot is in contact with the ground. Motion can take place in all planes.

Codman exercises: exercises for a stiff shoulder in which the patient is bent over at the waist (90 degrees) and the hand hangs like a pendulum toward the floor. A weight may be placed in the hand and the arm is then moved through various arcs to increase the range of motion (ROM) in that shoulder.

concentric contraction: muscle shortening with part moving in direction of muscle pull; also called **positive work.**

cross-training: a complex training regimen in which two or more sports or activities are combined into either a solitary or a cyclical program to exercise different muscle groups and to provide variety and protection from repetitive use syndromes.

DeLorme exercises: originally established on the basis of the 10 repetition maximum (RM), which is the maximal amount of resistance a muscle can lift through full ROM exercises 10 times; the term is frequently interchanged with progressive resistive exercises (PRE), which are designed to build strength and increase endurance through graduated resistance for a prescribed number of repetitions.

eccentric contraction: muscle lengthening during contraction, also called "negative work"; strengthening exercises in which the external force overcomes the actively contracting muscle, forcing the muscle to lengthen.

effleurage: a method of massage that uses a flowing motion with the hands over a tight muscle to relieve tightness.

endurance training: high repetition exercise designed to give maximum endurance for repeated muscle contraction.

gait training: the use of parallel bars, crutches, walkers, and canes with specific instructions to the patient. Weight-bearing may be described as non-weight-bearing (NWB), partial weight-bearing (PWB), or full weight-bearing (FWB). Ambulation with crutches is often described as three-point gait, and with walker, four-point gait.

isokinetic exercises: constant velocity; strengthening exercises requiring special equipment in which there is an accommodating resistance, resulting in a maximal force against the contracting muscle throughout its full ROM. Can be used for the spine as well as the upper and lower extremities.

isometric exercises: muscle contraction without joint movement in which the resistance may be provided by a fixed object (wall, stabilized bar) or the antagonistic muscle group (flexors versus extensors); a muscle-strengthening exercise that does not impel muscle to work through its range of motion; **constant angle exercise, static exercise.**

isotonic exercises: muscle contraction with movement of the joint through a specified ROM against a fixed amount of resistance; **constant force.**

joint manipulation: any skilled manual technique applied to a joint that moves one particular surface in relation to another.

joint mobilization: skilled passive movements applied to joint surfaces to restore "joint play" and range of motion or to treat pain.

joint play (accessory movement): involuntary movements of joint surfaces allowed by capsular elasticity that allow for normal, pain-free voluntary motion.

lumbar stabilization: exercise program to stabilize the torso by developing the "corset" muscles of the lumbar spine, particularly the abdominal muscles.

manual therapy: any treatment in which hands are used to manipulate, massage, or mobilize a part of the body.

McConnell taping: the technique of specific taping to correct abnormal tilt, glide, and rotation of the patella in patients with patellofemoral disorders.

McKenzie (extension) exercises: exercises performed to decrease the compression on the intervertebral disk.

muscle energy technique: manual technique that uses active contraction of a patient's muscle to correct joint dysfunction.

myofascial release: manual therapy technique that applies prolonged stretching to release restrictions in the muscle-fascia system.

open chain exercises: exercise that occurs when the distal segment of an extremity is free, such as performing a seated knee extension exercise. Non-weight-bearing and usually in one plane of motion; open kinetic chain.

pétrissage: a massage maneuver similar to kneading.

prehensile: the use of the thumb opposing the hand to grasp an object. The term prehensile implies function in which the thumb can be placed in opposition to the object. An atavistic hand lacks that capacity.

pulley exercises: a rope on pulley system used to increase ROM of a joint or strengthen muscles; resistance can be applied by another limb or by weights.

range of motion (ROM) exercises: designed to maintain or increase the amount of movement in a joint. They may be one of the following:

> *passive:* force is applied to bring about motion in a joint or joints by either a therapist or the patient, without any muscle function in these joints.

> *active-assistive:* exercise performed by the patient but requiring assistance from a therapist, another extremity, or a mechanical device because of muscle weakness or pain.

> *active:* exercise performed by patient without assistance or resistance; the therapist is only an instructor-observer.

resistive exercise table: commonly used for lower extremity problems, such as after knee surgery; resistance can be applied by weights (NK table in some locales) or by a graded hydraulic system.

spray and stretch: use of a vapocoolant, such as Fluori-Methane or ice, for treatment of trigger points in muscles. The vapocoolant is sprayed over a stretched muscle to increase range of motion.

strength training: exercise directed to achieve the maximum capacity of a muscle to pull in a single effort.

Swiss ball exercises: use of an inflatable gymnastic ball with various movements for mobility, strength, balance, coordination, and stabilization of the spine and the extremities.

tapotement: a method of massage that involves percussion such as used in chest therapy.

therapeutic massage: soft tissue manipulation using techniques such as friction, stroking, and kneading to reduce muscle spasm and edema, stimulate circulation, and encourage relaxation. Also used to stretch scar tissue.

Williams (flexion) exercises: for patients with low back pain; exercises are performed to open the lumbar intervertebral foramina and decrease the compression on the facet joints by flexing the lumbosacral spine, thereby stretching the extensors of the back and strengthening the abdominal muscles.

Tests and Measurements*

Given that the circulation is intact, the major parameters in assessing the function of a limb are range of motion, sensation, and strength. These can be tested directly by the application of forces to the muscle and stimuli to the skin or can be assessed indirectly by electrodiagnostic modalities such as electromyography. In muscle testing, strength is graded by the following scale as assessed directly by the examiner. ROM is measured with a goniometer, an instrument that measures joint motion in degrees.

---

*For more specific information on various tests and examinations, an excellent source is American Orthopaedic Association: *Manual of Orthopaedic Surgery*, ed 6, Chicago, 1985, The Association.

Key to Manual Muscle Evaluation

% of Normal Strength	Numerical Score	Letter Score	Muscle Strength Criteria
100%	5	N	Normal: Complete ROM against gravity with full resistance
75%	4	G	Good: Complete ROM against gravity with some resistance
50%	3	F	Fair: Complete ROM against gravity
25%	2	P	Poor: Complete ROM with gravity eliminated
10%	1	T	Trace: Evidence of contractility
0	0	0	Zero: No evidence of contractility
S			Spasm*
C			Contracture*

From Daniels L, Worthingham C: Muscle Testing: Techniques of Manual Examination by Comparison, ed 4, Philadelphia, 1980, WB Saunders.
*If spasm or contracture exists, place S or C after the grade of a movement incomplete for this reason.

dynamometer: an instrument to measure muscle strength and its effects from exercise, such as a handgrip d. that can be adjusted to test strength in different positions of grasp; or from a bicycle d. that measures muscular, respiratory, and metabolic effects of exercise, recording directly from a pressure gauge; **ergometer.**

computerized isokinetic dynamometer: an apparatus that can be used to test and record the maximal strength of a muscle as it acts on a joint through a full range of motion. The recording is used to evaluate the progress of a patient's condition during recovery or to confirm the existence and extent of injury.

Institute of Sports Medicine and Athletic Trauma (ISMAT) muscle testing: manual assessment of muscle strength with a small, handheld (by the examiner) force-measuring device.

osteokinetic movement: movement that occurs between two bones such as rotation, swing, or spin.

Sensory Testing

heat and cold testing: self-explanatory.

pinprick test: a gross test to check two variables: (1) the actual ability to feel a pinprick and (2) the ability to determine the difference between sharp and dull.

pressure testing: involves sensation produced by touch to a localized area using an instrument that indicates the pressure needed to produce sensation.

proprioceptive testing: tests the ability to sense the position of a body part with the eyes closed.

tendon reflex examination: graded from 0 to 4 and varies widely in meaning from examiner to examiner; the test is performed by striking the tendon briskly and watching muscle reaction.

two-point discrimination: ability to perceive difference between one or two points of touch at the fingertips or elsewhere; this test of fine sensation is measured in centimeters or millimeters.

vibrator sense examination: tests the patient's ability to feel vibrations with use of a tuning fork.

Electrical Testing

electromyography (EMG): an electrodiagnostic test conducted on a special machine that evaluates the capability of nerves and muscles to transmit and respond to normal or stimulated electric impulses. The muscle is evaluated by direct insertion of a small needle to which the muscle responds with characteristic contractile activity, which is referred to as "insertional activity." Once the muscle has acclimated to the presence of the needle, individual muscle fiber activity can be seen electrically on an **oscilloscope** and is described by the specific wave patterns. Disorders affecting the nerves, such as a herniated disk, will eventually cause changes in the wave pattern of the muscle. Other disorders commonly evaluated with this study include entrapment syndromes and other neuropathic and muscle disorders. **Conduction time** is the measurement of nerve stimulation applied through the skin, allowing the nerve to transmit impulses. The conduction time is increased in neurologic disorders, such as vitamin B_1 deficiency and carpal tunnel syndrome caused by local nerve pressure.

nerve conduction velocity (NCV): a diagnostic test often performed with the EMG, this is a test of the integrity of peripheral nerve(s) that involves placing an electric stimulator over the nerve and measuring the time required for an impulse to travel over a segment of nerve; useful in the diagnosis of nerve entrapment syndrome and polyneuropathies.

Occupational Therapy

Occupational therapists are skilled clinicians in the art of maximizing patient outcomes in a variety of settings. Through functional client-based treatment, occupational therapists enable patients to restore, reinforce, and enhance performance; facilitate new adaptation and learning; diminish or correct abnormalities; and promote and maintain health. By looking at the client holistically, as well as outside factors such as environment, therapists endeavor to apply the skills and adaptations needed to complete everyday activities of living.

The *licensed registered occupational therapist (OTR/L)* is a medical professional that has been educated in a baccalaureate, master's, or doctoral curriculum accredited jointly by the Committee on Allied Health Education, American Medical Association, and the American Occupational Therapy Association (AOTA). They have passed a national certification examination (NBCOT), hold state licensure for practice, and have completed clinical placements under supervision in settings ranging from hospitals and school systems to private clinics. A certified occupational therapy assistant (COTA) has satisfactorily completed an occupational therapy assistant curriculum approved by AOTA, has passed a national certification examination and works under the supervision of an OTR.

Occupational therapists can specialize in specific types of therapy and settings by receiving further training, certification, and education. Those holding the title of Certified Hand Therapist (CHT) have been trained extensively in hand and upper extremity rehabilitation and have passed a formal board examination as such. Other specialties can include neurology, sensory integration, intensive care, cardiac, oncology, and pediatrics.

As of 2005, all graduating occupational therapists are required to possess a master's degree or higher to help advance their roles as specialized practitioner, educator, or researcher. This allows clinicians to further venture into evidence-based practice wherein research provides rationale and helps to guide and justify treatment choices. Within the last decade, occupational therapists have pushed this imperative practice to the forefront of clinical application. As quantity and quality of research improve, therapists will be able to align occupational therapy practice with that of other medical arenas.

Specific Occupational Therapist Services

Specific occupational therapist services include but are not limited to the following:

- education and training in activities of daily living (ADL).
- administering and interpreting such tests as manual muscle and range of motion.
- design, fabrication, and application of slings and orthoses.
- developing perceptual-motor skills and sensory integrative functioning.
- restoration of hand functioning due to a disease process, after surgery, and/or a traumatic event.
- instruction in work simplification, energy conservation, and use of proper body mechanics during activity for work, leisure, and/or daily living.
- guidance in the selection and use of adaptive equipment.
- therapeutic activities to enhance functional performance.
- prevocational evaluation and training and physical capacity evaluation.
- consultation concerning adaptation to home or work environments.

Occupational Therapy Assessment

Services are provided to all age groups in a variety of settings, including hospitals, hand clinics, rehabilitation facilities, sheltered workshops, schools, extended care facilities, private homes, community agency clinics, and industrial settings.

Orthopaedists most frequently refer patients to occupational therapists for amputation, arthritis, hand trauma, fractures (hip, femur, tibia, ankle, humerus, radius, ulna, wrist), total joint replacement, sports injury, osteoporosis, elbow and shoulder arthroplasty, spinal cord injury, and chronic pain. One fourth of

AOTA's more than 40,000 members work with orthopaedic patients.

Before treatment is given, each potential patient's case is *screened* to determine the need for occupational therapy. This is followed by assessment, which consists of obtaining and interpreting data necessary for treatment, including that needed to plan for and document the evaluation process and treatment results. The occupational therapy evaluation includes assessment of functional abilities and deficits as related to the patient's needs.

Specific Evaluations, Tests, and Devices

Specific evaluations, tests, and devices used in the assessment process include but are not limited to the following:

Baltimore therapeutic equipment work simulator (BTE): a device used for evaluation and work hardening as well as regaining specific movement via attachments.

bulb dynamometer: a soft, cylindrical, rubber-filled squeeze bulb that measures gross isometric grasp and pinch, calibrated in pounds per square inch, measuring force in pounds by multiplying the reading by four.

Crawford small parts dexterity test: for fine eye-hand coordination and manipulation of small hand tools.

functional capacities assessment: simple rating scale on living skills, indicating progress according to 10 functional levels.

Jamar dynamometer: measures gross isometric grasp in five positions and records in either pounds or kilograms.

Jebsen-Taylor hand function test: consisting of seven subtests to measure major aspects of hand function related to activities of daily living.

LIDO lift and workset: provides rehabilitation and evaluation of physical work-related activities.

Martin Vigorimeter: to test handgrip strength.

Minnesota rate of manipulation test: measures dexterity from seventh grade to adult level.

O'Connor finger dexterity test: designed to measure fine motor ability.

Pennsylvania bimanual worksample: measures finger dexterity of both hands, gross movements of both arms, eye-hand coordination, ability to use both hands simultaneously.

pinch: three-point lateral and fingertip prehension tested with pinch gauge recorded in pounds or kilograms.

Purdue pegboard: measures gross movements of arm, hand, and fingers and fingertip dexterity.

Semmes-Weinstein monofilament (VonFrey hair test): a series of monofilaments with different ratings to determine amount of sensory loss.

Smith physical capacities evaluation (Smith PCE): objective test to measure ability of individual to perform selected aspects of occupations.

two-point discrimination: measured with calibrated metric aesthesiometer.

Valpar component work sample series: consisting of 16 work samples designed to measure 17 work behaviors by task analysis; developed for workers with industrial injuries.

volumeter set: accurately measures hand and distal forearm edema for objective monitoring of edema-reducing treatment modalities with water displacement.

VonFrey hair test (Semmes-Weinstein monofilament): a series of monofilaments with different ratings to determine amount of sensory loss.

WEST (work evaluation systems technology): evaluating work tolerance of upper extremities and/or total body, including ability to measure lifting capabilities and torque strength of hand.

Occupational Therapy Treatments

Occupational therapists are known for providing a "just right" fit with treatment, taking personal factors into account for each person. This client-centered approach allows clinicians to creatively target specific needs to further patient outcomes. This is especially important with patients who have a multitude of problems in different areas such as an orthopaedic patient who may have residual deficits from a neurologic event. Treatment refers to the use of specific activities or methods to develop, improve, or restore the performance of necessary functions, compensate for dysfunction, or minimize debilitation. The therapist plans for and documents treatment performance to show progression as well as where more work is needed. The following are categories of necessary functions treated in occupational therapy for orthopaedic problems*:

Activities of daily living/physical daily living skills (ADL/PDLS) are components of everyday activity, including self-care, work, and play/leisure activities. These may also be referred to as life skills or life tasks and consist of the following.

bathing: ability to obtain and use supplies and soap, rinse and dry all body parts, maintain bathing position, transfer to and from bathing position, use adapted bathing equipment such as bath mitt, tub bench, grab bars, scrub brush, and so forth.

dressing: ability to select appropriate clothing, obtain clothing from storage area, dress and undress in sequential fashion, fasten/unfasten clothes and shoes, and don and doff appliances, for example, glasses, prostheses, or orthoses.

feeding/eating: ability to set up food, use appropriate regular or adapted utensils and tableware, and bring food or drink from table to mouth.

functional communication: ability to use equipment or systems to enhance or provide communication, such as writing equipment, telephones, typewriters, communication boards, call lights, emergency systems, braille writers, augmentative communication systems, and computers.

functional mobility: ability to move from one position or one place to another as in bed mobility, wheelchair mobility, transfers (bed, chair, tub, toilet, car), and functional ambulation with or without adaptive aids, driving, or use of public transportation.

grooming: ability to obtain and use supplies to shave, apply and remove cosmetics, wash, comb, style, and

---

*Definitions taken from Cromwell FS, Brollier C: *Occupational Therapy Product Output Reporting System and Uniform Terminology for Reporting Occupational Therapy,* ed 2, Rockville, MD, p 415.

brush hair, care for nails, care for skin, and apply deodorant.

toilet hygiene: ability to obtain and use supplies, clean self, and transfer to and from and maintain toileting position on bedpan, toilet, and/or commode.

Work activities include home management tasks such as clothing care, cleaning, meal preparation and clean-up, household maintenance, care of others, and safety procedures. The latter is important in preventing falls in areas such as bathroom, kitchen, and stairs.

Vocational activities consist of vocational exploration, job acquisition, and timely and effective job performance.

Play or leisure involves choosing and engaging in activities for amusement, relaxation, spontaneous enjoyment, or self-expression.

sensorimotor skills: consist of performance patterns of sensory and motor behavior prerequisite to self-care, work, and play and leisure performance, such as:
range of motion (ROM)
gross and fine coordination
muscle control
coordination
dexterity
strength and endurance
sensory awareness, including
    tactile awareness
    stereognosis
kinesthesia
proprioceptive awareness

cognitive skills: necessary mental processes, including orientation, conceptualization/comprehension (concentration, attention span, memory), and cognitive integration (applying diverse knowledge to environmental situations, including ability to generalize and problem solve).

prevention and minimization of debilitation: refers to programs for persons with predisposition to disability, as well as for those who have already incurred a disability, and includes the following:

energy conservation: activity restriction, work simplification, time management, or organization of the environment to minimize energy output.

joint protection: procedures to minimize stress on joints, including use of proper body mechanics, avoidance of static or deforming postures, and avoidance of excess weight-bearing.

positioning: placement of body part in alignment to promote optimal functioning; or position of tasks and objects in a position to maximize performance.

therapeutic adaptations: design or restructuring of the physical environment to assist self-care, work, and play and leisure performance through selecting, obtaining, fitting, and fabricating equipment, as well as instructing client, family, and staff in its proper use and care, including making minor repairs and modifications for correct fit, position, or use.

Some categories of therapeutic adaptation are:

orthotics, splints, or slings: to relieve pain, maintain joint alignment, protect joint integrity, improve function, or decrease deformity.

dynamic splints: an orthotic device that achieves its effects by movement and force generated by the patient's own musculature or external forces such as springs and rubber bands.

functional fracture bracing (using thermoplastics): proximal or distal to fracture, in combination with hinge joint to provide motion and allowing weight-bearing to enhance osteogenesis.

static splints: an orthotic device that immobilizes all involved joints and surrounding musculature for protection and healing purposes (Fig. 12-1).

static progressive splints: a low-load stretch achieved through a changeable matrix; as a patient progresses, the splint can be advanced to provide more of a challenge to further advance movement and overall range of motion.

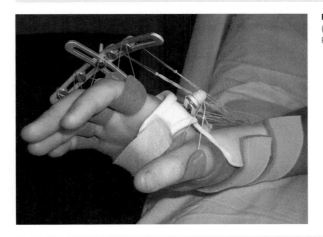

FIG 12-1 Dynamic splint for patient with high radial nerve lesion. (From Amanda Calhoon, Shady Grove Center for Sports Medicine, Rockville, MD.)

prosthetics: in this context, an artificial device used to replace a missing body part such as a limb, tooth, eye, or heart valve. Occupational therapists play a key role with said clients in adaptation and functional integration of prosthetic.

assistive/adaptive equipment: additions or devices that assist in performance or in structural or positional changes, such as installing ramps and bars, changing furniture heights, adjusting traffic patterns, and modifying wheelchairs. Some typical adaptive equipment examples for orthopaedics are reachers, sockdonners, elevated toilet seats, leg-lifter straps, and walker adaptations (platforms and walker bags).

Introduction: The Research Enterprise

13

Orthopaedic research encompasses a wide range of clinical, basic science, and epidemiologic investigation on the embryology, growth, development, and remodeling of the musculoskeletal system and of its response to disease and treatment. The single clinician/scientist working alone in a laboratory is becoming increasingly rare; most research efforts of recent years are interdisciplinary and take the form of teams of clinicians, basic scientists, engineers, epidemiologists, statisticians, and laboratory technicians.

A relatively small amount of the effort and time involved in biomedical research is taken up in actually performing the experiment and analyzing the results. Considerable effort is taken in the process of developing the research proposal, through which the investigators request permission and/or funds to conduct a study, and in reporting the results to the general scientific community.

The Research Proposal

Research proposals are submitted to internal, institutional bodies, to not-for-profit foundations, to corporations for extramural research, or to government agencies for extramural research, often in response to a **request for applications (RFA)** announced by the agency. By far the largest sources of orthopaedic research funding in the United States are the National Institutes of Health (**NIH**), an agency of the Department of Health and Human Services consisting of 19 separate institutes (e.g., **NIAMS**, the National Institute of Arthritis and Musculoskeletal and Skin Diseases).

The objective of the research proposal is to demonstrate to the reviewers that the proposed studies are necessary, reasonable, and feasible. The research proposal and the process of evaluating it differ between funding mechanisms and agencies, but most follow this general outline:

The investigators list **specific aims** for the proposed research, overall questions for which the research program is designed to provide general answers.

The investigators propose testable **hypotheses** associated with the specific aims, to which the proposed work will be addressed.

The **background and significance** of the research question is reviewed; what is known in the field, and what is controversial, are established and delineated.

The **materials and methods** of the proposed studies are outlined, as is a **plan for data analysis.**

Preliminary data (either supporting the proposed hypotheses, or demonstrating the ability to perform the proposed experiments) and a **sample size analysis** are presented.

Finally, a **budget** is proposed, with provisions for both **direct costs** (those actually involved in performing the study, including supplies, equipment, personnel, etc.) and **indirect costs** (usually a percentage of the direct costs, used for institutional overhead ["keeping the lights on"]).

Review processes differ between applications and institutions, but generally this task is given to a board of anonymous **peer reviewers** (scientists working in the same or closely related field). Many times, comments of the reviewers are forwarded to the investigators (in the case of the NIH, taking the form of the infamous **"pink sheets,"** which long ago stopped being pink), in the interests of improving the proposal for subsequent submissions. Often the task of evaluating a proposal is kept institutionally separate from the actual funding decisions. As a result, at times a research proposal may be approved but not funded.

Provisions for adequate protection and humane use of subjects must be addressed (in the case of human patients, by the **institutional review board [IRB]**; in the case of other animals by the **institutional animal care and use committee [IACUC]**). Local, institutional committees are also charged with reviewing the proposed use of radioisotopes, toxic material, or recombinant DNA; the concerns of these bodies must be addressed before the study is allowed to begin.

Reporting the Results

Usually the first step in reporting results to the scientific community takes the form of **abstracts** (poster presentations, or short podium presentations) at regional, national, or international meetings, such as those of the American Academy of Orthopaedic Surgeons (AAOS), the Orthopaedic Research Society (ORS), or the American Society for Bone and Mineral Research (ASBMR). Some of these venues provide anonymous peer reviews but with limited feedback to the investigators in the form of comments (in most cases, the investigators are told that the submitted abstract is either accepted or rejected, with no further comment). Published abstracts, with improved Internet applications, are becoming more available to those members of the community who do not personally attend the meetings, but these reports tend to be short, preliminary, and terse. The advantage of these venues is their relative speed and the opportunity for feedback from peers at the actual meeting.

Full **reports of original research,** to be published in journals (such as *Bone, Journal of Biomechanics,*

Journal of Orthopaedic Research, Journal of Bone and Mineral Research), the next step in the process, are fully analyzed and interpreted by the investigators. These are submitted to the editors of the journals, who then forward the manuscripts (often with authors and institutions redacted) to anonymous peer reviewers. Detailed feedback is provided to the investigators regarding methods and interpretations; often several iterations of the process are required before a paper is accepted for publication.

Review papers, often invited papers in journals by recognized leaders in a particular field, are designed to summarize the current state of the art and historical perspectives on a topic from many sources but generally do not include new data.

General Research Terminology

The following terms are likely to be found in many areas of research. They have been divided into statistics, biomechanics, techniques in measurements, and orthopaedic cell and tissue biology (general, cartilage, and bone).

Statistics and Epidemiology

accuracy: the property of a measurement denoting its proximity to some gold-standard "true" value. A measurement may be accurate without being precise (e.g., giving a wide range of test results, centered about the true value).

alpha value: the benchmark value that, *a priori*, is established to determine statistical significance. The alpha value is compared to the p value given by the data. If $p \leq \alpha$, then statistical significance has been established. In most cases, $\alpha = 0.05$.

ANOVA: analysis of variance, a method for evaluating differences in a continuous variable between multiple groups. The ANOVA may be further classified as to the number of grouping types being considered:

one-way ANOVA: considers only one categorical variable, which may itself have many possible values (e.g., gender, ethnicity, disease status). When the number of groups is two (e.g., male/female, young/old, diseased/not diseased), the one-way ANOVA reduces to a *t* test.

two-way ANOVA: (and more complex versions, involving three, four, or more "ways") considers simultaneously the effect of two or more categorical variables (e.g., the effect of gender and ethnicity on patient height would be properly addressed using a two-way ANOVA), along with the **interaction** between the variables.

Bayesian statistics (after Rev. Thomas Bayes, 1702–1761, British cleric): a family of statistical techniques in which the interpretation of the results of an experiment includes an evaluation of the results of similar, previous experiments to establish statistical significance. Used in some applications of evidence-based medicine.

categorical variable: a parameter characterized by having a limited number of possible values (e.g., male/female, old/middle-aged/young, right/left) (cf. continuous variable).

chi-square (χ^2) analysis: a test for determining whether the proportions of data described by two or more categorical variables is random (e.g., 51% of the people with a particular disease are men. Is the disease gender-related?).

confidence interval: an estimate of the range in which a particular percentage of values (usually 95%) may be found.

continuous variable: a parameter characterized by having an infinite number of possible values (e.g., height, weight, blood pressure, age) (cf. categorical variable).

correlation: the strength of the relationship between two continuous variables, with no assumption as to which of the variables may be causative (cf. **regression**). The method gives a p value and an **r value.** r values range between -1.000 (perfect negative relationship) and 1.000 (perfect positive relationship), with a value of 0.000 denoting no statistical relationship.

Fisher exact test (after Sir R.A. Fisher, 1890–1962, British statistician and agronomist): a test for determining whether the proportions of data described by two or more categorical variables is random. It is similar in concept to the χ^2 analysis but is more appropriate in cases in which the number of observations is small.

input variable (predictor variable, or independent variable; the X-axis): the parameter(s) that is/are varied experimentally (cf. output variable).

logistic regression: a special form of regression, in which the dependent variable is a categorical (usually binary) parameter. It is often used in outcomes research and epidemiology, in which the output variables are parameters such as diseased/not diseased, healed/not healed, and so forth.

nonparametric test: a distribution-free method (usually rank-ordered) of dealing with nonnormally distributed data (e.g., a Spearman rank-order test in place of a Pearson product-moment correlation; a Wilcoxon signed-rank test in place of a paired t test; a Kruskal-Wallis statistic in place of a one-way ANOVA).

normal distribution: a continuous parameter characterized by a frequency distribution that is Gaussian, that is, bell-shaped, symmetrical, with a maximum number of values at the average, 68% of the values found within one standard deviation of the mean, and 95% of the values found within 1.96 standard deviations of the mean. A normal distribution of the data is a basic assumption of a parametric test; if the data are decidedly nonnormal, then nonparametric tests should be used.

odds ratio (OR): the effect of a risk factor in increasing or decreasing the probability of an outcome, often determined by a logistic regression. By convention, if OR > 1, the outcome is more probable with addition of the risk factor (e.g., body mass index as a risk factor and osteoarthritis as the outcome); if OR < 1, the outcome is less probable with addition of the risk factor (e.g., regular exercise as the risk factor, and heart disease as the outcome).

output variable (dependent variable; the Y-axis): the variables that are measured to represent the response to changes in the input variable(s) (cf. input variable).

p value: the probability that a finding of a difference between groups, or of a correlation between parameters, is due to chance alone.

parametric test: statistical methods, such as linear regressions, ANOVAs, and t tests, which are based on estimates of the mean and variance of a population and which inherently assume a normal distribution of these values (Table 13-1).

***post-hoc* (multiple comparison) tests:** when an ANOVA provides evidence of a statistically significant effect of a particular parameter with three or

TABLE 13-1 Basic Parametric Statistical Techniques

	Input Variable	
Output variable	*Continuous*	*Categorical*
Continuous	Regression, Correlation	ANOVA *t* test
Categorical	Logistic, Regression	Chi-square, Fisher exact test

ANOVA, Analysis of variance.

more possible values (e.g., ethnicity, old/middle-aged/young), these tests are used in place of multiple *t* tests to determine which groups are different from which other ones. For instance, blood pressure may be significantly higher in a group of older patients than in the corresponding group of young patients, but neither may be significantly different from the values found in the middle-aged groups. Several methods are in common use, including the Tukey, Student-Newman-Kuels (SNK), Fisher least-squared difference, Duncan, and Bonferroni tests when making all pairwise comparisons; Dunnett's test when comparing test groups with a single control group, or McNemar's test as a nonparametric, pairwise test.

power: the probability that a finding of no difference between groups, or of no correlation between variables, is in fact true; alternatively, the probability of being able to statistically discern a significant difference between groups, or a correlation between variables, should one exist, given the existing sample size and variance. Generally, the minimum power for a definitive finding of no difference or no correlation is 0.80.

precision: the property of a measurement denoting its repeatability. A measurement may be precise without being accurate (e.g., tightly clustered about a value that is not correct).

pseudoreplication: statistical situation that occurs when more than one measurement is taken from a single individual. Such measurements cannot be considered as independent of one another. Special statistical tests are used in these cases, for example, the paired *t* test, the repeated-measures ANOVA, and the mixed-model ANOVA.

regression: a method of comparing two or more continuous variables, in which the relationship between the variables (usually in a linear form) is specifically described in terms of one or more independent, or causative variables, and a single dependent, or output variable. The method gives the geometric equation of the relationship (in the linear form, dependent variable = a **constant** + [a **slope** × independent variable]), a *p* **value** for both the constant (determining whether the constant is significantly different from zero) and for the slope (determining whether the slope is significantly different from zero), and an r^2 value, which is often interpreted as denoting the percentage of the variability in the data that is explained by the regression equation. The square root of the r^2 value is exactly the r value that would be obtained if a simple correlation between the variables were calculated.

sample size: in general, the sample size for a study, at best determined before the study is initiated, depends on:

- **the variability of the measurements:**
  - measurement accuracy and precision (which may be estimated by the standard error). The more accurate and precise the measurement, the smaller the sample size required.
  - variability within the population (which may be estimated by the standard deviation). The smaller the population variability, the smaller the sample size required.
- **the nature of the question to be addressed:**
  - for comparisons of data between categories (e.g., male vs. female, diseased vs. nondiseased), the difference between means of categories (quantified as the **effect size,** the difference between means, divided by the standard deviation). The larger the effect size, the smaller the sample size required.
  - for comparisons of continuous variables (e.g., age vs. blood pressure), the slope of the relationship between predictor and outcome variables, in a regression. The further the slope is from 0, the smaller the sample size required.
  - the chance of being wrong that the investigator is willing to accept (the alpha value, and the power). The higher the chance of being

wrong the investigator is willing to accept, the smaller the sample size required.

standard deviation (SD): a measure of the variability of a parameter in a population, equal to the positive square root of the variance. By definition, in a normally distributed population, 95% of the values of the parameter will be found within 1.96 standard deviations of the mean. Unlike standard error, the standard deviation is relatively insensitive to the sample size. It is always larger than the standard error.

standard error (standard estimate of the mean, SEM, or SE): a measure of the reliability of the mean of a parameter. By definition, if samples are taken of a normally distributed population, 95% of the time, the true mean will fall within 1.96 standard errors of the sample mean. The standard deviation is quite sensitive to the sample size; as the sample size approaches a census of the target population, the standard error by its very definition approaches zero. The standard error may be estimated as (the standard deviation) / (the square root of the sample size).

statistical errors: these are generally divided into two types:

type I error: in which a correlation between continuous variables or a difference between groups is asserted when such correlations or differences do not in fact exist. The probability of making a type I error is α.

type II error: in which a finding of no correlation between continuous variables, or no differences between groups is asserted, when such correlations or differences do in fact exist. The probability of making a type II error is 1-power, or β.

t test (Student's *t* test): a method for evaluating differences in a continuous variable between two groups. As such, it comprises a special case of the **one-way ANOVA**.

variance (s^2): a measure of the spread of the data. The formula for this measure is:

$$s^2 = \left(\left(\sum \chi^2\right) - \left(\left[\sum \chi^2\right]/n\right)\right)/(n - 1),$$

where $\sum \chi^2$ is the sum of all the squared values, $(\sum \chi^2)$ is the square of the summed values, and n is the number of observations.

TABLE 13-2 Evaluating Clinical Tests

	True Disease Status		
Test Result	*Positive*	*Negative*	*Negative*
Positive	a	b	a + b
Negative	c	d	c + d
Totals	a + c	b + d	a + b + c + d

Evaluating Clinical Tests

Assuming that there is some readily available "gold standard" of disease status, clinical tests may be evaluated using the terms found in Table 13-2.

Population Indices on the Columns

sensitivity: a/a + c (the part of the first column that is true).

specificity/selectivity: d/b + d (the part of the second column that is true).

Individual Indices on the Rows

positive predictive value: a/a + b (the part of the first row that is true).

negative predictive value: d/c + d (the part of the second row that is true).

Therefore, for example, if {Low Test Result} = Diseased and {High Test Result} = Not diseased, then

- make a test more sensitive (move the cutoff to the right in the example above, Fig. 13-1), and you will correctly classify more of the diseased population (more true positives). You will also falsely classify more of the nondiseased population as diseased (more false positives).

- make a test more specific/selective (move the cutoff to the left in the example above), and you will correctly classify more of the nondiseased population (more true negatives). You will also falsely clear more of the diseased population (more false negatives).

Study Design

Studies may be classified as a series of binary descriptors:

1. *experimental/interventional,* in which the investigator actively does something to change a risk factor (e.g., drug/placebo tests) compared with

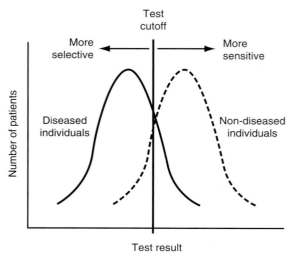

FIG 13-1 A comparison of the terms "sensitive" and "selective," for a test in which a low value implies disease and a high value implies no disease.

observational/effectiveness, in which the investigator takes no active role in the status of a risk factor.

2. *prospective,* in which the risk factor may or may not have occurred at the time of the study, but the outcome has not compared with
   retrospective, in which both the risk factor and the outcome have occurred at the time of the study.
3. *descriptive,* in which the outcomes are qualitatively reported compared with
   analytic, in which the outcomes are subjected to quantification and numerical analysis.

Study Groups

target population: the group to whom the results of the study will be inferred (e.g., all mammals, all people, all young people).

sample population: the specific part of the target population that the investigator has the ability to measure.

disease incidence: new cases per population at risk per time. This may be estimated with a *cohort* study, in which a group of subjects are followed, with multiple observations, over a defined period.

disease prevalence: cases per population at risk at one point in time (generally given as a percentage). This may be estimated with a *cross-sectional* study,

in which all observations are made, once per subject, at a defined time (e.g., next Thursday, or at first presentation).

Biomechanics

The field of biomechanics is concerned with the application of physical and engineering principles to issues of biologic interest.

acceleration: change in velocity per unit of time.
   angular acceleration (degrees, or radians/time^2): change in rotational velocity per time.
   linear acceleration (distance/time^2): change in velocity in a straight line/time.

adaptation: biologically mediated changes in mechanical properties of tissues associated with the mechanical milieu of the tissues.

anisotropy: the quality, usually of a material, of having varying mechanical properties (e.g., strength, stiffness) depending on the direction of applied forces (e.g., reflected in the grain in a piece of wood).

bending: deformation of a structure in response to a load applied to an unsupported portion of the structure.

bending moment, torque (N-m): the product of force applied and the distance from the point of application to the point of interest.

brittle: characterized by having a relatively small deformation before failure (e.g., glass) (cf. plastic or ductic).

center of mass (center of gravity): the point about which the mass of the object can be balanced.

centroid: the geometric center of a body. In an object of constant thickness, made of a homogeneous material, the centroid and the center of mass are at the same point.

coefficient of friction: ratio of tangential force to the interbody compressive force required to initiate motion between bodies.

compliance: deformation per load (inverse of stiffness).

compression: tending to push objects together. By convention, compressive forces or motions are considered to be negative in sign.

couple: a pair of equal and opposite parallel forces acting on a body and separated by some distance.

creep: deformation with time under a constant load (cf. stress relaxation).

degrees of freedom: the number of independent variables in a coordinate system required to completely define the position of an object in space.

displacement: a measurment of change in position in response to force; expressed in units of volume such as fluid displacement.

dynamic load: load that varies over time (cf. stress relaxation).

elastic: tending to return to original dimensions after the deforming force has been removed. By this definition, rubber bands might be considered elastic (nonlinearly elastic) but so might concrete (linearly elastic).

elongation: deformation caused by a tensile load, a measure of ductility.

energy (newton-meters, joules): the ability to do work, or the work added to a system by a force or a deformation.

equilibrium: the state of not accelerating, in which the sum of all forces acting on a body is zero.

factor of safety: ratio of structural or materials strength of a body to its load (structure) or stress (materials) encountered in normal service.

fatigue: failure or damage as a result of the cyclic application of multiple submonotonic-failure loads.

fatigue limit (endurance limit): the cyclic load a material or structure can endure indefinitely without damage.

finite element analysis (FE, FEA, or finite element modeling, FEM): a method of stress analysis, usually done on a computer. The geometry of the structure of interest is divided into regularly shaped elements, each with multiple nodes. The material of each element is defined in terms of its modulus and Poisson's ratio. Loading conditions (nodes of application and direction of loads) and constraints (limits on node motion) are defined. Changes in node-to-node distance are then calculated; from these can be calculated local stresses and strains.

free-body diagram (FBD): analytical technique in which a body and all the forces acting on it, and their points of application, are delineated. In its simplest form, an assumption is made of no net motion (equilibrium), although dynamic FBDs are also used.

helical axis of motion: a unique axis in space that completely defines a three-dimensional motion between two rigid bodies, analogous to instantaneous axis of rotation for planar motion.

hysteresis: consequence of cycling of a nonlinearly elastic material, or of post-yield, prefailure cycling of a linearly elastic material or structure, in which the stress-strain or force-deformation curves for increasing and decreasing deformations are not superimposed. The area of the stress-strain curve between the increasing and decreasing legs of the test represent the energy lost in the maneuver (Fig. 13-2).

impulse (units: N-s): a measure of impact properties.

inertia (units: kg): the property of a body that imparts **mass**; the tendency of a body at rest to remain at rest and of a body in motion to remain in motion.

instantaneous axis of rotation: when one body rotates about another, the distance from each point in the moving body to a single point in the stationary body remains constant. In more complex kinematics, the position of this point in the stationary body itself moves. The instantaneous axis of rotation is a line perpendicular to the plane of motion and passing through this point.

isotropy: the quality, usually of a material, of having constant mechanical properties (e.g., strength, stiffness) regardless of the direction of applied forces.

kinematics: the study of motion, without respect to energy input or output.

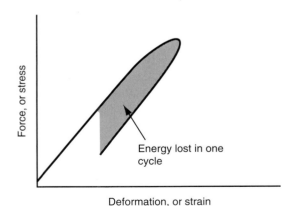

FIG 13-2 Energy loss (energy, or work = force × distance), due to hysteresis in one cycle.

kinesiology: the study of motion and of the forces that produce it.

kinetic energy (KE) (= 0.5 × mass × velocity^2): the energy possessed by a body in motion.

kinetics: the study of energy relationships with respect to motion.

load (= mass × acceleration): force applied to an object.

lubrication: any of a number of means towards reducing friction between surfaces (e.g., joint surfaces).

boundary lubrication: characterized by a thin layer (down to a single molecule thick) of fluid between surfaces.

film lubrication: in this type of lubrication, the opposing surfaces are kept completely apart by a thick layer of fluid.

elastohydrodynamic lubrication: lubrication that occurs when the bearing surfaces are relatively compliant and deform away from their opposing surface by the action of the lubricant.

squeeze film lubrication: characterized by a pressurized layer of fluid between surfaces.

hydrodynamic lubrication: in a relatively thicker layer of lubricant, hydrodynamic lubrication is created when the friction between lubricant molecules (related to the viscosity) acts to drag fluid into the space between surfaces. Generally most applicable during rapid joint movement.

weeping lubrication: lubrication caused by the extrusion of fluid from the matrix of the surfaces.

moment of inertia (MOI): one of several measurements of the distribution of material around an arbitrary plane or axis; in general, proportional to the structure's resistance to bending about that axis. Where m = the mass of a particle in the body, A = the area of that particle, x = the distance from that particle to the plane, and r = the distance from that particle to the axis.

area MOI: or second moment of the area: ($I = \Sigma Ax^2$), units in m^4; essentially the mass moment of inertia of a material whose density is 1 kg/m^2, but useful as a generalization or first approximation in which the density variability within the body is negligible or unknown.

mass MOI: ($I = \Sigma mx^2$), units in kg•m^2.

polar MOI: ($I = \Sigma mr^2$, or $I = \Sigma Ar^2$), units in kg•m^2 or m^4, respectively; useful in the special case of torsion about an axis.

momentum: a characteristic of a moving body, related to its ability to maintain its motion.

linear momentum (units N•s): the tendency of a moving body to pursue a straight path at a constant velocity.

angular momentum (mass moment of inertia × angular velocity, units N•m•s, or Planck): the tendency of a spinning body to continue spinning at a constant angular velocity.

normal (not the statistical definition): perpendicular to a surface.

plastic, or ductile: characterized by having a relatively large deformation before failure (e.g., a willow stick) (cf. brittle).

Poisson's ratio (ν, no units): ratio of lateral deformation to axial deformation (e.g., barreling in a compression test, necking in a tensile test).

potential energy (PE): the capacity of a body at rest to do work (e.g., by virtue of its height, PE = mass × acceleration due to gravity × height).

rheology: the study of fluid flow.

scalar: a parameter having only a quantity, with no directional information (cf. vector).

shear: a force or deformation oriented parallel to a surface.

stiffness (units differ, depending on the application): force/deformation, a structural property.

strain (units): strictly speaking, strain (deformation/original dimension) has no units. However, it is often expressed in microstrain (με), where 1με = a deformation/original dimension ratio of 1×10^{-6}. 10,000με = 1% deformation.

strength: maximum load (structure) or stress (materials) before yield or failure, depending on the specific application, occurs.

stress relaxation: viscoelastic decrease in load with time under constant deformation (cf. creep).

stress-strain curve: all mechanical tests, especially of objects of biologic origin, are tests of **structure** (e.g., whole-bone tests, tests of individual trabeculae), and most result in the development of a **force** (Y-axis)-**deformation** (X-axis) curve. Under certain conditions (e.g., milled specimens, continuum

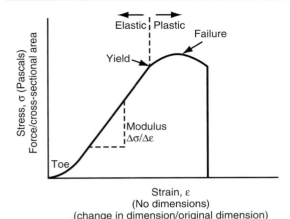

FIG 13-3 A classical stress-strain curve of a linearly elastic/plastic material, with the important components marked.

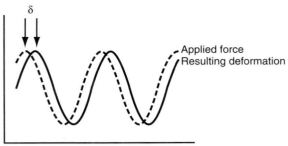

FIG 13-4 An example of the results of a dynamic mechanical analysis (DMA), with time on the horizontal axis. Delta (δ) represents the phase-angle difference (the "lag") between the applied stress and the resulting strain.

assumptions, or simplified geometry), a useful fiction is that of the **material** (or **materials**) test, in which the units are theoretically controlled for specimen size and shape (Fig. 13-3).

toe region: nonlinear region at the beginning of the test. Generally considered as an artifact of the testing machine-specimen gripping apparatus.

linear elastic region: region in which the increase in stress is directly proportional to the increase in strain.

yield point: point at which the strain begins to increase disproportionately to the increase in stress, in comparison to the ratio suggested by the modulus. Stress at the yield point is the yield strength of the material; associated with the onset of permanent damage and deformation.

plastic (post-yield) region: region between yield and failure.

failure point: point of maximum stress. Stress at the failure point is the **ultimate strength (Pa)** of the material. For some materials, plastic deformation can continue past the failure point.

modulus (Pa): material stiffness, defined as change in stress/change in strain.

energy, or work to yield, or to failure: energy put into the system (can be measured as the area under the stress-strain curve) from the beginning of the test to the yield point, or to the failure point, respectively.

tangent-delta, or Tan-δ (units radians): in an oscillatory viscoelastic test, a measure of the phase angle between an applied stress or strain and the resulting strain or stress, respectively (Fig. 13-4).

tension: tending to pull objects apart; by convention, tensile forces or motions are considered to be positive in sign.

tribology (or tiotribology): the study of friction, lubrication, and wear.

vector: a parameter having both a quantity and a direction (cf. scalar).

viscoelasticity: a materials or structural property, characterized by demonstrating a change in mechanical properties as a function of the speed of load application.

viscosity (units pascal-second, or kg/sm): a measure of the resistance of a fluid to flow.

wear: loss of surface material, associated with relative motion of interacting surfaces.

abrasive wear: wear due to contact between a relatively soft and a relatively hard material, resulting in a cutting of the softer material.

adhesive wear: wear due to formation of a temporary junction between one surface and another, pulling out fragments of the weaker material.

weight: (units N) mass times the local gravitational pull (on Earth, 9.81 m/s^2).

work: force times displacement (units Nm).

Measurements and Techniques

computed tomography (CT), or **computer-assisted tomography (CAT):** two- and three-dimensional imaging modality in which multiple x-ray absorption profiles are taken as the x-ray source and collection device are rotated about the patient or specimen. These are then constructed into two- and three-dimensional images by computer postprocessing.

quantitative CT (QCT): computed tomography in which the patient or specimen is imaged along with a set of solid or fluid calibration controls.

micro CT: extremely high resolution (on the order of μm) small-specimen CT.

dual-energy x-ray absorptiometry (DXA, or DEXA): two-dimensional imaging modality in which two simultaneous single-energy x-ray sources are passed over the patient or specimen. With appropriate computerized postprocessing, the resulting image can for instance give a measure of bone density that is independent of the overlying soft tissue densities.

electrophoresis and blotting: any of a number of techniques for separating molecules by their electric charge, in which the unseparated mixture is placed in a gel substrate and subjected to an electric field. The individual molecules then migrate until they reach their isoelectric point, at which point a combination of the molecular size and charge prevents further motion within the gel. The pattern of molecules is then transferred (blotted) by contact to nitrocellulose or nylon sheets.

Western blot: a method of measuring protein presence. A solution of many proteins is fractionated and transferred. The sheet is then exposed to an antibody specific to the protein in question, which is then imaged with autoradiography (a radiolabeled protein or antibody, exposed to photographic or radiographic film) or by stain-linked second antibodies.

Northern blot: a method of measuring gene expression. Single-stranded RNA is fractionated and transferred, and the sheet is exposed (*hybridized*) to a radiolabeled DNA probe, which, if the strands are complementary, stick together. The sheet is then washed and exposed to photographic or radiographic film. Areas in which hybridization has occurred, that is, in which the RNA is complementary to the probe, appear dark.

Southern blot: a method of measuring gene presence. Double-stranded DNA is fractionated and transferred, and the sheet is exposed to a radiolabeled DNA probe. The sheet is then washed and exposed to photographic or radiographic film. Bands that contain DNA that is complementary to the probe appear dark.

There is no Eastern blot.

enzyme-linked immunosorbent assay (ELISA): a competitive binding assay using an immunoglobulin attached to an enzyme-generated chromophoric substance that, when the complex attaches to a specific antigen, will reveal and quantitate (when read by a photosensor) the amount of antigen present.

flow cytometry: device and techniques for sorting particles (usually cells) by differential fluorescence. Particles in a suspension are stained with a fluorescent dye. The particles are the run past a laser fluorescent excitatory and emission detector in single file.

force plate: a device used in kinetics and kinematics, generally consisting of a flat plate with multiple piezoelectric sensors underneath. The forces imparted by interaction between the test subject and the plate (for instance, while running across the plate) can then be measured, as a function of time, in the X (in the direction of motion), Y (in the lateromedial direction), and Z (normal to the plate) directions.

high-performance (or high-pressure) liquid chromatography (HPLC): a means of making rapid separation of solutes with the use of small-bead ion-exchange or gel-filtration columns under high pressure.

in vitro: ("in glass") (also, **ex vivo**) analysis of a process that takes place outside the living body (e.g., cell culture, dissection), often written in italics.

in vivo: ("in the live") analysis of a process within a living animal, often written in italics.

magnetic resonance imaging (MRI): two- and three-dimensional imaging modality, based on the magnetic spin characteristics of molecules (for the most part, water) within a tissue.

mechanical testing: devices and techniques for applying controlled loads and/or deformations to structures and materials and for measuring resulting deformations and/or loads, respectively.

microarray (or genome chip): a glass or nylon substrate, to which has been adhered nucleic acid probes for known genes or gene products in spots of 200-μm diameter or less. When an unknown sample in solution is placed in contact with this chip and subjected to standard hybridization techniques (miniaturized), the state of expression of thousands of genes can be determined simultaneously and quickly.

microscopy: devices and techniques for preparing specimens, magnifying images, and measuring features on the resulting images.

backscatter electron microscopy (BSE): scanning electron microscopy (SEM) in which the energy of the resulting photons is analyzed for characteristics of the elements present within the sample.

bright-field microscopy: classical laboratory unit, in which a light is passed through a condenser, then transmitted through a thinly sliced specimen (embedded in wax [paraffin] or plastic [commonly polymethylmethacrylate]), then through an objective lens, and finally through an ocular lens to the user or to a camera. With oil immersion lenses, resolution of 0.2 μm is possible.

confocal scanning microscopy (CSM): computerized bright-field microscopy (usually used in conjunction with fluorescence), in which the focus point is altered automatically during the imaging process, resulting in a longer depth of field.

dark-field microscopy: a means of imaging living microscopy, in which the light source is directed parallel to the microscope slide, and the scattered light is collected by the lenses.

differential interference contrast microscopy (DIC, Nomarski): a means of imaging living cells, in which the brightness of the image is proportional to the gradient in refraction index of the material.

fluorescence microscopy: bright field microscopy, in which a fluorescent dye (one which absorbs light at one frequency, causing it to emit light at a different frequency) is applied to tissues being studied. Two filters are used, one which limits the light entering the specimen to the **excitation frequency,** and one that limits the light after it passes through the specimen to the **emission frequency.**

Fourier transform infrared (FTIR) spectroscopy and microscopy: a means of imaging material based on the reflection and analysis of infrared portion of the spectrum.

histomorphometry: any of a number of methods, both manual and automated, for measuring the size and shape of objects as they appear on a histologic section.

microradiography: high-resolution (<1 μm) x-ray imaging of thin specimens, imaged with bright-field microscopy.

phase contrast microscopy: a means of imaging living cells, complementary to DIC, in which the brightness of the image is proportional to the refractive index of the material.

polarized light microscopy: bright-field microscopy, in which two polarizing filters are placed in the light path, one above and one the specimen. Often used to determine the general direction of populations of collagen molecules.

Raman spectroscopy and microscopy: a means of imaging material based on the Raman effect, in which a certain number of photons directed at a surface are reflected inelastically, that is, a loss of energy is recorded, generally as a function of the molecular bond length and vibration status.

scanning electron microscopy (SEM): in this imaging modality, the surface of a structure is bombarded at a discrete point in a raster pattern by an electron beam, and the electrons that are scattered by this interaction are counted by a detector. The brightness of the corresponding point on an imaging device (usually a cathode-ray tube) is set proportionally to the number of electrons counted. The electron beam on both the specimen and on the imaging device are then moved, and the process is repeated.

transmission electron microscopy (TEM): the principles of TEM are not unlike those of bright-field microscopy; the illumination source used is the accelerated electron, the specimens are much thinner, and the resolution is improved to the angstrom range.

microsphere: small glass or polystyrene beads, injected intravenously or intra-arterially for studies involving vascularization and local ischemia.

motion analysis: any of a number of techniques for quantifying kinematics and kinetics, usually involving light or radiographic imaging, as well as measurements of joint angles **(goniometry),** force plate analysis and electrical evidence of muscle activity **(electromyography, EMG).**

photogrammetry: technique for motion analysis, in which two or more images are taken with the image collection devices at known positions. The relative positions of known points that are present on both images can then be calculated. **Radio-photogrammetry** is photogrammetry accomplished with x-ray equipment.

polymerase chain reaction: a method for amplifying selected DNA (for instance, from a particular gene of interest) to measurable amounts from small samples by repeated gentle heating (to separate DNA strands), cooling (annealing) with hybridization with known DNA primers, and polymerization with the four DNA bases in the presence of a DNA polymerase. A reverse polymerase chain reaction can measure the presence of mRNA in the cell.

radioactive tracers: a variety of compounds are used in orthopaedic research to follow specific biologic activity. The most common tracers used are:

^{45}Ca	^{67}Ga
^{3}H (tritium)	^{99m}Tc
^{51}Cr	^{85}Sr
$^{35}SO_4$	

stress-generated potentials (SGP): any electrical potential (voltage) produced by mechanical deformation.

  piezoelectric: a potential that is developed on the molecular surface of a material when that material is deformed.

  streaming (zeta): a potential that is created by the passage of charged ions in fluids passing by fixed surface charges.

strain gauge (or gage): a device for measuring deformation. Designs and construction differ between applications, but generally these consist of a miniature conductor printed on a thin piece of plastic, which is then glued to the structure of interest. As the structure is deformed, there is a change in the resistance of the conductor, which can then be amplified and calibrated through a **Wheatstone bridge** circuit, and converted into units of strain.

transgenic animals: animals in which particular genes have been added to **(knockins)** or removed from **(knockouts)** the germ line.

Units of Measurement

The basic International System (SI) units for length, mass, time, and temperature are, respectively, the meter, gram, second, and degree Celsius (centigrade), and are listed below, along with their English system equivalents. The dalton is used as a measure of molecular mass. Force and pressure are derived quantities (Table 13-3).

The triple point of water is $0.01°$ C (that point at which water may exist as a gas, liquid, and solid in thermodynamic equilibrium at standard atmospheric pressure); $-273.16°$ C (0 Kelvin) is defined as absolute zero, and water boils at standard atmospheric pressure at $100°$ C.

One **hertz (Hz)** is defined as one cycle per second.

Orthopaedic Cell and Tissue Biology
General

adipogenesis: the process of producing adipose, or fatty tissue.

agarose: purified plant protein gel, used in electrophoresis as the matrix through which the molecules travel.

angiogenesis: the process of creating new blood vessels.

apoptosis: programmed cell death, in which the cell and nucleus are systematically condensed and fragmented in a well-defined series of molecular events. Cf. **necrosis,** in which the cells swell and burst.

biglycan: core protein with two glycosaminoglycan (GAG) chains.

caspase: any of a group of cysteine proteases, crucial for apoptosis.

cathepsin: any of a number of lysosomal enzymes that can degrade the components of the extracellular matrix.

cell components: substructures within the cell. The ones most commonly described in orthopaedic research include:
centriole
endoplasmic reticulum
filaments

TABLE 13-3 SI Units of Measurement

Magnitude	Length	Mass	Time	Force	Pressure
10^{-15}	Femtometer, fm	Femtogram, fg	Femtosecond, fs		
10^{-12}	Picometer, pm	Picogram, pg	Picosecond, ps		
10^{-10}	Angstrom, A				
10^{-9}	Nanometer, nm	Nanogram, ng	Nanosecond, ns		
10^{-6}	Micron, micrometer, μm	Microgram, μg	Microsecond, μs		
10^{-3}	Millimeter, mm	Milligram, mg	Millisecond, ms		
10^{-2}	Centimeter, cm				
10^{0}	Meter, m (39.37 inches)	Gram, g(0.0352 ounces); *Dalton*, Da (1/12 the mass of a C_{12} atom)	Second, s	Newton, N(1 kg accelerated 1 m/s^2; 0.225 lb on Earth)	Pascal, Pa(1 N/m^2); 1.45×10^{-4} lb/square inch
10^{3}	Kilometer, km	Kilogram, kg; Kilodalton, kD		Kilonewton, kN	Kilopascal, KPa
10^{6}					Megapascal, MPa
10^{9}					Gigapascal, GPa
10^{12}					Terapascal, TPa

Golgi apparatus
lysosome
microsome
microtubule
mitochondria
nucleolus
nucleus
plasma (or cell) membrane
polyribosome
ribosome
vesicle

cell cycle: referring to several sequential phases in a cell's life, centered around cell proliferation. Most cells proceed slowly through the cycle or remove themselves from the cycle to enter the G_0 phase at some stage of their lives.

> ***G_0 phase:*** nonproliferative, "resting" (only in terms of cell division).
>
> ***G_1:*** the interval between the end of mitosis and the beginning of DNA synthesis.
>
> ***S ("synthesis"):*** DNA synthesis stage.
>
> ***G_2:*** the interval between the end of DNA synthesis and the beginning of cell division.

> ***M ("mitosis"):*** active mitosis and cell division (Fig. 13-5).

circadian: pertaining to a 24-hour biologic cycle.

collagen: any of at least 18 forms of extracellular proteins, which account for at least 30% of the protein in the mammalian body. It consists of a structure of small amino acids (glycine 35%, alanine 11%) and permanently "kinked" amino acids (proline 12%–25%, hydroxyproline 9%), in which every third protein

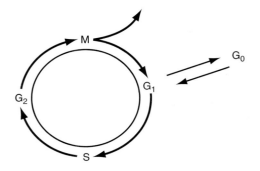

FIG 13-5 Cell cycle.

is glycine, in a pattern glycine-X-proline, glycine-proline-X, or glycine-X-hydroxyproline. The mixture of the amino acid X determines the collagen type. Usually seen as a stable triple helix, held together with hydrogen bonds, and a few covalent crosslinks. Major types found in the mammalian body include:

Type I: bone, skin, cornea, sclera, tendon, ligament.

Type II: cartilage, intervertebral disk, vitreous humor.

Type III: skin, blood vessels, repair tissue.

Type IV, VI: basement membrane.

Type X: growth plate, repair tissue, embryonic tissue.

cyclooxygenase: a common enzyme in the synthesis pathway of prostaglandins, prostacyclines, and thromboxanes from arachidonic acid.

cytokine: extracellular peptide or protein used in cell-to-cell communication, differentiated from a **hormone** in that its action is local to the area of secretion.

decorin: small proteoglycan, thought to modulate collagen fibril assembly and cross-linking in bone.

defensins: a group of short, naturally produced antimicrobial proteins important in naturally occurring bacterial contamination such as in and around the gums.

fibromodulin: noncollagenous protein found in articular cartilage, associated with fibril assembly, and found in greater abundance away from the chondrocytes.

gene expression: messenger RNA production, which is necessary but not sufficient for protein production.

ischemia: local decrease in oxygen tension, often due to damage to blood supply.

lysosomal protease: degradative enzymes found in lysosomes, generally active at acid pH, may be associated with extracellular matrix breakdown.

metalloproteinases (metalloproteases, or matrix metalloprotease, MMP): protein-cleaving enzymes that often have an association with a Zn ion. Some of the major musculoskeletal MMPs include:

collagenases: (MMP I and MMP XIII).

gelatinase: (MMP II, which cleaves specific collagens, fibronectin, and proteoglycans).

stromelysin: (MMP III, which cleaves core protein and, thereby, aggrecan from hyaluronic acid).

mitogen-activated protein (MAP) kinase: serine/threonine-specific protein kinase cascade that responds to extracellular stimuli to regulate *gene expression, mitosis, differentiation,* and cell survival/*apoptosis,* and that are well conserved across species.

neuropeptides: neuroactive peptides, 2-40 amino acids long, which can act as hormones, neurotransmitters, or neuromodulators (e.g., substance P, luteinizing hormone releasing hormone [LHRH], somatostatin).

proteomics: the identification and characterization of gene protein products.

reactive oxygen species: highly transient and chemically reactive species of oxygen atom; includes oxygen ions, free radicals, and peroxides. Important in some cell signaling mechanisms, increased levels can result in significant damage to subcellular structures (oxidative stress).

small interfering RNA (siRNA): a method by which genes can be selectively turned off in cell culture or in live animals without resort to transgenic methods, by hybridizing small complementary strands of RNA to messenger RNA. This blocks the ability of the RNA to transcribe a protein.

stem cell: pluripotential cell; a subset of these, **Mesenchymal stem cells** can differentiate into osteocytes, chondrocytes, or adipocytes.

tissue inhibitor of metalloproteinases (TIMP): a specific protein that inhibits MMPs.

transforming growth factor (TGF): a family of cytokines associated with growth and development, which includes the BMPs.

Cartilage

ADAMTS: proteases characterized by *A D*isintegrin-like *A*nd *M*etalloprotease domain (reprolysin-type) with *T*hrombo*S*pondin type I motifs; ADAMTS 4 and ADAMTS 5 are also called aggrecanase 1 and 2, respectively.

cartilage: smooth, relatively low-cellularity tissue, consisting of chondrocytes in lacunae, and a large amount of extracellular matrix composed of water, collagen, and proteoglycans.

hyaline cartilage: found at the articular surface of joints, tracheal rings, at the distal end of ribs. Blue-white, shiny, smooth.

elastic cartilage: found in the ligamentum nuchae, epiglottis, external ear. Yellow, flexible.

fibrocartilage: found in intervertebral disks, symphyses, and repair tissue of damaged hyaline cartilage. Histologically shows a herringbone fiber pattern.

physeal cartilage: forming the growth plate of endochondral ossification. Appears much like hyaline cartilage, and in some species (e.g., reptiles) the two are often coincident.

calcified cartilage: forming the thin layer of cartilage between the hyaline articular cartilage and the subchondral bone.

Hierarchy of Cartilage Structure

aggrecan: large matrix molecule composed of a hyaluronic acid backbone with numerous proteoglycan chains covalently attached via link proteins.

chondrocyte: the major type of cell found in cartilage. Generally encased in a cartilage **lacuna.**

chondroitin sulfate: a sulfated sugar with 40 to 60 repeating units of *n*-acetylgalactosamine and glucuronic acid, part of the glycosaminoglycan seen in cartilage.

core protein: the central protein of the proteoglycan subunit, to which the GAGs are associated.

fibril: several strands of tropocollagen held together with crosslinks.

fiber: an assembly of several fibrils.

glucosamine: one of the components of GAG; a glucose with a nitrogen-containing group.

glycosaminoglycan (GAG): linear carboxylated and sulfated sugar polymers, covalently attached to a small peptide.

hyaluronic acid: nonsulfated GAG of glucuronic acid and *N*-acetylglucosamine that makes up the backbone of the aggrecan molecule in cartilage.

keratin sulfate: a GAG with 5 to 20 repeating units of galactose and *N*-acetylglucosamine.

link protein: a 44- to 55-kD protein that associates the core protein to the hyaluronic acid chain.

perichondrium: the fibrous tissue on the outside (nonarticular) border of cartilage or continuous with periosteum in the case of a physis.

proteoglycan (mucopolysaccharide): a polymer consisting of a core protein associated with multiple GAGs.

procollagen: triple-helical form of collagen immediately after extracellular polymerization of intracellularly-produced **tropocollagen α-chains** into **procollagen** and subsequent cleavage of terminal peptides.

tidemark: border in articular cartilage between calcified and uncalcified cartilage layers.

Bone

alkaline phosphatase: a serum marker for bone formation.

bone morphogenic protein (BMP): a family of at least 18 proteins involved in the stimulation of bone formation, part of the TGF superfamily.

Bone Cells

osteoblast: cells of mesenchymal origin, capable of laying down bone matrix (**osteoid,** which is mostly collagen), which then calcifies extracellularly.

osteoclast: multinucleate cells of monocyte origin, whose major role is in the removal of bone.

osteocyte: osteoblasts encased in **lacunae,** which communicate (quite possibly, information about mechanical strain) with one another and with bone lining cells, via cell processes encased in **canaliculi** or tunnels within the bone matrix.

Bone Lining Cell

basic multicellular unit (BMU): the combination of osteoclasts and osteoblasts, working in concert in the remodeling of bone.

calbindin (calcium binding protein): a protein involved in cytoplasmic transport of calcium.

calcitonin: a short-chain protein hormone that is involved in bone accretion. The activity of this hormone can reduce the level of serum calcium by its effect on new bone formation.

calcium hydroxyapatite: $Ca_{10}(PO_4)_6(OH)_2$, the major mineral form found in bone.

cancellous (or trabecular) bone: thresholds differ between authors, but generally bone with a porosity of more than 40%, usually found toward the ends of long bones and in the body of vertebrae.

cement line (or reversal line): the outer edge of a BMU, which stains dark under toluidine blue, representing the furthest extent of osteoclastic activity during the remodeling process that resulted in the BMU.

compact (or cortical) bone: thresholds differ between authors, but generally bone with a porosity of less than 40% is usually found in the diaphysis and metaphysis of long bones, and in the shells of vertebrae.

diaphysis: the tubular, central section of a long bone.

endochondral ossification: process of bone development in which bone replaces a cartilage anlage. Usually characterized by the presence of a physis (e.g., most long bones, vertebrae).

epiphysis: the portion of a long bone between the physis and the end of the structure.

Haversian system (after Clopton Havers, 17th-century British microscopist): a secondary osteon with its associated canal.

Howship's lacuna (after John Howship, 19th-century British surgeon): the surface (or, in some definitions, the space bordered by the surface) of bone after osteoclastic activity has begun and before osteoblastic refilling as begun. Characterized by scalloped edges, in which individual osteoclasts have been actively resorbing bone. Often, osteoclasts are present at these surfaces.

intramembranous ossification: process by which bone is formed without a pre-existing cartilage anlage, for example, most of the bones of the skull, and the increase in width of long bone diaphyses.

lamellar bone: bone that is laid down in orderly sheets, in which the collagen fibers are parallel to one another.

matrix vesicle: extracellular depot of enzymes near osteoblasts that are involved in the initiation of bone mineral formation.

metaphysis: the cone-shaped portion of a long bone between the physis and the diaphysis.

modeling: placement of bone material where there was none earlier; does not require osteoclastic activity.

osteon: circumferential pattern of lamellar bone around an Haversian canal containing blood vessels.

primary osteon: osteon that is laid down *de novo,* without previous osteoclastic activity (thus, no cement line), usually as a result of periosteal expansion.

secondary osteon: osteon that is the result of remodeling (osteoclastic and subsequent osteoblastic activity, thus, a cement line is present).

osteocalcin: the most abundant noncollagenous protein in bone, important in the mineralization of new bone and as a chemoattractant for bone cells.

osteopontin: noncollagenous bone matrix protein, possibly involved in cell attachment to the matrix and in force transduction.

osteonectin (secreted protein, acidic, rich in cysteine, SPARC): noncollagenous bone matrix protein involved in mineralization, binding of growth factors, regulation of bone formation, and matrix control of metastasis.

osteoprotegerin (OPG): a protein inhibitor of osteoclastogenesis.

parathyroid hormone (PTH): polypeptide hormone involved in elevation of serum calcium, bone resorption, and renal calcium retention.

periosteum: the fibrous tissue covering on the nonarticular, nonligament/tendon attachment surfaces of a bone.

physis: the growth plate, a highly organized cartilaginous structure in which most long bone growth occurs.

plexiform bone: lamellar bone, often seen in ungulates, formed by filling in a surface trabecular network.

receptor activator of nuclear factor κ–β (RANK)/ RANK Ligand (RANKL): osteoclast precursors expressing RANK on their cell surfaces interact with osteoblasts or with stromal cells expressing RANKL on their cell surfaces, an important step in osteoclastogenesis and in bone resorption.

remodeling: removal and replacement of bone material; requires osteoclastic as well as osteoblastic activity.

vitamin D: alternatively considered a vitamin or a hormone, it is produced in the skin on exposure to ultraviolet (UV) light and altered in the kidney and liver. It acts by affecting the intestinal absorption of calcium, renal retention of calcium, and the remodeling process at the bone surface. Related terms include **1,25-dihydrocholecalciferol, 1,25-dihydroxyvitamin D3, 25-hydroxycholecalciferol,** and **24,25-dihydroxycholecalciferol.**

Wolff's law (after Julius Wolff, 19th-century German surgeon and pathologist): the clinical observation that bone will model and remodel in response to and in the direction of the forces acting on it.

woven bone: bone that is placed in a relatively disorganized fashion, with no clear order under polarized light microscopy; generally laid down quickly, as in the early stages of fracture repair (callus) or in rapid growth phases of ungulates, and replaced later with **lamellar** bone.

Appendix: Orthopaedic Abbreviations

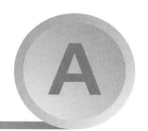

The Joint Commission on Accreditation of Healthcare Organizations (JCAHO) has directed that each hospital establish a standard list of abbreviations and acronyms that are known by all specialties. Listed here are those approved by the JCAHO, but also many more that are used by the orthopaedic physician to expediently document patient records in a clinical situation. These additional abbreviations and acronyms are included as a compendium for recognition as a reference only.

Table A-1 at the end of this appendix has specific abbreviations that **should not be used** for drug measure, usage, and names.

Care must be taken when using abbreviations. In some cases, a single abbreviation may refer to several words. For example, the abbreviation "quad" could refer to quadrilateral (hip), quadriceps (musculature), and quadriplegic (paralysis). Therefore, always consider the context of the material being read to determine which word is used. References vary widely in the use of capitalization of abbreviations.

AA: active-assistive (range of motion)
AA: advancement ulnar arm of arcuate ligament
AAL or ant ax line: anterior axillary line
AAOS: American Academy of Orthopaedic Surgeons
AAROM: active assisted range of motion
abd: abdomen; abdominal (pad)
ABD: abduction; abdomen
abd poll: abductor pollicis
ABOS: American Board of Orthopaedic Surgery
AC: acromioclavicular (joint); before meals

ac: before meals
ACCF: anterior cervical corpectomy and fusion
ACDF: anterior cervical discectomy and fusion
ACID PO4: acid phosphatase
ACS: acetabular cup system
AD: assistive devices
ADD: adduction
add poll: adductor pollicis
ADL: activities of daily living
ad lib: as desired
adm: admission
ADQ/ADM: abductor digiti quinti (or minimi)
AE: above elbow
AEA: above elbow amputation
AFO: ankle-foot orthosis
AG: antigravity
AGE: angle of greatest extension
AGF: angle of greatest flexion
AIDS: acquired immunodeficiency syndrome
AIIS: anterior inferior iliac spine
AJ: ankle jerks
AK: above knee
AKA: above-knee amputation
ALB: albumin
ALIF: anterior lumbar interbody fusion
ALPSA: anterior labrum periosteum shoulder arthroscopic lesion
ALRI: anterolateral rotatory instability (knee)
ALS: amyotrophic lateral sclerosis; anterolateral sclerosis
ALT: same as serum glutamic pyruvic transaminase (SGPT)
AML: anatomic medullary locking

AML: anatomic medullary locking (total hip replacement)

amp: ampule

ANA: antinuclear antibody

Anes: anesthesia

ANF: antinuclear factor

ANOVA: analysis of variance

ANS: autonomic nervous system

AO: Arbeitsgemeinschaft für Osteosynthesaefragen

AOA: American Orthopaedic Association

AP: anteroposterior (view)

APB: abductor pollicis brevis

APC: anteroposterior compression (pelvic fracture)

APL: abductor pollicis longus

APRL: Army Prosthetics Research Lab

aq, aqu: aqueous; water solution

ARDS: acute respiratory distress syndrome

ARIF: arthroscopically assisted reduction and internal fixation

AROM: active range of motion

AS: arteriosclerosis; aortic stenosis

ASAP: as soon as possible

ASES: American Shoulder and Elbow Surgeons (scales and ratings)

ASI: acromial spur index

ASIS: anterosuperior iliac spine

AV: arteriovenous; atrioventricular

AVF: arteriovenous fistula

AVM: arteriovenous malformation

BB to MM: belly button to medial malleolus (examination)

BE: below elbow

BFO: balanced forearm orthosis

BID: twice a day (ii)

BIL: biceps interval lesion

BJ: biceps jerks

BK: below knee

BKA: below knee amputation

BMD: bone mineral density

BMI: body mass index

BMP: bone morphogenic protein

BP: blood pressure

Bx: biopsy

C: centigrade

C/E angle: center edge angle

c/o: complaint of

C-1 through C-7: cervical vertebrae or nerve roots

C1-C7: cervical vertebrae

C3-4 through C6-7: intervertebral disk spaces between cervical vertebrae

C7-T1: intervertebral disk space between seventh cervical and first thoracic vertebra

C8: eighth cervical nerve root

Ca: calcium

CA: carcinoma

CAD-CAM: computer-assisted design–computer-assisted manufacturing

Ca lig: coracoacromial ligament

CAMBA: calcaneal axis first metatarsal base angle

CASH: cruciform anterior spinal hyperextension orthosis

CAT-CAM: contour-adducted trochanteric–controlled alignment method

CAT scan (CT): computed axial tomography

CC: chief complaint

CCK: constrained condylar knee

CG: contact guarding

CHF: congestive heart failure

CID: carpal instability dissociative

CIND: carpal instability, nondissociative

CLIP: capitolunate instability pattern

CMC: carpometacarpal

CMF: chondromyxoid fibroma

CPM: continuous passive motion

CNS: central nervous system

CO: certified orthotist; complaint of

COA: Canadian Orthopaedic Association

CP: cerebral palsy

CP: certified prosthetist

CPA: condylar-plateau angle

Cpd: compound

CPO: certified prosthetist and orthotist

CPPD: calcium pyrophosphate deposition (disease)

CPR: cardiopulmonary resuscitation

CPT: Current Procedural Terminology

CREST: *c*alcinosis, *R*aynaud, *e*sophageal, *s*clerodactyly, *te*langiectasia

CROW: Charcot restraint orthotic walker

CRP: cross reactive protein

CRT: cathode-ray tube

CSF: cerebrospinal fluid

C-spine: cervical spine

CT: computed tomography
CTO: cervicothoracic orthosis
CTR: carpal tunnel release
CTS: carpal tunnel syndrome
CTSO: cervical thoracolumbosacral orthosis
CV: cardiovascular
CVA: cerebrovascular accident (stroke)
cva: costovertebral angle
CX: culture
CXR: chest x-ray examination
D1, D2: dorsal vertebrae 1, 2, etc.
Da: Dalton
DANA: designed after natural anatomy (prosthesis)
DBS: Denis Browne splint
dc, D/C: discontinue
DC: dorsal capsulodesis
DCP: dynamic compression plate
DDH: developmental dysplasia of the hip
DEA: Drug Enforcement Agency
decub: decubitus position; lying down
dev: deviation
DEXA/DXA: dual x-ray absorptiometry
DIE: died in emergency room
dig: digitorum
DIP: distal interphalangeal (joint); DIPJ
disch: discharge
DISH: diffuse idiopathic skeletal hyperostosis
DISI: dorsal intercalated segment instability
Disl: dislocation
Distal/3 or D/3: distal third
DJD: degenerative joint disease
DKB: deep knee bends
DM: diabetes mellitus
DNR: do not resuscitate
DOA: date of admission; dead on arrival
DOE: date of examination
DOMS: delayed-onset muscle soreness
DP: distal phalanx
DP: dorsalis pedis pulse
DPA: dual photon absorptiometry
DPC: distal palmar crease
DPD: dual photon densitometry
dr: dram (4 ml)
DRUJ: distal radioulnar joint
DSA: digital subtraction angiography
D-spine: dorsal spine; thoracic spine

DTR: deep tendon reflex
DTRs: deep tendon reflexes
DVT: deep vein thrombosis
Dx or diag: diagnosis
Dz: disease
EBL: estimated blood loss
EBV: Epstein-Barr virus
ECF: extended care facility
ECG, EKG: electrocardiograph(gram)
ECRB: extensor carpi radialis brevis
ECRL: extensor carpi radialis longus
ECU: extensor carpi ulnaris
ED: elbow disarticulation; emergency department
EDB: extensor digitorum brevis
EDC: estimated date of confinement
EDC: extensor digitorum communis
EDL: extensor digitorum longus
EDQ/EDM: extensor digiti quinti (or minimi)
EDS: Ehlers-Danlos syndrome
EEG: electroencephalograph(gram)
EIP: extensor indicis proprius
EJ: elbow jerks
ELISA: enzyme-linked immunosorbent assay
ELPS: excessive lateral pressure syndrome
EMG: electromyography
EOM: extraocular movement
EPB: extensor pollicis brevis
EPL: extensor pollicis longus
EPP: end-plate potential (depolarization of muscle)
ERE: external rotation in extension
ERF: external rotation in flexion
ESIN: elastic stable intramedullary nailing
ESO: electrospinal orthosis
ETOH: alcohol
EULAR: European League Against Rheumatism
expir: expiration
EXT: extremities
F: Fahrenheit
FA: false aneurysm
FAAOS: Fellow, American Academy of Orthopaedic Surgeons
FABER: flexion in abduction and external rotation
FADIR: flexion in adduction and internal rotation
FB: foreign body
FCR: flexor carpi radialis
FCU: flexor carpi ulnaris

FDI: first dorsal interosseous (hand or foot)
FDL: flexor digitorum longus
FDP: flexor digitorum profundus
FDQB: flexor digiti quinti brevis
FDS: flexor digitorum sublimis (or superficialis)
FES: functional electrical stimulation
FF: further flexion
FFC: fixed flexion contracture
FFP: fresh frozen plasma
FH: family history
fl: fluid
FPB: flexor pollicis brevis
FPL: flexor pollicis longus
FQF: four-quadrant fusion
FRA: femoral ring allograft
fract or Fx: fracture
FRCS: Fellow, Royal College of Surgeons
FTA: femorotibial angle
FUO: fever of undetermined origin
FWB: full weight-bearing
g: gram (15 grain)
GAG: glycosaminoglycans
GB: gallbladder
Gd-DTPA: gadopentetate dimeglumine
GHL: glenohumeral ligament
GI: gastrointestinal
Gla: γ-carboxyglutamic acid
Glut: gluteal
Gm: gram
Gpa: gigapascal
gr: grain (60 milligram)
GSH: Green-Seligson Henry (nail)
gt: drop
gtt: drops (0.05 ml)
GU: genitourinary
H&P: history and physical (examination)
H: per hypodermic
H/H: hemoglobin and hematocrit
HA: hallux abductus
Hct: hematocrit
HCTU: home cervical traction unit
HD: heloma durum (hard corn)
HD: hip disarticulation
HEENT: head, ears, eyes, nose, throat (examination)
Hg: mercury

Hgb: hemoglobin
HIV (HTLV): human immunodeficiency virus
HLAM: hemilaminectomy
HM: heloma molle (soft corn)
HMO: health maintenance organization
HNP: herniated nucleus pulposus
HP: hot packs
HPI: history of present illness
HPLC: high-performance (pressure) liquid chromatography
hs: at bedtime
HT: hammertoe
HT: Hubbard tank
HV: hallux valgus
Hx: history
Hz: hertz
I&D: incision and drainage
I&O: intake and output
ICD: International Classification of Diseases (WHO Classification)
ICD-9-CM: International Classification of Diseases, 9th Revision, Clinical Modification
ICDA: International Classification of Diseases (U.S. classification)
ICS: intercostals space (ribs)
ICT: intermittent cervical traction
IDK: internal derangement of the knee
IHW: inner heel wedge
IM: intramuscular; intermuscular; intramedullary (rod)
IMF: intramedullary fixation
Inf: inferior
INFH: ischemic necrosis of femoral head
Inj: injection
IP: interphalangeal (joint)
IPJ: interphalangeal joint
IPK: intractable plantar keratosis
IPSF: immediate postsurgical fitting
IR: infrared (light)
IRE: internal rotation in extension
IRF: internal rotation in flexion
IS: interspace
ISIS: integrated shape imaging system
ISMAT: Institute of Sports Medicine and Athletic Trauma
ITB: iliotibial band

ITT: internal tibial torsion; iliotibial torsion

IV: intravenous

IV: intravenous (injection)

IVP: intravenous pyelogram

JBJS: *Journal of Bone and Joint Surgery.*

JCAH: Joint Commission on Accreditation of Hospitals

JCAHO: Joint Commission on Accredited Healthcare Organizations

Jct: junction

JRA: juvenile rheumatoid arthritis

K: potassium

KB: knee bearing

Kg: kilogram (1000 gram)

KJ: knee jerks

KMFTR: Kotz modular femur and tibia resection (system)

Kp: Kilopond

KUB: kidney, ureter, and bladder view of abdomen

KVO: keep view open (for IV fluids)

L: liter

L&W: living and well

L1-L5: lumbar vertebrae

LAC: long-arm cast

LAC: scapholunate advanced collapse

LAD: ligamentous anterior dislocation

LAM: laminectomy

LAMI: laminotomy

LANC: long-arm navicular cast

LAS: long-arm splint

LASER: light amplification by stimulated emission of radiation; lower case in context

lat: lateral

lat men: lateral meniscus or meniscectomy

LBP: low back pain

LBQC: large-based quad cane

LC/DCP: limited-contact dynamic-compression (plate)

LCP: Legg-Calvé-Perthes (disease)

LCS mb: low-contact stress meniscal bearing

LCS rp: low-contact stress rotating patella

LE: lupus erythematosus (SLE also for systemic lupus erythematosus); lower extremity

LFA: low friction arthroplasty

LHD: left-hand dominant

LIFO: locked intramedullary fracture osteosynthesis

lig: ligature; ligament

Liq: liquid

LISS: less invasive spine surgery

LLC: long-leg cast

LLD: leg-length discrepancy

LLE: left lower extremity

LLL: left lower limb

LLQ: left lower quadrant

LLS: long-leg splint

LLWC: long-leg walking cast

LOM: limitation of motion

LP: lumbar puncture

LS: lumbosacral spine

LSK: liver, spleen, and kidneys

LSP: lumbosacral orthosis

L-spine: lumbar spine

LSS: lumbosacral spine

LUE: left upper extremity

LUL: left upper limb

LUQ: left upper quadrant

MAC: monitored anesthesia care

MACS: MAST-associated compartment syndrome

MAL: midaxillary line

MARS: modular acetabulum reconstruction system

MAST: medical antishock trousers

MC: metacarpal; midcarpal

MCI: midcarpal instability (volar, palmar, extrinsic)

MCL: midclavicular line

MCP: metacarpophalangeal (joint)

MD: muscular dystrophy

Med: medial or medical

MED: multiple epiphyseal dysplasia

med: medicine

MEDLARS: Medical Literature Analysis Retrieval System

med men: medial meniscus or meniscectomy

MENS: microamperage electrical nerve stimulation

MESS: mangled extremity severity score

mg: milligram (1/60 grain)

MHW: medial heel wedge

MI: myocardial infarction

Middle/3 or M/3: middle third

MIS: minimally invasive surgery

MISS: minimally invasive spine surgery

M/L: medial lateral (narrow M/L)

MLD: median lethal dose (radiation)

ml: milliliter

mm: millimeter

mm: muscles; mucous membrane

MMT: manual muscle testing

MP: middle phalanx (or metaphalangeal) joint

MPC: midpalmar crease

MPJ: metaphalangeal joint

MPV: metatarsus primus varus

MRI: magnetic resonance imaging

MRSA: methicillin resistant *Staphylococcus aureus.*

MS: multiple sclerosis

MSD: microsurgical discectomy

MSL: midsternal line

MT: muscle testing

MTA: metatarsus adductus

MT bar: metatarsal bar

MTJ: midtarsal joint

MTP: metatarsophalangeal (joint)

MTV: metatarsus varus

MUA: manipulation under anesthesia

MVA: motor vehicle accident

mx: management

NaCl: sodium chloride

NB: note well

NC: neuroma-in-continuity

NCV: nerve conduction velocity

Neg: negative

NKA: no known allergies

NMR: nuclear magnetic resonance

NOS: not otherwise specified

NPO: nil per os (nothing per mouth)

NSAID: nonsteroidal anti-inflammatory drug

NSNA: normal shape, normal alignment

NV: neurovascular

NWB: non-weight-bearing

NYU: New York University (inserts)

OA: osteoarthritis

OAWO: opening abductory wedge osteotomy

obl: oblique

OCD: osteochondritis dissecans

OD: oculus dexter (right eye); overdose

ODQ/ODM: opponens digiti quinti (or minimi)

OI: osteogenesis imperfecta

OKC: Oklahoma City cable (system)

OP: opponens pollicis

OPD: outpatient department

OR: operating room; open reduction

ORIF: open reduction/internal fixation

ORTHO: orthopaedic

OS: oculus sinister (left eye); also abbreviated OL

OSHA: Occupational Safety and Health Administration

OT: occupational therapy

OU: both eyes

OW: open wedge (osteotomy)

Oz: ounce (8 dram, 30 ml)

P&A: percussion and auscultation

p: after

P: passive; phosphorous

PA: pascal (expressed as Newtons/square meter)

PA: psoriatic arthritis

PA: posteroanterior

PAL: posterior axillary line

PASS: passive

Path: pathology

PB: paraffin baths

PB: peroneus brevis

pc: after meals

PCA: patient-controlled anesthesia

PCA: porous-coated arthroplasties

PCA: porous-coated anatomic (total hip replacement)

PCE (Smith): physical capacities evaluation

PCP: primary care provider

PE, Px: physical examination

PE: pulmonary embolism

PEMF: pulsating electromagnetic fields

PEMF: pulsed electromagnetic fields

PERRLA: pupils equal, round, regular to light accommodation

PEX: physical examination (also Px)

Pf: plantar flexion

PFC: pelvic flexion contracture

PFFD: proximal femoral focal deficiency

PH: past history

phal: phalanx or phalanges

PI: present illness

PID: pelvic inflammatory disease

PIP: proximal interphalangeal (joint); PIPJ

PL: palmaris longus

PLIF: posterior lumbar interbody fusion; posterolateral interbody fusion

PLRI: posterolateral rotary instability

PMA: progressive muscle atrophy

PMD: progressive muscular dystrophy

PMHx (PMH): past medical history

PMMA: polymethylmethacrylate

PMRI: posteromedial rotary instability

PNF: proprioceptive neuromuscular facilitation

PNS: peripheral nervous system

PO: per os; per oral

POC: plan of care

polio: poliomyelitis

Post: posterior

Post-op: postoperatively

pp: after meals (postprandial)

PP: proximal phalanx

PPM: parts per million

PPO: passive prehension orthosis

PQ: pronator quadratus

PR: pelvic rock

pr: per rectum

pre-op: preoperatively

prep: preparation

PREs: progressive resistive exercises

PRN: whenever necessary, as often as necessary; ad lib

prog: prognosis

prox/3 or P/3: proximal third

PSIS: posterosuperior iliac spine

PSS: progressive system scoliosis

pt: patient

PT: physical therapy

PT: pronator teres

PTA: prior to admission

PTB: patella tendon bearing; pretibial bearing (socket type)

PTB: patellar tendon bearing (cast, orthosis, prosthesis)

PTBO: patellar tendon bearing orthosis

PTBS: patellar tendon bearing suspension

PTB-SC: patellar tendon-bearing-supracondylar

PTB-SP: patellar tendon-bearing-suprapatellar

PTH: parathyroid hormone

PTP: posterior tibial pulse

PTS: patellar tendon socket

PTT: patellar tendon transfer; partial prothrombin time

PVC: premature ventricular contraction

PVD: peripheral vascular disease

PVS: peripheral vascular surgery

PVS: peripheral vascular system

PW: plantar wart

PWB: partial weight-bearing

q: every

q3h: every 3 hours

qam: every morning

qct: quantitative computed tomography

qd: every day

qh: every hour

qid: four times a day (iiii)

qod: every other day

qoh: every other hour

qs: as much as suffices; quantity sufficient

QSAC: quadrant-sparing acetabular component

qt: quart (32 oz, 0.946 liter)

quad: quadriceps; quadrilateral; quadriplegic

quant: quantity

R: roentgen unit, x-ray examination

Ra: radium

RA: rheumatoid arthritis

rad: radiology, radiation absorbed dose

RC: radiocarpal

rem: roentgen-equivalent-man

RGO: reciprocating gait orthosis

RHD: right-hand dominant

Rheum: rheumatology

RICE: rest, ice, compression, elevation

RLE: right lower extremity

RLL: right lower limb

RLQ: right lower quadrant

RM: repetition maximum

R/O: rule out

ROM: range of motion

ROS, SR: review of systems

RR: recovery room; relative risk

RRE: round, regular, and equal

RSD: reflex sympathetic dystrophy

RTC: return to clinic

RUE: right upper extremity

RUL: right upper limb; right upper lobe

RUQ: right upper quadrant

RV: return visit

S1-S5: sacral vertebrae

SAC: short-arm cast

SACH: solid ankle cushioned heel

SAFE: stationary ankle flexible endoskeletal (foot)

SANC: short-arm navicular cast

SAPHO: synovitis-acne-pustulosis-hyperostosis-osteomyelitis syndrome

SAS: short-arm splint

SBQC: small base quad cane

SC: sternoclavicular (joint)

SC: supracondylar

SCFE: slipped capital femoral epiphysis

SCOPE: Sacramento, California orthotic-prosthetic evaluation

SCSP: supracondylar-suprapatellar

SD: shoulder disarticulation

SDD: sterile dry dressing

SDR: surgical dressing room

Sed Rate: erythrocyte sedimentation rate

Segs: segmented white cells

SEM: scanning electron microscopy

SGOT: serum glutamic oxalacetic transferase

SGP: stress-generated potentials

SGPT: serum glutamic pyruvic transferase

SH: social history

SI: Système International d'Unités (Fr.); International System of Units (extension of metric system)

SI: sacroiliac (joint)

SIG: let it be labeled; directions

SIS: Standard International System

SL: serious list

SLAP: superior labrum anterior to posterior (shoulder lesion)

SLC: short-leg cast

SLE: systemic lupus erythematosus

SLR: straight leg raise

SLS: short-leg splint

SMA: spinal muscular atrophy

SMPS: sympathetic maintained pain syndrome

SNF: skilled nursing facility

SOAP: Subjective, Objective Assessment Plan; a problem-oriented medical record-keeping system

sol, soln: solution

SOMI: sternal-occiput-mandibular immobilization (orthosis)

SOS: if necessary, repeat once if need exists

SP: suprapatellar

SPC: suprapatellar cuff

SPECT: single photon emission computed tomography

SPGR: spoiled grass (image)

ss: ½ (e.g., gt ss = ½ drop)

SSEP: somatosensory-evoked potentials

SSI: segmental spinal instrumentation

staph: *Staphylococcus* or implies *Staphylococcus aureus* species

STAT: immediately

STEN: stored energy

STIR: short tau inversion recovery

STJ: subtalar joint

strep: *Streptococcus.*

STSG: split-thickness skin graft

Sub-Q, SQ, SC: subcutaneous (under the skin)

Sub-Q: subcutaneous

sup: superior

surg: surgical; surgery

SWD: shortwave diathermy

sympt or Sx: symptoms

T: temperature

T1-T12: thoracic vertebrae

tabs: tablets

TAL: tendon Achilles lengthening

TAMBA: talar axis first metatarsal base angle

TARA: total articular replacement arthroplasty

TASTM: The American Society for Testing Metals (and Alloys)

TB: tuberculosis

TC: total condylar

TEM: transmission electron microscopy

TENS: transcutaneous electrical nerve stimulation

TEV: talipes equinovarus

TFCC: triangular fibrocartilage complex

TFD: target-film distance

TG: tendon graft

THA: total hip arthroplasty

THF: triquetrohamate fusion

THR: total hip replacement

TIA: transient ischemic attack

TID: three times a day (iii)

TIMP: tissue inhibitor of metalloproteinase

TJ: triceps jerks

TJR: total joint replacement

TKA: total knee arthroplasty

TKR: total knee replacement

TLIF: transforaminal lumbar interbody fusion

TLR: triquetrohamate ligament reconstruction

TLSO: thoracic lumbosacral orthosis

TMJ(s): temporomandibular joint (syndrome)

TMT: talometatarsal (angle)

Tomo: tomogram

TPC: thenar palmar crease

TPN: total parenteral nutrition (IM, IV, subcutaneous, intramedullary)

TPR: temperature, pulse, respiration

TSD: target-scan distance

T-spine: thoracic spine

TSS: toxic shock syndrome

TT: tendon transfer

TT: tilt table

TTAP: threaded titanium acetabular prosthesis

Tx: traction; treatment, transfusion

UCB: University of California (Berkeley) orthosis (additional abbreviations within the chapter)

UCL: ulnar collateral ligament

UE: upper extremity

UHMWPE: ultrahigh molecular weight polyethylene

UN: ulnar nerve (finger spreader)

URI: upper respiratory (tract) infection

US: ultrasound

ut dict: as directed

UTI: urinary tract infection

UV: ultraviolet (light)

VATER: *v*ertebral, *a*nd *t*racheoesophageal, *e*sophageal, *r*adial, and *r*enal

VC: volar capsulodesis

VDDR: vitamin D–dependent rickets

VDRR: vitamin D–resistant rickets

VISI: volar intercalated segment instability

VS: vertical shear (pelvic fractures)

VSL: very serious list

VTED: venous thromboembolic disease

VWF: vibratory white finger (Raynaud phenomenon)

WBC: white blood cell count

WC: wheelchair

WD: wrist disarticulation

WD, WN: well developed, well nourished

WEST: work evaluation systems technology

WFE or Wms flex ex: Williams flexion exercises

WNL: within normal limits

WPB: whirlpool bath

Wt: weight

XIP: x-ray in plaster (examination)

XMATCH: cross match

XOP: x-ray out of plaster (examination)

Yr: year

c̄: with; cum

p̄: after

s̄: without

‖ bars: parallel bars

x̄: except

⊖ or ō: negative

+ or ⊕: positive

Δ: difference, deltoid muscle

↑: increase

↓: decrease

>: greater than

<: less than

♂: male

♀: female

1°: primary

2°: secondary

3°: tertiary

℞ (Latin): to take; recipe

dr, ℨ: dram (4 ml)

oz, ℥: ounce (8 dram, 30 ml)

s̄s̄: ½ (e.g., gt s̄s̄ = ½ drop)

TABLE A-1

Abbreviation/Dose Expression	Intended Meaning	Misinterpretation	Correct Usage
cc	Cubic centimeter	Mistaken for units when poorly written	Write mL for milliliters
Q.D.	Once daily	Mistaken for Q.O.D.	Write daily
Q.O.D.	Every other day		Spell out every other day
S.C. or S.Q.	For subcutaneous	Mistaken as SL for sublingual or "5 every"	Write "sub-Q" "subQ," or "subcutaneously"
Trailing zero (X.0 mg), lack of leading zero (.X mg)		Decimal point is missed	Never write a zero by itself after a decimal point (X mg), and always use a zero before a decimal point (0.X mg)
U	Units	Mistaken for a zero, resulting in a ten-fold dosing overdose	Spell out "units"
μg	Microgram	Mistaken for mg (milligrams) resulting in one thousand-fold overdose	Spell out microgram or use "mcg"
&	And		Spell out "and"
IU	International Unit	Mistaken as IV (intravenous) or 10 (ten)	Written out "international unit"
No abbreviated drug names are allowed	All drug names		Spell out complete drug name
MS or MSO_4	Morphine sulfate		Write out "morphine sulphate"
$MgSO_4$	Magnesium sulfate		Write "magnesium sulphate"

Appendix: Anatomic Positions and Directions

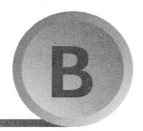

In orthopaedics, anatomic positions and directions are routinely used to provide an accurate description of specific anatomic locations. These basic directions may be compared to looking at a map to determine the longitude and latitude of an area. Humans are three-dimensional subjects with points of reference made in the orthograde (upright) position. The surface locations and anatomic planes are described as follows.

Surface Location

The location of a structure is described in reference to a standing person facing the examiner with outstretched hands in a palms-up position. The basic directional terms are:

anterior (ventral): forward or front surface (Fig. B-1).
posterior (dorsal): back surface.
lateral: sides, away from midline.
medial: middle, toward the midline.
superior: upper area, above, toward the head.
inferior: lower area, below, toward the tail end.

These reference points may be combined to give a more precise location to a specific region on a surface or in structures deep within the body, for example, the exposed hip in a surgical procedure. When these terms are compounded and hyphen omitted, the combining forms may be:

anterosuperior: front and above.
anteromedial: front and to inner side.
anterolateral: front and to outer side.
anteroposterior: front and toward back.
anteroinferior: front and below.

These can be used in combination with locations in reverse order, such as

posterosuperior: back to front toward head.
posteromedial: back to inner side.
posterolateral: back to outer side.
posteroinferior: back to below.

In some cases, dorsal (back) may be used for posterior (e.g., dorsolateral).

Anatomic Planes

The term *plane* comes from the Latin word, planus, meaning a flat, level surface. There are three directions of planes, all in reference to a standing person facing the examiner: vertical anterior to posterior (sagittal), vertical side to side (coronal or longitudinal), and horizontal (transverse).

anteroposterior planes
median (midsagittal) plane: vertical plane directly through the midline of the body, transecting the nose, navel, and spine, and dividing body into left and right halves.

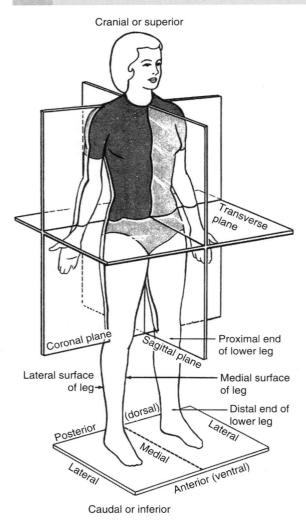

Cranial or superior

Transverse plane

Coronal plane

Sagittal plane

Proximal end of lower leg

Lateral surface of leg

Medial surface of leg

Distal end of lower leg

(dorsal)

Lateral

Posterior

Medial

Lateral

Anterior (ventral)

Caudal or inferior

FIG B-1 Anterior view of human figure demonstrating meaning of terms used in describing the body. (From Anthony CP, Kolthoff N: *Textbook of Anatomy and Physiology*, ed 9, St Louis, 1975, Mosby.)

median or sagittal plane: any of the anteroposterior planes through the midaxis, dividing body in half; the term sometimes implies the median plane only. If the word sagittal is used to denote the median plane, then other sagittal planes are called parasagittal planes.

vertical side to side planes

    coronal (frontal plane): a plane parallel with long axis of body at right angles to median sagittal

plane going through coronal sutures of the skull (approximately center of body) and dividing body into front and back parts.

    longitudinal: lengthwise and parallel with long axis of body or part; any of the vertical side to side planes. Coronal and longitudinal planes have been used interchangeably to describe each other. In this case, the context of the sentence will indicate the reference point of the plane.

horizontal (transverse) plane: any of the horizontal planes across the body at right angles to coronal and sagittal planes parallel to baseline.

neutral plane: the plane of a structure around which bending occurs.

Specific Locations

When describing limb anatomy, the nomenclature is very specific. The four appendages are correctly referred to as the upper and lower limbs, two forelimbs, and two hind limbs. The **thigh** indicates that portion above the knee and the **shank** the portion between the knee and ankle. The **calf** is the posterior aspect and the **shin** the anterior aspect of the leg. The sole (bottom) of the foot is called the **plantar surface,** and the top is the **dorsal surface.** The **brachium** refers to that portion of the arm above the elbow and below the shoulder. The **antebrachium** refers to the portion of the arm below the elbow but above the wrist. The **ventral side** of the hand is the palm or **volar surface,** with the opposite side being the **dorsum** or **dorsal surface.** The forearm is similarly divided into volar and dorsal aspects.

Joint Motions* (Fig. B-2)

Ranges of joint motion refer to the extent of movement within a given joint. Joint motion may be active, passive, or active assistive. The major joint areas involve

---

*Further information about the assessment and recording of joint motions is obtainable from American Academy of Orthopaedic Surgeons: *Joint motion—method of measuring and recording,* Chicago, 1985, The Academy.

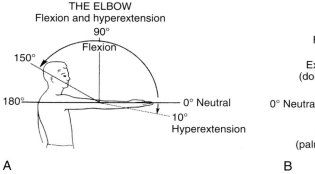

THE ELBOW
Flexion and hyperextension

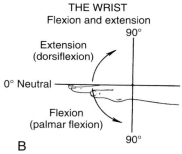

THE WRIST
Flexion and extension

A

B

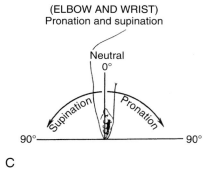

(ELBOW AND WRIST)
Pronation and supination

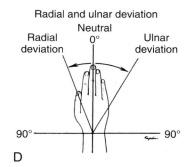

Radial and ulnar deviation

C

D

FIG B-2 A, Elbow. *Flexion:* 0 to 150 degrees. *Extension:* 150 degrees to 0 (from angle of greatest flexion to 0 position). *Hyperextension:* measured in degrees beyond the 0 starting point. This motion is not present in all individuals; when it is, it may vary from 5 to 15 degrees. **B,** Elbow and wrist, *Pronation:* 0 to 80 or 90 degrees. *Supination:* 0 to 80 or 90 degrees. *Total forearm motion:* 160 to 180 degrees. **C,** Wrist. *Flexion* (palmar flexion): 0 to about 80 degrees. *Extension* (dorsiflexion): 0 to about 70 degrees, **D,** Wrist. *Radial deviation:* 0 to 20 degrees. *Ulnar deviation:* 0 to 30 degrees. (From American Academy of Orthopaedic Surgeons: *Joint Motion—Method of Measuring and Recording,* Chicago, 1985, The Academy.)

the shoulder (glenoid), elbow (cubitus), hip (coxa) (Fig. B-3), and knee (genu).

All the hinge joints have motion described in terms of **flexion** and **extension.** Except for the ankle, the 0-degree position occurs when the limb is held out straight, and the degree of flexion is then stated in terms of degrees from the 0-degree extended position. The knee and elbow will occasionally extend beyond the 0-degree limit, and this motion is expressed in degrees of **hyperextension.** The wrist has approximately 90 degrees of extension and 90 degrees of flexion (dorsiflexion and palmar flexion).

The Neutral Zone Method is used for measuring joint motion. The anatomic position of the joint defines the starting position at zero, and motion is measured in degrees of a circle. Other measured motions include:

circumduction: a maneuver or movement of a ball-and-socket joint in a circular motion; for example, the shoulder can circumduct 180 degrees with six movements possible.

flexion: to bend from the joint as in flexion movements of the spine at the waist (anterior or lateral). In the foot or hand is expressed as:

dorsiflexion: the toe-up motion of the ankle expressed in degrees from the 0-degree position of the foot at rest on the ground in standing position.

THE HIP

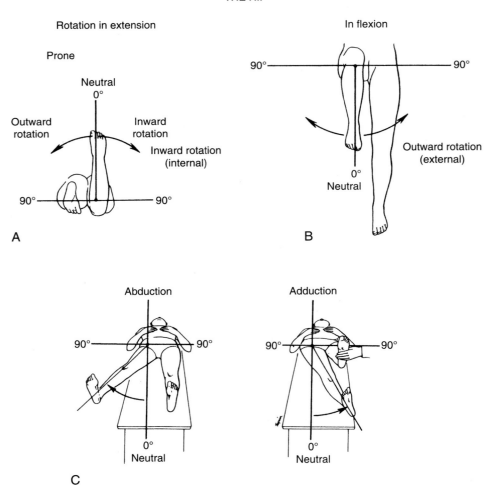

FIG B-3 The hip. **A,** *Inward rotation:* measured by rotating leg outward. *Outward rotation:* measured by rotating leg inward. **B,** *Inward rotation (internal):* measured by rotating leg away from midline of trunk with thigh as the axis of rotation, thus producing inward rotation of the hip. *Outward rotation (external):* measured by rotating leg toward midline of trunk with thigh as the axis of rotation, thus producing outward rotation of the hip. **C,** *Abduction:* outward motion of the extremity is measured in degrees from 0 starting position. *Adduction:* to measure, examiner should elevate opposite extremity a few degrees to allow leg to pass under it. (From American Academy of Orthopaedic Surgeons: *Joint Motion—Method of Measuring and Recording,* Chicago, 1985, The Academy.)

plantar flexion: the toe-down motion of the foot at the ankle expressed in degrees from 0-degree position of the foot at rest on the ground in standing position.

palmar flexion: of the wrist with palm up in flexion.

extension: extending distally away from body as in the limbs, or bending back posteriorly as in the spine.

pronation: palm-down position of hand with elbow at a 90-degree angle, brought about by the motion of the radius around the ulna (posterior rotation). In the foot, the plantar surface is turned down.

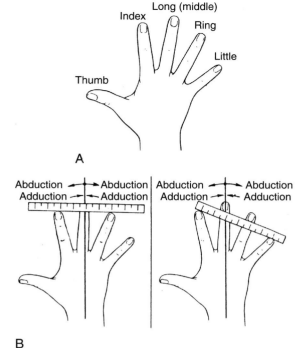

A

B

FIG B-4 A, Nomenclature of fingers. To avoid mistakes, fingers and thumb are referred to by name rather than by number. **B,** Finger spread in abduction and adduction can be measured in centimeters or inches from the tip of index finger to tip of little finger. Individual fingers spread from tip to tip of indicated fingers. (From American Academy of Orthopaedic Surgeons: *Joint Motion—Method of Measuring and Recording,* Chicago, 1985, The Academy.)

supinate, supination: palm-up position of the hand with elbow flexed at a 90-degree angle, brought about by motion of the radius around the ulna (anterior rotation). In the foot, the plantar surface is turned inward.

ulnar deviation: of the hand at the wrist such that the hand is directed in an ulnar direction; measured in degrees from 0 with hand in midline.

radial deviation: of the hand at the wrist such that the hand is directed radially; measured in degrees from 0 with hand in midline.

abduction: movement away from midline of body in frontal plane; applied to hip, shoulder, fingers, thumb, and foot. The midline reference point is a central line in the body for proximal joints and the central part of a limb for distal joints (Figs. B-4, B-5).

adduction: movement toward the midline in frontal plane as in abduction. On verbal transcription in clinical notes the person dictating will sometimes say "a-b-duction" or "a-d-duction" to clarify distinction between *abd*uction and *add*uction (Fig. B-4).

anteversion: to lean forward at an angle; in reference to the neck of humerus or femur, an anterior rotation.

anteroflexion: bending forward.

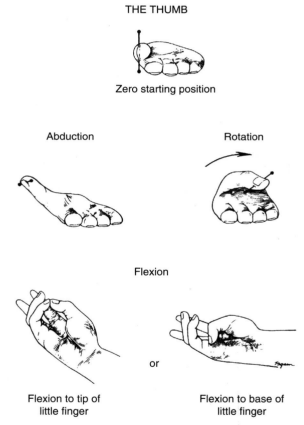

FIG B-5 Thumb opposition. The motion is a composite of three elements: abduction, rotation, and flexion. This motion is considered complete when tip, or pulp, of thumb touches tip of fifth finger or, according to some surgeons, when tip of thumb touches base of the fifth finger. (From American Academy of Orthopaedic Surgeons: *Joint Motion—Method of Measuring and Recording,* Chicago, 1985, The Academy.)

eversion: turning outward, when applied to the heel, describes the degree of motion of the heel pushed outward with ankle in neutral position; when applied to the foot, describes the combined motions of dorsiflexion, pronation, and abduction (Fig. B-6).

inversion: when applied to the heel, describes the degree of motion of the heel pushed inward with ankle in neutral position; when applied to the foot, describes the combined motions of plantar flexion, supination, and adduction (Fig. B-6).

retroflexion: bending backward.

retroversion: turned toward the back; in reference to the neck of femur or humerus, a posterior rotation.

apposition: contact of two adjacent parts; bringing together as in a finger movement, the thumb to index finger.

opposition: applied mostly to the thumb but also to little finger; describes the motion required to bring about opposition, or the setting opposite, of thumb against little finger (pulp surfaces). For the thumb, opposition is the combined action of abduction, rotation, and flexion.

external rotation: in frontal plane is away from midline.

internal rotation: in a frontal plane is toward the midline.

valgus: turned outward; the distal part is bent away from the midline; for example, genu valgus (bow-legged).

varus: turned inward; the distal part is toward the midline; for example, genu varus (knock-kneed).

Anatomic Associated Terms

The following are other associated terms referring to directions of anatomy or physical signs.

a, an: no, not, against.

AAL: anterior axillary line.

ab: away from (*ab*duct).

ad: toward (*ad*duct).

AGE: angle of greatest extension.

AGF: angle of greatest flexion.

alignment: linear position of one part of an extremity compared with another; to bring into a straight line.

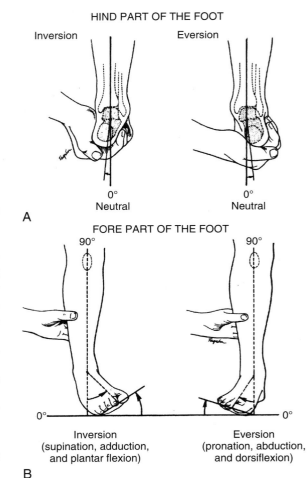

FIG B-6 **A,** Hindpart of the foot. *Inversion:* heel is grasped firmly in cup of examiner's hand. Passive motion is estimated in degrees, or percentages of motion, by turning heel inward. *Eversion:* motion is estimated by turning heel outward. **B,** Forepart of the foot. *Active inversion:* foot is directed medial. This motion includes supination, adduction, and some degree of plantar flexion; can be estimated in degrees or expressed in percentages as compared with the opposite foot. *Active eversion:* sole of foot is turned to face laterally. This motion includes pronation, abduction, and dorsiflexion. (From American Academy of Orthopaedic Surgeons: *Joint Motion—Method of Measuring and Recording,* Chicago, 1985, The Academy.)

ambi: on both sides.

ambidextrous: using both right and left hands effectively.

amph-, amphi-: both ways, all around, both sides.

an-: not, against, without.

anatomic axis: the true axis of an extremity measured by lines.

angle: the figure or space outlined by the diverging of two lines from a common point or by the meeting of two planes; a projecting or sharp corner.

angulation: deviation from the norm; sharp bend of a structure to form an angle.

aniso: unequal, asymmetrical, dissimilar.

annulus: any circular structure, ring-shaped.

ante-: forward, before.

antecedent: to precede, or go before.

anteflexion: to bend forward.

anterior: front view, ventral side, face surface, superior.

antero-: before, in front of.

anteversion: tipping forward.

anticus: foremost, in the front.

antimere: the right or left half of the body; a segment of an animal body formed by planes, cutting the axis of the body at right angles.

apex: top, tip, point of activity, summit, vertex (refers to C2).

apical: pertaining to apex; situated near point of reference.

apo-: away from.

asymmetric: lacking symmetry; uneven, as one limb to another.

axis: line of symmetry, rotation, or revolution; pivot dividing line; also second vertebra.

axis of rotation: circular arcs of limb segments that move in a line of right angles to the plane.

basal, basilar: base of a part.

bilateral: both sides.

cata-: prefix meaning down, against, or according to.

caudal, caudad: toward the lower end of the erect trunk or tail, inferior to or bottom point of reference.

centri-: center.

cephalic: toward the head; uppermost point of reference.

circumference: around, outer circular boundary.

circumflex: describes an arc of a circle; winding around.

co-, com-, con-: together, with.

concave: rounded, depressed surface.

contralateral: opposite side.

convex: rounded, elevated surface.

coronal: a plane dividing the body with front and back portions; in the direction of the coronal suture; a longitudinal plane passing through the body at right angles to the median plane.

craniad: toward the head.

curvilinear: curved away from straight line.

de-: away, from, down.

deep: depth from surface.

delta: triangle (deltoid).

dexter: right.

dia-: between, through, across, apart.

diffuse: widely distributed.

dis-: apart from.

distal: away from, furthest point of reference.

dorsal: back or posterior aspect.

ec-: out, out from.

ectopic: located away from normal position; out of place.

em-, en-: in, within.

endo-: within, in.

epi-: on, above, over.

eso-: in, inward, inside.

ex-, exo-: out, outside.

external: outside, describing walls, cavities, or hollow viscera.

extra-: beyond, outside, without.

facet: flat surface.

flexure: curved or bent.

fore: in front of, before.

hyper-: over, above, excessive.

hypo-: under, below, deficient.

in-, ino-: into, within.

inferior: below point of reference, underneath.

infra: below or under.

in situ: in its natural place or position.

inter-: between.

intercalary: middle.

internal: inside; describing walls, cavities, or hollow viscera.

interspace: the space between two similar parts (e.g., the vertebrae, ribs).

interstitial: spaces within a structure.

intra-: within.

intro-: into, beginning.

ipsilateral: same side.

iso-: equal, symmetrical.

juxta-: prefix for close to, near, in apposition, side by side (e.g., juxtaposition).

lat, latero-, lateral: sides, right and left; away from median plane, outer surface.

latus: broad.

length: the linear distance between two joints. The International System (SI) unit of length is measured in meters (m).

levo: left.

linea aspera: linea (line) and aspera (rough).

linear: elongated, straight line.

longitudinal: lengthwise, parallel to the long axis of a part (coronal or frontal planes).

MAL: midaxillary line.

medi-, medial: middle or median plane, toward midline, inner surface, link making halves.

megalo-: large.

meso-: middle intermediate.

met-, meta-: beyond, from one place to another, point of change.

multiangular: many angles.

neutral axis: the longitudinal line of a structure around which torsion occurs; the longitudinal line in a long structure where normal axial stresses are zero when structure is subjected to bending.

oblique: slanted, inclined.

oblongata: oblong.

orthograde: upright position, as in a standing person.

palmar: side of hand surface, face up.

para-, par-: beyond, beside.

parallel: equal in lines or surface; in the same direction.

pars: a division or part; a particular part of a greater structure (e.g., pars interarticularis).

patent: open, unobstructed, apparent, evident.

peri-, peripheral: immediately around, sphere.

perpendicular: exactly upright; being at right angles to a given line or plane.

pivot: to turn as in a circular motion.

plantar: sole, bottom of the foot.

posterior, postero-, post-: after, behind, tail end, back, inferior to surface.

prone: face down (lying face down).

protract: pull forward.

proximal: close to nearest point of reference.

quadratus: four-sided.

re-: back, again.

recurvatum: bending backward; a flexure or hyperextension.

residual: left behind.

retract: pull back.

retrad: backward, toward back part.

retro-, retrograde, retroflex: bending backward, behind.

rotation: turning in a circular motion.

sinister: left.

striate: having transverse lines (muscles).

sub-: under.

subjacent: lying underneath (sub—under + jacent—to lie).

summit: top.

super-, supra-: above, beyond, upon, over.

superficial: near the surface.

superior, sup.-: uppermost side, above point of reference, toward head (cephalic).

supine: lying on back, face up.

sym-, syn-: together.

symmetric: exhibiting symmetry, even, alike.

terminal: end.

trans-, transverse: through, across, horizontal.

ultra: beyond.

unilateral: one side.

ventral: belly side (abdomen), anterior, front, face up.

vertex: the top or summit, apex.

vertical: perpendicular to the plane of the horizon (vertex).

volar: underneath surface, palm or sole side up.

Appendix: Etymology of Orthopaedics

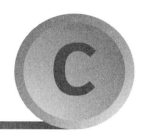

The word "etymology" comes from the Latin *etymon,* meaning genuine or true, plus *logos,* word. Etymology is the study of the origin of words (*origo,* beginning).

In ancient times, the classic language was Greek and Latin in origin and nonmedical in use. Scientific language was attributed to early physicians and writers such as Hypocrites, Aristotle, and Galen. Latin terms were introduced by Galen, a Greek physician who moved to Rome, and the Flemish anatomist, Vesalius. Celsus, Areatus, Pliny, and Chaucer were among many others who contributed to the scientific vocabulary.

Galen gave the first account of musculi by describing more than 300. In 1543 BC, Vesalius abandoned the system of naming muscles and accurately numbered them. In the 16th century, Jacque Dubois renamed muscles after parts to which they were attached, for example, tibialis, peroneus, and others were named by shape (rhomboid), size (longus, brevis), substance (membranous), or from the number of heads (biceps, triceps). Borelli added to names the action of muscles (pulley, lever, wheel). In the 18th century, Winslow, Albinus, Cowper, Douglas, and Riolan named muscles as we know them today. Leonardo da Vinci lettered his illustrations and occasionally gave a muscle a special name.

Centuries later, scholars preferred using the languages of Latin and Greek in science over other languages for a number of reasons, mainly because of the ease in which words could be used interchangeably in combining forms based on roots, prefixes, and suffixes. Anglo-Saxon English has a limited capacity for compounding words and often requires numerous words to make a point. Therefore, Latin and Greek were retained as the main structure of scientific language as we know it today. Scholars for generations have studied word origins and discovered full histories for most words, found mostly in the authoritative Oxford English Dictionary.

As mentioned previously, anatomy is a very descriptive science. Many words that are of nonmedical origin describe sizes and shapes (deltoid, lamboid, piriformis) or plants (sesamoid, sesame seed; nucleus, little nut; pisiform, pea-shaped) or are taken from living creatures (lupus, wolf; musculus, little mouse; cauda equina, horse's tail; lumbrical, worm). Often, the Greek and Latin words having the same meaning are very different; for example, clavicle (L, dim. of *clavis,* a key) and *cleido* (Gr, a fastener or key), that is used in combining form (sternocleidomastoid).

Anglo-Saxon (A-S) English, on the other hand, favors monosyllabic words such as hand, foot, back, leg, arm, and so forth and is augmented by many words from other languages such as Latin (L), Greek, (Gr), French (Fr), Italian (It), Spanish (Sp), Middle English (ME), German (Ger), and other nonclassical origins.

A knowledge of word derivation is the best way to accurately use words in their proper form. A brief description of the origin of orthopaedic terminology is given here to assist in the understanding of this specialty.

a, an: (G) negative prefix before a word that signifies the thing named is deprived of its quality (e.g., anaerobic, anorexic); not, without.

abdomen: (L) belly, the area between the chest and pelvis.

abduct: (L) abducens, led away; *ab-* from *ducere,* to lead.

accident: (L) from *accidens,* a happening; *accidere,* to happen; (G) *cado,* to fall. An unexpected happening.

acetabulum: (L) *acetum,* vinegar cup + *bulum,* little cup, dim. of *abrum,* a holder or receptacle. Cup-shaped depression of the ilium (true hip) for holding head of femur.

acromion: (G) *akron* or *akros,* summit, peak + *−omos,* shoulder; outermost tip of scapula.

acute: (L) *acutus,* sharp, from *acuere,* to sharpen (cf. *acus,* needle).

adduct: (L) *adductus,* to bring toward median plane.

adhesion: (L) *ad,* to bring in + *haerere,* to stick; *adhaesio,* stuck to.

adipose: (L) *adeps, adipis,* fat. Term used to describe animal fat.

adventitia: (L) *adventicius. Ad,* to + *veniere,* to come. An adventitious bursa is one formed from surrounding tissues in an unusual situation (e.g., tailor's bursa, student's elbow). A tunica adventitia is applied to the outer covering of a structure or organ (artery).

agonist: (G) *agonistes,* a rival or combatant, a prime mover; a muscle concerned with carrying out a movement (contraction) as compared with antagonist (opposite).

ala, alar: (L) wing-like structure; alar ligament of first cervical vertebra, and sacral ala, the lateral portion.

allograft: (G) *allos,* other + (L) *graphium,* grafting knife. To transplant tissue from same species.

amphiarthrosis: (G) *amphi,* on both sides + *arthron,* a joint. Limited mobility with movement in all directions. Diarthrosis and synarthrosis refer to incomplete joints (intervertebral disks).

amputation: (L) *amputare,* to cut around + amputation, a pruning. Hippocrates recommended this operation at the joint.

analgesia: (G) *an,* not + *algos,* pain. Absence of pain.

anaphylaxis: (G) *ana,* up + phylaxis, *protection.*

anapophysis: (G) *ana,* back + *apophysis,* an offshoot. An accessory spinal process of a vertebra.

anastomosis: (G) an opening. Created by a natural, pathologic, or surgical communication between two normally distinct spaces or organs.

anatomy: (G) *ana,* apart + *tome,* a cutting; *anatome,* dissection. Hippocrates (420 BC) used word for a branch of medical education. The oldest treatise known on anatomy is an Egyptian papyrus (1600 BC) on dissecting bodies for medical purposes. The science was based on dissection, from which it got its name.

anconeus: (G) *ancon,* a bend, especially the elbow (cf. angle).

anesthesia: (G) *an,* against + *aesthesis,* sensation.

ankle: (A-S) from (L) *angulus,* an angle, corner, or bend; (G) bend.

ankylosis: (G) *ankyl,* stiff + *osis,* condition. Ancient term for stiffening of joints, loss of mobility.

annulus: (L) ring-shaped structure; annular fibrosis of intervertebral disks.

anomaly: (G) anomalia *an,* against + *omaly,* ordinary. Abnormality or deviation from normal, whether in structure, form, location, or function.

antagonist: (G) anti- or *an,* against, opposite + *tagon,* a struggle; *agonistes,* a rival. A muscle that opposes the action of another muscle (agonist).

anterior: (L) *ante-,* before, more in front; from *anterus,* positive form of anterior. Antero- used in combining form.

apex: (L) tip.

aplasia: (G) *a,* against + *plasia,* to mold or form. A failure in tissue formation.

aponeurosis: (G) *apo,* away from + *neuron,* tendon. Before Aristotle (c. 350 BC) introduced the word neura for nerves, everything of a fibrous nature was called a neuron. Galen (c. 180 AD) was first to use the word aponeurosis to refer to the insertion of a muscle that was not by flesh fibers but terminated in the white sheath.

apophysis: (G) *apo,* from + *physis,* growth; offshoot. Outcropping, but not end of bone, but rather the outgrowth of bone without an independent center of ossification. A place for tendinous attachment.

appendages: (L) *appendere,* to hang to, an extremity (pl. appendices).

arachnoid: (G) *arachne,* spider-like + *eidos,* form, shape; resembling a web; cerebellum and spinal cord covering.

arcuate: (L) *arcualis,* arch-shaped, bowed. Refers to arcuate line of rectus sheath and arcuate ligament of wrist.

artery: (G) *aer,* air + *terso,* to carry; arteries were believed to be air carriers in vessels. Later referred to arteries carrying blood.

arthritis: (G) *arthro,* joint + *-itis,* inflammation.

arthrodesis: (G) *arthro,* joint + *desis,* binding; fusion of a joint.

arthrology: (G) *arthro,* joint + *-ology,* treatise or discourse. Galen recorded two main orders of joints: diarthrosis (articulation with movement) and synarthrosis (articulation without movement). He then divided the diarthroses into enarthroses, arthrodies, and ginglymus. Synarthroses were divided into suture, symphysis, and gomphosis.

articulatio: (L) *articulus,* little joint, dim. of *artus,* fitted close. Artus was used for limbs, thus, articulatus, jointed. Galen, Pliny, and Celsus preferred the Latin "articulus" to the Greek "arthro"; however, both continue to be used.

artifact: (L) *ars,* art + *facere,* to make anything artificially produced.

aspera: (L) *asper,* rough. Linea aspera is a roughened ridge on the femur associated with insertion of the adductor group of muscles.

asthenia: (G) *asthenis,* without strength; loss of strength, myasthenia—loss of muscle strength.

atlas: (G) from *atlao,* endure or sustain. Galen (c. 180 AD) called the atlas, protos spondylos, the first cervical vertebra, and second vertebra, epistropheus, to rotate on. The term was later changed to refer to the axis.

atrophy: (G) *atrophia,* a wasting; *a,* lacking + *trophia,* nourishment. A decrease in size of an organ or tissue, commonly a muscle.

autogenous: (G) *autos,* self + *genous,* to produce; self-produced or originating within the body.

autonomic: (A-S) *auto,* self + *nomos,* law; functioning independently.

auxe: (G) enlargement, increase; auxetic, to promote proliferation of leukocytes and other cells.

avulsion: (L) *avulsio,* to separate by force. From (G) *ab,* away from + (L) *vellere,* to pull.

axilla: (L) armpit. Uncertain origin, but thought to be a compound word from axis alae, meaning axle of a wing, where arm revolves at this point.

axis: (L) a line, real or imaginary, that runs through center of a body; or a pivot, about which a part revolves.

bacterium (pl. bacteria): (G) *bakterion,* rod; rod-shaped one-celled organism.

biceps: (L) *bi,* two + *ceps,* head; caput; bicipital, having two heads. Refers to the biceps brachii and biceps femora muscle groups.

bifida: *bi,* two + *findere,* to cleave; having two parts, e.g., spina bifida.

biopsy: (G) *bio,* life + *op,* vision. Excision of living tissue for microscopic examination.

blasts:(G) suffix meaning germ; used in reference to cells that make other cells, such as the osteoblasts, bone-making cells.

bone: (A-S) from (L) *os* and (G) *osteon.*

boss: (Fr) *boce,* a swelling; a rounded eminence, e.g., carpal bossing. Bosselated refers to having many small prominences.

brachium: (L) arm, from (G) *brakhion,* shorter; *brachy,* short, Brachialis muscle of arm.

brevis: (L) short. Refers to short flexor of fingers (flexor digitorum brevis).

brisement: (Fr) crushing as in breaking by force; pronounced breez-mon.

bruise: (Fr) *bruiser,* to break. Broken vessel.

bruit: (Fr) noise; pronounced broo-ee.

bunion: (G) bunion, bugnone, a lump; bouvos, a hill or eminence; (L) *bunia,* enlargement.

bursa: (G) *bursula,* a pouch or sac, a purse; (L) pouch, wine skin. A sac between tendons, tendon and bone, muscle and bone that acts as a gliding surface at pressure points where friction can occur. Named in association with their anatomic location.

cadaver (pl. cadavera): (L) *cadere,* to fall, die.

calcar: (L) a spur, calcarine, spur-shaped; small spiny projection of bone.

calcaneus: (L) *calx,* a heel; os calcis, heel bone.

calcification: (L) *calx,* lime + *facere,* to make.

calcium: (L) *calx,* lime.

calisthenics: (G) *kalos,* beautiful + *sthenos,* strength.

callus: (G) *kalon,* callositas, dry wood; (L) *callum,* hard skin; (A-S) callus, new bone formation at site of fracture.

callous: hard thickened skin, e.g., the foot.

canal: (L) *canalis,* channel. Conduit for vessels, nerves.

cancellous: (L) *cancelli,* lattice work. A resemblance of cancellous tissue in bone to lattice work.

capitate: (L) *caput,* head-shaped; having a rounded extremity, Refers to small bone on distal row of hand; triquetrocapitate is the ligament.

capitellum: (L) *capitella,* small head. Knob-like protrusion of lateral condyle of the distal humerus.

capsule: (L) dim. of *capsa,* capsula, a little box; from *capio,* I receive.

caput: (L) a head; (G) *capitulum,* a little head. Modified to -ceps, as in biceps and triceps.

carotid: (G) *karos,* deep sleep; refers to main arteries of head and neck.

carpus: (L) *carpus, carpi,* wrist; (G) *karpos, karphyos,* dry bits of wood.

cartilage: (L) cartilage, gristle; (G) chondro.

cauda: (L) a tail, from *cadere,* to fall. Hence, cauda equina, termination of the spinal cord, was believed to resemble a plaited horse's tail.

cell: (L) *cella,* a chamber.

cervical: (L) cervico, cervicalis; pertaining to the neck.

cheiro: (G) *chiro,* hand; (L) *manus,* to grasp.

chirurgery: (G) hand + work; one who works with his hands, a chirurgeon.

chondral: (G) from *chondros,* cartilage or gristle; (L) cartilage, gristle.

chronic: (G) *chronos,* time; of long duration.

circulation: (L) *circulatio,* movement in a circular course.

claudication: (L) *claudicare,* to limp or be lame. Disturbance of circulation.

clavicle: (L) *claviculum,* dim. of *clavis,* a key. Was probably related to *claudere,* to shut or close; (G) *cleido-* as in sternocleidomastoid. Both Latin and Greek use meant a key, bolt, fastener. The collar bone was likened to a key because it locks the shoulder girdle to the breast bone and because of its shape.

clinic: (G) *klinikos,* to recline, a bed.

clonus: (G) *klonos,* turmoil; convulsing movements of epileptics. Now refers to spasm in which rigidity and relaxation alternate.

coccyx: (G) cuckoo's beak, from *kokkyx, coccygeus,* a cuckoo. Coccyx, tip of spine.

collagen: (G) *kolla,* glue + *gennan,* to produce; a glue-like substance that holds connective tissues together. Colloid, kollodes, glutinous.

collateral: (L) *con,* together + *lateralis,* latus, side. Secondary, accessory.

comitans: (L) companion. *Comes* (sing.), *cometes* (pl.). A blood vessel that accompanies a nerve trunk.

communis: (L) common, a vessel; that supplies several branches of the hand.

comminuted: (L) *com,* together + *minuere,* to crumble. To break into pieces, crushed.

concussion: (L) *concussus,* a shaking, from *concutio,* shake violently. An old term for thunder.

condyle: (G) *kondylos,* knuckle, knob; projections at the end of bones.

conjoined: (Fr) to meet, touch, overlap; refers to the aponeurotic tendon.

contusion: (L) *contusio,* a bruise; from *contundere*: *con,* together + *tundere,* to break.

coracoid: (G) *korax,* a crow + *oeides,* shape; (L) *corvus.* Anything hooked or pointed like a raven's beak. Variant of coronoid.

corpus: (L) *corporis,* body; (G) *somatos, soma.*

corpuscle: (L) *corpusculum,* small, rounded body. Former term for blood cell.

cortex: (L) *corticis,* rind; outer hard layer of compact bone.

cortical: (L) cortex, a rind, outer layer.

costo: (L) costa, from *costarum,* ribs. Refers to costovertebral cartilage.

coxa: (L) kaksha, the hip bone.

cranium: (L) skull.

crepitus: (G) *krepis,* a little noise, creaking; from *crepitare,* to crackle.

cribriform: (L) *cribrum,* a sieve + *forma,* form, sievelike; anything perforated with holes (e.g., cribriform plate of ethmoid bone).

cricoid: (G) *krikos,* a ring + *oeides,* shape. Refers to cricoid cartilage shaped like a signet ring.

cruciate: (L) crux, shaped like a cross; refers to the two intra-articular ligaments of the knee joint that cross and give strong support to the knee.

cubitus: (L) elbow, from *cubo,* lying down (cf. decubitus). Cuboid is cube-shaped; (G) kyboides, cube.

cuneiform: (L) *cuneus,* a wedge + *forma,* shape. Anything wedge-shaped.

curettage: (Fr) curette, a cleanser; scraping out a cavity. Also called debridement.

cutaneous: (L) *cutis,* skin.

dactylos: (G) a digit, of the fingers or toes.

debridement: (Fr) de + bridle; thus, unbridling. Originally, to cut away as restricting bands, and later to include tissue.

decubitus: (L) lying down; position of lying down, decubitus ulcer may occur.

dehiscence: (L) *dehiscere,* to gape; to burst open as in a wound.

deltoid: (G) *delta* (fourth letter of Greek alphabet); triangular-shaped.

dermas: (L) skin; *cutis vera,* true skin; corium, integumentary.

dermatome: (G) *derma,* skin + *tome,* incision. Refers to dermatome distribution of spinal cord segments and nerve distribution.

desmoid: (G) from *desmos,* band, a ligament.

desiccant: to dry up, as in a wound; desiccans (e.g., osteochondritis desiccans).

diagnosis: (G) *dia,* through + *gnosis,* knowledge; to discern.

diaphragm: (G) *dia,* through + *phragm,* a partition, wall. Any partition of the body; more specifically, the abdominal diaphragm.

diaphysis: (G) *dia,* through + *physis,* growth. To grow through, produce. Refers to center of ossification for shaft of long bones situated between growing regions at end of bone (epiphysis, metaphysis).

diarthrosis: (G) a joint, a movable articulation; freely movable hinge joint.

diastase: (G) *dia,* through + *stase,* to stand. A standing apart, separation. Now refers to complete separation of bone.

diathermy: (G) *dia,* through + *therme,* heat.

digitorum: (L) digitus, fingers or toes.

diplegia: (G) *di,* two + *plegia,* stroke; paralysis affecting one side only.

disk: (L) *discus,* plate; flat, round, plate-like structure (intervertebral d.).

disease: (Fr) *desaise; des,* from + *aise,* depart from normal.

dislocation: (L) *dis,* apart + *locus* or *locare,* to place; dislocatio. Refers to separation of bone at joint area; formerly called a subluxation.

doctor: (L) from *docere,* to teach.

dorsum: (L) the back of a part.

dysfunction: (G) *dys,* difficult, painful + *functio* (L), a performance. Abnormal, impaired function.

dysplasia: (G) *dys,* bad + *plasien,* to form. Abnormal growth process.

dura: (L) hard. Refers to dura mater, the outermost and toughest of three membranes enclosing the spinal cord and brain. Syn. pia mater, soft.

dystrophy: (G) *dys,* bad, defective + *troph,* nourishment. Deficient by way of nutrition or metabolism; shortening of a muscle.

ebonation: (L) *e,* out + (A-S) *ban,* bone. Removal of bony fragments from a wound.

eburnate: (L) *eburnus, ivory,* refers to changes in bone density to an ivory-like structure in a process called eburnation.

ecchymosis: (G) *ek,* out + *chymos,* juice + *osis,* condition; *ecchy,* extravasation + *mosis,* to pour, shed. Extravasation of blood into tissue.

edema: (G) *oedema,* a swelling. Hippocrates referred to fluid buildup in tissue as oedematous, and the term continues to this day.

elbow: (A-S) from *elboga; eln,* forearm + *boga,* bend. From *ell,* a measure of length used in early times from shoulder to fingers; *boga* was a bending or bow.

embolus: (G) plug.

enarthrosis: (G) *en,* in + *arthron,* joint; a ball-and-socket joint.

enchondroma: (G) *en,* within + *chondro,* cartilage + *oma,* tumor; tumor within cartilage.

endoskeleton: (G) *endo,* within + (A-S) *skeleton*; the bony and cartilaginous parts of the skeleton that develop from mesoderm and not ectoderm and that are buried within the soft parts.

endosteum: (G) *endo,* within; medullary cavity of bone.

ensiform: (L) *ensis,* sword + *forma,* shape. Part of breastbone (xiphoid).

epicondyle: (G) *epi,* upon + *kondylos,* a knuckle, knob. Prominence on bone above or upon a condyle.

epidermis: (L) *epi,* upon + *dermis,* skin. Outer layer of skin.

epilepsy: (G) *epi,* upon + *lepsy,* falling sickness. Ancient term referring to infliction, seizures. The French terms are petit mal (short) and grand mal (large).

epimysium: (G) *epi*, upon + *mys*, muscle. The fibrous sheath enclosing a muscle.

epiphysis: (G) *epi*, upon + *physis*, outgrowth. Center of ossification where a part of the process ossifies separately before making an osseous union with the main portion of bone.

epithelium: (G) *epi*, upon + *thele*, nipple. Areas with nipple-like papillae. Term usually applied for the skin. The cognate word "endothelium" is usually applied to blood vessel inner lining and "mesothelium" to visceral lining such as the lung pleura and lining of the peritoneal cavity.

eponychium: (L) from *onyx*, nail; the structure from which the nail develops.

equina: (L) from *equus*, horse; refers to equinovarus and valgus (a form of clubfoot).

erythema: (G) *erythros*, red + *ema*, condition. To redden, to blush.

erythropoietic: (G) *erythros*, red + *poietic*, suffix for making or producing.

ethmoid: (G) *ethmos*, a sieve + *oeides*, form, shape, resembles. Cribriform, sieve-like. Perforations of the ethmoid plate.

etiology: (G) aetiology; refers to studying causes of disease.

eversion: (L) out + *ventere*, to turn the foot out at the ankle between the talus and calcaneus.

exacerbate: (L) *ex*, out + *acerbus*, harsh, bitter; from *exacerbare* and exasperate, an increase in symptoms, a flare-up, to make worse.

exostosis: (G) *ex*, out + *os*, bone + *osis*, condition. A bony outgrowth.

extrinsic: (L) *extrinsecus*, coming from; *extra*, outside + *secus*, otherwise.

fabella: (L) dim. of *faba*, a bean; a bean-shaped sesamoid fibrocartilage that may develop in the lateral head of the gastrocnemius muscle behind the knee joint.

facet: (Fr) *facette*, little face; refers to the small, smooth articular surface of bone as in facet joints of the spine.

falciform: (L) *falx*, sickle + *forma*, shape; triangular ligament of ischium (inguinal ligament).

falx: (L) sickle-shaped structure; denotes a ligamentous opening, e.g., conjoined tendon.

fascia: (L) a band, bandage. Anatomic fasciae denote sheath-like fibrous connective tissue that supports, separates, and covers muscles, joints, and other tissues of the body.

femur: (L) dim. of *ferendum*, bearing; bearing weight as in the thigh bone.

fenestra: (L) a window; to open or make a window; fenestrate, fenestration.

fiber: (L) *fibra*, thread-like; (G) fibrin, fibroid.

fibula: (L) a small clasp, or needle-like point, a broach, buckle; (G) anything pointed or piercing. Long, thin bone of lower limb behind the tibia.

fissure: (L) *fissura*, a cleft or groove; any groove in bone or fascia.

flap: (Dutch) *flappens*, to strike; named for a pedicle graft covering bone after resection.

flavum: term for yellow; refers to band of yellow elastic tissue of laminae of spine, called yellow ligament or ligamentum flavum.

flexor: (L) *flectere*, to bend; any muscle that flexes or bends a joint; flexion.

foramen: (L) *forare, foro*, to pierce; a natural opening or passageway in bone or fascia or vessels or nerves to pass through (e.g., obturator foramen).

fossa: (L) *fovea*, pit or hollow; (Fr) *fodere*, to dig. Any hollow depression in bone.

fracture: (L) *fractura*, a break; (Fr) *frangere*, to break.

ganglion: (G) *ganglia*, a knot, mass, tumor swelling.

gastrocnemius: (G) *gaster*, belly + *kneme*, leg. Refers to the large superficial calf muscle of the posterior lower limb.

gemellus: (L) for twin; one of two muscles inserted in the obturator internus tendon.

genu: (L) to bend. Geniculum referred to a knot or node. (G) *gony, gonu*, knee; genu recurvatum, valgus, and varus.

gladiolus: (L) dim. of *gladius*, a sword; main part of sternum.

glenoid: (G) *glene*, shallow socket + *oeides*, shape. Cup-shaped depression of scapula of shoulder.

glia: (G) glue; supporting tissue of spinal cord.

gluteal: (G) *gloutos*, a rump, buttock; any rounded eminence; gluteus maximus.

gout: (L) *gutta*, a drop, meaning poison falling drop by drop into a joint as a cause of pain and disease. Hippocrates described gout in the foot as podagra.

gracilis: (L) thin, lean, slender; a muscle of the thigh.

hallux: (G) *hallus, allomai,* to leap; (L) great toe, halluces.

hamate: (L) *hamatus, hamatum,* hook-like process; hamate bone of wrist.

hamstring: (A-S) ham, back of thigh; flexor tendons behind knee that stand out like cords.

hang nail: (A-S) *angnaegl,* from *ange,* troublesome + *naeagl,* nail.

hemiplegia: (G) *hemi-,* half + *plege,* a stroke. Paralysis affecting one side of body.

histology: (G) *histos,* woven web + *logos,* a treatise; histo refers to any woven material, a web, and in Homer, the sail of a ship. The tissue structure of an organism or part.

humerus: (L) ossa humeri that involved the scapula, clavicle, and humerus. Later changed to mean only upper arm bone.

hyaline: (G) *hyalos,* glass; hyaloid, glass-like that denotes clear matrix (e.g., hyaline cartilage of joint surfaces).

hyoid: (G) U-shaped; from Greek letter upsilon.

idiopathic: (G) *idios,* own, peculiar to oneself + *pathos,* disease. Refers to a condition or disease state without known cause.

index: (L) from *dico,* to point out, a pointer; hence, the forefinger (pl. indices).

ilium: (L) flank, from ilia, soft parts, because the iliac bone supports the gut. It is the wide portion of bone of the pelvis.

incarnatus: to grow, as in to grow a fingernail or toenail.

infection: (L) *infectum,* from *inficere,* to taint or tinge; to alter by invasion of a pathogenic agent, to infect.

inflammation: (L) *inflammatic,* from *inflammare,* to burn, or flame within. In the 18th century, Sauvages introduced suffix "-itis" to refer to inflammation.

infraspinatus: *infra-,* beneath + *spina,* thorn; beneath scapular spine.

innervation: (L) *in,* into + *nervus,* a nerve. Reciprocal innervation refers to muscles moving a joint.

innominate: (L) innominatus, from *in,* without + *nomen,* name. Given to three bones of the pelvis where compound bone was not named.

interossei: *inter,* between + *ossei,* bone; situated between bones, such as specific muscles of the hands and feet.

intramedullary: (L) within + *medullaris,* marrow. Within marrow cavity of bone.

intrinsic: (L) *intrinsecus,* situated inside; thus, intrinsic muscles have their origin and insertion entirely within a structure and thereby are limited to it.

insertion: (L) *in,* into + *serere,* to plant. Place of attachment of a muscle into a bone that it moves.

interstitial: lying between; spaces within an organ or tissue.

inversion: (L) *ventere,* to turn; to turn foot inward at the ankle.

involucrum: from *volvere,* to wrap; a covering of newly formed bone enveloping the sequestreum in infection of bone.

ischemic: (G) *isch,* to keep back + *aemia,* blood. Deficiency of blood to a part, ischemia.

ischium: (G) *ischion,* hip, meaning strength; lowermost bone of innominate bones forming the bony pelvis, seat bone; (L) coxa.

joint: (L) *junctura, junctio,* from *jungere,* to join; the point of articulation between two bones.

juxtaposition: (L) near, close proximity + *positio,* place. Adjacent to or side by side.

kinematics: (G) *kinematos,* movement; relates to biomechanics and muscle movements.

knuckle: (Ger) *knokel;* (L) *articulus,* joint segment. Prominence of the distal heads of the metacarpals or dorsal aspect of any of the phalangeal joints.

kyphosis: (G) *kypho,* hump + *-osis,* condition. Convex prominence of spine.

lacuna: (L) a pit, hollow space; refers to microscopic resorption areas in bone, cartilage, or cementum. Lacunula, small or minute lacuna.

lamella: (L) a little plate, dim. of lamina; layer of bone or ground substance of osseous tissue situated in places within bone.

lamina: (L) flat plate; refers to flattened part of either side of the vertebral arch when used alone.

latissimus: (L) *latus,* broad; refers to latissimus dorsi back sheath muscle.

leio: (G) *leios,* smooth; prefix that refers to muscles.

lepto: (G) *leptos,* slender; e.g., leptodactyly, abnormally slim fingers.

levator: (L) *levo,* to lift, a lifter; refers to levator musculi.

ligamentum: (L) *ligare,* to tie, bind + *mentum,* a bandage. Fibrous band of tissue connecting articular ends of bone serving to bind them together to facilitate or limit motion, or to support viscera.

limbus: (L) edge, fibrocartilaginous rim of a joint; refers to glenoid (shoulder) and acetabulum (hip).

linea aspera: (L) *linea*, line + *aspera*, rough. Roughened ridge on femur for insertion of adductus group of muscles.

lipos: (G) *lipos*, fat; lipoid, resembling fat.

lordosis: (G) *lordo*, curved, to bend; an exaggeration of the normal forward convexity in the lumbar region of the spine.

lumbar: (L) *lumbus*, loin; refers to lumbar region.

lumbrical: (L) *lumbricus*, worm; refers to the four small worm-like muscles of the palm of the hand and foot.

lunate: (L) *luna*, moon; crescent-shaped bone in wrist.

lunula: (L) dim. of *luna*; refers to half-moon-shaped white area at base of nail.

lupus: (L) wolf; named for gradual skin disease, lupus erythematosus.

luxation: (G) *luxatio*, dislocation, from *luxo*, to dislocate; subluxate is a partial dislocation.

lymph: (L) *lympha*, water; clear, transparent fluid found in lymphatic vessels.

magnum: (L) large or great; capitate bone, formerly called os magnum, the largest of carpal bones

malacia: (G) *malakia*, softening; as of abnormal tissue softening.

malaise: (Fr) discomfort; indisposed, not well.

malleolus: (L) *malleus*, small hammer; refers to bony eminences on either side of the ankle.

manubrium: (L) a handle, from *manus*, hand + *hibrium* or *habeo*, to hold. Named for uppermost part of sternum (manubrium sterni) that is similar to the handle of a sword.

manus: (L) the hand; (G) *cheir*.

marrow: (A-S) *mearh*, unknown origin; (L) medulla. The spinal cord was formerly called the spinal marrow (14th c.). Now, any soft central part of bone.

matrix: (L) *mater*, mother tissue; refers to intercellular substance of tissue, the formative portion of a structure.

mediastinum: (L) *medius*, middle + *stare*, to stand; taken from *per medium tensum*, that which is tight down the middle. (The term is applied to partitions and in no way is connected to the word *mediastinus* of Latin origin.)

medicine: (L) *medicina*, the art of healing; *medicor* meant to heal or cure. From 13th century, medicus applied to anyone associated with the art of healing in the care and treatment of patients.

medullary: (L) *medullaris*, marrow, from medius, middle (medio ossis); refers to the medullary cavity, medulla.

meninges: (G) *meninx*, a membrane; refers to membranes investing the spinal cord and brain.

melia: (G) *melos*, limb; refers to absence of a limb, e.g., hemimelia.

meniscus: (G) *meniskos*, crescent-shaped, dim. of *mene*, moon; the medial and lateral crescent-shaped intraarticular fibrocartilage in the knee.

metabolic: (G) *metaballein*, to change; refers to metabolism.

metacarpus: (G) *meta*, beyond + *karpus*, wrist. Five bony rays distal to the wrist.

metaphysis: (G) *meta*, beyond + *physis*, growth. The line of junction of the epiphysis and the diaphysis.

metaplasia: (G) *meta*, beyond + *plasia*, to form. Virchow described connective tissue group changes into another tissue of the same group, such as cartilage into bone.

metatarsal: (G) *meta*, beyond + *tarsos*, ankle. Five bony rays distal to the tarsal bones of the foot.

mnemonic: (G) memory; a very old system for remembering, dating back to 477 BC.

monostotic: (G) *mon*, single + *osteon*, bone; refers to a single bone.

mucous: (L) *muco*, slimy exudate from membrane.

muscle: (L) little mouse, dim. of *mus*, mouse and (G) *myo*; probably derived from the way muscles move under the skin.

myelos: (G) marrow, the pith of plants; refers to the marrow cavity of the spinal cord.

navicular: (L) *navicula*, little boat, dim. of *navis*, a ship; boat-shaped structure hollowed out in form. Both navicular and scaphoid are used for the boat-shaped carpal and tarsal bones.

necrosis: (G) *nekrosis*, state of death; sequestrum of bone, sloughing of soft tissue. Insufficient blood supply to a part resulting in death of tissue.

nerve: (L) *nervus,* sinew and (G) *neuron,* sinew; refers to the nerve cells.

neurolemma: (G) *neuro,* nerve + *lemma,* sheath, husk. A thin membranous sheath covering a nerve fiber.

nodule: (L) *nodulus,* a knot; refers to a small node or collection of cells.

nuchae: (L) nucha, back of neck; refers to neck area.

nucleus: (L) *nux,* nut, a little nut; the central part of a cell.

obturator: (L) *obturare/obturo,* to stop up, obstruct, or occlude; a membrane that covers an opening (e.g., obturator foramen).

occult: (L) from *occulere,* to hide or cover over; occultus, hidden, concealed.

odontoid: (G) *ondon,* tooth + *oid,* resembles; toothlike process of second cervical vertebra.

olecranon: (G) *olenes kranon, kranos,* helmet, olekranon, point of the elbow; elbow process at the proximal end of the ulna.

omo: (G) *omos,* shoulder; used in combining form, e.g., omovertebral.

omohyoid: (G) *omos,* shoulder + *hyoeides,* U-shaped. Shoulder muscle formerly called omohyoid because the muscle was attached to the scapula at one end and the hyoid bone at the other.

onco: (G) *onkos,* bulk, mass; used in combining form, e.g., oncogene, a gene associated with tumors.

onychia: (G) *onychos, onyx,* nail; (L) *unguis.* Inflammation of nail bed.

opponens: (L) opposing; applied to the muscles of the hand and foot.

organ: (G) *organon,* (L) *organum,* viscus, viscera.

orifice: (L) *orificium,* a natural opening.

orthopaedic: (G) *orthos,* straight + *paes,* a child. Literally means straightening of children. First introduced in 1741 by Nicholas Andry, French physician, who published the first book on orthopaedics. He proposed to prevent and correct deformities in children by exercise, diet, and mechanical means. His was the first work specifically devoted to the subject.

os: (L) *os, ossis,* bone; ossicle, ossiculum, small bone. (G) *oste,* allows for use in combining form.

ossification: (L) *os,* bone + *facere, to* make. Process of bone formation.

osteoblast: (G) *osteo,* bone + *blast,* a germ or sprout. A bone-producing cell.

osteoclast: (G) *osteo,* bone + *klasis,* to break up. Concerned with absorption and removal of unwanted tissue.

osteogenesis: (G) *osteo,* bone + *genesis,* origin. Bone production.

osteophyte: (G) *osseo,* bone + *phyte,* outgrowth; bony excrescence branched in shape.

pain: (L) *poena,* a fine, a penalty.

palmaris: (L) palm, hand; palmaris longus and brevis muscles of hand.

palpate: (L) *palpare, palpabilis,* to touch; perceptible by feel, touch.

palsy: (Fr) *paralysie,* (ME) *parlesie;* term palsy appeared in 1300.

paralysis: (G) *para,* besides + *lysis,* to loosen, *paralyein,* to disable. Disabling limb condition.

paraplegia: (G) *para,* besides + *plegia,* a stroke. Formerly meant stricken on one side, and now refers to paralysis of both limbs and maybe the trunk.

paratenon: *para,* around + *tenon,* tendon; fatty tissue surrounding tendon to fill in spaces.

paresis: (G) *parienai,* to let fall or pass; referred to muscle weakening and now includes partial paralysis.

pars: (L) a part of a larger structure; the pars interarticularis bridges the spine between articular facets.

paronychia: (G) *para,* besides + *nychia,* a nail. Refers to infection of marginal area of nail.

patella: (L) a saucer, small pan, dim. of *patera,* a round plate, and *patere,* to lie open or exposed; the kneecap.

patency: (L) *patens,* open, evident.

pathology: (G) *pathema,* disease + *logos,* word, reason. Study of the nature and cause of disease.

pectineus: (L) *pecten,* comb; muscle that flexes and adducts the thigh.

pectoralis: (L) from *pectus,* the breast; ancient term for an ornamental breast plate that was later included in medicine to mean the pectoralis major and minor muscles of the chest.

pedicle: (L) *pes, pedis,* foot, and *pediculus,* a little foot, stem; referred to stalks of plants originally, and later to structures of anatomy.

pelvis: (L) a basin, (G) tub or wooden bowl; any basin-shaped structure or cavity. Named for the large three innominate bones.

periosteum: (G) *peri,* around + *osteon,* bone. Hard protective fibrous membrane covering bone.

peritoneum: (G) *peri,* around + *teinein,* to stretch. Serous membrane that supports the abdominal cavity.

peroneal: (G) *perone,* pin, sewing needle, anything pointed for piercing; (L) fibula, brooch. Peroneal relates to the fibula; peroneus, perone, relates to one of three muscles of the leg causing motion of the foot.

pes: (L) *pedis,* a foot or foot-like projection; applied to different structures such as pes cavus (hollow), pes planus (flat), pes anserinus (goose foot).

phalanges: (G) *phalanx,* a band of soldiers; (L) *internodia,* because joints of fingers and toes were called nodes in close knit row. Refers to the distal, medial, and proximal phalanges of the hands and feet.

phlebo: (G) *phleps, phlebos,* vein; combining form for vein.

physician: (Fr) *physicien;* one who has successfully completed a prescribed course of studies in medicine.

physis: (G) *phyein,* to generate growth; portion of long bone involved in growth, e.g., diaphysis and epiphysis.

pinna: a static wing-like projection.

piriformis: (L) *pium,* a pear + *forma,* shape; piriformis muscle.

pisiform: (L) *pisum,* pea + *forma,* shape. Pea-shaped bone of wrist and smallest of carpal bones, proximal row, ulnar side.

placebo: (L) for "I shall please"; imitation therapeutic agent.

plantar: (L) *planta,* sole of foot, and (G) *platus, planus,* flat; from (L) *plantaris,* a sprout, twig, plant.

plaster: (G) *emplastron,* to form, mould. Hippocrates and Galen wrote extensively on the subject. Pliny described it in making casts. Originally, bandages were made of starch and paste, lime, and egg white. The gypsum variety was made in Paris, thus plaster of Paris.

pleura: (G) a rib. Now applied to serous membrane lining the chest wall.

plexus: (L) a braid, plait, entanglement; a complex, especially of blood and lymphatic vessels, and nerves (e.g., brachial plexus).

pollicis: (L) thumb, from *polleo,* strong; (pl. pollices); refers to the pollicis longus and brevis of the hand (formerly called pollex).

popliteal: (L) *poples,* the ham; ancient term from *plicare,* to fold. Refers to the popliteus muscle behind the knee between the hamstrings that flexes the leg and aids in rotation.

profundus: (L) deep seated; refers to source located deeper than indicated reference point (e.g., profundus tendon). Opposite of sublimis.

pronator: (L) *pronatus,* prone (face down), from *pronare,* to bend forward and *pronus,* turned, inclined; pronator muscle that allows pronation. Vesalius used pronum and supinum to refer to muscles.

proprioceptive: (L) *proprius,* one's own, special + *capere,* to take, seize. A perception of sensations that creates awareness of what's going on within the body.

prosthesis: (G) prosthesis, an addition.

proximal: (L) nearest point of reference.

pseudo: (G) false.

psoas: (G) *psoa;* one of two muscles of the loins.

pubis: (L) grown up; anterior part of innominate bone, anterior pelvic bone.

pulse: (L) *pulsus,* beating; pulsate, *pulsare,* throb.

quadriceps: (L) *quadri,* four + *caput,* head. Four-headed as a quadriceps muscle.

rachio: (G) *rhachis,* spinal column; used in combining form.

radius: (L) a staff, rod, spoke of a wheel; (G) *radix,* a ray. The distal radius rotates around the distal ulna through a radius of 180 degrees.

ramus: (L) rami, branch; a branch of any given artery or nerve of the spine, extension.

ray: (L) radius; in orthopaedics, refers to the five rays of bones in the hands and feet.

rectus: (L) straight; refers to rectus abdominus muscle of the abdomen.

reflex:(L) *reflexus,* to bend back and (G) *reflectere,* to turn back; used to describe muscle movements of the body.

resection: (L) *resectio,* a cutting off; partial excision of a bone.

retinaculum: (L) halter, a tether, from *retinere,* to restrain; restraining fibers of fascia that hold a part in place, e.g., the patellar retinaculum, fibers that surround the knee cap and knee, and the flexor and extensor retinacula of the palm of the hand.

retroversion: (L) *retro,* back + *versio,* a turning.

rheumatoid: (G) *rheuma,* discharge + *oid,* resembling. Resembling rheumatism.

rhomboids: (G) rhombus, kite-shaped; a four-sided figure with all sides equal. Refers to the rhomboid muscles, greater and lesser.

sacrum: (L) *sacer,* sacred, holy. In ancient times, the sacrum was used in sacrificial rites because it was the last bone to decay, and it was believed that the body would reform around it. Largest of vertebral bones, it protects and supports the lower organs.

sagittal: (L) *sagitta,* an arrow; the sagittal suture resembles an arrow. The sagittal plane is the medial vertical plane in line with the suture (i.e., the median plane of the body).

saphenous: (Arabic) *al safin,* hidden; saphenous vein.

sarcolemma: (G) *sarx,* flesh + *lemma,* sheath. The delicate membranous sheath surrounding each individual muscle fiber.

sartorius: (L) *sartor,* a tailor; refers to a muscle whose action is to bring the leg into a flexed, adducted, and laterally rotated cross-legged sitting position habitually adopted by tailors.

scaleneus: (G) *scalenos,* uneven; refers to a triangle with unequal sides, and named for the neck muscle group of unequal length composed of the medius, minimus, and anterior m.

scaphoid: (G) *skaphe,* a small boat, and (L) *scapha,* skiff; scooped out, hence, boat-shaped bones in the hands and feet.

scapula: (L) *scapulae,* resembling a trough or digging tool and (G) *spathula,* broad implement, resembling a spade; the large, flat, triangular bone of the shoulder that articulates with the clavicle and humerus, shoulder blades.

sciatic: (L) *sciaticus,* and (G) *ischion,* a hip joint; refers to pain in the loins and hip, and is associated with the large sciatic nerve.

sclerosis: German in origin; meant degeneration of tissue. Later, referred to a hardening process.

scoliosis: (G) a curvature. In early times, meant anything bent or curved. Now refers specifically to a lateral curvature of the spine.

semilunar: (L) *semi,* half + *luna,* moon. The crescent-shaped lunate bone of carpus, lunate bone.

septum: (L) *saeptum,* a partition.

sequestrum: (L) *sequestrare,* to separate, set aside; fragment of necrosed bone that has detached from surrounding tissue.

serratus: (L) *serra,* a saw, serrated, having a sawtooth edge; serratus anterior muscles, anterior (chest) and posterior (back).

sesamoid: (G) *sesamon,* sesame plant + *-oid,* resembling. In Arabic, is *sem sem,* a sesame seed. Seed-shaped bones or fibrocartilage situated in tendons that move over a bony surface.

skeleton: (G) *skeletos,* a dried up body; the framework of the body consisting of 206 bones.

soleus: (L) *solea,* a flat fish; the flat, triangular-shaped muscle that inserts into the tendocalcaneus of the lower limbs.

spasm: (G) *spasmos,* convulsion, to draw out or pluck; refers to tonic or clonic muscle spasms.

spica: (L) ear of grain. Compares the overlapping of a cast to an ear of corn.

spina: (L) a thorn, (G) *spondylos.* In anatomy, thorn-like projections were called spines dating back to the 14th century; the vertebral column with its spinous processes.

spinalis: (L) a muscle attached to a spinal process of a vertebrae.

splay foot: (ME) *splayen,* to spread out + (A-S) foot. Flatfoot, pes planus.

splenius: flat muscle on either side of the back of the neck and upper thoracic region.

spondylo: (G) spine; used in combining form to refer to the vertebrae.

sprain: (L) *exprimere,* to press, squeeze, strain; (Fr) *espraindre,* to wring.

spur: (A-S) a pointed instrument. Refers to calcaneus of heel and femoral neck of femur (medial and underside where spurs are likely to occur).

stenosis: (G) *stenos,* narrow, a stricture; narrowing of a passageway.

sternum: (G) *sternon,* breast, chest + *steros,* hard, solid, and palpable. Thus, the breastbone is composed of the manubrium (top portion), gladiolus (body), and ensiform orxiphoid process (lower portion).

stethoscope: (G) *stethos,* chest + *skopein,* to examine. Instrument used to mediate the sounds produced within the body.

styloid: (G) *stylos,* pillar and (L) *stilus,* any long, pointed instrument; the ulnar styloid is the large prominence of bone at the back of the wrist.

sublimis: (L) uplifted, up in the air; applied to physical position, such as sublimus tendon near the surface.

subclavian: (L) *sub,* under, below + *clavis,* key. Refers to muscle, artery, or vein under the clavicle (collar bone).

subscription: (L) *subscriptus,* written under.

sulcus: (L) groove; plural sulci. The sulci cutis are the ridges on the skin of the palmar surface of fingers that comprise the fingerprints.

superficialis: (L) superficial. Denotes an artery, vein, or nerve close to the surface.

supination: (L) *supinatio,* turning face upward; supinator muscle of forearm, or that of leg, turning leg or foot outward.

supraspinatus: (L) *supra,* above + *spinatus,* spines or thorn-shaped. Refers to the supraspinatus muscle above the spine of the scapula.

sural: (L) *sura,* calf; refers to calf muscle group, triceps surae (gastrocnemius, plantaris, and soleus muscles).

surgeon: (G) from *chirurgeon, cheir,* meaning the hand + *ergon,* to work. One who works with the hands.

symphysis: (G) *syn,* together + *phyein,* to grow, growing together; a natural union. Refers to the symphysis pubis, two articular bones joined by fibrocartilage.

symptom: (G) *symptoma,* occurrence.

synarthrosis: (G) *syn,* together + *arthrosis,* a joint. An immovable joint.

syndesmosis: (G) *syn,* together + *desmos,* a band. A joint in which two bones are held together by ligaments.

syndrome: (G) concurrence, running together; clinical picture of a disease made by the presence of several typical signs and symptoms.

synergists: (G) *syn,* together + *ergon,* work, to cooperate. Refers to the smooth coordinated way in which muscles work together in the execution of movement, such as the synergist muscle group, organs, or parts acting in unison.

synostosis: (G) *syn,* together + *osteon,* bone. The union of two bones by osseous tissue such as the diaphysis and epiphysis of a long bone at the end of the growth period.

synovium: (G) *syn,* together + *oon,* egg, (L) ovum, egg white. Refers to the egg white appearance of fluid present in movable joints.

tabatiere anatomique: (Fr) anatomic "snuff box"; refers to space at the base of the thumb.

talipes: (L) *talipedare,* to be weak on the feet, to totter. Hence, talipes, club foot.

talus: (L) from Cicero, *ludere talis,* to play at dice, and *taxillus,* dice; bone resembling dice because dice were carved from the calcaneus of a horse. Talus, ankle bone.

tarsus: (G) from *tarsomai,* to become dry, tarsos; referred to anything flat or spread out. Thus, applied to the flat part of the feet.

tendon: (L) *tendere,* to stretch out; (Gr) *tenon,* a tightly stretched band; the elongated end of a muscle. Syn. sinew.

tensor: (L) *tendere,* tensum, to stretch; named for muscle that tenses or stretches and does not alter the direction of a part (e.g., tensor fascia).

teres: (L) from *terere,* to rub or grind smooth, well turned or rounded off; refers to the ligamentum teres, round ligament of the hip.

thecal: (G) sheath, capsule; relates to a tendon sheath, theca.

thenar: (G) from *theino,* to strike; referred to flat part of hand used to strike. Now refers to muscles of the palm divided into groups called thenar (major group) and hypothenar (lesser group).

thoraco: (G) thorax, chest, breast plate, stethos. In classical Greek, the thorax was armor (breastplate) to protect the chest and abdomen.

therapy: (G) *therapeia,* treatment, remedy, cure. First referred to the noun, *therapeutae,* healers, and later included treatment.

tibialis: (L) a pipe or flute, shin bone, variant of *tubia,* tube. In ancient times, musical instruments were made from shin bones of animals and objects of tubular form. Tibia, the larger anterior bone of the lower limb.

tourniquet: (Fr) *tournier,* to turn. Originally applied to a stick that turned to tighten a bandage or apply pressure over a large artery to stop blood flow.

trabecula: (L) little beam, dim. of *trabs, trapes,* timber; any large wooden beam, such as the rib of a boat or strands of supporting fibers. Refers to beam-like pattern or arrangement of bony lamellae in cancellous bone and muscle bundles raised up beneath ventricular endocardium of heart.

trapezoid: (L) an irregular, four-sided figure; referred to a four-sided geometrical figure with two sides parallel to two sides divergent. Named for a carpal wrist bone (os magnum), the muscle was also called musculus cucullaris, because together with its fellow of the opposite side, it resembled a monk's cowl or hood.

trapezius: (L) the flat, triangular muscle covering the posterior surface of the neck and shoulders.

trauma: (G) *tro,* to wound or hurt + *ma,* results of action. Any wound or injury to the body by exterior forces inflicted or by physical agent.

triceps: (G) *tri,* three + (L) *tres,* three + *ceps,* head; a three-headed muscle with a single insertion (e.g., triceps brachii in the arm and triceps surae of the lower limb that combines the gastrocnemius and soleus muscles).

triquetrum: (L) *triquetrus,* having three corners; refers to the wedge-shaped cuneiform bone of the wrist.

trochanter: (G) *trochos,* a wheel or runner; two bony processes below the neck of the femur for muscle attachment. Galen applied term to greater and lesser trochanters and bony protuberance because of the way it moved in the act of running.

trochlea: (L) *trochilsa,* a pulley and (G) *trochos,* a wheel; refers to trochlea of humerus, an articular cylinder around which the ulna moves, similar to a pulley, but cylinder does not turn. A structure having the function of a pulley, a ring through which a tendon or muscle projects.

tubercle: (L) *tuberculum,* a little swelling; in orthopaedics, bony prominences that provide ligamentous attachment.

tuberosity: (L) tuberosities, to roughen; any roughened areas of bone for muscle attachment (e.g., greater tuberosity of the humerus).

ulna: (L) from *ell,* a measure of length; (Gr) *olene,* the elbow. In earlier times, the word denoted the whole arm, and now refers to the inner and larger bone of the forearm and elbow opposite the thumb side.

unguis: (L) claw, talon, nail; the toe or fingernails under the nail bed.

uniceps: (L) *unus,* one + *ceps,* head. Having a single head or origin.

unilateral: (L) *unus,* one + *latus,* side; occurring on one side.

valgus: (L) bent outward, bow-legged; also, talipes valgus; hallux valgus, distal to a point outward, genu valgus.

varus: (L) bent, turned inward; talipes varus (foot), genu varum (knock-kneed).

vascular: (L) *vas,* a vessel or dish; hence, a vascular organ is one with a profuse blood supply.

vastus: (L) vast, wide and great; refers to the three large muscle groups of the thigh (v. lateralis, v. medialis, v. intermedius).

vena: (L) vein, vessel; refers to the vena cava, the large vein leading to the heart with an upper and lower distribution.

vertebrae: (L) joint, from *vertere,* to turn and *vertebratus,* jointed or articulated. Refers to the 33 bony segments of the spinal column.

viability: (L) *vita,* life + *habilis,* fit. The ability to live, grow, and develop.

vinculum: (L) a band, cord, or anything that binds; from *vincio,* I bind; ring-like ligaments of the wrists and ankles; blood vessel bridges to the flexor tendons (brevis and longus), vinculae.

viscera: (L) *vis,* strength, casing, cavity; internal organs enclosed in the abdominal cavity and thorax.

volar: (L) *vola,* palm of hand or sole, from vola manus, hollow of hand; (Gr) *ballo,* to hurl. Palma referred to outstretched open hand.

vulnerable: (L) *vulnerare,* to wound; easily wounded.

whitlow: (ME) *whitflawe,* white flow; suppurative inflammation at the end of a finger or toe, deep-seated or superficial. Paronychia, felon.

wound: (A-S) *wund;* trauma to tissue.

xiphoid: (Gr) *xiphos,* a sword + *oeides,* shape, sword-shaped; sword-shaped bone of the inferior tip of the sternum to which ribs attach, ensiformis.

Appendix: ICD Codes for Eponymic Musculoskeletal Disease Terms

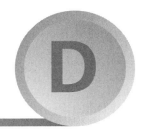

The following is intended for quick reference to International Classification of Diseases (ICD) codes that may be hard to find because of the use of eponymic terminology. It is recommended that the specific number be cross-checked with the coding system you are using, as a second decimal digit is sometimes required by insurance companies. In the preparation of the assignment of codes to these eponymic terms we used as a supplemental resource *The 3-In-1 Code Book for Orthopaedics and Neurosurgery,* Alexandria, VA, 1993, St. Anthony Publishing.

Fractures are coded primarily for closed (skin not broken) fractures. Closed fractures usually have a .0 and then a fifth digit if required. Open fractures are usually .1 with a fifth digit for location if required.

Many conditions affect joints. The fifth digit (second to the right of the decimal) assigns the portion of bone involved. In general, the shoulder is 1, elbow 2, wrist 4, hip 5, knee 6, and ankle and foot 7.

Some insurers insist on a fifth digit, which is usually served by adding a zero if the given code is only four digits.

The code for open fractures is given to the right of the closed fracture code.

Addison's keloid 701.0
Ainhum 136.0
Albert achillodynia 729.5
Albes-Schönberg disease 756.52
Albright-McCune-Sternberg syndrome 756.59
Allman clavicle fractures classification 810.02 or .03 (open 810.12 or .13)

Anderson and d'Alonzo classification 805.02 (open 805.12)
Apert disease 755.55
Arnold-Chiari 741.0
Ashurst classification 824.3
aviator's astragalus 825.21 (.31 for open f.)
Baastrup syndrome 721.5
Babinski-Frohlich syndrome 253.8
backfire fracture 813.42 (open f.: 813.52)
backpack palsy 955.7
Badelon classification 812.42 (open f.: 812.52)
Bado 813.03 (open f.: 813.13)
Baker cyst 727.51
Bamberger-Marie disease 731.2
Bankart lesion 718.31
Barton fracture 813.42 (open f.: 813.52)
baseball elbow 726.31
baseball finger 816.02 (open f.: 816.12)
Bechterew's disease 720.0
Behçet syndrome 136.1
Bell palsy 351.0
Bennett dislocation 834.01 (open d.: 834.11)
Bennett fracture 815.01 (open f.: 815.11)
black dot heel 924.20
black heel syndrome 924.20
Blount disease 732.4
blue toe syndrome (varies with source of embolism)
Boeck sarcoid 135
boot top fracture 823.2X (open f.: 823.3X)
    X .20 or .30 tibia alone
    X .21 or .31 fibula alone

X .22 0r .32 both tibia and fibula

Bosworth fracture 824.2 (open f.: 824.3)

Bouchard node 715.14

boutonnière deformity 736.21

boutonnière deformity finger 736.21

bowler's thumb 727.05

boxer's elbow 813.01 (open f.: 813.11)

boxer's fracture 815.04 (open f.: 815.14)

Boyd and Griffin 820s (depending on location)

Brailisford's disease 732.3

breaststroker's knee 717.7

Brendt and Harty fracture classification 825.21 (open f.: 825.31)

Brodie abscess 730.1X (depending on location)

Brown-Sequard syndrome 344.89

Buchanan disease 732.1

Bucholtz fracture classification 808s

bucket handle meniscus tear
    medial 717.0
    lateral 717.41

Buerger disease 443.1

bump, runners 726.71

bumper fracture (depends on bone involved)

Burns disease 732.3

butterfly fracture (depends on bone involved)

Caffey disease 756.59

caisson disease 993.3

cartilage hair hypoplasia 756.9

cartwheel fracture 821.22 (open f.: 821.32)

cast syndrome 557.1

cauda equina syndrome 344.6X

Chadwick and Bentley fracture 823.8X (open f.: 823.9X)

chalk bone 756.52

Chance fracture 805.4

Chandler disease 732.7

Charcot disease 356.1

Charcot joint 713.5

Charcot-Marie Tooth disease 356.1

charley horse
    quadriceps or hamstring 843.8
    calf 844.8

chauffeur fracture 813.42 (open f.: 813.52)

chisel fracture 813.05 (open f.: 815.15)

Chopart amputation 897.0

Chopart dislocation 838.02 (open d.: 838.12)

clawfoot 754.71
    acquired 736.74

clawhand 755.59
    acquired 736.06

clawtoes 754.71
    acquired 735.5

clay shoveler's fracture 812.44 (open f.: 812.54)

Codman tumor M9230/0

collar button abscess 682.4

Colles fracture 813.41 (open f.: 813.51)
    reverse 813.41 (open f.: 813.51)

Colonna fracture classification 820s (depending on location)

Colton fracture classification 813.01 (open f.: 813.11)

Cotton fracture 824.8 (open f.: 824.9)

CREST (CRST) 710.1

Cushing disease 255.0

Danis-Weber classification 824.2 (open.3)

Darrock-Hughston-Milch fracture 813.42 (open f.: 813.52)

dashboard fracture 808.0 (open 808.1)

Delbet fracture classification 820s depending on location

de Quervain disease 727.04

de Quervain fracture 814.01 (open f.: 814.11)

de Quervain syndrome 727.04

Desault dislocation 833.02 (open 833.12)

Diaz disease 732.5

Diaz fracture classification 824s

direct fracture (by region)

DISH 721.6

DISI 842.01

diver disease 993.3

Down syndrome 758.0

Duchenne muscular dystrophy 359.1

Dupuytren contracture 728.6

Dupuytren fracture
    ankle 824.4 (open f.: 824.5)
    radius 813.42 (open f.: 813.52)

Duverney fracture 808.41 (open 808.51)

Ehlers-Danlos syndrome 756.83

Ellis-van Creveld 756.55

Engelmann disease 756.59

Epstein dislocation classification system 808s and 820s

Epstein fracture classification system 808s and 820s

Erb disease 359.1

Erb-Goldflam disease 358.0

Erb paralysis 767.6X

Essex-Lopresti fracture 813.05 (open f.: 813.15) or 833.01 (open f.: 833.12)

Essex-Lopresti (os calcis fractures)

Evans femur fracture classification 820s (based on location)

Ewing tumor M9260/3

Fairbanks changes in x-ray 719s

Fairbanks dysostosis 756.50

Fanconi anemia 284.0X

Fanconi syndrome 270.0

Felix disease 732.1

Felty syndrome 714.1

Ferkel-Cheng classification talus OCD and fracture 825.21 (open f.: 825.31) or 732.5

Ferkel-Sgaglione classification of OCD and talus fracture 825.21 (open f.: 825.31) or 732.5

Fielding fracture classification system 820.22 (open f.: 820.32)

Freiberg disease 732.5

Frieberg infarction 732.5

Friedrich ataxia 334.0

Frohlich adiposogenital dystrophy 253.8

frozen shoulder 726.0

Frykman fracture classification system 813.4/.5 (fifth digit by specific type)

Galeazzi fracture 813.42 f.: (open 813.52)

gamekeeper thumb 842.12

Garden fracture classification system 820.0 (fifth digit by region)

gargoylism 277.5

Garré, chronic sclerosing osteomyelitis 730.1 (depending on location)

Garrod disease 728.79

Gartland fracture classification 812.41 (open f.: 812.51)

Gaucher disease 272.7

golfer elbow 726.31

Gosselin fracture 824.8 (open f.: 824.9)

Gower muscular dystrophy 359.1

greenstick fracture (by region)

Guillain-Barré syndrome 357.0

Gustillo (open) fracture (depends on location)

Haglund deformity
    congenital 755.67

acquired 732.72

Haglund disease 732.5

Hand-Schüller-Christian disease 277.8X

handlebar palsy 354.2

hangman fracture 805.02

Hass disease 732.3

hatchet head deformity 718.31

Hawkins fracture classification system 825.21/.31

Haygarth node 714.0

Heberden node 715.04

Henderson-Jones chondromatosis 727.82

Herbert and Fisher fracture classification system 814.02 (open f.: 814.11)

Hermodsson fracture 718.31

herpetic whitlow 054.6

Hill-Sachs fracture 718.31

Hill-Sachs lesion 718.31

hip pointer 843.0

Hodgkin tumor M9650/3 (varies by cell type)

Hohl fracture classification system 823.0X (open f.: 823.1X)

horseshoe abscess 682.4

hot cross bun skull 268.1 (rickets)

housemaid's knee 726.65

hump, dowager (general term)

Hunter syndrome 277.5

Hurler syndrome 277.5

Ideberg fracture classification 811.03 (open f.: 811.13)

Iselin disease 732.5

Jaccoud's syndrome 714.4

Jacksonian epilepsy 345.5X

Jaffe disease
    hereditary multiple exostosis 756.4
    osteoid osteoma M9191/0

javelin thrower elbow 726.31

Jefferson fracture 805.02

Jensen fracture classification 820.21 (open f.: 821.31)

Johansson classification system 820s, 821s

joint mice 727.82

Jones fracture 825.25 (open f.: 825.35)

jumper knee 726.69

Kaschin-Beck disease 716.0 (fifth digit by region)

Kawasaki disease 446.1

keloid, Addison 701.0

keratoma 701.1

Key and Conwell fracture classification 808s

Kidner lesion 755.69
Kienböck disease 732.3
Kienböck dislocation 833.03 (open d.: 833.13)
Kilfoyle fracture classification 812.43 (open f.: 812.53)
kissing spine 721.5
Klippel disease 723.8
Klippel-Feil disease 756.16
Kocher fracture 812.44 (open f.: 812.54)
Kohler disease 732.5
Konig disease 732.7
Kummel disease 721.7
Kyle fracture classification system 820.21 (open f.: 820.31)
kyphoscoliosis 737.30
Landouzy-Dejerine disease 359.1
Lange-Hansen classification fracture 824s
Le Fort fracture 824.2 (open f.: 824.3)
leadpipe fracture (by bone involved)
Legg-Calvé-Perthes disease 732.1
Legg-Calvé-Waldenstrom disease 732.1
Legg-Perthes disease 732.1
Letterer-Siwe disease M9722/3
Letts Vincent Gouw classification fracture 821s, 822s
Letournel and Judet fracture classification 808s
Levine fracture classification 805.02 (open f.: 805.12)
linebacker arm 728.12
Lisfranc amputation 897.0
Lisfranc dislocation 838.0X
Lisfranc fracture 825.25 (open f.: 825.35)
little leaguer's elbow 718.82
little leaguer's shoulder 718.81
lobster-claw deformity 755.58
loose bodies 717.6
lorry driver fracture 813.42 (open f.: 813.52)
Lou Gehrig's disease 335.20
Madelung deformity 755.54
Maffucci syndrome 756.4
Maisonneuve fracture 823.01 (open f.: 823.11) 837.0 (open f.: 837.1)
Malgaigne fracture 808.43 (open f.: 808.53)
mallet finger (if tendon only) 736.1
mallet fracture 816.02 (open f.: 816.12)
mallet toes 736.79
Mallory fracture classification E878.1
marathoner toe 703.8
marble bones 756.52

march fracture 825.25
Marfan syndrome 759.82
Marie-Bamberger disease 731.2
Marie-Charcot-Tooth disease 356.1
Marie-Strumpell disease 720.0
Maroteaux-Lamy syndrome 277.5
Mason fracture classification system 813.05 (open f.: 813.15)
Mast, Spiegel, and Pappas classification 823.8X of 823.9X
Mauclaire disease 732.3
Mayo 813.01 (open f.: 813.11)
McCune-Albright syndrome 756.59
Meyers and McKeever 823.0X (open f.: 823.1X)
milk-alkali disease/syndrome 999.1
milkmaid's dislocation 832.09
milkmaid's elbow 832.09
milkman syndrome 268.2
Milroy's disease 757.0
Monckeberg sclerosis 440.2X
mongolism 758.0
Monteggia dislocation 835.03 (open d.: 835.13)
Monteggia fracture-dislocation 813.22 (open f.-d.: 813.32)
Montercaux fracture 823.01 (open f.: 823.11) 837.0 (open f.: 837.1)
Moore fracture 813.41 (open f.: 813.51)
Morel syndrome 733.3
Morquio syndrome 277.5
Morton neuroma 355.6
Morton toe 726.7X
Mouchet's disease 732.5
Naffziger syndrome 353.0
nail-patella syndrome 756.81
Namaqualand hip dysplasia 732.1
Neer fracture classification 812.0s (open f.: 812.1s)
nightstick fracture 813.22 (open 813.32)
Ogden fracture classification system (by bone involved)
Ogden fracture classification 823.0X (open f.: 823.1X)
Ollier disease 756.4
opera glass hand 715.14
Osgood-Schlatter disease 732.4
Otto pelvis 715.35
Paget disease 731.0
Panner disease 732.3
paratrooper fracture 824.8 (open f.: 824.9)

parrot-beak meniscus tear 717.1–717.4 (depends on location)

Parsonage-Aldren-Turner syndrome 353.5

Parsonage-Turner syndrome 353.5

Pauwels 820s

Pellegrini-Steida disease 726.62

Perthes disease 732.1

Piedmont fracture 813.21 (open f.: 813.31)

Pierson disease 732.1

Pipkin fracture classification system 820.09 (open f.: 820.19)

pitcher elbow 718.82

Poland fracture classification system (by bone)

Pott disease 730.88 and/or 015.0

Pott fracture 824.4 (open f.: 824.5)

Preiser disease 733.09

"pump bump"
    congenital 755.67
    acquired 732.72 invalid

Quénu and Küss modified fractures-dislocations classification 825s, 838s

Raynaud disease 443.0X

Raynaud phenomenon 443.0X

Reiter syndrome 099.3

reverse Colles fracture 813.41 (open f.: 813.51)

reverse tennis elbow 726.31

ring fracture 808s

ring man shoulder 733.99

Riseborough and Radin fracture classification system 812.4X (open f.: 812.5; fifth digit by region)

rocker-bottom foot 754.61

Rockwood classification 840.0

Rolando fracture 815.01 (open f.: 815.11)

Rowe and Lowell classification system for fracture-dislocations 808.0 (open f.-d.: 808.1)

Rüedi and Allgöwer 823.8X (open f.: 823.9X)

rugger jersey (spine) 268.2

runner bump (depends on location)

runner knee (depends on cause)

Russel-Taylor classification 820s

Salter-Harris fractures (involving the physis in children) (code number varies by fracture location)

Samilson classification 715.11

Sanfilippo syndrome 277.5

Schatzker 823s

Scheie syndrome 277.5

Scheuermann disease 732.0

Schmorl node 722.30
    thoracic 722.31
    lumbar 722.32

Schwann tumor M9560/0, malignant/3

Segond fracture 823.00 (open f.: 823.10)

Seinsheimer fracture classification system 820.22 (open f.: 822.32)

Sever disease 732.5

Shepard fracture 825.21 (open f.: 825.31)

shepherd crook deformity 756.54

shoulder pointer 840.8

silver-fork deformity 813.41 (open d.: 813.51)

Sinding-Larsen-Johansson disease 732.4

skeletal amyloidosis 277.3X

skier injury 823.22 (open f.: 823.32)

Skillern's fracture 813.44 (open f.: 813.54)

Smith dislocation 838.03 (open d.: 838.13)

Smith fracture 813.41 (open f.: 813.51)

snapping hip 719.65

Stewart-Morel syndrome 733.3

Stickler syndrome 756.4

Stieda fracture 821.21 (open f.: 821.31)

stiff man syndrome 333.91

Streeter bands 762.9

Stewart and Milford 820.09 (open f.: 820.19)

Sudeck atrophy not specified 337.20
    of upper limb 337.21
    of lower limb 337.22
    of other specified site 337.29

swan-neck deformity General term

tackler arm 728.12

TAR syndrome 284.0 (thrombocytopenic component), 754.8X

teardrop fracture 805–806

tennis elbow 726.32
    reverse 726.31

tennis leg 844.8

tennis toe 703.8

Thiemann disease 732.5

Thompson and Epstein fracture classification system 808s 820s, 835s

thrower elbow 726.31

thumb
    bowler 727.05
    gamekeeper 842.12

TIA 435.9

Tietze syndrome 733.6

Tile classification 808s

Tillaux Kleiger fracture 824.8 (open f.: 824.9)

TMJ syndrome 524.6X

toe

    mallet 736.79

    marathoner 703.8

    tennis 703.8

Torode and Zieg 808s

trigger finger 727.03 (congenital: 756.89)

triplane fracture 824.8 (open f.: 824.9)

Tronzo fracture classification system 820.21 (open f.: 820.31)

Trunkey fracture classification system 808s

Tscherne classification 823s

Turner syndrome 758.6

van Necks disease 731.1

VATER association 759.8X

VDDR 275.3

VDRR 275.3

VISI 842.10

Volkmann contracture 958.6

Volkmann deformity 755.37

Volkmann fracture 824.8 (open f.: 824.9)

Voorhoeve disease 756.4

wagon wheel fracture 821.22 (open f.: 821.32)

Wagstaff fracture 824.2 (open f.: 824.3)

Waldenström disease 732.3

Watson-Jones 823.0X (open f.: 823.1X)

weaver bottom 726.5

Weber (Danis-Weber) classification 824s

whiplash (assuming neck) 847.0

whitlow, herpetic 054.6

willow fracture (by bone)

Winquist-Hansen 820.3X

wrist and fore arms, fractures of 813s and 814s

wryneck (wry neck) 754.1 (congenital)

Y fracture (by bone)

Young fracture classification 808s

Zickle fracture classification system 820.22 (open f.: 820.32)

Bibliography

General

American Academy of Orthopaedic Surgeons, Heck CV, editor: *Fifty Years of Progress (1922-1983)*, Chicago, 1983, The Academy.

American Medical Association: *International Classification of Diseases 9th Revision Clinical Modification*, Dover, DE, 1997, American Medical Association.

American Medical Association: *Manual of Style*, ed 8, Baltimore, 1989, Williams & Wilkins.

American Orthopaedic Association: History of orthopaedics. In *Manual of Orthopaedic Surgery*, Chicago, 1985, AAOS, pp 1–8.

Anthony C, Kolthoff N: *Textbook of Anatomy and Physiology*, ed 9, St Louis, 1975, The CV Mosby Co.

Brashear RH, Raney RB: *Handbook of Orthopaedic Surgery*, ed 10, St Louis, 1986, The CV Mosby Co.

Canale ST: *Campbell's Operative Orthopaedics*, ed 10, CD-ROM, 4-volume set.

Cozen L: *Office Orthopaedics*, ed 4, Springfield, Ill, 1975, Charles C Thomas.

Cyriax J: *Textbook of Orthopaedic Medicine: Diagnosis of Soft Tissue Lesions*, ed 8, vol 1, Philadelphia, 1984, Bailliere Tindall.

Dorland's Illustrated Medical Dictionary, ed 30, Philadelphia, 2003, WB Saunders Co.

Glanz WD, et al: *Mosby's Medical and Nursing Dictionary*, ed 2, St Louis, 1986, The CV Mosby Co.

Hilt NE, Cogburn SB: *Manual of Orthopaedics*, St Louis, 1977, The CV Mosby Co.

Hoppenfeld S, Zeide MS: *The Orthopaedic Dictionary*, Philadelphia, 1994, JB Lippincott.

International Organization for Standardization ISO 8548-1: Prosthetics and Orthotics Limb Deficiencies, Part I: Method of describing limb deficiencies present at birth, Geneva, Switzerland, International Organization for Standardization.

Reider B: *The Orthopaedic Physical Examination*, Chicago, 2005, WB Saunders.

Simpson JA, Weiner ESC, eds: *The Oxford English Dictionary*, ed 2, Oxford, New York, 1989, Clarendon Press/Oxford University Press.

Stedman's Medical Dictionary, ed 25, Baltimore, 1990, Williams & Wilkins.

Thomas CL: *Taber's Encyclopedic Medical Dictionary*, ed 16, Philadelphia, 1989, FA Davis.

Turek SL: *Orthopaedics: Principles and Their Applications*, ed 4, vol 1, 2, Philadelphia, 1984, JB Lippincott.

Webster's II New Riverside University Dictionary, Boston, 1988, Houghton Mifflin.

Fractures

Allman FL: Fractures and ligamentous injuries of the clavicle and its articulation. *J Bone Joint Surg* 49A(4):774–784, 1967.

Anderson IF: Osteochondral fractures of the dome of the talus. *J Bone Joint Surg* 71A:1143–1152, 1989.

Anderson LD, D'Alonzo RT: Fractures of the odontoid process of the axis. *J Bone Joint Surg* 56A(8):1663–1674, 1974.

Ashurst APC: Classification and mechanism of fractures of the leg bones involving the ankle: based on a study of three hundred cases from the Episcopal Hospital. *Arch Surg* 4:51–129, 1922.

Badelon O, Bensahel H, Mazda K, Vie P: Lateral humeral condylar fractures in children: a report of 47 cases. *J Pediatr Orthop* 8 (1):31–34 1988.

Bado JL: The Monteggia lesion. *Clin Orthop Rel Res* 50:71–86, 1967.

Boyd HB, Griffin LL: Classification and treatment of trochanteric fractures. *Arch Surg* 58:853–866, 1949.

Buckholtz RW: Pathomechanics of pelvic ring disruptions. *Adv Orthop Surg* 10:167, 1987.

Cabenela ME, Morrey BF: Fractures of the proximal ulna and olecranon. In Morrey BF (ed): *The Elbow and Its Disorders*, Philadelphia, 1993, WB Saunders.

Canale ST, Kelly FB Jr: Fractures of the neck of the talus: Long-term evaluation of seventy-one cases. *J Bone Joint Surg Am* 60 (2):143–156, 1978.

Chadwick CJ, Bentley G: The classification and prognosis of epiphyseal injuries. *Injury* 18:157–168, 1987.

Colonna PC: Fracture of the neck of the femur in children. *Am J Surg* 6:793–797, 1929.

Colton CL: Fractures of the olecranon in adults: classification and management. *Injury* 5:121–129, 1973.

Crenshaw AH: Fractures of shoulder girdle, arm and forearm. In Crenshaw AH (ed): *Campbell's Operative Orthopaedics*, ed 8 St Louis, 1991, Mosby-Year Book.

DePalma AF:In Connelly JF (ed): *The Management of Fractures and Dislocations: An Atlas*, ed 3, vols 1-2, Philadelphia, 1981, WB Saunders.

Dias LS, Tachdjian MO: Physeal injuries of the ankle in children. *Clin Orthop Rel Res* 136:230–233, 1978.

Essex-Lopresti P: The mechanism, reduction technique, and results in fractures of the os calcis. *Br J Surg* 39:395–419, 1952.

Evans EM, Wales SS: Trochanteric fractures. *J Bone Joint Surg* 33B(2):192–204, 1951.

Ferkel RD, Cheng MS, Applegate GR: *A new method of arthroscopic staging of osteochondral lesions of the talus*, Presented at the American Academy of Orthopaedic Surgeons, Orlando, Fla, February 17, 1995.

Ferkel RD, Sgaglione NA, Del Pizzo W, et al: Arthroscopic treatment of osteochondral lesions of the talus: technique and results. *Othop Trans* 14:172–173, 1990.

Fielding JW, Magliato HJ: Subtrochanteric fractures. *Surg Gyn Obs* 122:555–560, 1966.

Frykman G: Fracture of the distal radius including sequelae-shoulder-hand-finger syndrome, disturbance in the distal radio-ulnar joint and impairment of nerve function: a clinical and experimental study. *Acta Orthop Scand* 108(suppl):1, 1967.

Garden RS: Malreduction and avascular necrosis in subcapital fractures of the femur. *J Bone Joint Surg* 53B(2):183–197, 1971.

Gartland JJ: Management of supracondylar fractures of the humerus in children. *Surg Gynecol Obstet* 109:145–154, 1959.

Gustilo RB: *The Fracture Classification Manual*, St Louis, 1991, Mosby-Year Book, Inc.

Gustilo RB, Mendoza RM, Williams DN: Problems in the management of type III (severe) open fractures. *J Trauma* 24:742, 1986.

Gustilo RB, Merkow RL, Templeman D: The management of open fractures. *J Bone Joint Surg* 72A:299–304, 1990.

Hardcastle PH, Reschauer R, Kutscha-Lissberg E, Schoffmann W: Injuries to the tarsometatarsal joint: incidence, classification, and treatment. *J Bone Joint Surg* 64B(3):349–356, 1982.

Hawkins LG: Fracture of the neck of the talus. *J Bone Joint Surg* 52A(5):991–1002, 1970.

Helfet DL, Howey T, et al: Limb salvage versus amputation. *Clin Orthop Rel Res* 256:80–86, 1990.

Herbert TJ, Fisher WE: Management of the scaphoid fracture using a new bone screw. *J Bone Joint Surg* 66B:114–123, 1984.

Hohl M, Moore TM: Articular fractures of the proximal tibia. In Evarts M (ed): *Surgery of the Musculoskeletal System*, ed 2, New York, 1990, Churchill Livingstone.

Hoppenfeld S, Zeide MS: *The Orthopaedic Dictionary*, Philadelphia, 1994, JB Lippincott.

Ideberg R: Fractures of the scapula involving the glenoid fossa. In: *Surgery of the Shoulder*, Toronto, 1984, BC Decker, pp 63–66.

Jensen JS: Classification of trochanteric fractures. *Acta Orthop Scand* 51:803–810, 1980.

Johansson JE, McBroom R, Barrington TW, Hunter GA.: Fracture of the ipsilateral

femur in patients with total hip replacement. *J Bone Joint Surg* 63A:1435–1442, 1981.

Judet R, Judet J, Letournel E: Fractures of the acetabulum: classification and surgical approaches for open reduction: preliminary report. *J Bone Joint Surg* 46A (8):1615–1646, 1675, 1964.

Judet and Letournal acetabular fracture classification. *J Bone Joint Surg* 73A:639–645, 1991.

Key JA, Conwell HE: *Management of Fractures, Dislocations and Sprains*, St Louis, 1951, CV Mosby.

Kilfoyle RM: Fractures of the medial condyle and epicondyle in children. *Clin Orthop Rel Res* 41:43–50, 1965.

Klafs CE, Arnheim DD: *Modern Principles of Athletic Training*, ed 5, St Louis, 1981, The CV Mosby Co.

Kulund DN: *The Injured Athlete*, Philadelphia, 1982, JB Lippincott.

Kyle RF, Gustilo RB, Premer RF: Analysis of six hundred and twenty-two intertrochanteric hip fractures. *J Bone Joint Surg* 61A (2):216–221, 1979.

Lauge-Hansen N: Fractures of the ankle. II. Combined experimental-surgical and experimental-roentgenologic investigations. *Arch Surg* 60:957–985, 1950.

Letts M, Vincent N, Gouw G: The "floating knee" in children. *J Bone Joint Surg* 68B:442–446, 1986.

Levine AM, Edwards CC: The management of traumatic spondylolisthesis of the axis. *J Bone Joint Surg* 67A(2):217–226, 1985.

Mallory TH, Kraus TJ, Vaughn BK: Intraoperative femoral fractures associated with cementless total hip arthroplasty. *Orthopaedics* 12 (2):231–239, 1989.

Mason ML: Some observations on fractures of the head of the radius with a review of one hundred cases. *Br J Surg* 42:123–132, 1954.

Mast JW, Spiegel PG, Pappas JN: Fractures of the tibial pilon. *Clin Orthop Relat Res* 230:68–82, 1988.

Meyers MH, McKeever FM: Followup notes: fracture of the intercondylar eminence of the tibia. *J Bone Joint Surg* 52A (8):1677–1684, 1970.

Milch H: Fractures and fracture dislocations of the humeral condyles. *J Trauma* 4:592–607, 1964.

Müller ME, Allgöwer M, Schnieder R: *Manual of Internal Fixation*, ed 3, Berlin, 1991, Springer-Verlag, pp 152–157.

Müller ME, Nazarian S, et al: *The Comprehensive Classification of Fractures of Long Bones*, Berlin, 1990, Springer-Verlag.

Neer CSI: Displaced proximal humeral fractures. Part I: Classification and evaluation. *J Bone Joint Surg* 52A(6):1077–1089, 1970.

Neer CSI, Howrowitz BS: Fractures of the proximal humeral epiphyseal plate. *Clin Orthop Rel Res* 41:24–31, 1965.

Oestern HH, Tscherne H: Pathophysiology and classification of soft tissue injuries associated with fractures. In Tscherne H, Gotzen L eds: *Fractures with Soft Tissue Injuries*, Berlin, 1984, Springer-Verlag, pp 1–8.

Ogden JA: Skeletal growth mechanism injury patterns. *J Pediatr Orthop* 2:371–377, 1982.

Ogden JA, Tross RB, Murphy MJ: Fractures of the tibial tuberosity in adolescents. *J Bone Joint Surg* 62A(2):205–215, 1980.

Owen R, Goodfellow J, Bullough P: *Scientific Foundations of Orthopaedics and Traumatology*, London, 1980, William Heinemann Medical Books, Ltd.

Pauwels F: *Der Schenkenholsbruck, em mechanisches Problem Grundlagen des Heilungsvorganges Prognose und kausale Therapie*, Stuttgart, 1935, Beilageheft zur Zeitschrift fur Orthopaedische Chirurgie, Ferdinand Enke.

Peterson L: *Sports Injuries*, Chicago, 1986, Year Book Medical Publishing.

Pipkin G: Treatment of grade IV fracture-dislocation of the hip. *J Bone Joint Surg* 39A(5):1027–1042, 1957.

Poland J: *Traumatic Separation of the Epiphysis*, London, 1898, Smith, Elder and Company.

Riseborough EJ, Radin EL: Intercondylar T fracture of the humerus in the adult: a comparison of operative and non-operative treatment in twenty-nine cases. *J Bone Joint Surg* 51A(1):130–141, 1898.

Rockwood CA: Subluxations and dislocations about the shoulder. In: *Fractures in Adults*, Philadelphia, 1984, JB Lippincott, pp 1192–1198.

Rockwood CA, Green D, Buckholtz: *Fractures in Adults*, 3rd ed, vol 1-2, Philadelphia, 1984, JB Lippincott.

Rockwood CA, Wilkins KE, King RE: *Fractures in Children*, vol 3, Philadelphia, 1984, JB Lippincott.

Rowe CR, Lowell JD: Prognosis of fractures of the acetabulum. *J Bone Joint Surg* 43A:30–59, 1962.

Rüedi T, Allgöwer M: Fractures of the lower end of the tibia into the ankle joint. *Injury* 1:92, 1969.

Russell TA: Fractures of the hip and pelvis. In Crenshaw AH (ed): *Campbell's Operative*

Orthopaedics, ed 8, St Louis, 1991, Mosby-Year Book.

Salter RB, Harris WR: Injuries involving the epiphyseal plate. *J Bone Joint Surg* 45A:587–622, 1963.

Samilson RL, Preito V: Dislocation arthropathy of the shoulder. *J Bone Joint Surg* 65A (4):456–460, 1983.

Schatzker J, McBroom R, Bruce D: The tibial plateau fracture: the Toronto experience 1968–1975. *Clin Orthop Rel Res* 138:94–104, 1979.

Schultz RJ: *The Language of Fractures*, Huntington, NY, 1976, RE Krieger Publishing Co.

Seinsheimer FI: Subtrochanteric fractures of the femur. *J Bone Joint Surg* 60A (3):300–306, 1978.

Seligson D, Pope M: *Concepts in External Fixation*, New York, 1982, Grune & Stratton.

Stewart MJ, Milford LW: Fracture-dislocation of the hip: an end result study. *J Bone Joint Surg* 36A:315–342, 1954.

Thompson VP, Epstein HC: Traumatic dislocation of the hip: a survey of 204 cases covering a period of twenty-one years. *J Bone Joint Surg* 33A(3):746–778, 1951.

Tile M: Pelvic ring fractures, should they be fixed. *J Bone Joint Surg* 70B:1–12, 1988.

Torode I, Zieg S: Pelvic fractures in children. *J Pediatr Orthop* 5:76, 1985.

Tronzo RG: Special considerations in management. *Orthop Clin North Am* 5(3):571–583, 1974.

Watson-Jones: *Fractures and Joint Injuries*, Edinburgh, 1955, E and S Livingston.

Weber BG: Die Verletzungen des oberen Spurnggelenkes. In Bern: *Aktuelle Probleme in der Chirurgie, 1966*, Verlag Han Huber.

Winquist RA, Hansen ST: Comminuted fractures of the femoral shaft treated by intramedullary nailing. *Orthop Clin North Am* 11(3):633–647, 1980.

Young JW, Burgess AR, Brumback RJ, Poka A: Pelvic fractures: value of plain radiography in early assessment and management. *Radiology* 160:445–451, 1986.

Zickle RE: An intramedullary fixation device for the proximal part of the femur: nine years experience. *J Bone Joint Surg* 58A:866–872, 1976.

Diseases

Aegerter E, Kirkpatrick JA: *Orthopaedic Diseases: Physiology, Pathology, Radiology*, ed 4, Philadelphia, 1975, WB Saunders.

Albright JA, Brand RA: *Scientific Basis of Orthopaedics*, New York, 1979, Appleton-Century-Crofts.

American Academy of Orthopaedic Surgeons and the International Society for the Study of the Lumbar Spine: *Glossary on Spinal Terminology*, document 675-680, Chicago, 1980, The Academy.

Bogumill GP, Schwamm HA: *Orthopaedic Pathology: A Synopsis with Clinical and Radiographic Correlation*, Philadelphia, 1984, WB Saunders.

Dietz FR, Matthews KD: Update on genetic bases of disorders with orthopaedic manifestations. *J Bone Joint Surg* 78A:1583–1598, 1996.

Enneking WF: A system of staging musculoskeletal neoplasms. *Clin Orthop* 204:9–24, 1986.

Enzinger FM, Weiss SW: *Soft Tissue Tumors*, ed 2, St Louis, 1988, CV Mosby.

Fitzgerald RH, et al: *Orthopedic Knowledge Update*, 1987, American Academy of Orthopedic Surgeons.

Frantz CH, O'Rahilly R: Congenital Limb Deficiencies. *J Bone Joint Surg* 43 (8):1202–1224, 1961.

Frassica FJ, Thompson RC: Evaluation, diagnosis and classification of benign soft-tissue tumors. *J Bone Joint Surg* 78A:126–140, 1996.

Gartland JJ: *Fundamentals of Orthopaedics*, ed 5, Philadelphia, 1991, WB Saunders.

Levesque J: *A Clinical Guide to Primary Bone Tumors*, Philadelphia, 1998, Lippincott, Williams & Wilkins.

Mercier LR: *Practical Orthopaedics*, ed 3, St Louis, 1991, Mosby-Year Book.

The Merck Manual of Diagnosis and Therapy, ed 16, Rahway, NJ, 1992, Merck Research Laboratories.

Mirra JM: *Bone Tumors: Clinical, Radiographic, and Pathologic Correlations*, ed 2, Philadelphia, 1989, WB Saunders.

Mourad LA: *Orthopaedic Disorders*, St Louis, 1991, Mosby-Year Book.

Praemer, Furner, Rice: *AAOS Musculoskeletal Conditions in the U.S.*, Chicago, 1999, AAOS.

Salter RB: *Textbook of Disorders and Injuries of the Musculoskeletal System*, ed 2, Baltimore, 1984, Williams & Wilkins.

Schajowicz F, Ackerman IV, Sissons HA: Histological typing of bone tumors. *International Classification of Tumors*, vol 6, Geneva, 1972, World Health Organization.

Steinberg ME, Hayken GD, Steinberg DR: A quantitative system for staging avascular necrosis. *J Bone Joint Surg* 77B:34–41, 1995.

X-Ray Imaging

Ewald FC: Knee Society total knee arthroplasty roentgenographic evaluation and scoring system. *Clin Orthop* 248:9–13, 1989.

Greulich WW, Pyle SI: *Atlas of the Development of the Hand and Wrist*, ed 2, Stanford, Calif, 1959, Stanford University Press.

Tanner JM, et al: *Assessment of Skeletal Maturity and Prediction of Adult Height (TW2) method*, ed 2, London, 1983, Academic Press.

Todd TW: *Atlas of Skeletal Maturity*, St Louis, 1937, The CV Mosby Co.

Test, Signs, & Maneuvers

American Academy of Orthopaedic Surgeons: *Joint Motion: Method of Measuring and Recording*, ed 6, Chicago, 1985, The Academy.

Gerhardt JJ: *Measuring and Recording of Joint Motion: Instrumentation and Techniques*, ed 2, Toronto/Lewiston, NY, 1990, Hogrefe & Huber.

Hoppenfeld S: *Physical Examination of the Spine and Extremities*, New York, 1976, Appleton-Century-Crofts.

Lliang MH, Katz JN, Phillips C, et al: The American Academy of Orthopaedic Surgeons Task Force on Outcome Studies: the total hip arthroplasty evaluation form of the American Academy of Orthopaedic Surgeons. *J Bone Joint Surg* 73B:816, 1991.

Polly HF, Hunder GG: *Physical Examination of the Joints*, ed 2, Philadelphia, 1978, WB Saunders.

Reider B: *The Orthopaedic Physical Examination*, ed 2, Philadelphia, 2005, WB Saunders.

Trumbly CM: *Physical Disabilities*, ed 2, Baltimore, 1983, Williams & Wilkins.

Laboratory

Henry JB, ed: *Clinical Diagnostic Management by Laboratory Methods*, ed 18, Philadelphia, 1991, WB Saunders.

Kjeldsberg CR, Knight JA: *Body Fluids*, ed 2, 1987, American Society of Clinical Pathologists.

Schumacher HR. Synovial fluid analysis and synovial biopsy. In: Kelly WW, Harris ED, Ruddy S, and Sledge CB eds. *Textbook of Rheumatology*, ed 3, Philadelphia, 1989, WB Saunders.

Casts, Splints, and Dressings

American Academy of Orthopaedic Surgeons: *Emergency Care and Transportation of the Sick and Injured*, ed 6, Chicago, 1997, The Academy.

Schmeisser GA: *A Clinical Manual Of Orthopedic Traction Techniques*, Philadelphia, 1963, WB Saunders.

Schneider RF: *Handbook for the Orthopaedic Assistant*, ed 2, St Louis, 1976, The CV Mosby Co.

Simon RR, Koenigsknecht SJ: *Emergency Orthopaedics: The Extremities*, ed 2, Norwalk, Conn, 1987, Appleton & Lange.

Prosthetics and Orthotics

American Academy of Orthopaedic Surgeons: *Atlas of Orthotics*, ed 2, St Louis, 1985, CV Mosby Co.

American Academy of Orthopaedic Surgeons: *Atlas of Limb Prosthetics: Surgical, Prosthetic, and Rehabilitation Principles*, ed 2, St Louis, 1992, Mosby-Year Book.

Bunch WH, Keagy RD: *Principles of Orthotic Treatment*, St Louis, 1976, The CV Mosby Co.

Goldberg, Bertram, Hsu John D eds: *Atlas of Orthotics and Assistive Devices*, ed 3, AAOS, St Louis, 1997, Mosby.

Redford JB: *Orthotics Etcetera*, ed 3, Baltimore, 1986, Williams & Wilkins.

Smith DG, Michael JW, Bowker JH eds: *Atlas of Amputations and Limb Deficiencies: Surgical, Prosthetic, and Rehabilitation Principles*, Chicago, 2004, American Academy of Orthopaedic Surgeons.

Anatomy and Surgery

American Orthopaedic Association: *Manual of Orthopaedic Surgery*, Chicago, 1985, The Association.

Burchardt H: The biology of bone graft repair. *Clin Orthop* 174:28, 1983.

Casscells SW: *Arthroscopy: Diagnostic and Surgical Practice*, Philadelphia, 1984, Lea & Febiger.

Crenshaw AH (ed): *Campbell's Operative Orthopaedics*, ed 10, vols 1-4, St Louis, 2002, Mosby-Year Book, Inc.

Epps CH Jr: *Complications in Orthopaedic Surgery*, ed 3, vols I and II, Philadelphia, 1994, JB Lippincott.

Friedlaender G: *Allografting*, St Louis, 1992, Mosby-Year Book.

Friedlaender GE: Immune responses to osteochondral allografts: current knowledge and future directions. *Clin Orthop* 174:58, 1983.

Haimovici H: *Vascular Surgery: Principles and Techniques*, New York, 1984, Appleton-Century-Crofts.

Moore KL: *Clinically Oriented Anatomy*, ed 2, Baltimore, 1985, Williams & Wilkins.

Reckling F, Reckling JA, Mohn M: *Orthopaedic Anatomy and Surgical Approaches*, St Louis, 1990, Mosby-Year Book.

Robertson PA: Prediction of amputation after severe lower limb trauma. *J Bone Joint Surg* 73A:639–645, 1991.

Rutherford RB (ed): *Vascular Surgery*, ed 2, Philadelphia, 1984, WB Saunders.

Shahriaree H (ed): *O'Connors Textbook of Arthroscopic Surgery*, ed 2, Philadelphia, 1992, JB Lippincott.

Tomford WW, Friedlaender GE: Bone banking procedures. *Clin Orthop* 174:15, 1983.

Weiland AJ: Current concepts review: vascularized free bone transplants. *J Bone Joint Surg* 63A:166, 1981.

The Spine

Weinstein JN, Rydevik BL, and Sonntag VKH eds: *Essentials of the Spine*, Raven Press, NY, 1995, Lippincott, Williams & Wilkins.

Hand and Wrist

DiDio LJA: *Synopsis of Anatomy*, St Louis, 1970, The CV Mosby Co.

Doyle JR, Blythe W:In: *American Academy of Orthopaedic Surgeons: Symposium on Tendon Surgery in the Hand*, St Louis, 1975, The CV Mosby Co.

Edmonson AS and Crenshaw AH eds: *Campbell's Operative Orthopaedics*, ed 9, vol 1, St Louis, 1996, Mosby.

Green DP (ed): *Operative Hand Surgery*, ed 2, New York, 1988, Churchill-Livingstone.

Lichtman DM: *The Wrist and Its Disorders*, Philadelphia, 1988, WB Saunders.

Mackinnon SE, Dellon AL: *Surgery of the Peripheral Nerve*, New York, 1988, Thieme Medical Publishers.

Scher RK, Daniel CR III eds: *Nails: Therapy, Diagnosis, Surgery*, Philadelphia, 1990, WB Saunders.

Steichen JB (ed): *Comprehensive Atlas of Hand Surgery*, Chicago, 1989, Year Book Medical Publishers.

Foot and Ankle

Jahss MH: *Disorders of the Foot,* vols I and II, Philadelphia, 1982, WB Saunders.

Mann RA: *Surgery of the Foot*, ed 5, St Louis, 1986, CV Mosby.

Occupational Therapy and Physical Therapy

American Occupational Therapy Association Commission on Practice Uniform Reporting System Task Force: *Uniform terminology system for reporting occupational therapy services*, Rockville, Md., 1986, The Association.

Kamenetz HL: *Dictionary of Rehabilitation Medicine*, New York, 1983, Springer.

Magee DJ: *Orthopaedic Physical Assessment*, ed 3, Philadelphia, 1997, WB Saunders.

Research

Brighton CT, Black J, Pollack S: *Electrical Properties of Bone and Cartilage*, New York, 1979, Grune & Stratton.

Frankel V: *Orthopedic biomechanics*, Philadelphia, 1970, Lea & Febiger.

Hoppenfeld S, deBoer P: *Surgical Exposures in Orthopaedics: The Anatomic Approach*, ed 3, Philadelphia, 2003, Lippincott, Williams & Wilkins.

Orthopaedic Research Laboratory, Good Samaritan Medical Center, West Palm Beach, FL.

Poole AR: Cartilage in health and disease. In McCarthy D, Koopman W eds: *Arthritis and Allied Conditions. A Textbook in Rheumatology*, ed 12, Philadelphia, 1992, Lea & Febiger, pp 279–333.

Suggested Readings

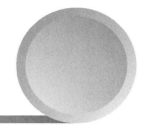

Journals and Tapes

AAOS Instructional Course Lectures (Park Ridge, Ill).
ACTA Chirurgiae Orthopaedicae et Traumatologiae Cechoslovaca (Praha).
ACTA Orthopaedica Scandinavica.
Aktuelle Probleme in Chirurgie und Orthopadie (Bern).
Advances in Ortho Surg 1985 (Baltimore).
American Journal of Emergency Medicine (Philadelphia).
American Journal of Knee Surgery (Thorofare, NJ).
American Journal of Sports Medicine (Waltham, Mass).
Archives of Orthopaedic and Traumatic Surgery (Berlin).
Archives of Physical Medicine and Rehabilitation (Chicago).
Archivio Putti di Chirurgia Degli Organi di Movimento (Firenze).
Arthritis and Rheumatism (Philadelphia).
Arthroscopy (New York).
Audio Digest Foundation (AAOS Ortho Tapes) (Chicago).
Beitrage zur Orthopadie und Traumatologie (Berlin).
Bone (New York).
Bone Marrow Transplant (United Kingdom).
Bone and Mineral (Amsterdam).
Buck CJ: 2006 ICD-9-CM Volume 1 and 2, St Louis, 2006, Elsevier.
Bulletin of the Hospital for Joint Diseases Orthopaedic Institute (New York).
Chirurgia Degli Organi di Movimento (Bologna).
Chirurgia Narzadow Ruchu I Ortopedia Polska (Warszara).
Clinical Orthopaedics and Related Research (Philadelphia).

Clinics in Sports Medicine (Philadelphia).
Continuing Education in Ortho Surg (Recert) (AAOS) (Chicago).
Foot and Ankle (Baltimore).
Hand Clinics (Philadelphia).
Hip (Philadelphia).
Instructional Course Lectures; AAOS (Chicago).
International Orthopaedics (NY).
Italian Journal of Orthopaedics and Traumatology (Bologna).
JAMA (Chicago).
Journal of the American Medical Association (Chicago).
Journal of the American Podiatric Medical Association (Bethesda, MD).
Journal of Arthroplasty (New Brunswick, NJ).
Journal of Bone and Joint Surgery, American Volume (Boston).
Journal of Bone and Joint Surgery, British Volume (London).
Journal of Bone and Mineral Research (New York).
Journal of Foot Surgery (Baltimore).
Journal of Hand Surgery (St Louis).
Journal of Hand Therapy (Philadelphia).
Journal of Orthopaedic Research (New York).
Journal of Orthopaedic and Sports Physical Therapy (Baltimore).
Journal of Orthopaedic Trauma (New York).
Journal of Pediatric Orthopaedics (New York).
Journal of Prosthetics and Orthotics (Alexandria, VA).
Journal of Rheumatology (Buffalo, NY).
Journal of Sports Medicine and Physical Fitness (Torino, Italy).
Journal of Trauma (Baltimore).
Magyar Traumatologia, Orthopaedia es Helyreallito Sebeszet (Budapest).
New England Journal of Medicine (Boston).

Nippon Seikeigeka Gakkai Zasshi. Journal of the Japanese Orthopaedic Association (Tokyo).
Orthopaedic Audio-Synopsis (AAOS) (Chicago).
Orthopaedic Clinical Update Monograph (AAOS) (Chicago).
Orthopade (Berlin).
Orthopaedic Nursing (Pitman, NJ) (NAON).
Orthopaedic Review (Lawrenceville, NJ).
Orthopaedic Survey (Chicago).
Orthopaedics (Thorofare, NJ).
Orthopedic Clinics of North America (Philadelphia).
Ortopediia Travmatologiia I Protezirovanie (Kharkov).
Pediatric Clinics of North America (Philadelphia).
Physical Therapy Journal (Alexandria).
Revue de Chirugie Orthopedique et Reparatrice de l'Appareil Moteur (Paris).
Skeletal Radiology (Berlin).
Spine (Hagerstown, Md).
Sports Medicine.
Yearbook of Orthopaedic Trauma & Surgery (Chicago).
Yearbook of Orthopaedic and Traumatic Surgery (St Louis).
Yearbook of Orthopaedics (abstracts) (St Louis).
Yearbook of Sports Medicine (Chicago).
Yearbook of Sports Medicine (St Louis).
Zeitschrift fur Orthopadie und ihre Grenzgebiete (Stuttgart).

Osteopathic Medicine

Journal of the American Osteopathic Association (Chicago).

Index